IN VIVO IMAGING OF CANCER THERAPY

CANCER DRUG DISCOVERY AND DEVELOPMENT

BEVERLY A. TEICHER, SERIES EDITOR

In Vivo Imaging of Cancer Therapy, edited by *Anthony F. Shields and P. Price*, 2007
Oncogene-Directed Therapies, edited by *Janusz Rak*, 2003
Cell Cycle Inhibitors in Cancer Therapy: Current Strategies, edited by *Antonio Giordano and Kenneth J. Soprano*, 2003
Chemoradiation in Cancer Therapy, edited by *Hak Choy*, 2003
Flouropyrimidines in Cancer Therapy, edited by *Youcef M. Rustum*, 2003
Targets for Cancer Chemotherapy: Transcription Factors and Other Nuclear Proteins, edited by *Nicholas B. La Thangue and Lan R. Bandara*, 2002
Tumor Targeting in Cancer Therapy, edited by *Michel Pagé*, 2002
Hormone Therapy in Breast and Prostate Cancer, edited by *V. Craig Jordan and Barrington J.A. Furr*, 2002
Tumor Models in Cancer Research, edited by *Beverly A. Teicher*, 2002
Tumor Suppressor Genes in Human Cancer, edited by *David E. Fisher*, 2001
Matrix Metalloproteinase Inhibitors in Cancer Therapy, edited by *Neil J. Clendeninn and Krzyszt of Appelt*, 2001
Farnesyltransferase Inhibitors in Cancer, edited by *Saïd M. Sebti and Andrew D. Hamilton*, 2001
Platinum-Based Drugs in Cancer Therapy, edited by *Lloyd R. Kelland and Nicholas P. Farrell*, 2000
Apoptosis and Cancer Chemotherapy, edited by *John A. Hickman and Caroline Dive*, 1999
Signaling Networks and Cell Cycle Control: The Molecular Basis of Cancer and Other Diseases, edited by *J. Silvio Gutkind*, 1999
Antifolate Drugs in Cancer Therapy, edited by *Ann L. Jackman*, 1999
Antiangiogenic Agents in Cancer Therapy, edited by *Beverly A. Teicher*, 1999
Anticancer Drug Development Guide: Preclinical Screening, Clinical Trials, and Approval, edited by *Beverly A. Teicher*, 1997
Cancer Therapeutics: Experimental and Clinical Agents, edited by *Beverly A. Teicher*, 1997

IN VIVO IMAGING OF CANCER THERAPY

Edited by

ANTHONY F. SHIELDS

Karmanos Cancer Institute
Wayne State University School of Medicine
Detroit, MI

PAT PRICE

Manchester Molecular Imaging Center
Christie Hospital NHS Trust
Academic Department of Radiation Oncology
The University of Manchester Wolfson Molecular Imaging Centre
Manchester, UK

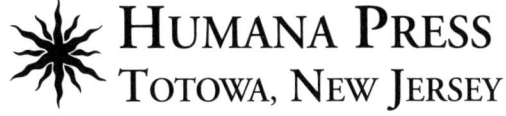

© 2007 Humana Press Inc.
999 Riverview Drive, Suite 208
Totowa, New Jersey, 07512
www.humanapress.com

All rights reserved. No part of this book may be reproduced, stored in a retrevial system, or transmitted in any form or by any means, electronic, mechanical, photocopying, microfilming, recording, or otherwise without written permission from the Publisher.

All articles, comments, opinions, conclusions, or recommendations, are those of the author(s), and do not necessarily relfect the views of the publisher.

Due diligence has been taken by the publisher, editors, and authors of this book to assure the accuracy of the information published and to describe generally accepted practices. The contributors herein have carefully checked to ensure that the drug selection and dosages set forth in this text are accurate and in accord with the standards accepted at the time of publication. Notwithstanding, as new research, changes in government regulations, and knowledge from clinical experience relating to drug therapy and drug reactions constantly occurs, the reader is advised to check the product information provided by the manufacturer of each drug for any change in dosages or for additional warnings and contraindications. This is of utmost importance when the recommended drug herein is a new or infrequently used drug. It is the responsibility of the treating physican to determine dosages and treatment strategies for individual patients. Futher it is the responsibility of the health care provider to ascertain the Food and Drug Administration status of each drug or device used in their clinical pratice. The publisher, editors, and authors are not responsible for errors or omissions or for any consequences from the application of the information presented in this book and make no warranty, express or implied, with respect to the contents in this publication.

This publication is printed on acid-free paper. ∞
ANSI Z39.48-1984 (American National Standards Institute)
Permanence of Paper for Printed Library Materials

Cover illustration: Fig. 4 from Chapter 15.

For additional copies, pricing for bulk purchases, and/or information about other Humana titles, contact Humana at the above address or at any of the following numbers: Tel.: 973-256-1699; Fax: 973-256-8341l; Email: humanapr.com; or visit our Website: http://www.humanapress.com.

Photocopy Authorization Policy:

Authorization to photocopy items for internal or personal use, or the internal or personal use of specific clients, is granted by Humana Press Inc., provided that the base fee of US $30.00 per copy is paid directly to the Copyright Clearance Center at 222 Rosewood Drive, Danvers, MA 01923. For those organizations that have been granted a photocopy license from the CCC, a separate system of payment has been arranged and is acceptable to Humana Press Inc. The fee code for users of the Transcriptional Reporting Service is: [978-1-58829-633-7 $30.00].

10 9 8 7 6 5 4 3 2 1

Library of Congress Control Number: 2006940361

ISBN: 978-1-58829-633-7   e-ISBN: 978-1-59745-341-7

FOREWORD

In vivo medical imaging involves administering a known amount of energy to the body and measuring, with spatial localization, the energy that is transmitted through, emitted from, or reflected back from various organs and tissues. The difference between the administered and the recorded energy provides information about some property of the matter with which the energy interacted. The energy most commonly used is some form of electromagnetic energy, such as X-rays or light, but occasionally other forms are used, such as mechanical energy for ultrasound scans. For most of the past century, the property of matter that has generally been inferred from the energy recorded during medical imaging is physical structure or anatomy. This has been, and continues to be, enormously important in clinical medicine, including oncology. For example, dramatic improvements have occurred in the past 25 years such that modern computed tomography (CT) and magnetic resonance imaging (MRI) scanners can now depict anatomic detail at submillimeter resolution. However, as clinical medicine moves into the molecular era, the property of matter about which clinicians will increasingly need to know is the biochemical makeup of normal and abnormal tissues.

There are a variety of imaging methods used to obtain information about a patient's biochemistry, and no single modality is superior to all others. Collectively these methods are referred to as molecular imaging. *In vivo* molecular imaging can be thought of as a form of *in vivo* assay. Some *in vivo* imaging methodologies, such as magnetic resonance spectroscopy and optical spectroscopy, allow us to make direct inferences about underlying biochemistry simply from administering energy and analyzing the recorded energy. However, the extent of biochemical information that can be obtained from energy alone is currently limited. Therefore, we commonly give patients diagnostic drugs, referred to as contrast agents or molecular probes, which interact in a specific way with the patient's underlying biochemistry and thereby alter the recoded energy in a way that tells us more about the patient's biochemistry than we could learn from administered energy alone.

In vivo imaging assays cannot currently provide the extensive breadth and resolution of genomic, proteomic, and other phenotypic information that can be obtained from various *in vitro* assays on biopsied tissue or body fluids. However, *in vivo* imaging has at least three potentially important advantages that complement information from *in vitro* tests. First, imaging provides spatially localized information over large volumes of tissue or the entire body, whereas *in vitro* tests are usually performed on a very small volume of tissue. *In vivo* imaging is therefore sometimes referred to "regional proteomics" that can better reflect the heterogeneity of cancer. Second, *in vivo* imaging can be performed serially or continuously for periods of time, thereby providing dynamic information. *In vitro* assays provide information from a single time point. Third, *in vivo* imaging depicts information from a tumor in its usual milieu or microenvironment. *In vitro* assays, on the other hand, will reflect the changes in gene expression patterns that occur very quickly after tissue is removed by biopsy. Information from *in vivo* and *in vitro* studies is therefore complementary, and both are essential in modern oncology research and clinical care.

Investigators in drug development need *in vivo* assays indicate whether a given patient has the appropriate molecular phenotype to benefit from a targeted therapy, to indicate whether the drug has hit its molecular target, to determine whether the drug has been given in the optimal biological dose, and to ascertain whether the tumor is responding. Clinicians increasingly will have a series of targeted therapies to choose from for any given tumor, and will need *in vivo* assays to obtain an early determination as to whether their patient is responding to the chosen therapy. Early predictive assays will be important so that clinicians can change therapy quickly, thereby obviating unnecessary toxicity and expense, and increasing the chances of matching the patient to an effective therapy. In addition to simply knowing whether a given biochemical event is occurring, researchers and clinicians will increasingly need objective, quantitative information about the biochemical events and will need to monitor them quantitatively over time, before and after interventions. That level of quantification is generally not yet available in clinical imaging methods, but is an area of active research and development.

This comprehensive textbook covers the entire spectrum of *in vivo* imaging for oncology, including current approaches to detailed anatomic measurements, MR and optical spectroscopy, and molecular imaging techniques requiring exogenously administered imaging agents. The challenges and approaches to quantification are also outlined. The authors describe technologies and methods that are currently clinically available, and many that are still in a developmental stage or useful only in animal studies. However, it is important to realize that the majority of imaging devices now offered for sale by the major imaging equipment manufacturers did not exist as recently as 3 or 4 years ago. Thus the pace of technology development is such that techniques described here as laboratory or investigational will likely be in clinical use within a few years. *In vivo* imaging will continue to have profound effects on how we think about, detect, diagnose, treat, and monitor cancer.

Daniel C. Sullivan, MD

Preface

Cancer treatment is an area of medicine that has flourished over the last couple of decades, taking advantage of rapid developments in molecular biology and pharmacology. The perspective on cancer and its treatment has changed dramatically not only among those in the public but within the medical profession as well. The diagnosis of cancer used to be thought of as an automatic death sentence and the treatments were considered extremely toxic and futile. Fellow physicians would often ask those of us in medical and radiation oncology why we chose to work in such a depressing area of research and practice. This was an interesting perspective, since such thoughts were expressed by cardiologists and pulmonologists who spent their days taking care of patients with severe congestive heart failure or emphysema; diseases with equally poor prognoses. Clearly cancer was thought of as a particular curse. Family members would urge us to withhold information from sick loved ones, fearing that they would lose all hope if they knew the truth. Those in the public eye would also hide information about the diagnosis from the press. Patients even feared being shunned because some thought that cancer was contagious.

Fortunately, much has changed in the last couple of decades. The public now readily hears about and discusses the disease and has gained much more, but still very incomplete, insight into it causes and treatments. Clearly much of this change in attitude reflects the ability to provide improved curative treatment for those with early stages of cancer. Even those with advanced disease can now gain significant months and years of life with treatment that has tolerable side effects. For example, while a decade ago it was debated if any treatment should be offered those with advanced lung cancer, we now have first, second and third line treatments that have been demonstrated to prolong patient's lives. The agents employed included older and newer cytotoxic drugs along with targeted agents that attack pathways involved in tumor growth and angiogenesis. The future holds many more fortuitous options.

With the availability of a multiplicity of new agents has come a growing need to evaluate the success or failure of each treatment. When no treatment is useful, one clearly has no real need to develop methods to decide which agent to use or for how long. When a number of agents or approaches are available for a given type of cancer we need to assess the patient's prognosis, predict treatment response and then measure the outcome. The initial and still standard approach to measuring outcome relied on determining the size of the tumor. This approach is still very useful, despite its limitations, as is described within this book. The advent of new molecular imaging techniques allows the researcher and clinician to make use of a growing array of imaging devices to peer into tumors in vivo and measure their biochemistry. These include optical, X-ray, magnetic resonance, and nuclear approaches. All of these provide different bits of information about the tumors pathways and metabolism that can be used to understand and predict the best treatment methods and monitor their outcomes. These techniques are now regularly employed in the laboratory and in clinical research to assist in the development of existing new molecular agents. The new methods of molecular biology have provided a remarkable list of targets and agents that need to be evaluated. At the same time the cost of such testing and development has skyrocketed. While imaging technologies are rather expensive, drug development costs have made such investments seem very reasonable. One clearly needs new ways to understand how agents are working and to figure out what schedule should be used, in which combination, and in which disease, since cancer is not one disease but over one hundred. In fact, the new studies in molecular biology seem to prove that almost each cancer is unique. Hence, each patient must be evaluated to determine the best treatment. The conjunction of these stars has brought together these new therapies and imaging modalities at a critical time in the evolution of modern cancer treatment. This book is aimed at furthering the understanding of how these two fields now work together and will require the close collaboration of those practicing both arts.

As in any book of this type this has been the combined effort of many collaborators. We want to thank our co-authors for their studied contributions to the fields over many years and their efforts to distill their knowledge into a very readable text. We want to thank Janice Akoury and James Cullen, from Detroit and Manchester respectively, for keeping us organized and focused on the tasks needed to complete this effort and for their editing assistance. The support and assistance of Paul Dolgert at Humana Press and Dr. Beverly Teicher made this book possible. We want to thank those who have spent many years teaching use and working with us in the laboratory and clinics to further the fields of cancer therapy and imaging, whose work helped make our careers and this book possible. We want to thank our parents for their guidance and confidence that led to our career paths. Finally, we both want to thank our spouses Drs. Fayth Yoshimura and Terry Jones, both for their encouragement to pursue scientific rigor and years of support.

Anthony F. Shields, MD, PhD
P. Price, MD

Contents

Foreword by *Daniel C. Sullivan* v

Preface vii

Contributors xi

1   Role of Imaging in Cancer Treatment 1
Anthony F. Shields and P. Price

2   Preclinical Models of Tumor Growth and Response 13
Patrick McConville, William L. Elliott, Alicia Kreger, Richard Lister, Jonathan B. Moody, Erin Trachet, Frank Urban, and W.R. Leopold

3   Anatomical Measure of Tumor Growth with Computed Tomography and Magnetic Resonance Imaging 33
Stephen J. Gwyther

4   Positron Emission Tomography Imaging of Blood Flow and Hypoxia in Tumors 47
Joseph G. Rajendran and David A. Mankoff

5   Magnetic Resonance Measurement of Tumor Perfusion and Vascularity 73
Jeffrey L. Evelhoch

6   Computed Tomography Measurements of Perfusion in Cancer Therapy 85
Ken Miles

7   [^{18}F]Fluorodeoxyglucose Positron Emission Tomography Assessment of Response 103
Wolfgang A. Weber

8   Measurement of Tumor Proliferation with Positron Emission Tomography and Treatment Response 121
Anthony F. Shields

9   Estrogen-Receptor Imaging and Assessing Response to Hormonal Therapy of Breast Cancer 143
Farrokh Dehdashti and Barry A. Siegel

10 Quantitative Approaches to Positron Emission Tomography 155
Adriaan A. Lammertsma

11 Position Emission Tomography Measurement of Drug Kinetics 169
Azeem Saleem and P. Price

12 Imaging Genes for Viral and Adoptive Therapies 205
Inna Serganova, Vladimir Ponomarev, Phillipp Mayer-Kuckuk, Ekaterina Doubrovina, Michael Doubrovin, and Ronald G. Blasberg

13 *In Vivo* Magnetic Resonance Spectroscopy in Clinical Oncology 241
Arend Heerschap

14 Magnetic Resonance Probes for Tumor Imaging 259
Alexander S.R. Guimaraes and Ralph Weissleder

15 Fluorescent Imaging of Tumors 281
Kamiar Moin, Oliver J. McIntyre, Lynn M. Matrisian, and Bonnie F. Sloane

16 Imaging of Apoptosis 303
Francis G. Blankenberg and H. William Strauss

Index 317

CONTRIBUTORS

FRANCIS G. BLANKENBERG MD • Department of Radiology/Division of Pediatric Radiology, Lucile Salter Packard Children's Hospital, Stanford, CA

RONALD G. BLASBERG MD • Departments of Neurology and Radiology, Memorial Sloan Kettering Cancer Center, New York, NY

FARROKH DEHDASHTI MD • Division of Nuclear Medicine, Mallinckrodt Institute of Radiology, Washington University School of Medicine, St. Louis, MO

MICHAEL DOUBROVIN MD, PhD • Department of Neurology, Memorial Sloan Kettering Cancer Center, New York, NY

EKATERINA DOUBROVINA MD, PhD • Department of Pediatrics, Memorial Sloan Kettering Cancer Center, New York, NY

WILLIAM L. ELLIOTT PhD • MIR Preclinical Services, Ann Arbor, MI

JEFFREY L. EVELHOCH PhD • Amgen, Inc., Thousand Oaks, CA

ALEXANDER S. R. GUIMARAES MD, PhD • Center for Molecular Imaging Research, Massachusetts General Hospital, Harvard Medical School, Charlestown, MA

STEPHEN J. GWYTHER MBBS, FRCS, FRCR • Department of Medical Imaging, East Surrey Hospital, Surrey, United Kingdom

AREND HEERSCHAP PhD • Department of Radiology, Radboud University, Nijmegen Medical Center, Nijmegen, The Netherlands

ALICIA KREGER BS • MIR Preclinical Services, Ann Arbor, MI

ADRIAAN A. LAMMERTSMA PhD • Department of Nuclear Medicine and PET Research, VU University Medical Center, Amsterdam, The Netherlands.

W. R. LEOPOLD PhD • MIR Preclinical Services, Ann Arbor, MI

RICHARD LISTER BS • MIR Preclinical Services, Ann Arbor, MI

DAVID A. MANKOFF MD, PhD • Division of Nuclear Medicine, Department of Radiology, University of Washington, Seattle, WA

LYNN M. MATRISIAN PhD • Department of Cancer Biology, Vanderbilt University, Nashville, TN

PHILLIPP MAYER-KUCKUK PhD • Department of Neurology, Memorial Sloan Kettering Cancer Center, New York, NY

PATRICK MCCONVILLE PhD • MIR Preclinical Services, Ann Arbor, MI

OLIVER J. MCINTYRE PhD • Department of Cancer Biology, Vanderbilt University, Nashville, TN

KEN MILES MD • Brighton and Sussex Medical School, University of Sussex, Brighton, United Kingdom

KAMIAR MOIN PhD • Department of Pharmacology and Karmanos Cancer Institute, Wayne State University School of Medicine, Detroit, MI

JONATHAN B. MOODY PhD • MIR Preclinical Services, Ann Arbor, MI

VLADIMIR PONOMAREV MD, PhD • Department of Radiology, Memorial Sloan Kettering Cancer Center, New York, NY

P. PRICE MD • Manchester Molecular Imaging Center, Christie Hospital NHS Trust, Academic Department of Radiation Oncology, The University of Manchester Wolfson Molecular Imaging Centre, Manchester, UK

JOSEPH G. RAJENDRAN MD • Division of Nuclear Medicine, Department of Radiology, University of Washington, Seattle, WA

AZEEM SALEEM PhD • Manchester Molecular Imaging Center, Christie Hospital NHS Trust, Manchester, United Kingdom

INNA SERGANOVA PhD • Department of Neurology, Memorial Sloan Kettering Cancer Center, New York, NY

ANTHONY F. SHIELDS MD, PhD • Karmanos Cancer Institute, Wayne State University School of Medicine, Detroit, MI

BARRY A. SIEGEL MD • Division of Nuclear Medicine, Mallinckrodt Institute of Radiology, Washington University School of Medicine, St. Louis, MO

BONNIE F. SLOANE PhD • Department of Pharmacology, Karmanos Cancer Institute, Wayne State University School of Medicine, Detroit, MI

H. WILLIAM STRAUSS MD • Department of Radiology/Section of Nuclear Medicine, Memorial Sloan Kettering Cancer Center, New York, NY

DANIEL C. SULLIVAN MD • Cancer Imaging Program, National Cancer Institute, National Institutes of Health, Bethesda, MD

ERIN TRACHET BS • MIR Preclinical Services, Ann Arbor, MI

FRANK URBAN MS • MIR Preclinical Services, Ann Arbor, MI

WOLFGANG A. WEBER MD • Departments of Molecular and Medical Pharmacology, Ahmanson Biological Imaging Center, UCLA David Geffen School of Medicine, Los Angeles, CA

RALPH WEISSLEDER MD, PhD • Center for Molecular Imaging Research, Massachusetts General Hospital, Harvard Medical School, Charlestown, MA

1 Role of Imaging in Cancer Treatment

Anthony F. Shields, MD, PhD, and P. Price, MD

CONTENTS
  INTRODUCTION
  SCREENING
  STAGING
  IMAGING

1. INTRODUCTION

Cancer therapy and cancer imaging are scientific and clinical companions. Most cancers are initially detected by an imaging technique, either through the routine screening of at-risk populations or by the evaluation of patients presenting with symptoms. Imaging the human body began as part of routine clinical care with the development of X-ray imaging by Roentgen. While X-rays still play an important role in cancer evaluation, the imaging technologies have expanded greatly over the past 30 years. Computerized tomographic (CT) imaging has added immeasurably to the clinician's ability to find, measure, and monitor cancers. The algorithms originally developed by Hounsfield to produce tomographic images with X-rays have also been extended to nuclear medicine for use with positron emission tomography (PET) and single photon emission computed tomography (SPECT). The development of magnetic resonance imaging (MRI) has provided high levels of contrast with superb resolution in many areas of the body. These techniques have been complemented by ultrasound (US) imaging and more recently by the introduction of new optical approaches. Each technique has its strengths and limitations, leading clinicians to compare the results and data from the various approaches to determine the optimal imaging modalities to use for a given indication. Clinical presentation often leads a physician to obtain a series of images as an evaluation progresses or changes. For example, one might initially detect a suspicious lesion with a simple chest X-ray, more completely evaluate its characteristics and extent with a CT scan, and use PET to help stage the tumor within the thorax and abdomen or MRI to detect lesions within the brain. In fact, new devices are beginning to combine modalities, such as PET and CT, to take advantage of the strengths of each approach (Fig. 1).

From: *Cancer Drug Discovery and Development
In Vivo Imaging of Cancer Therapy*
Edited by: A.F. Shields and P. Price © Humana Press Inc., Totowa, NJ

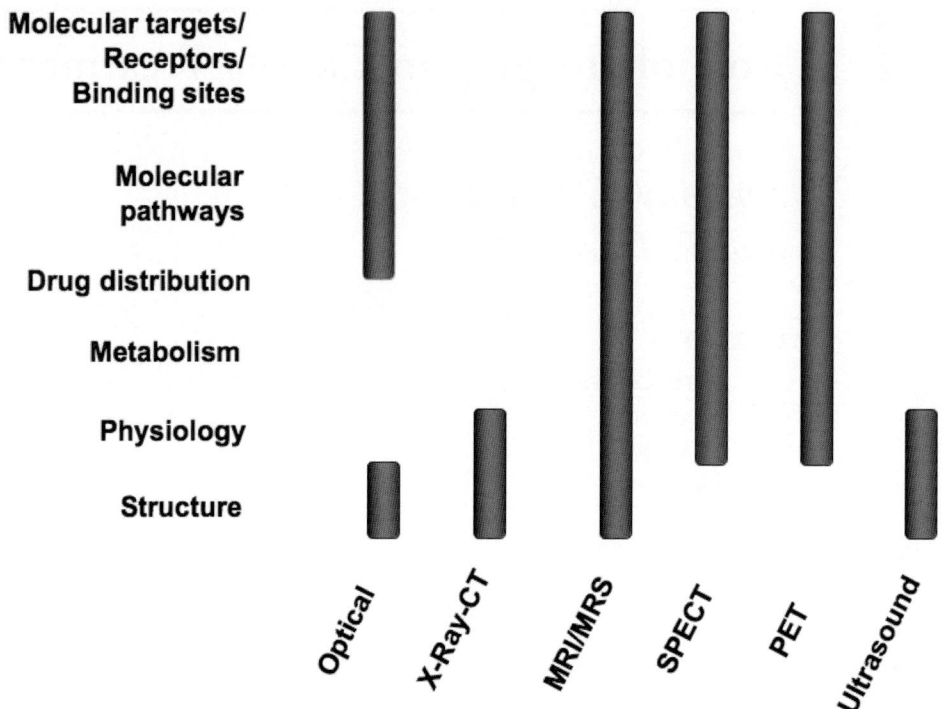

Fig. 1. Imaging modalities and measurements obtained.

The newer imaging approaches also provide visualization of tumor metabolism and physiology that add information to that obtained with anatomic images. In reality it is possible to deduce some physiologic information from even the now standard anatomic imaging obtained with CT and MRI. For example, differences in contrast can be used to suggest areas that are necrotic and those containing viable tumor. The injection of contrast media into arteries leading to a tumor has also provided information about the architecture and detail of the tumor's blood supply, including measurements of flow and perfusion. Such measurements can be obtained using PET and $^{15}O[H^2O]$, dynamic contrast enhanced MRI (DCE MRI), and similar CT techniques.

Expanding from the simple (or not so simple) measurements of tumor perfusion, a wide variety of metabolic measurements of tumors are now available. Generally, these are limited to research uses, but they are moving into the clinical realm. At present, the most commonly used method is PET imaging with ^{18}F-labeled fluorodeoxyglucose ([^{18}F]FDG), routinely used for the detection of tumors as part of the staging and restaging. As described in this volume (Chapter 7) a number of studies have also examined its use in the measurement of tumor response. While this approach is very promising, further work to refine this technique is considered standard-of-care in the treatment of any malignancy. In fact, while the main focus of this text is on the assessment of tumor response, almost all the chapters present ongoing research in this area, whether considering CT, MR, PET, or optical approaches. The only technique that is used as part of routine clinical practice is anatomic measurement of tumor size. Even phase I, II, and III clinical studies of new drugs primarily use such anatomic measures to assess the efficacy of newer agents. More frequently, new imaging techniques are finding use in the development of new therapeutic compounds. The authors highlight these uses from a number of unique perspectives. Hopefully, as such techniques are tested in the early clinical trials, investigators will find that they offer utility for clinicians and patients as part of routine care.

2. SCREENING

This book will focus on the use of imaging for treatment response, but appropriate diagnosis and staging play a critical role in the choice of treatment. The earlier the diagnoses of a tumor the more likely it is to be at a stage amenable to surgical removal and cure. It is important to understand the role imaging plays in this realm. The only tumor where screening with imaging is widely accepted and utilized is in the detection of breast cancer. Mammography is regularly used in the developed world and, depending on the study, from 40% to 80% of women of the appropriate age in the United States are being screened *(1, 2)*. Mammography screening is a major public health effort in many countries and studies have shown that mammography detects cancer at an early stage and decreases the death rate from breast cancer *(3)*. This technique can still miss cancers until they are fairly large and this has led to the development and testing of new approaches to tumor detection. These include MRI, which has been found to be of use in women at high genetic risk for the disease *(4)*. Approaches with US and PET are also being developed, but are not yet used as part of routine screening. In many cases, these other techniques are used in the follow-up of suspicious lesions found on routine mammogram, as well as lumps found by the patient or during a routine examination.

Chest X-rays are one of the most commonly used imaging techniques and have been tested for the early detection of lung cancer *(5)*. Unfortunately, the current studies have not shown a benefit to this approach. The use of low-dose spiral CT is now being pursued. Early results have demonstrated that this approach yields a higher rate of tumor detection, but the effect on patient outcome remains to be seen *(6)*. The other imaging technique that is now being evaluated for tumor detection is CT colonography, also known as virtual colonoscopy *(7)*. While a number of different methods for early colon cancer detection are used in clinical practice, including fecal occult blood testing and sigmoidoscopy, the most accurate test has been the complete endoscopic evaluation of the entire colon. The use of total colonic evaluation by barium enema has been regularly practiced in the past, but has fallen out of favor in more recent years. This is due in part to the need for the same cleansing of the bowel that is required for colonoscopy, but the technique is less accurate and requires a separate colonoscopy for abnormal findings *(8)*. The high cost of the colonoscopy and restricted availability of the technique have limited its usage. CT colonography requires an appropriate scanner and software. At present, a patient still requires bowel evacuation for the test, but new methods to contrast tag the stool may make the use of purgatives unnecessary. One further advantage of CT colonography is that it also assists in staging the patient if a lesion is found.

In each of these instances, early detection is being pursued to detect tumors at an early stage. In fact, in colon cancer screening the physician wishes to detect adenomatous polyps before they have even become malignant. In general, patients with tumors detected by screening will have a better prognosis than those presenting with more advanced disease. This is the whole point of such an endeavor. Furthermore, treatment may be simpler and less toxic to the patient.

3. STAGING

Improved screening has the goal of detecting tumor of lower stage and thus leading to improved outcomes. However, the declared stage of a patient depends on the accuracy of the evaluation. Staging takes into account the local invasion and tumor size (T-stage), spread to regional lymph nodes (N-stage), and distant spread (M-stage). Staging gives the physician and patient prognostic information, but it is not a perfect measure. As technology and analysis techniques improve so does the accuracy of staging. Improvements can include laboratory tests, such as tumor markers; pathologic examinations, like new immunocytologic detection of tumor spread to lymph nodes; and also superior imaging techniques, such as PET detection of previous unsuspected distant disease. Even within a given stage the extent of disease may have prognostic importance and alter the plan of treatment. For example, PET has been used to restage colon cancer patients with a small number of resectable liver metastases *(9)*. Patients staged by PET had a 58% 5-year survival rate, while previous historical controls had a survival rate of about 30%. This is the result of PET detecting additional lesions, both in and outside the liver, that preclude resection for cure. Those patients remaining in the surgical group have improved survival. This is generally not the result of improved treatment, just better patient selection. This is called the Will Rogers' effect, after the American humorist who commented that the migration of a group of poor farmers from Oklahoma to California "raised the average intelligence level in both states." Improved staging can be seen with new MRI techniques for detecting lymph node involvement in prostate cancer *(10)* and PET staging of esophageal cancer *(11)*. Combining techniques can also improve staging, for example, PET/CT improves localization of areas of increased activity found on PET *(12)*. This has led to more accurate assessment of tumor extent and altered therapy. In each case, the outcome is likely to be changed as improved staging leads to better defined groups of patients for treatment.

4. IMAGING

4.1 Basic Principles of Imaging Treatment Response

Imaging treatment response in individual patients requires a treatment with at least some level of efficacy, a method to image the tumor at baseline, and a change that is reflected in the imaging modality/technique after therapy in some of the patients. In patients with advanced disease or those receiving neoadjuvant treatment, imaging over the course of therapy is a standard practice to assess the response to therapy. Patients receiving adjuvant therapy for resected cancer regularly ask "how can we tell that the treatment is working?" Unfortunately in that situation there is no way to assess response in an individual patient; the efficacy can be determined in large groups of patients only by comparing results of patients treated with different approaches. The recent emphasis on neoadjuvant therapy provides increased opportunities to use imaging to determine the efficacy of treatment prior to surgical resection. Neoadjuvant treatment is now regularly used in patients with head and neck, esophageal, breast, and rectal cancer. It is occasionally used in patients with lung and pancreatic cancer, especially in those with locally advanced disease. In each of these situations an imaging approach must provide accurate information on the result of therapy and this information must be incorporated into the pathway of cancer treatment.

The type of therapy, its response, and the best method and timing of imaging can vary greatly depending on the clinical situation. At present the common approach to imaging response in patients receiving standard cytotoxic therapy for advanced disease is to obtain anatomic images with CT or MRI about every 2 months. The size of the tumor is measured using either the sum of perpendicular diameters (the original WHO approach) or more recently using the sum of the largest diameters (RECIST) *(13)*. These approaches are described in more detail in Chapter 6. This approach has the advantage that cross-sectional anatomic imaging is widely available and that basic measurements can be made using a cursor on the computer or a ruler on X-ray film. The major limitations of this approach include the difficulty in quantitating diffuse and multiple tumors and the inability to determine the viability of a lesion that has been detected. This has led to the exploration of a number of different metabolic approaches to tumor imaging that are described in this text, including magnetic resonance spectroscopy, PET imaging, and optical approaches. These approaches to measurement of tumor response have been the focus of research for many years and are just approaching routine use in clinical care.

The best approach to imaging treatment response in any given patient will vary greatly depending on the tumor being evaluated and the treatment being employed. For each case and clinical circumstance one or another imaging technique may provide the most useful information. Imaging before treatment can also be especially valuable in choosing treatment, though clearly the response is not being measured at this point. As indicated above the staging information is valuable in determining prognosis. New imaging techniques may also provide predictive information. For example, the uptake of a labeled drug, such as 5-fluorouracil, may predict the likelihood of treatment response (as discussed in Chapter 11) *(14)*. Or the distribution of estrogen receptors measured with *in vivo* imaging may provide information superior to that obtained with a single, small biopsy in predicting the response to antiestrogenic therapy *(15)*.

After the start of therapy, the optimal timing of imaging can vary greatly (Table 1). Anatomic imaging of tumor response is routinely done every 2 months in most clinical trials. But it can sometimes take a number of months before progression or shrinkage becomes evident. Metabolic approaches may demonstrate evidence of response within hours or days of therapy. For example, antivascular therapy with combretastatin can be imaged to measure changes in tumor blood flow within hours after treatment, while

Table 1
Common Imaging Techniques and Timing after Treatment

Imaging measurement	*Timing from start of treatment*
Blood flow (MR, PET, CT)	<1 week
Receptor interference (PET)	
Metabolic changes (PET, MR)	3–4 weeks
Proliferation	
Tumor size	2–6 months
Restage (CT, MR)	
Tumor viability (MR, PET)	
Restage	>6 months
Assess recurrence	

therapy of gastrointestinal stromal tumors with imatinib has been shown to alter tumor metabolism within days of therapy *(16)*. After cytotoxic therapy it may be necessary to wait for 2–4 weeks to detect changes in tumor metabolism. After some treatments, such as radiation therapy of brain tumors, imaging months later may be needed to differentiate progression from necrosis *(17)*. The best time for imaging will depend on the technique employed and which therapy was given to the patient. The timing of imaging will also depend on when clinical information will be most useful in directing therapy. For example, a patient may receive a single dose of chemotherapy once a month. It would be desirable to know prior to the next dose if the patient is responding to treatment, but it may not be of clinical significance if this is known in the hours after treatment or 3 weeks later. What is of importance is the accuracy of the assessment in determining the ultimate patient outcome. In early research studies, phase I and II, one is generally looking for any evidence of efficacy. In such a situation a high sensitivity for detecting evidence of long term tumor control is needed. It should be kept in mind that with newer targeted agents, such control may mean lack of tumor growth rather than actual decreased tumor size. In a clinical situation, early imaging must be accurate in determining treatment failure. The ability to predict that the treatment will fail up to 80% of the time may not be sufficient to stop therapy. Many treatments work to decrease tumor size only 20% of the time, so a higher accuracy is needed to allow the clinician to stop therapy. This is one of the most difficult issues that imagers will have to face. Ultimately this will require randomized trials to demonstrate that early imaging, by providing early predictions of therapeutic response, can favorably alter patient outcome and substantially decrease cost and toxicity.

Some tumors are not well measured by any present imaging technique. For example, a patient may present with pleural involvement that can result in an effusion containing tumor cells. Measuring the amount of fluid tells us little about the status of the underlying cancer. Another issue that is presently insurmountable is the evaluation of patients receiving adjuvant treatment after tumor resection. To measure the response of a tumor to therapy it is necessary to have a baseline test able to measure some aspect of the tumor. While this sounds obvious, patients receiving adjuvant therapy are problematic. In a single patient it can never be proved that adjuvant therapy was essential for success, since the patient may have been cured without such treatment. Imaging is often of use in demonstrating the failure of adjuvant treatment, since recurrence of a tumor is regularly detected or proven using imaging.

4.2 Imaging in Radiotherapy Treatment

New imaging modalities are increasingly being considered for the radiotherapy management of patients. There are a number of areas where they may play a significant role: improved disease staging and tumor volume delineation (TVD); tumor phenotype definition, response assessment, and as a research tool for the development of radiotherapy techniques.

A great deal of research interest has focused on investigating whether additional tumor biological information provided by PET imaging—largely using [^{18}F]FDG—can improve cancer staging, refine TVD for radiotherapy, and have an effect on subsequent disease outcome. Precise definition of the gross tumor volume (GTV) is essential to the process of effective radiotherapy. This ascertains accurate staging and ensures that the necessary therapeutic dose of ionizing radiation is delivered to tumor tissue while minimizing irradiation of normal tissue. Once the GTV is defined, the planning target volume (PTV)—the area to which radiation will be delivered—can subsequently be delineated. This encompasses areas of potential microscopic tumor infiltration and additional margins to incorporate possible inaccuracies and patient/organ motion. Traditionally, the radiation treatment plan is based on anatomical imaging data produced by CT and MRI. Tumor visualization is therefore based on variation of tissue density, intensity, volume effects, and contrast enhancement. However, these changes are not characteristics confined to tumor tissue. They may also be observed in nontumor tissue owing to pathological conditions such as necrosis, inflammation, or the effects of anticancer therapy. The complex nature of a tumor site may itself also limit the effectiveness of anatomical imaging techniques for TVD. Although PET lacks the anatomical resolution provided by CT, it does offer the additional advantage of providing both biological and anatomical information, affording evidence of disease spread. When combined with the detailed CT anatomical information, PET therefore has the potential to substantially refine tumor detection and localization. With the advent of combined PET-CT scanners, the role of PET imaging for improved TVD for radiotherapy treatment planning (RTP) is now under consideration.

Although research is still ongoing, FDG-PET has been associated with improvements in GTV delineation in a number of tumor types. For example, studies carried out in lung cancer have concluded that FDG-PET adds essential information to CT results to improve TVD, with significant consequences for refined disease staging and GTV and PTV delineation *(18, 19)*. Several further observations were also made: FDG-PET was noted to improve the accuracy of staging lymph node involvement; the interobserver variability of GTV and PTV definition was often significantly reduced when using FDG-PET for RTP; and improved delineation of malignant tissue from atelectasis using FDG-PET was demonstrated, leading to significant reductions of radiotherapy target volumes. The improved accuracy conferred by FDG-PET for GTV delineation in lung cancer has led to its recommendation as a standard method to be used in combination with CT imaging for all future dose escalation studies *(20)*.

The impact of FDG-PET for TVD for RTP was also investigated in studies of head and neck cancer, which showed that FDG-PET could result in significant changes to GTV delineation *(21–25)*. However, its use is complicated in head and neck cancer by false-positive FDG-PET results. These have been observed to result from inflammatory lymph nodes and in some structures such as tonsils and salivary glands, where FDG uptake may be increased.

In general, in other tumor types, such as gastrointestinal tract cancer (including esophageal cancer), gynecological cancer, and lymphomas, FDG-PET can have a significant impact on improved tumor detection and nodal involvement, allowing accurate contouring of the gross tumor mass and thus staging and GTV. However, information concerning the impact and value of FDG-PET for TVD for RTP is more limited for other tumor types. The broad conclusions to date are that there are commonly discordances between conventional imaging (CT or MRI) and functional imaging (FDG-PET). This results in altered PTVs (increases and decreases) for some patients *(18, 19)*. More research is required to determine the potential value of imaging methods for improved RTP, particularly for tumor sites other than the lung, and to help define their clinical capacity.

Molecular imaging holds great promise for allowing biologically adapted radiotherapy. Techniques such as PET, molecular resonance spectroscopy (MRS), and MRI can increase our understanding of the biological mechanisms underlying the heterogeneity of tumor response to radiotherapy. In turn, this will enable the definition of biological target volumes (BTVs) that can be specifically targeted for dose escalation. Methods are under development to facilitate imaging of biological processes known to have special significance for tumor response to radiotherapy, such as hypoxia, blood flow, proliferation, angiogenesis, apoptosis, and DNA repair. By visualizing these events in tandem with the anatomical information provided by traditional radiological techniques, different areas of a nonhomogeneous tumor mass can be identified. Radiation dose can then be adapted both to the morphology and the biology of the tumor. For example, hypoxia is a well-recognized factor that limits the curability of radiotherapy, negatively affecting patient outcome. A number of PET probes are being developed for measuring hypoxia, of which [^{18}F]fluoromisonidazole ([^{18}F]FMISO) is the most widely studied. It has a potential clinical role as a tool to define hypoxic subregions (BTVs) that could benefit from targeted dose escalation. This image-guided, functional radiotherapy approach could revolutionize the future biological individualization of radiation therapy.

As well as using PET technology to allow biologically adapted RTP, PET imaging also holds great potential as a useful tool for radiobiology and radiotherapy research. By utilizing the ability of various PET tracers to assess biological factors known to influence radiotherapy response, such as hypoxia (e.g., [^{18}F]MISO), proliferation (e.g., [^{18}F]FLT), and perfusion (e.g., [^{15}O]H$_2$O), PET studies can be designed so that the dynamics of these biological process can be evaluated *in vivo* both during and after a fractionated course of radiotherapy. In this way, various fractionation schedules, escalated doses, boost volumes, hypoxic cell radiosensitizers, and other methods aimed at improving the efficacy of radiotherapy can be investigated, with the aim of attaining maximal therapeutic gain.

A further role for PET exists as a means for monitoring treatment and assessing radiotherapy response, and is presently under investigation. Currently, response to anticancer treatment is determined by a decrease in anatomical tumor size, but this tends to occur late in the treatment course. PET studies could be used to assess whether biological responses occur earlier in the treatment course. This would facilitate optimal patient management and ultimately influence disease outcome and survival. Due to the inherent problems of postradiotherapy inflammation contaminating the FDG-PET signal, it is speculated that alternative PET probes (e.g., for proliferation markers) may prove to be more effective in this context.

4.3 Imaging and Anticancer Drug Development

Molecular imaging modalities have the ability to provide crucial support to the development of new cancer treatments, and are predicted to radically alter the drug development process. By providing direct information of underlying *in vivo* normal tissue and tumor pharmacology, early proof-of-principle and efficacy-of-action studies can be carried out *(26, 27)*. Imaging studies can help to increase the understanding of a drug's behavior within the body (pharmacokinetics) and of its effects (pharmacodynamics). This type of information offers the means to aid rational modifications in the drug development process, hence saving time and money *(28)*.

Compounds aimed at inhibiting cellular processes can be directly assessed. For example, by using radiolabeled thymidine as a biomarker, PET imaging can be used to demonstrate inhibition of the thymidylate synthase pathway *(29)*. Studies can be designed so that downstream functional effects expected of a therapeutic agent, such as changes in blood flow, metabolism, or proliferation, can be monitored during drug delivery to determine expected mechanism of action. Examples include the use of radiolabeled water ($[^{15}O]H_2O$-PET), used to assess tissue perfusion, and to demonstrate the efficacy of the antivascular agent combretastatin *(30)*.

By directly radiolabeling an anticancer agent, its biodistribution in the human body and individual tissue pharmacokinetics can be measured through the quantitative imaging offered by PET. The sensitivity of this technology is such that the amount of compound needed is at most a thousandth of that of an initial phase I dose; typically a dose of around 1 µg is needed, which removes concerns of toxicity. This offers the opportunity to examine a range of potential agents in the quest to optimize delivery to and retention by a tumor relative to normal tissue. Initial reports of this imaging microdosing procedure have focused on the radiolabeling of well-established cancer drugs such as 5-FU *(31, 32)* and BCNU *(33, 34)*. This has since been followed by the labeling of drugs during and even prior to phase I trials *(35)*. Magnetic resonance spectroscopy can also be used to investigate drug pharmacokinetics. For example, MRS has been used to demonstrate tumor uptake of 5-FU in colorectal metastases *(36–38)*. It has the advantage of chemical resolution and does not need radiolabeled compounds, but does not have the sensitivity of PET. The advent of higher energy MRS machines may provide greater sensitivity and so allow expansion of this opportunity.

In the future it is expected that PET imaging probes will be developed to bind specifically to selective molecular therapeutic targets. As these would be administered intravenously, resulting images will relate both to the presence and the accessibility of those targets from the bloodstream. This could allow *in vivo* assay of binding sites within a particular tumor. In turn, this could define the density of the therapeutic target for an individual tumor and hence the case for administering an agent specific for that target.

The potential advantages that molecular imaging can offer rational drug design are huge, with consequences for reduced time and increased successful outcomes for the drug development and testing process in prephase I and phase I–III clinical trials. However, it is important to acknowledge that there are formidable challenges to overcome. A molecular imaging probe needs to be specific for the molecular pathway or binding site to which it is targeted. It also has to penetrate endothelial barriers and undergo minimal metabolism (otherwise, for instance, PET images will be contaminated with radiolabeled metabolites); therefore a good drug does not necessarily produce a good imaging probe. Methods also need to be developed to analyze the recorded image data in a meaningful manner. There then remains the need to characterize or validate the derived functional data against a reference; currently in oncology the principal means of characterization will be by comparison to tumor biopsy material, but future developments of pharmaceutical mediators of tumor selective binding sites are expected to offer further means for validation.

4.4 Imaging as a Translational Link among Academic Research, the Pharmaceutical Industry, and the Clinic

It is evident that molecular imaging is of considerable interest to drug developers within the pharmaceutical industry. Providing early proof-of-concept of treatment in patients is clearly seminal as it is estimated that 50–60% of anticancer drugs fail at the point of phase III clinical trials *(39–41)*. Throughout development, decisions need to be made on whether or not a drug should progress through the increasingly expensive phases of clinical trials. Early evidence derived from molecular imaging studies concerning the expression of molecular targets, appropriate biodistribution, and tumor drug delivery, as well as data on mechanisms and efficacies of action, would be invaluable to this process.

Links between the pharmaceutical industry and clinical academic centers are likely to develop as they both share the motivation to advance molecular imaging in order to gain further insights into human tumor biology to support the development of new therapies. As a result, there is mutual interest in the pursuit of more specific imaging probes for targeted tumor biological processes, molecular pathways, and binding sites. Pharmaceutical companies are the custodians of large libraries of molecules and have the ability to custom synthesize many more. To undertake imaging research with these new probes, it will be important for scientists from the pharmaceutical and biotech industries to collaborate with multidisciplinary clinical academic centers. These centers will provide access to significant populations of cancer patients, and equipped with the required imaging facilities and suitable range of expertise, such environments would provide the opportunity to bring together all the resources necessary to support the role of molecular imaging as a key component of effective anticancer drug discovery.

REFERENCES

1. Eisner EJ, Zook EG, Goodman N, Macario E. Knowledge, attitudes, and behavior of women ages 65 and older on mammography screening and Medicare: Results of a national survey. *Women Health* 2002;36:1–18.
2. Harrison RV, Janz NK, Wolfe RA, Tedeschi PJ, Huang X, McMahon LF Jr. 5-Year mammography rates and associated factors for older women. *Cancer* 2003;97:1147–1155.
3. Elmore JG, Armstrong K, Lehman CD, Fletcher SW. Screening for breast cancer. *JAMA* 2005;293: 1245–1256.
4. Kriege M, Brekelmans CT, Boetes C, Besnard PE, Zonderland HM, Obdeijn IM, Manoliu RA, Kok T, Peterse H, Tilanus-Linthorst MM, Muller SH, Meijer S, Oosterwijk JC, Beex LV, Tollenaar RA, de Koning HJ, Rutgers EJ, Klijn JG. Efficacy of MRI and mammography for breast-cancer screening in women with a familial or genetic predisposition. *N Engl J Med* 2004;351:427–437.
5. Bach PB, Kelley MJ, Tate RC, McCrory DC. Screening for lung cancer: A review of the current literature. *Chest* 2003;123:72S–82S.
6. Gohagan JK, Marcus PM, Fagerstrom RM, Pinsky PF, Kramer BS, Prorok PC, Ascher S, Bailey W, Brewer B, Church T, Engelhard D, Ford M, Fouad M, Freedman M, Gelmann E, Gierada D, Hocking W, Inampudi S, Irons B, Johnson CC, Jones A, Kucera G, Kvale P, Lappe K, Manor W, Moore A, Nath H, Neff S, Oken M, Plunkett M, Price H, Reding D, Riley T, Schwartz M, Spizarny D, Yoffie R, Zylak C. Final results of the Lung Screening Study, a randomized feasibility study of spiral CT versus chest X-ray screening for lung cancer. *Lung Cancer* 2005;47:9–15.
7. Pickhardt PJ, Choi JR, Hwang I, Butler JA, Puckett ML, Hildebrandt HA, Wong RK, Nugent PA, Mysliwiec PA, Schindler WR. Computed tomographic virtual colonoscopy to screen for colorectal neoplasia in asymptomatic adults. *N Engl J Med* 2003;349:2191–2200.

8. Winawer SJ, Stewart ET, Zauber AG, Bond JH, Ansel H, Waye JD, Hall D, Hamlin JA, Schapiro M, O'Brien MJ, Sternberg SS, Gottlieb LS. A comparison of colonoscopy and double-contrast barium enema for surveillance after polypectomy. National Polyp Study Work Group. *N Engl J Med* 2000;342:1766–1772.
9. Fernandez FG, Drebin JA, Linehan DC, Dehdashti F, Siegel BA, Strasberg SM. Five-year survival after resection of hepatic metastases from colorectal cancer in patients screened by positron emission tomography with F-18 fluorodeoxyglucose (FDG-PET). *Ann Surg* 2004;240:438–447; discussion 447–450.
10. Harisinghani MG, Barentsz J, Hahn PF, Deserno WM, Tabatabaei S, van de Kaa CH, de la Rosette J, Weissleder R. Noninvasive detection of clinically occult lymph-node metastases in prostate cancer. *N Engl J Med* 2003;348:2491–2499.
11. Kato H, Miyazaki T, Nakajima M, Takita J, Kimura H, Faried A, Sohda M, Fukai Y, Masuda N, Fukuchi M, Manda R, Ojima H, Tsukada K, Kuwano H, Oriuchi, N, Endo K. The incremental effect of positron emission tomography on diagnostic accuracy in the initial staging of esophageal carcinoma. *Cancer* 2005;103:148–156.
12. Syed R, Bomanji JB, Nagabhushan N, Hughes S, Kayani I, Groves A, Gacinovic S, Hydes N, Visvikis D, Copland C, Ell PJ. Impact of combined (18)F-FDG PET/CT in head and neck tumours. *Br J Cancer* 2005;92:1046–1050.
13. Therasse P, Arbuck SG, Eisenhauer EA, Wanders J, Kaplan RS, Rubinstein L, Verweij J, Van Glabbeke M, van Oosterom AT, Christian MC, Gwyther SG. New guidelines to evaluate the response to treatment in solid tumors. European Organization for Research and Treatment of Cancer, National Cancer Institute of the United States, National Cancer Institute of Canada. *J Natl Cancer Inst* 2000;92:205–216.
14. Dimitrakopoulou-Strauss A, Strauss LG, Schlag P, Hohenberger P, Mohler M, Oberdorfer F, van Kaick G. Fluorine-18-fluorouracil to predict therapy response in liver metastases from colorectal carcinoma. *J Nucl Med* 1998;39:1197–1202.
15. Linden HM, Stekhova S, Link JM, Gralow JR, Livingston RB, Ellis GK, Peterson LM, Schubert EK, Petra KA, Krohn KA, Mankoff DA. HER2 expression and uptake of 18F-fluoroestradiol predict response of breast cancer to hormonal therapy. *J Nucl Med* 2004;45(Suppl):85–86p.
16. Jager PL, Gietema JA, van der Graaf WT. Imatinib mesylate for the treatment of gastrointestinal stromal tumours: Best monitored with FDG PET. *Nucl Med Commun* 2004;25:433–438.
17. Langleben DD, Segall GM. PET in differentiation of recurrent brain tumor from radiation injury. *J Nucl Med* 2000;41:1861–1867.
18. Gambhir SS, Czernin J, Schwimmer J, Silverman DH, Coleman RE, Phelps ME. A tabulated summary of the FDG PET literature. *J Nucl Med* 2001;42:1S–93S.
19. Grosu A-L, Piert M, Molls M. Experience of positron emission tomography for target localisation in radiation oncology. *Br J Radiol* 2005;28(Suppl):18–32.
20. Chapman JD, Bradley JD, Eary JF, Haubner R, Larson SM, Michalski JM, Okunieff PG, Strauss HW, Ung YC, Welch MJ. Molecular (functional) imaging for radiotherapy applications: An RTOG symposium. *Int J Radiat Oncol Biol Phys* 2003;55:294–301.
21. Ciernik IF, Dizendorf E, Baumert BG, Reiner B, Burger C, Davis JB, Lutolf UM, Steinert HC, Von Schulthess GK. Radiation treatment planning with an integrated positron emission and computer tomography (PET/CT): A feasibility study. *Int J Radiat Oncol Biol Phys* 2003;57:853–863.
22. Rahn AN, Baum RP, Adamietz IA, Adams S, Sengupta S, Mose S, Bormeth SB, Hor G, Bottcher HD. [Value of 18F fluorodeoxyglucose positron emission tomography in radiotherapy planning of head-neck tumors]. *Strahlenther Onkol* 1998;174:358–364.
23. Nishioka T, Shiga T, Shirato H, Tsukamoto E, Tsuchiya K, Kato T, Ohmori K, Yamazaki A, Aoyama H, Hashimoto S, Chang TC, Miyasaka K. Image fusion between 18FDG-PET and MRI/CT for radiotherapy planning of oropharyngeal and nasopharyngeal carcinomas. *Int J Radiat Oncol Biol Phys* 2002;53:1051–1057.
24. Paulino AC, Koshy M, Howell R, Schuster D, Davis LW. Comparison of CT- and FDG-PET-defined gross tumor volume in intensity-modulated radiotherapy for head-and-neck cancer. *Int J Radiat Oncol Biol Phys* 2005;61:1385–1392.
25. Daisne JF, Duprez T, Weynand B, Lonneux M, Hamoir M, Reychler H, Gregoire V. Tumor volume in pharyngolaryngeal squamous cell carcinoma: Comparison at CT, MR imaging, and FDG PET and validation with surgical specimen. *Radiology* 2004;233:93–100.

26. Saleem A, Aboagye EO, Price PM. In vivo monitoring of drugs using radiotracer techniques. *Adv Drug Deliv Rev* 2000;41:21–39.
27. Saleem A. Potential of positron emission tomography (PET) in oncology and radiotherapy. *Br J Radiol* 2005;28(Suppl):6–16.
28. Kelloff GJ, Sigman CC. New science-based endpoints to accelerate oncology drug development. *Eur J Cancer* 2005;41:491–501.
29. Wells P, Aboagye E, Gunn RN, Osman S, Boddy AV, Taylor GA, Rafi I, Hughes AN, Calvert AH, Price PM, Newell DR. 2-[11C]Thymidine positron emission tomography as an indicator of thymidylate synthase inhibition in patients treated with AG337. *J Natl Cancer Inst* 2003;95:675–682.
30. Anderson HL, Yap JT, Miller MP, Robbins A, Jones T, Price PM. Assessment of pharmacodynamic vascular response in a phase I trial of combretastatin A4 phosphate. *J Clin Oncol* 2003;21:2823–2830.
31. Harte RJ, Matthews JC, O'Reilly SM, Tilsley DW, Osman S, Brown G, Luthra SJ, Brady, F, Jones T, Price PM. Tumor, normal tissue, and plasma pharmacokinetic studies of fluorouracil biomodulation with N-phosphonacetyl-L-aspartate, folinic acid, and interferon alfa. *J Clin Oncol* 1999;17:1580–1588.
32. Saleem A, Yap J, Osman S, Brady F, Suttle B, Lucas SV, Jones T, Price PM, Aboagye EO. Modulation of fluorouracil tissue pharmacokinetics by eniluracil: In-vivo imaging of drug action. *Lancet* 2000;355:2125–2131.
33. Mitsuki S, Diksic M, Conway T, Yamamoto YL, Villemure JG, Feindel W. Pharmacokinetics of 11C-labelled BCNU and SarCNU in gliomas studied by PET. *J Neurooncol* 1991;10:47–55.
34. Tyler JL, Yamamoto YL, Diksic M, Theron J, Villemure JG, Worthington C, Evans AC, Feindel W. Pharmacokinetics of superselective intra-arterial and intravenous [11C]BCNU evaluated by PET. *J Nucl Med* 1986;27:775–780.
35. Saleem A, Harte RJ, Matthews JC, Osman S, Brady F, Luthra SK, Brown GD, Bleehen N, Connors T, Jones T, Price PM, Aboagye EO. Pharmacokinetic evaluation of N-[2-(dimethylamino)ethyl]acridine-4-carboxamide in patients by positron emission tomography. *J Clin Oncol* 2001;19:1421–1429.
36. Findlay MP, Leach MO, Cunningham D, Collins DJ, Payne GS, Glaholm J, Mansi JL, McCready VR. The non-invasive monitoring of low dose, infusional 5-fluorouracil and its modulation by interferon-alpha using in vivo 19F magnetic resonance spectroscopy in patients with colorectal cancer: A pilot study. *Ann Oncol* 1993;4:597–602.
37. Kamm YJ, Heerschap A, van den Bergh EJ, Wagener DJ. 19F-magnetic resonance spectroscopy in patients with liver metastases of colorectal cancer treated with 5-fluorouracil. *Anticancer Drugs* 2004;15:229–233.
38. Presant CA, Wolf W, Waluch V, Wiseman CL, Weitz I, Shani J. Enhancement of fluorouracil uptake in human colorectal and gastric cancers by interferon or by high-dose methotrexate: An in vivo human study using noninvasive (19)F-magnetic resonance spectroscopy. *J Clin Oncol* 2000;18:255–261.
39. Gilbert J, Henske P, Singh A. Rebuilding big pharma's business model. IN VIVO: *Bus Med Rep* 2003;17:73.
40. Lesko LJ, Woodcock J. Translation of pharmacogenomics and pharmacogenetics: A regulatory perspective. *Nat Rev Drug Discov* 2004;3:763–769.
41. Reichert JM. Trends in development and approval times for new therapeutics in the United States. *Nat Rev Drug Discov* 2003;2:695–702.

2 Preclinical Models of Tumor Growth and Response

Patrick McConville, PhD, William L. Elliott, PhD, Alicia Kreger, BS, Richard Lister, BS, Jonathan B. Moody, PhD, Erin Trachet, BS, Frank Urban, MS, and W.R. Leopold, PhD

CONTENTS
>
> INTRODUCTION
> TYPES OF TUMOR MODELS
> ENDPOINTS AND MEASUREMENTS
> SUMMARY AND FUTURE DIRECTIONS

1. INTRODUCTION

Experimental models of cancer have played an important role in cancer drug discovery for more than 60 years. The same models have proven critical as tools for the elucidation of the molecular basis of neoplastic transformation, the processes involved in tumor progression and metastasis, and the determinants of therapeutic success or failure. More recently, transgenic models in particular have been used to "validate" and prioritize new strategies for therapeutic intervention. *In vivo* cancer models can be considered to fall within two broad classes, transplantable models, and *in situ* models, each with a number of subtypes (Fig. 1). For pragmatic reasons, transplantable models as a group are the most commonly used for drug evaluation, while *in situ* models such as cancer-prone transgenic mice provide a rich source of information on cancer etiology. It should be noted that each transplantable model represents the tumor of a single patient, not a tumor type. This discussion is centered on the application of both model types, and the potential impact of imaging technologies for cancer drug discovery. However, with recent advances in preclinical imaging technologies, these models are also proving useful in the development and testing of new imaging techniques and contrast agents. Increasingly, with the expanding role of drugs tied to specific molecular

From: *Cancer Drug Discovery and Development*
In Vivo Imaging of Cancer Therapy
Edited by: A.F. Shields and P. Price © Humana Press Inc., Totowa, NJ

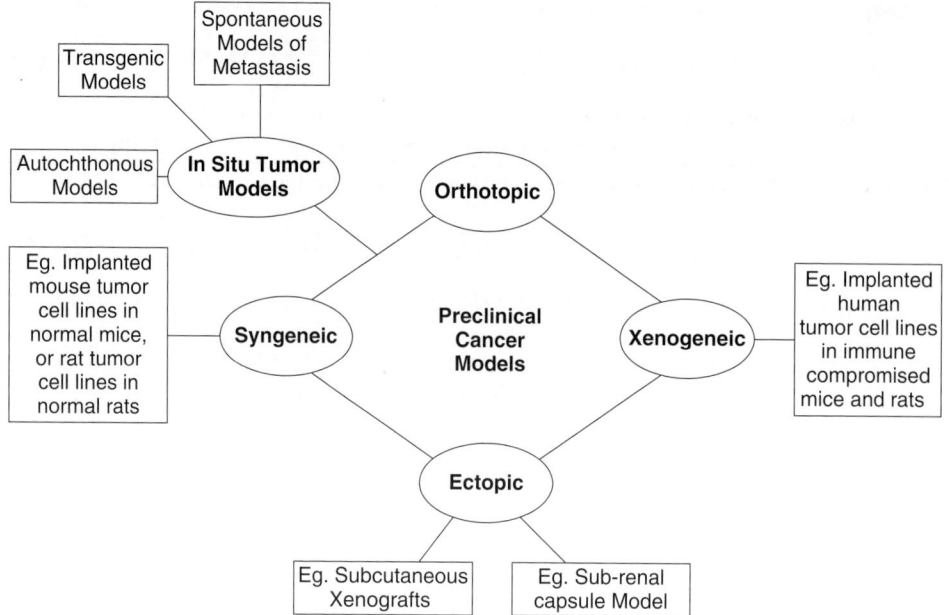

Fig. 1. Schematic representation of the broad categories of preclinical cancer models in use today. *In situ* tumor models can be subcategorized by the method for induction of the tumor. Transplantable tumor models are commonly subcategorized according to whether the tumor is implanted in the organ in which the cell line originated (orthotopic versus ectopic) and in the species in which it originated (syngeneic versus xenogeneic).

targets, these models are also being used to optimize and validate clinical imaging strategies. Finally, molecular imaging techniques are finding a critical role preclinically in the simultaneous confirmation of mechanism of action and assessment of efficacy. This is particularly true in orthotopic or transgenic model systems.

2. TYPES OF TUMOR MODELS

2.1 Transplantable Syngeneic Models

Transplantable syngeneic leukemia and solid tumor models were developed from spontaneous or induced tumors subsequently adapted to serial *in vivo* passage in the same animal strain. The majority of early syngeneic models were leukemias, the most familiar of which are P388 and L1210 *(1–4)*. Syngeneic transplantable solid tumor models were developed in the 1960s and 1970s by exposure of rodents to chemical carcinogens. This provided a variety of tumor histotypes and tumors with different growth rates within each histotype *(5–11)*. Development of these tumor models was pioneered by investigators such as Fidler *(12, 13)*, Morris *(5, 14)*, Skipper *(15–17)*, Schabel *(18–20)*, Griswold *(21–23)*, and Corbett *(7, 8, 24–26)*.

Early drug screening strategies often involved an initial experiment against a murine leukemia with life span as the measured endpoint *(27)*. Active compounds typically then moved into a solid tumor screening panel *(15, 16, 18, 19, 28, 29)* wherein solid tumor fragments were implanted into the subcutaneous space, and therapy was assessed by caliper measurement *(27)*. Advantages of these models include their low cost and reproducibility. Imaging was generally not needed for assessment of tumor response in these easily accessible and observable tumors. However, many investigators have used such models in the development and testing of new imaging approaches. In addition, the tumors grow in an immune-competent host, making these models appropriate for the study of immune modulation and vaccine approaches. However, the genetics of murine cancer are not always identical to their human counterparts, reducing the expectation of a direct correlation with clinical experience. The lack of progress in treatment of the major human solid tumors led to the conclusion that screening strategies with leukemias as the first triage point may not be appropriate *(30)*. Subsequently, many investigators adopted screening strategies that involved direct testing against a panel of solid tumors.

2.2 Spontaneous and Autochthonous Models

There has been a resurgence in autochthonous models *(31–33)*, such as mammary *(34)* and colon tumors *(35)* induced in rats with a carcinogen. The major theoretical advantage of both spontaneous and autochthonous models is that they may be more relevant to the development of human disease because the tumors reside in the tissue appropriate for the histotype. However, studies against tumors induced in this fashion are difficult because of low tumor incidence, variable and delayed onset of tumor growth, and deep tissue location of the tumors. Often treatment is initiated on an animal-by-animal basis as tumors arise and assessment of tumor burdens is performed by terminal sacrifice, complicating treatment and data collection. Lastly, autochthonous model systems require the handling and administration of known potent human carcinogens.

2.3 Human Tumor Xenografts

Syngeneic models, however well characterized, are not human. Xenotransplantation is the transplantation of tissues or organs from one species into a different species. The application of xenotransplantation techniques to the growth of human tumors in experimental animals was a major breakthrough in cancer biology and drug discovery research.

2.3.1 Subrenal Capsule

One of the first of these models sought to take advantage of the immunologically privileged status of the subrenal capsule (SRC) *(36, 37)*. Human tumor fragments implanted under the SRC are not subject to immediate rejection. Changes in tumor volume during therapy are determined by invasive measurements with an ocular micrometer. Unfortunately, the SRC xenograft assay is labor intensive and both tumor growth and response to therapy are often highly variable.

2.3.2 Human Tumor Xenografts in Immunodeficient Animals

A major breakthrough in the *in vivo* evaluation of novel agents against human tumors was the identification and characterization of immunodeficient mice and rats. These animals have genetic immune deficiencies that minimize or prevent the rejection of the grafted tissues from other species. The difficulty in using immune compromised animals is that they are highly susceptible to viral, bacterial, and fungal infections. These infections can alter the outcome and reproducibility of experiments. Therefore, immunodeficient animals are maintained in specific pathogen-free (SPF) environments, dramatically increasing research costs *(38, 39)*.

Nude, *scid*, *xid*, and *beige* mice are the four primary types of immune-deficient mice. Each type of immunodeficient mouse has one or more mutations that diminish the animal's capacity to reject transplanted allografts and xenografts. None of the mutations completely eliminates the immune system function *(40–50)*. *Nude* and *scid* mice are predominantly used for cancer drug evaluation. Xenografted tumors often exhibit a more neoplastic phenotype in *scid* mice than in nudes, presumably because of the more severe immune deficiency of *scid* mice. These animals are often crossed with *beige* and/or *xid* mice to further suppress immune function. The availability of these animals transformed drug discovery paradigms. However, the costs of purchasing and maintenance of these animals is many fold higher than that of conventional animals.

2.3.3 Methods for Xenograft Studies in Immunodeficient Mice

2.3.3.1 Subcutaneous Xenografts. Subcutaneous xenografts are human tumor xenografts (cells, brei, or fragments) that are injected underneath an immune-deficient animal's skin and not into the underlying tissue or cavities. These models are cost effective, and provide a direct assessment of efficacy against a human cancer through simple, noninvasive caliper measurement of tumor size. The accessibility of the tumor is also an advantage for harvesting of tumor tissue. Several publications have suggested that human tumor xenograft models are better predictors of clinical activity than syngeneic models *(51–55)*. Although the use of human tumor xenografts has many advantages, there are also a number of disadvantages. Human cells are placed in a murine environment creating interactions that may not faithfully reflect the human disease process (e.g., differences in the local cellular environment, cytokine, chemokine, and growth factor incompatibility, differences in immunologic state, etc.). Moreover, the subcutaneous environment of the xenograft may also fail to recapitulate normal interaction of the tumor and stroma. Other disadvantages of this model include occasional tissue ulcerations, loss of metastatic potential, and dedifferentiation of the tumor. In addition, the genomic instability of human cancer requires that considerable care be taken to avoid unintended change of the model over time and multiple passages. Despite these potential shortcomings, human tumor xenograft testing remains the mainstay of *in vivo* anticancer therapeutics evaluation.

2.3.3.2 The Hollow Fiber Assay. The hollow fiber assay *(56)* utilizes polyvinylidene fluoride hollow fibers inoculated with human tumor cell lines *(57)*. The fibers are then sealed and implanted into the intraperitoneal cavity or subcutaneous space of an immunodeficient mouse for 3–10 days. After treatment, the fibers are removed and live cells are counted. Advantages of this method are that multiple cell lines can be tested simultaneously in one animal contributing to low cost and high throughput. Disadvantages are that the technique requires survival surgery, the tumor cells are unable to interact with the normal stroma, and the cells have no opportunity to develop a blood supply. Hence, this assay does not reflect treatment-induced changes in stroma-tumor interactions and vascular effects.

2.4 Orthotopic Models

An orthotopic model involves the implantation of a tumor into the organ from which it arose. This is an increasingly popular assay format. A theoretical advantage of this format is that the tumor cells grow in the "context" of their native *in situ* environment *(58–60)*. Orthotopic models have additional advantages over subcutaneous and hollow fiber systems besides cell context. These advantages may include retention of differentiated structures within the tumor, vascular growth differences, more realistic tissue pharmacokinetics at the tumor site, and metastatic spread. However, tumor implantation for orthotopic models requires potentially complex survival surgery. Observation of tumor growth in internal organs typically requires serial sacrifice of cohorts of animals, tumor take rates and growth can be highly variable, and it may be difficult and costly to harvest tumor tissue for pharmacodynamic and pathological analyses. These factors increase cost and decrease throughput. The use of imaging technologies can dramatically enhance the efficiency of orthotopic models. Although it is generally accepted that orthotopic implants often better preserve various aspects of tumor biology, demonstrations that they give different or more predictive assessments of therapeutic potential are lacking. The recent focus on signal transduction pathways (where context may be important) as targets for cancer drug discovery has renewed interest in the relevance of this assay format.

2.5 Models of Metastasis

While the general stability of the tumor tissue in the models discussed above can be an advantage, they often lack key features of human cancer, such as metastasis to secondary organ sites. Prevention of the metastatic process and specific targeting of metastatic lesions offers opportunities for therapeutic intervention. However, reproducible animal models of metastasis that recapitulate all aspects of the metastatic cascade are rare.

Clinically, metastases to the lungs, regional lymph nodes, liver, and brain are most common. A major determinant of the metastatic site is simply location of the primary tumor and the next capillary bed capable of trapping blood-borne tumor emboli. However, the process of metastasis is also critically dependent on the ability of cells that metastasize to promote angiogenesis and proliferate in the new organ environment, giving rise to the "seed and soil" hypothesis *(61–64)*.

Several models of metastasis employ direct or systemic injection techniques. The choice of the site or route of injection is generally based on vascular proximity to the target organ. For example, liver metastases models often rely on intrasplenic injection, lung metastases can be reproducibly obtained from tail vein injection, and bone metastases from intracardiac injection. While direct injection models generally provide the most reproducible and cost-effective models, they have the limitation of not encompassing the entire metastatic process.

Spontaneous models of metastasis, including subcutaneous, transgenic, orthotopic, and autochthonous models provide a better representation of the entire metastatic process than direct injection models, and are specifically suited to the testing of therapeutics for prevention of metastasis. The most common of these relies on continuous passage of metastatic lesions arising from subcutaneous tumors to maintain target organ specificity and metastatic potential. However, these models require longer staging periods and generally have poorer reproducibility and organ specificity than direct injection methods. In addition, these models may require excision of the primary tumor.

Regardless of the model, the study of metastatic lesions has traditionally required inefficient experimental designs that involve serial sacrifice of cohorts of animals. However, *in vivo* imaging technologies can dramatically facilitate these assessments and are finding increased use.

2.6 Transgenic Tumor Models

The massive shift of drug discovery efforts toward inhibition of specific oncogene or suppressor gene related targets has led to increased interest in the use of transgenic models for target validation and the evaluation of drug candidates *(65–70)*. Transgenic tumor models are created by the introduction of heritable (germ line) or somatic mutations that are implicated in neoplastic transformation. Target genes can be replaced by new alleles, conditionally expressed, conditionally turned off, or mutated. A key advantage of transgenic models is that the etiology of tumor development closely mimics that in humans. The animals can be treated with therapeutic agents at any stage of tumor development to further elucidate therapeutic efficacy and the mechanism of action *(71)*.

Three examples of transgenic mouse models with germline mutations are the TRAMP (transgenic adenocarcinoma of the mouse prostate) model, and the p53 and PTEN knockout mice. The TRAMP model was created by linking the prostate-specific probasin promoter to the SV40 large T antigen. These animals develop variably differentiated tumors that metastasize primarily to the lungs and lymph nodes *(71, 72)*. This model has been used to study late events in prostate tumorigenesis and mechanisms of angiogenesis. p53 is the most commonly mutated gene in human cancer. In the p53 knockout mouse, the p53 tumor suppressor gene is inactivated by mutation to create a model of the human Li-Fraumeni familial cancer predisposition syndrome. These mice are more susceptible to spontaneous and carcinogen-induced tumors in many organs *(70)*. The average tumor latency for a homozygous p53 (−/−) mouse is about 4.5 months with an increased latency period for heterozygous p53 (−/+) animals *(73)*. The PTEN heterozygous knockout mouse is predisposed to many tumor types, including colon carcinomas, leukemia, germline tumors, and T cell lymphomas *(71, 74)*. Elimination of one PTEN allele results in the inactivation of proapototic pathways possibly contributing to drug resistance. The PTEN double null (−/−) is an embryonic lethal mutation.

Transgenic models driven by germline mutations can be problematic. Mutations of interest are often embryonic lethal. Additionally, unwanted physiological or toxic effects during development may occur that render the model unusable. Organ specificity can also be difficult to control and the study of multiple gene defects can require complex breeding efforts. Lastly, these animal models are often characterized by long tumor latency periods.

Somatic cell modification strategies offer advantages over germline modification strategies that include improved tissue specificity of transgene expression, avoidance of embryonic lethal events, and opportunities for introduction of sequential multigene defects. An example of a transgenic mouse model created by somatic cell mutation strategies is the TVA model, which is based on retroviral gene transfer. A transgenic animal is created that expresses the avian leukosis virus (ALV) receptor 1 (TVA) from a tissue-specific promoter. These animals are not predisposed to develop cancer without further manipulation. The target gene construct of interest is cloned into a replication-

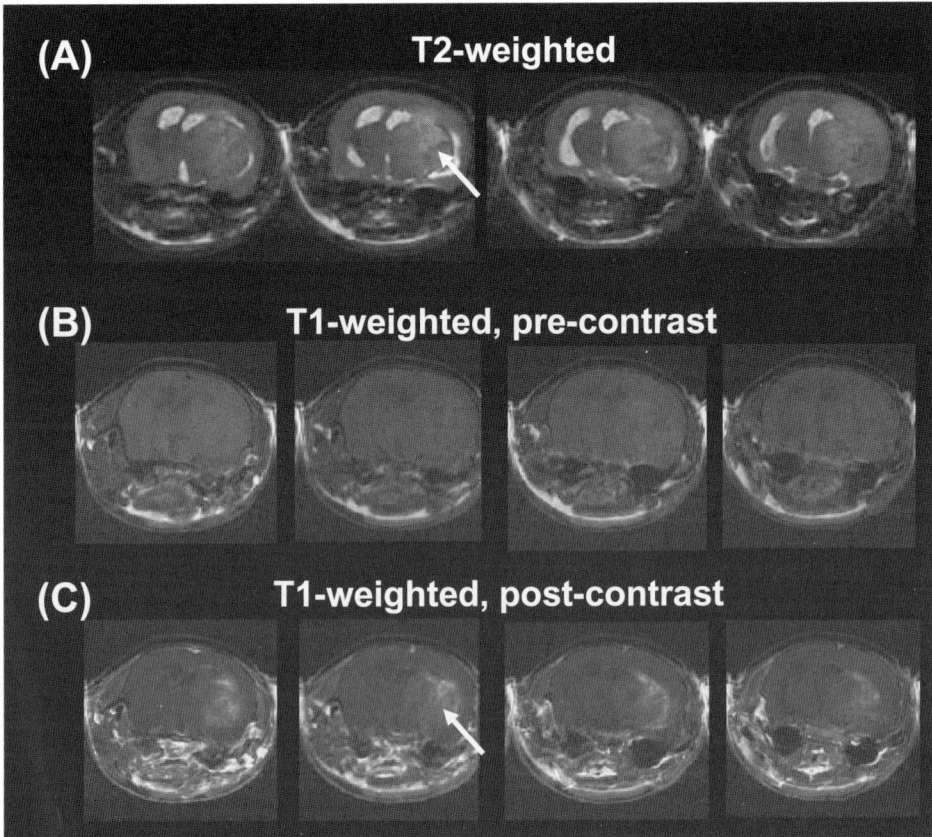

Fig. 2. MRI of PDGF-induced glioma in a Ntv-a mouse (76). The same four contiguous slices are shown for (A) T2-weighted scans showing the tumor as a hyperintense region in the right upper cortex, and T1-weighted scans (B) before, and (C) after administration of Gd-DTPA. The T1-weighted scans highlight localized, heterogeneous contrast enhancement in the tumor. The MRI appearance of glioma in this model is typical of that of human glioma.

competent ALV splice-acceptor (RCAS) vector followed by direct injection of the modified virus or virus-infected cells into the TVA-expressing tissue *(75)*. The TVA/RCAS system has been used in mouse models of induction of gliomas *(76)* (Fig. 2) and ovarian cancer *(77, 78)*.

3. ENDPOINTS AND MEASUREMENTS

Diverse types of information may be gleaned from any of the tumor models described above. Historically, with the exception of transgenic systems, these models have been used primarily to simultaneously assess the response of tumors to drug treatment and the potential for host toxicity (therapeutic index). Imaging technologies are routinely used for anatomical detection of tumors, particularly in orthotopic, metastatic, and transgenic models. However, trends toward molecular-targeted therapies are increasing the use of imaging technologies for quantifying drug-induced changes in physiology. Such methods can enable the use of endpoints that are tied to target modulation, in addition to more traditional growth-based endpoints.

3.1 Detection or Diagnosis of Tumors

The basic method of tumor detection and quantitation is visual observation. Traditionally this involves palpation followed by caliper measurements. Calculation of tumor volume and an assumption of unit density generate an estimate of tumor burden. Caliper measurements have proven representative when compared to actual weights of excised tumors. This detection method is cost effective but primarily limited to subcutaneous tumors.

Increased interest in orthotopic and transgenic systems has created a demand for imaging-based methods for tumor diagnosis or detection. A broad array of imaging modalities and techniques is available for *in vivo* detection of tumors in mouse cancer models. These include bioluminescence imaging (BLI) and *in vivo* fluorescence imaging, magnetic resonance imaging (MRI), magnetic resonance spectroscopy imaging (MRSI), X-ray computed tomography (CT), positron emission tomography (PET), and single photon emission computed tomography (SPECT). Additional technologies not discussed in this chapter include ultrasound imaging and optical coherence tomography.

Bioluminescence imaging and fluorescence imaging—in vivo: BLI is a recently developed optical imaging method that allows visualization of luciferase-driven light emitted from within an animal *(79, 80)*. In the most basic application, mice are inoculated with tumor cells that have been stably transfected with the luciferase gene, and the constitutive expression of luciferase allows assessment of tumor burden after systemic injection of substrate (luciferin). High sensitivity and the ability to quantify tumor burden make BLI ideally suited to detection of the spread and growth of metastases and *in situ* tumor models. Throughput is also high since image acquisition is generally rapid and several mice may be imaged simultaneously. Low spatial resolution is a limitation of BLI. In addition, since the images are commonly two dimensional, images from several animal positions may be necessary to unambiguously identify the anatomical location of a given signal.

In vivo fluorescence imaging can also be used to detect and monitor tumor growth in small animals *(81–83)*. The fluorescent signal is emitted following excitation with monochromatic light of fluorescent proteins or dye-labeled biological molecules. Unlike BLI, fluorescence imaging does not require the injection of exogenous substrate. In addition, the high fluorescence signal allows image acquisition on a millisecond time scale, compared to minutes for BLI. Signal attenuation in deep tissues and a high background of autofluorescence can be problematic for standard fluorescent compounds, however, newer imaging agents provide fluorescent emission at the near-infrared wavelengths that minimizes these effects *(84)*.

Magnetic resonance imaging: MRI of preclinical tumor models combines outstanding soft tissue contrast with high spatial resolution *(85–87)*. Due to differential MR relaxation properties, tumors can usually be distinguished from normal tissue in rapid anatomical scans (Fig. 2). Another common approach to detection of tumors is with a contrast agent such as gadolinium diethylenetriaminepentaacetic acid (Gd-DTPA). Differential uptake of the contrast agent by the tumor compared with surrounding normal tissue, allows the tumor to be delineated in MR images (Fig. 2). MRI has been used in mouse models to detect tumors in the brain, lung, liver, and pancreas, among others *(87)*. Tumors as small as 0.5 mm in diameter can be detected and monitored *in vivo* using MRI.

Magnetic resonance spectroscopic imaging: MRSI involves the combination of MR imaging techniques with conventional NMR spectroscopic methods (commonly proton or phosphorus based) to provide spatially localized spectra. Pathological tumor biology provides unique spectral signatures of various metabolites that distinguish tumors from normal tissue. For example, metabolites such as choline, creatine, lactate, ATP, lipid, and lysine can differentiate certain tumor types from surrounding normal tissue, as well as distinguish between benign and malignant disease in some cases *(85, 88)*.

Computed tomography: The application of high-resolution X-ray CT to preclinical cancer models has recently become feasible, particularly for detection of lesions in bone, lung, and mammary glands *(89)*. Three-dimensional images with resolution on the order of a 10–50 µm are produced. With the use of CT contrast agents and blood pool agents, soft tissues such as liver, pancreas, spleen, and kidney, as well as vasculature can also be imaged *(89)*.

Positron emission tomography: PET is increasingly used to study tumor biology. Equipment design and sensitivity have improved, allowing higher image resolution and animal throughput. Tumor detection using micro-PET takes advantage of pathological changes in tumor cells that promote enhanced uptake of positron-emitting radiotracers. PET tracers have been developed to measure cellular glucose metabolism ($[^{18}F]$fluoro deoxyglucose, FDG), cellular proliferation ($[^{18}F]$fluorothymidine, FLT), protein synthesis ($[^{11}C]$methionine, MET; $[^{18}F]$tyrosine), as well as transgene expression *(90–96)*. An alternative method $[^{124}I]$ uses radioimmunotracers targeting tumor-specific antigens that provides distinction between normal and malignant tissues *(97, 98)*.

3.2 Assessments of Change in Tumor Burden

Change in tumor burden, usually in response to drug treatment, has historically been measured directly with calipers, by weight of an excised tumor mass, or by inference from measurement of host lifespan *(1, 27)*. Excised tumor masses and tumors measured *in situ* contain both viable and dead tissue, and gross assessment of their mass is not equivalent to determination of the surviving fraction. The surviving fraction can be estimated for excised tumor masses by *in vitro* determination of clonogenic survival *(99)*.

By far the most common format for the determination of therapeutic effect involves the estimation of tumor burden from caliper measurements of subcutaneous tumor masses. A number of mathematical treatments of these types of data have been developed, but two are dominant. The most common assesses response to therapy by comparison of control and treated tumor burdens as simple ratios of tumor mass (T/C) at a single point in time. Alternatively, ratios of the change in mass over the course of treatment ($\Delta T/\Delta C$) are generated *(100, 101)*. This method is quick and economical, but it is also prone to severe variability, and the results are not directly comparable between experiments or across models. In addition, the same data set can give different estimates of therapeutic effect depending on the day of measurement, making the data highly subjective. Finally this method cannot give a quantitative estimate of the number of tumor cells surviving treatment. An alternative approach, pioneered by the group at Southern Research Institute, uses more data points to assess a therapy-induced tumor growth delay ($T-C$) from which estimates of net change in tumor burden are derived

(27). The advantages of this more rigorous method are that it produces data that are *quantitatively* comparable between experiments and across models.

As the use of transgenic, orthotopic, and metastasis models increases, all of the imaging modalities described above are being increasingly utilized for detection of tumor masses and measurement of the effect of therapeutic intervention. Imaging can greatly increase the efficiency of these models and provide a more accurate assessment of tumor burden than traditional determination after serial sacrifice. However, imaging can be associated with increased cost and decreased throughput. In certain cases, the use of a contrast agent or labeled molecule may also be required for image-based assessment of tumor burden, which may further increase the complexity of the assay.

3.3 Pharmacokinetics

Pharmacokinetic analysis quantifies the processes of absorption, distribution, metabolism, and elimination (ADME) of compounds over time. Often this is accomplished through serial collection and analysis of body fluids or tissues, or by autoradiography to generate a concentration–time profile. These traditional methods typically consume large numbers of animals, time, and resources.

In autoradiography, animals are systemically exposed to radiolabeled compounds and sacrificed at specific time points. Frozen tissue sections are exposed to imaging plates to produce high-resolution images directly from tissue samples *(102)*. Two-dimensional images can then be stacked to form a three-dimensional image *(103)*. However, this technology is time and labor intensive and relies on the use of potentially hazardous and long-lived radioisotopes.

As imaging modalities have advanced, a number of techniques have been applied to the determination of pharmacokinetic profiles. Positron emission tomography and SPECT have shown particular promise in this respect. These imaging technologies can be used to track movement of compounds, formation of metabolites, tissue concentrations, and drug half-lives. These are noninvasive imaging modalities that image radiotracer distribution after systemic injection into the animal. However, quantification can be problematic due to tissue scattering of emitted photons. While PET is 10- to 20-fold more sensitive with better image resolution than SPECT *(104)*, the generally shorter half-lives of PET isotopes can make the generation and use of labeled compounds challenging. Both imaging modalities are broadly applicable in clinical and preclinical settings.

3.4 Drug Effects at the Molecular Target

The dramatic shift of cancer drug discovery efforts toward a focus on specific molecular targets over the past decade has prompted an increased interest in pharmacodynamic analysis of drug function. These analyses confirm target modulation and can allow quantitative correlation of target modulation with both pharmacokinetics and preclinical efficacy *(105–107)*. Pharmacodynamic analyses can also be used productively to enhance the efficiency of the discovery process by preempting doomed efficacy determinations. Pharmacodynamic analyses to determine the extent and duration of target modulation are typically rapid (1–2 days), and they require minimal drug supplies and only a few animals. By comparison to efficacy testing against a xenograft model, a pharmacodynamic analysis consumes 10- to 25-fold fewer resources. It can allow efficient "drop" decisions for weak compounds and enable an informed design (with respect to dose selection and treatment schedule) of efficacy experiments for compounds with strong potential. Optimization of *in vivo* function for target modulation prior to efficacy determination is becoming the discovery paradigm of choice for targeted programs. These correlations can also be used to set decision-making thresholds for biomarker analyses in phase I clinical trials. Failure to reach a predetermined threshold for target modulation at tolerated dose levels would prompt a decision to terminate development of the targeted compound.

Pharmacodynamic analysis traditionally has involved harvest of tumor tissue from treated animals and quantitative assessment of target modulation with techniques that include Western or Northern blot analysis, biochemical assays for enzyme activity, or immunohistochemistry. More recently *in vivo* imaging-based assays have been developed to measure changes in enzyme activity, substrate or reaction product concentrations, and protein interactions. Imaging-based pharmacodynamic analyses using modalities such as bioluminescence, fluorescence, PET, and SPECT are becoming more widely used. They offer simultaneous evaluation of drug function at the molecular level and efficacy at the whole animal level, dramatically increasing efficiency, reducing animal use, and generating tighter correlations.

Extensions of the basic BLI experiment include various strategies for coupling the expression or activation of luciferase to molecular events within the cell, so that the event is signaled by light production of the active luciferase *(79, 108)*. For example, BLI has been used to image DNA damage *in vivo* with a transgenic mouse that harbors an Mdm2-Luc cassette. Events that induce DNA damage cause stabilization of p53 wherein it accumulates approximately 100-fold, followed by induction of p53 transcriptional activity, leading to activation of the Mdm2 promoter. Subsequent luciferase expression can be detected by BLI. This has been used to demonstrate the radio-sensitizing effect of 5-fluorouricil in mice (A Rehemtulla *et al.*, University of Michigan, 2003, personal communication).

3.5 Drug-Induced Physiological Changes

Direct assessment of drug function at the molecular target is often difficult or impossible. This is particularly true in the clinic, where the requisite biopsies may not be possible. In these situations, surrogate or indirect measures of drug-induced changes in physiology can be useful. Perhaps the best examples are assessments of drug-induced changes in tumor blood flow, vascular density, and vascular permeability now popularly applied to the development of antiangiogenic agents *(109–111)*. However, a key difference between most clinical and preclinical imaging applications is the preclinical use of anesthesia such as isoflurane or ketamine/xylazine. The potential influence of anesthesia on the signal of interest must be carefully considered *(112)*. Examples of changes in drug-induced physiology that can be measured with imaging technologies include the following.

Blood flow (MRI/PET): Blood flow, blood volume, and vascular permeability can be assessed in tumors using a variety of MRI-based techniques such as dynamic contrast-enhanced MRI (DCE MRI) *(113, 114)*, arterial spin labeling *(115, 116)*, and iron-oxide-based contrast MRI *(117)*. These methods have been widely used to detect response to antiangiogenic therapies in mouse cancer models *(118)*. Tumor blood flow measurements have also been performed using clinical PET imaging of $^{15}O[H_2O]$ *(119)*, and may show future widespread use in preclinical PET. Imaging of tumor perfusion and vascularity by PET and MRI is described in more detail in Chapters 4 and 5, respectively.

Apoptosis (BLI/SPECT/PET/MRI: Imaging of apoptosis provides a means of assessing the extent of tumor response to cytotoxic therapy. Several *in vivo* approaches have been developed utilizing BLI, MRI, PET, and SPECT *(120–124)*. One technique using BLI makes use of tumor cells that have been transfected with a hybrid recombinant reporter consisting of luciferase linked to the estrogen receptor (ER) regulatory domain via a cleavage site for caspase-3 (DEVD) *(120)*. The presence of ER in the hybrid reporter renders the luciferase inactive. On activation of caspase-3 during apoptosis, the DEVD site is cleaved and the luciferase becomes active, signaling the onset of apoptosis in the presence of luciferin. Other strategies for *in vivo* imaging of apoptosis are described in Chapter 16.

Metabolism. PET scans using [^{18}F]FDG provide a common approach to *in vivo* assessment of energy metabolism. Since tumors generally have elevated glucose metabolism, [^{18}F]FDG can be used to diagnose tumors as well as monitor changes in tumor metabolism in response to therapy *(125)*. However, these types of images must be interpreted with care because elevated glucose metabolism may be associated with other physiological processes such as macrophage activity and inflammation. Methods such as MRI or MRSI can be used to quantify the levels of metabolites such as choline, lactate, and lipids using ^{1}H-MR, and ATP and phosphocreatine using ^{31}P MR *(126, 127)*.

3.6 Assessment and Early Prediction of Response

Conventional imaging methods for evaluating tumor response to therapy have generally been limited to simple morphological criteria such as an apparent reduction in tumor volume *(128)*. Determination of these endpoints can take weeks or months, hindering timely detection of failed therapies and delaying opportunities to shift to potentially more efficacious treatment. Clearly the development of highly prognostic indicators of therapeutic benefit would be a meaningful advance; FDG-PET has proven to be useful for assessing response to therapy at early time points in cancers such as lung, colorectal, cervical, and esophageal carcinomas *(129–131)*. Assessment of response is achieved in these cases by following the relative change in FDG uptake during tumor treatment. Other PET tracers that are associated with cellular proliferation and protein synthesis have also been used to evaluate tumor response to therapy. Further discussion may be found in Chapters 4, 7, 8, and 9.

Diffusion MRI (dMRI) has been widely used in the clinic to assess acute stroke patients *(132, 133)*, but is being increasingly used in oncology applications for the early evaluation of tumor response to therapy. It provides a measure of the apparent diffusional mobility of water in tissue. The apparent diffusion of tissue water is influenced by diffusion barriers such as cytoplasmic structures, organelles, cell membranes, and the extracellular matrix. These break down in response to treatment. Measurement of water diffusivity by dMRI yields images or maps of the apparent diffusion coefficient (ADC). Several studies of different tumor types and models have shown that ADC within the tumor is correlated with tissue cell density *(134–137)*. When a tumor responds to therapy, an early change in ADC can be observed, often before a measurable decrease in tumor volume *(138)*. This has been interpreted as a decrease in tumor

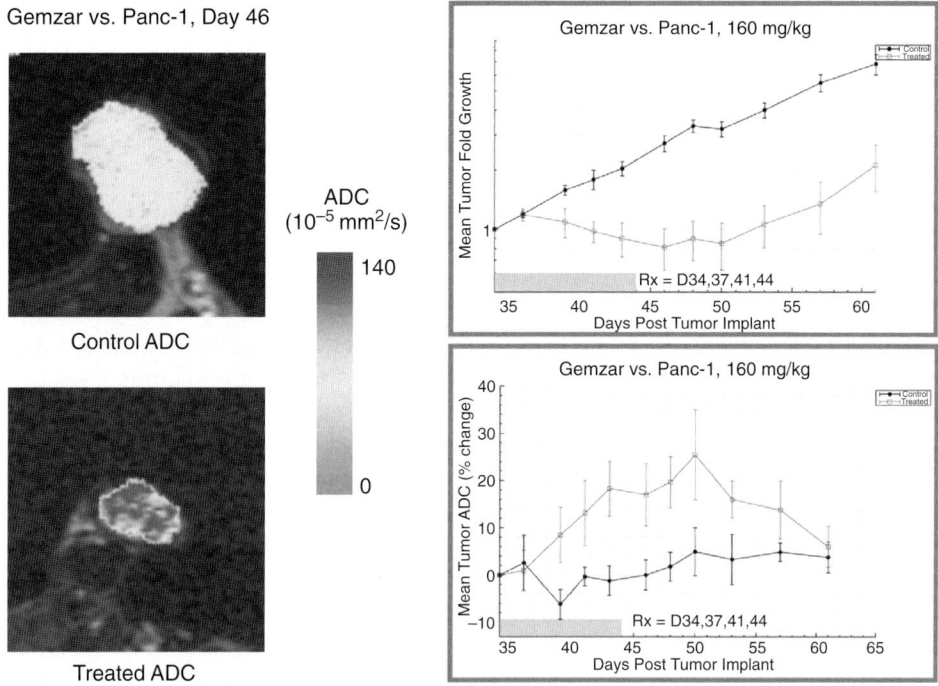

Fig. 3. Diffusion MRI of Panc-1 subcutaneous xenograft treated with Gemzar (160 mg/kg Q3D × 4 IP). On the left, ADC maps are shown of a single slice on day 46 for control (vehicle) and treated tumors from two different animals. Control tumor ADC values are approximately 75×10^{-5} mm^2/sec; the treated tumor has focal regions with ADC values approaching 130×10^{-5} mm^2/sec. Tumor burden (mean fold growth) is plotted in the upper right panel, and mode tumor ADC change relative to pre-treatment values in the lower right panel. Open symbols are means of treated animals ($N = 4$) and closed symbols are means of control animals ($N = 4$).

cell density and increase in necrotic fraction *(135, 136)* (Fig. 3). In preclinical tumor models, this change in tumor ADC may be correlated with cell kill, providing an earlier indication of the activity of the therapeutic agent without the requisite measurement of tumor regrowth. Relative changes in ADC may also be used to optimize combination therapies or dose schedules. Recent clinical trials suggest a positive prognostic value for early ADC change in brain tumors *(139)*. Advantages of dMRI include the following: (1) it is directly translatable to the clinic, (2) it does not require injection of contrast agents or tracers, and (3) it can be carried out with standard MRI equipment and very short scan times.

4. SUMMARY AND FUTURE DIRECTIONS

A wide range of *in vivo* tumor models is available. Although most have been criticized for poor correlation with clinical outcomes, compelling evidence exists indicating that for several types of models, the absence of preclinical *in vivo* anticancer activity is a negative indicator of clinical utility *(53–55)*. The well-recognized shift to drug discovery strategies targeting specific molecules thought to cause or support the transformed phenotype has led to increased interest in the use of orthotopic and transgenic tumor models. These discovery strategies are also facilitated by correlation of drug effect at the molecular target with efficacy. Fortunately, recent advances in preclinical imaging technologies offer enhanced opportunities for noninvasive analysis of drug function in addition to basic tumor biology at anatomic, physiologic, and mechanistic levels. These technologies are especially well suited to the use of the increasingly relevant transgenic and orthotopic models.

With the shift toward therapeutic targeting of cancer-specific molecular defects, confirmation of the interaction of the drug with its target and analyses of downstream effects (drug-induced changes in physiology) are also frequently sought. Imaging technologies are increasingly used to this end. However, imaging at the resolution required in small animals presents many challenges. While MRI is a relatively mature modality that is now used routinely for small animal imaging, modalities such as micro-PET, micro-SPECT, and *in vivo* optical imaging have only seen widespread use in the past decade, and they pose greater challenges in terms of sensitivity and resolution. Related to these issues is the image time required, or "throughput." Improvements in animal imaging throughput are critical in enabling meaningful and efficient animal studies that involve sufficient animal numbers and multiple time points to provide statistical power and biological relevance *(140)*. With future technological advancements that improve sensitivity, resolution, and throughput, clinical protocols that are already used routinely in nuclear imaging, CT and MRI, will be successfully translated to true quantitative imaging in the preclinical arena. Similarly, advances in novel preclinical imaging technologies and imaging agents will be translated to clinical trial.

Quantitative imaging can offer correlations of efficacy and therapeutic index with either target modulation at the molecular level or surrogate markers of drug function. These correlations can then be used to establish decision-making thresholds for measurable endpoints in early clinical trials. Hence, the future of imaging in preclinical tumor models lies in the development and validation of image-based biomarkers and surrogate markers for tumor response that will be used in clinical trials. These technologies will be used increasingly in the earlier stages of preclinical development of new therapies as correlates for growth-based determination of efficacy.

REFERENCES

1. Dykes D, Waud W. Murine L1210 and P388 leukemias. In: Teicher B, ed. Tumor Models in Cancer Research. Totowa, NJ: Humana Press, Inc., 2002:23–40.
2. Venditti JM, Humphreys SR, Goldin A. Investigation of the activity of cytoxan against leukemia L1210 in mice. *Cancer Res* 1959;19:986–995.
3. Law LW, Potter M. Further evidence of indirect induction by x-radiation of lymphocytic neoplasms in mice. *J Natl Cancer Inst* 1958;20(3):489–493.
4. Burchenal JH. Murine and human leukemias. *Bibl Haematol* 1975(40):665–677.
5. Morris HP, Slaughter LJ. Historical development of transplantable hepatomas. *Adv Exp Med Biol* 1977;92:1–19.
6. Double JA, Ball CR, Cowen PN. Transplantation of adenocarcinomas of the colon in mice. *J Natl Cancer Inst* 1975;54(1):271–275.
7. Corbett TH, Griswold DP Jr, Roberts BJ, Peckham JC, Schabel FM Jr. Biology and therapeutic response of a mouse mammary adenocarcinoma (16/C) and its potential as a model for surgical adjuvant chemotherapy. *Cancer Treat Rep* 1978;62(10):1471–1488.
8. Corbett TH, Griswold DP Jr, Roberts BJ, Peckham JC, Schabel FM Jr. Tumor induction relationships in development of transplantable cancers of the colon in mice for chemotherapy assays, with a note on carcinogen structure. *Cancer Res* 1975;35(9):2434–2439.

9. Langdon SP, Gescher A, Hickman JA, Stevens MF. The chemosensitivity of a new experimental model –the M5076 reticulum cell sarcoma. *Eur J Cancer Clin Oncol* 1984;20(5):699–705.
10. Shay H, Aegerter EA, *et al.* Development of adenocarcinoma of the breast in the Wistar rat following the gastric instillation of methylcholanthrene. *J Natl Cancer Inst* 1949;10(2):255–266.
11. Stewart HL, Hare WV, *et al.* Adenocarcinoma and other lesions of the glandular stomach of mice, following intramural injection of 20-methylcholanthrene. *J Natl Cancer Inst* 1949;10(2):359; Discussion, 99–403.
12. Fidler IJ. Selection of successive tumour lines for metastasis. *Nat New Biol* 1973;242(118):148–149.
13. Fidler IJ. Biological behavior of malignant melanoma cells correlated to their survival in vivo. *Cancer Res* 1975;35(1):218–224.
14. Morris HP. Studies on the development, biochemistry, and biology of experimental hepatomas. *Adv Cancer Res* 1965;9:227–302.
15. Skipper HE. Drug evaluation in experimental tumor systems: Potential and limitations in 1961. *Cancer Chemother Rep* 1962;16:11–18.
16. Skipper HE, Schmidt LH. A manual on quantitative drug evaluation in experimental tumor systems. I. Background, description of criteria, and presentation of quantitative therapeutic data on various classes of drugs obtained in diverse experimental tumor systems. *Cancer Chemother Rep* 1962;17:1–143.
17. Skipper HE. Cancer chemotherapy is many things: G.H.A. Clowes Memorial Lecture. *Cancer Res* 1971;31(9):1173–1180.
18. Schabel FM Jr. Screening, the cornerstone of chemotherapy. *Cancer Chemother Rep* 2 1972;3(1):309–313.
19. Schabel FM Jr, Corbett TH. Cell kinetics and the chemotherapy of murine solid tumors. *Antibiot Chemother* 1980;28:28–34.
20. Schabel FM Jr, Montgomery JA, Skipper HE, Laster WR Jr, Thomson JR. Experimental evaluation of potential anticancer agents. I. Quantitative therapeutic evaluation of certain purine analogs. *Cancer Res* 1961;21:690–699.
21. Griswold DP Jr, Casey AE, Weisburger EK, Weisburger JH, Schabel FM Jr. On the carcinogenicity of a single intragastric dose of hydrocarbons, nitrosamines, aromatic amines, dyes, coumarins, and miscellaneous chemicals in female Sprague-Dawley rats. *Cancer Res* 1966;26(4):619–625.
22. Griswold DP, Corbett TH. A colon tumor model for anticancer agent evaluation. *Cancer* 1975;36(6 Suppl):2441–2444.
23. Griswold DP, Skipper HE, Laster WR Jr, Wilcox WS, Schabel FM Jr. Induced mammary carcinoma in the female rat as a drug evaluation system. *Cancer Res* 1966;26(10):2169–2180.
24. Corbett TH, Roberts BJ, Leopold WR, *et al.* Induction and chemotherapeutic response of two transplantable ductal adenocarcinomas of the pancreas in C57BL/6 mice. *Cancer Res* 1984;44(2):717–726.
25. Roberts BJ, Fife WP, Corbett TH, Schabel FM. Response of five established solid transplantable mouse tumors and one mouse leukemia to hyperbaric hydrogen. *Cancer Treat Rep* 1978;62(7):1077–1079.
26. Tapazoglou E, Polin L, Corbett TH, al-Sarraf M. Chemotherapy of the squamous cell lung cancer LC-12 with 5-fluorouracil, cisplatin, carboplatin or iproplatin combinations. *Invest New Drugs* 1988;6(4):259–264.
27. Schabel FM, Griswold DP, Laster WR, Corbett TH, Lloyd HH. Quantitative evaluation of anticancer agent activity in experimental animals. *Pharmacol Ther Part A: Chemother Toxicol Metabol Inhibit* 1977;1(4):411–435.
28. Venditti JM, Wesley RA, Plowman J. Current NCI preclinical antitumor screening in vivo: Results of tumor panel screening, 1976–1982, and future directions. *Adv Pharmacol Chemother* 1984;20:1–20.
29. Zee-Cheng RK, Cheng CC. Screening and evaluation of anticancer agents. *Methods Find Exp Clin Pharmacol* 1988;10(2):67–101.
30. Jackson RC. The problem of the quiescent cancer cell. *Adv Enzyme Regul* 1989;29:27–46.
31. DiGiovanni J. Modification of multistage skin carcinogenesis in mice. *Prog Exp Tumor Res* 1991;33:192–229.
32. Konishi Y, Tsutsumi M, Tsujiuchi T. Mechanistic analysis of pancreatic ductal carcinogenesis in hamsters. *Pancreas* 1998;16(3):300–306.

33. Miller MS, Leone-Kabler S, Rollins LA, et al. Molecular pathogenesis of transplacentally induced mouse lung tumors. *Exp Lung Res* 1998;24(4):557–577.
34. Russo J, Russo IH. Experimentally induced mammary tumors in rats. *Breast Cancer Res Treat* 1996;39(1):7–20.
35. Nakagama H, Ochiai M, Ubagai T, et al. A rat colon cancer model induced by 2-amino-1-methyl-6-phenylimidazo[4,5-b]pyridine, PhIP. *Mutat Res* 2002;506–507:137–144.
36. Aamdal S, Fodstad O, Pihl A. Human tumor xenografts transplanted under the renal capsule of conventional mice. Growth rates and host immune response. *Int J Cancer* 1984;34(5):725–730.
37. Bogden AE. The subrenal capsule assay (SRCA) and its predictive value in oncology. *Ann Chir Gynaecol Suppl* 1985;199:12–27.
38. Simmons ML, Richter CB, Tennant RW, Franklin J. Production of specific pathogen-free rats in plastic germfree isolator rooms. In: Symposium on Gnotobiotic Life in Medical and Biological Research, 1968.
39. (U.S.) IoLAR, NetLibrary I. Guide for the care and use of laboratory animals. National Research Council, 1996.
40. Custer RP, Bosma GC, Bosma MJ. Severe combined immunodeficiency (SCID) in the mouse. Pathology, reconstitution, neoplasms. *Am J Pathol* 1985;120(3):464–477.
41. Dorshkind K, Keller GM, Phillips RA, et al. Functional status of cells from lymphoid and myeloid tissues in mice with severe combined immunodeficiency disease. *J Immunol* 1984;132(4):1804–1808.
42. Eaton GJ. Hair growth cycles and wave patterns in "nude" mice. *Transplantation* 1976;22(3):217–222.
43. Flanagan SP. "Nude", a new hairless gene with pleiotropic effects in the mouse. *Genet Res* 1966;8(3):295–309.
44. Bosma GC, Custer RP, Bosma MJ. A severe combined immunodeficiency mutation in the mouse. *Nature* 1983;301(5900):527–530.
45. Bosma GC, Davisson MT, Ruetsch NR, Sweet HO, Shultz LD, Bosma MJ. The mouse mutation severe combined immune deficiency (scid) is on chromosome 16. *Immunogenetics* 1989;29(1):54–57.
46. Clark EA, Shultz LD, Pollack SB. Mutations in mice that influence natural killer (NK) cell activity. *Immunogenetics* 1981;12(5–6):601–613.
47. Mahoney KH, Morse SS, Morahan PS. Macrophage functions in beige (Chediak-Higashi syndrome) mice. *Cancer Res* 1980;40(11):3934–3939.
48. Roder J, Duwe A. The beige mutation in the mouse selectively impairs natural killer cell function. *Nature* 1979;278(5703):451–453.
49. Saxena RK, Saxena QB, Adler WH. Defective T-cell response in beige mutant mice. *Nature* 1982;295(5846):240–241.
50. Scher I, Frantz MM, Steinberg AD. The genetics of the immune response to a synthetic double-stranded RNA in a mutant CBA mouse strain. *J Immunol* 1973;110(5):1396–1401.
51. Kerbel RS. Human tumor xenografts as predictive preclinical models for anticancer drug activity in humans: Better than commonly perceived–but they can be improved. *Cancer Biol Ther* 2003;2(4 Suppl 1):S134–139.
52. Suggitt M, Bibby MC. 50 years of preclinical anticancer drug screening: Empirical to target-driven approaches. *Clin Cancer Res* 2005;11(3):971–981.
53. Voskoglou-Nomikos T, Pater JL, Seymour L. Clinical predictive value of the in vitro cell line, human xenograft, and mouse allograft preclinical cancer models. *Clin Cancer Res* 2003;9(11):4227–4239.
54. Jackson RC, Sebolt JS, Shillis JL, Leopold WR. The pyrazoloacridines: Approaches to the development of a carcinoma-selective cytotoxic agent. *Cancer Invest* 1990;8(1):39–47.
55. Johnson JI, Decker S, Zaharevitz D, et al. Relationships between drug activity in NCI preclinical in vitro and in vivo models and early clinical trials. *Br J Cancer* 2001;84(10):1424–1431.
56. Decker S, Hollingshead M, Bonomi CA, Carter JP, Sausville EA. The hollow fibre model in cancer drug screening: The NCI experience. *Eur J Cancer* 2004;40(6):821–826.
57. Hall LA, Krauthauser CM, Wexler RS, Slee AM, Kerr JS. The hollow fiber assay. *Methods Mol Med* 2003;74:545–566.

58. Fidler IJ, Wilmanns C, Staroselsky A, Radinsky R, Dong Z, Fan D. Modulation of tumor cell response to chemotherapy by the organ environment. *Cancer Metastasis Rev* 1994;13(2):209–222.
59. Killion JJ, Radinsky R, Fidler IJ. Orthotopic models are necessary to predict therapy of transplantable tumors in mice. *Cancer Metastasis Rev* 1998;17(3):279–284.
60. Singh RK, Tsan R, Radinsky R. Influence of the host microenvironment on the clonal selection of human colon carcinoma cells during primary tumor growth and metastasis. *Clin Exp Metastasis* 1997;15(2):14–50.
61. Hart IR. "Seed and soil" revisited: Mechanisms of site-specific metastasis. *Cancer Metastasis Rev* 1982;1(1):5–16.
62. Fidler IJ. The pathogenesis of cancer metastasis: The "seed and soil" hypothesis revisited. *Nat Rev Cancer* 2003;3(6):453–458.
63. Paget S. The distribution of secondary growths in cancer of the breast. *Lancet* 1889;1:571–573.
64. Radinsky R. Modulation of tumor cell gene expression and phenotype by the organ-specific metastatic environment. *Cancer Metastasis Rev* 1995;14(4):3–38.
65. Clarke AR, Hollstein M. Mouse models with modified p53 sequences to study cancer and ageing. *Cell Death Differ* 2003;10(4):44–50.
66. Kavanaugh CJ, Desai KV, Calvo A, *et al*. Pre-clinical applications of transgenic mouse mammary cancer models. *Transgenic Res* 2002;11(6):61–133.
67. Kwak I, Tsai SY, DeMayo FJ. Genetically engineered mouse models for lung cancer. *Annu Rev Physiol* 2004;66:647–663.
68. Lakhtakia R, Panda SK. Transgenic mouse models and hepatocellular carcinoma: Future prospects. *Trop Gastroenterol* 2000;21(3):91–94.
69. Lowy AM. Transgenic models of pancreatic cancer. *Int J Gastrointest Cancer* 2003;33(1):71–78.
70. Lubet RA, Zhang Z, Wiseman RW, You M. Use of p53 transgenic mice in the development of cancer models for multiple purposes. *Exp Lung Res* 2000;26(8):58–93.
71. Kasper S, Smith JA Jr. Genetically modified mice and their use in developing therapeutic strategies for prostate cancer. *J Urol* 2004;172(1):12–19.
72. Gingrich JR, Barrios RJ, Morton RA, *et al*. Metastatic prostate cancer in a transgenic mouse. *Cancer Res* 1996;56(18):4096–4102.
73. Macleod KF, Jacks T. Insights into cancer from transgenic mouse models. *J Pathol* 1999;187(1):43–60.
74. Deng CX, Brodie SG. Knockout mouse models and mammary tumorigenesis. *Semin Cancer Biol* 2001;11(5):38–94.
75. Fisher GH, Orsulic S, Holland EC, *et al*. Development of a flexible and specific gene delivery system from production of murine tumor models. *Oncogene* 1999;18:5253–5260.
76. McConville P, Hambardzumyan D, Moody JB, Leopold WR, Kreger AR, Woolliscroft MJ, Rehemtulla A, Ross BD, Holland EC. MRI determination of tumor grade and early response to temozolomide in a genetically engineered mouse model of glioma. *Clin Cancer Res* 2007, in press.
77. Orsulic S. An RCAS-tva-based approach to designer mouse models. *Mammalian Genome* 2002;13:543–547.
78. Orsulic S, Li Y, Soslow RA, Vitale-Cross LA, Gutkind JS, Varmus HE. Induction of ovarian cancer by defined multiple genetic changes in a mouse model. *Cancer Cell* 2002;1:53–62.
79. Contag CH. Bioluminescence imaging of mouse models of human cancer. In: Holland EC, ed. Mouse Models of Human Cancer. Hoboken, NJ: John Wiley & Sons, Inc., 2004:363–373.
80. Edinger M, Cao YA, Hornig YS, *et al*. Advancing animal models of neoplasia through in vivo bioluminescence imaging. *Eur J Cancer* 2002;38(16):2128–2136.
81. Choy G, Choyke P, Libutti SK. Current advances in molecular imaging: Noninvasive in vivo bioluminescent and fluorescent optical imaging in cancer research. *Mol Imaging* 2003;2(4):303–312.
82. Choy G, O'Connor S, Diehn FE, *et al*. Comparison of noninvasive fluorescent and bioluminescent small animal optical imaging. *Biotechniques* 2003;35(5):1022–1026.
83. Contag CH, Bachmann MH. Advances in in vivo bioluminescence imaging of gene expression. *Annu Rev Biomed Eng* 2002;4:235–260.
84. Jaffer FA, Weissleder R. Molecular imaging in the clinical arena. *JAMA* 2005;293(7):855–862.
85. Benaron DA. The future of cancer imaging. *Cancer Metastasis Rev* 2002;21(1):45–78.

86. Muruganandham M, Koutcher JA. Magnetic resonance imaging in mouse cancer models. In: Holland EC, ed. Micro-Computed Tomography of Mouse Cancer Models. Hoboken, NJ: John Wiley & Sons, Inc., 2004:349–362.
87. Pautler RG. Mouse MRI: Concepts and applications in physiology. *Physiology (Bethesda)* 2004; 19:168–175.
88. Swindle P, McCredie S, Russell P, et al. Pathologic characterization of human prostate tissue with proton MR spectroscopy. *Radiology* 2003;228(1):144–151.
89. Weichert JP. Micro-computed tomography of mouse cancer models. In: Holland EC, ed. Mouse Models of Human Cancer. Hoboken, NJ: John Wiley & Sons, Inc., 2004:339–348.
90. Spence AM, Mankoff DA, Muzi M. Positron emission tomography imaging of brain tumors. *Neuroimaging Clin North Am* 2003;13(4):717–739.
91. Shields AF, Grierson JR, Dohmen BM, et al. Imaging proliferation in vivo with [F-18]FLT and positron emission tomography. *Nat Med* 1998;4(11):1334–1336.
92. Shields AF, Mankoff DA, Link JM, et al. Carbon-11-thymidine and FDG to measure therapy response. *J Nucl Med* 1998;39(10):1757–1762.
93. Jager PL, Que TH, Vaalburg W, Pruim J, Elsinga P, Plukker JT. Carbon-11 choline or FDG-PET for staging of oesophageal cancer? *Eur J Nucl Med* 2001;28(12):184–189.
94. Jager PL, Vaalburg W, Pruim J, de Vries EG, Langen KJ, Piers DA. Radiolabeled amino acids: Basic aspects and clinical applications in oncology. *J Nucl Med* 2001;42(3):432–445.
95. Furumoto S, Takashima K, Kubota K, Ido T, Iwata R, Fukuda H. Tumor detection using 18F-labeled matrix metalloproteinase-2 inhibitor. *Nucl Med Biol* 2003;30(2):119–125.
96. Gambhir S, Herschman H, Cherry S, et al. Imaging transgene expression with radionuclide imaging technologies. *Neoplasia* 2000;2(1–2):118–138.
97. Lee FT, Hall C, Rigopoulos A, et al. Immuno-PET of human colon xenograft- bearing BALB/c nude mice using 124I-CDR-grafted humanized A33 monoclonal antibody. *J Nucl Med* 2001;42(5):764–769.
98. Sundaresan G, Yazaki PJ, Shively JE, et al. 124I-labeled engineered anti-CEA minibodies and diabodies allow high-contrast, antigen-specific small-animal PET imaging of xenografts in athymic mice. *J Nucl Med* 2003;44(12):1962–1969.
99. Rockwell S. Tumor cell survival. In: Teicher B, ed. Tumor Models in Cancer Research. Totowa, NJ: Humana Press, Inc., 2002:617–631.
100. Dykes DJ, Abbott BJ, Mayo JG, et al. Development of human tumor xenograft models for in vivo evaluation of new antitumor drugs. *Contrib Oncol* 1992;42:1–22.
101. Plowman J. Human tumor xenograft models in NCI drug development. In: Teicher B, ed. Anticancer Drug Development Guide: Preclinical Screening, Clinical Trials, and Approval. Totowa, NJ: Humana Press, 1997:10–25.
102. Coe RA. Quantitative whole-body autoradiography. *Regul Toxicol Pharmacol* 2000;31(2 Pt 2): S1–3.
103. Malandain G, Bardinet E, Nelissen K, Vanduffel W. Fusion of autoradiographs with an MR volume using 2-D and 3-D linear transformations. *Neuroimage* 2004;23(1):111—27.
104. Fischman AJ, Alpert NM, Rubin RH. Pharmacokinetic imaging: A noninvasive method for determining drug distribution and action. *Clin Pharmacokinet* 2002;41(8):581–602.
105. Sebolt-Leopold JS, Dudley DT, Herrera R, et al. Blockade of the MAP kinase pathway suppresses growth of colon tumors in vivo. *Nat Med* 1999;5(7):810–816.
106. Mendel DB, Laird AD, Xin X, et al. In vivo antitumor activity of SU11248, a novel tyrosine kinase inhibitor targeting vascular endothelial growth factor and platelet-derived growth factor receptors: Determination of a pharmacokinetic/pharmacodynamic relationship. *Clin Cancer Res* 2003;9(1): 327–337.
107. Fry DW, Harvey PJ, Keller PR, et al. Specific inhibition of cyclin-dependent kinase 4/6 by PD 0332991 and associated antitumor activity in human tumor xenografts. *Mol Cancer Ther* 2004; 3(11):1427–1438.
108. Ross BD, Chenevert TL, Moffat BA, et al. Use of magnetic resonance imaging for evaluation of treatment response. In: Holland EC, ed. Mouse Models of Human Cancer. Hoboken, NJ: John Wiley & Sons, Inc., 2004:377–390.
109. Willett CG, Boucher Y, di Tomaso E, et al. Direct evidence that the VEGF-specific antibody bevacizumab has antivascular effects in human rectal cancer. *Nat Med* 2004;10(2):145–147.
110. Galbraith SM, Maxwell RJ, Lodge MA, et al. Combretastatin A4 phosphate has tumor antivascular activity in rat and man as demonstrated by dynamic magnetic resonance imaging. *J Clin Oncol* 2003;21(15):2831–2842.

111. Galbraith SM. Antivascular cancer treatments: Imaging biomarkers in pharmaceutical drug development. *Br J Radiol* 2003;76(Spec No 1):S83–S86.
112. Toyama H, Ichise M, Liow JS, et al. Evaluation of anesthesia effects on [18F]FDG uptake in mouse brain and heart using small animal PET. *Nucl Med Biol* 2004;31(2):251–256.
113. Taylor JS, Tofts PS, Port R, et al. MR imaging of tumor microcirculation: Promise for the new millennium. *J Magn Reson Imaging* 1999;10(6):90–97.
114. Leach MO, Brindle KM, Evelhoch JL, et al. Assessment of antiangiogenic and antivascular therapeutics using MRI: Recommendations for appropriate methodology for clinical trials. *Br J Radiol* 2003;76(Spec No 1):S87–S91.
115. Moffat BA, Chenevert TL, Hall DE, Rehemtulla A, Ross BD. Continuous arterial spin labeling using a train of adiabatic inversion pulses. *J Magn Reson Imaging* 2005;21(3):290–296.
116. Sun Y, Schmidt NO, Schmidt K, et al. Perfusion MRI of U87 brain tumors in a mouse model. *Magn Reson Med* 2004;51(5):893–899.
117. Moffat BA, Reddy GR, McConville P, et al. A novel polyacrylamide magnetic nanoparticle contrast agent for molecular imaging using MRI. *Mol Imaging* 2003;2(4):324–332.
118. Miller JC, Pien HH, Sahani D, Sorensen AG, Thrall JH. Imaging angiogenesis: Applications and potential for drug development. *J Natl Cancer Inst* 2005;97(3):172–187.
119. Anderson H, Price P. Clinical measurement of blood flow in tumours using positron emission tomography: A review. [Article]. *Nucl Med Commun* 2002;23(2):131–138.
120. Laxman B, Hall DE, Bhojani MS, et al. Noninvasive real-time imaging of apoptosis. *Proc Natl Acad Sci USA* 2002;99(26):16551–16555.
121. Jung HI, Kettunen MI, Davletov B, Brindle KM. Detection of apoptosis using the C2A domain of synaptotagmin I. *Bioconjug Chem* 2004;15(5):983–987.
122. Hakumaki JM, Brindle KM. Techniques: Visualizing apoptosis using nuclear magnetic resonance. *Trends Pharmacol Sci* 2003;24(3):146–149.
123. Collingridge DR, Glaser M, Osman S, et al. In vitro selectivity, in vivo biodistribution and tumour uptake of annexin V radiolabelled with a positron emitting radioisotope. *Br J Cancer* 2003;89(7):1327–1333.
124. Zhao M, Beauregard DA, Loizou L, Davletov B, Brindle KM. Non-invasive detection of apoptosis using magnetic resonance imaging and a targeted contrast agent. *Nat Med* 2001;7(11):1241–1244.
125. Phelps ME. Inaugural article: Positron emission tomography provides molecular imaging of biological processes. *Proc Natl Acad Sci USA* 2000;97(16):9226–9233.
126. Maxwell RJ, Nielsen FU, Breidahl T, Stodkilde-Jorgensen H, Horsman MR. Effects of combretastatin on murine tumours monitored by 31P MRS, 1H MRS and 1H MRI. *Int J Radiat Oncol Biol Phys* 1998;42(4):891–894.
127. Kristensen CA, Askenasy N, Jain RK, Koretsky AP. Creatine and cyclocreatine treatment of human colon adenocarcinoma xenografts: 31P and 1H magnetic resonance spectroscopic studies. *Br J Cancer* 1999;79(2):278–285.
128. Therasse P, Arbuck SG, Eisenhauer EA, et al. New guidelines to evaluate the response to treatment in solid tumors. European Organization for Research and Treatment of Cancer, National Cancer Institute of the United States, National Cancer Institute of Canada. *J Natl Cancer Inst* 2000;92(3):205–216.
129. Stahl A, Ott K, Schwaiger M, Weber WA. Comparison of different SUV-based methods for monitoring cytotoxic therapy with FDG PET. *Eur J Nucl Med Mol Imaging* 2004;31(11):1471–1478.
130. Stahl A, Wieder H, Piert M, Wester HJ, Senekowitsch-Schmidtke R, Schwaiger M. Positron emission tomography as a tool for translational research in oncology. *Mol Imaging Biol* 2004;6(4):214–224.
131. Stahl A, Wieder H, Wester HJ, et al. PET/CT molecular imaging in abdominal oncology. *Abdom Imaging* 2004;29(3):388–397.
132. Xavier AR, Qureshi AI, Kirmani JF, Yahia AM, Bakshi R. Neuroimaging of stroke: A review. *South Med J* 2003;96(4):367–379.
133. Roberts TP, Rowley HA. Diffusion weighted magnetic resonance imaging in stroke. *Eur J Radiol* 2003;45(3):185–194.
134. Chenevert Tl, Stegman LD, Taylor JMG, et al. Diffusion magnetic resonance imaging: An early surrogate marker of therapeutic efficacy in brain tumors. *J Natl Cancer Inst* 2000;92(24):2029–2036.

135. Chenevert TL, McKeever PE, Ross BD. Monitoring early response of experimental brain tumors to therapy using diffusion magnetic resonance imaging. *Clin Cancer Res* 1997;3(9):1457–1466.
136. Lyng H, Haraldseth O, Rofstad EK. Measurement of cell density and necrotic fraction in human melanoma xenografts by diffusion weighted magnetic resonance imaging. *Magn Reson Med* 2000;43(6):828–836.
137. Sugahara T, Korogi Y, Kochi M, *et al.* Usefulness of diffusion-weighted MRI with echo-planar technique in the evaluation of cellularity in gliomas. *J Magn Reson Imaging* 1999;9(1):53–60.
138. Ross BD, Moffat BA, Lawrence TS, *et al.* Evaluation of cancer therapy using diffusion magnetic resonance imaging. *Mol Cancer Ther* 2003;2(6):581–587.
139. Moffat BA, Chenevert TL, Lawrence T, *et al.* Functional diffusion map: A noninvasive MRI biomarker for early stratification of clinical brain tumor response. *Proc Natl Acad Sci USA* 2005;102(15):5524–5529.
140. McConville P, Moody JB, Moffat BA. High-throughput magnetic resonance imaging in mice for phenotyping and therapeutic evaluation. *Curr Opin Chem Biol* 2005;9(4):413–420.

3 Anatomical Measure of Tumor Growth with Computed Tomography and Magnetic Resonance Imaging

Stephen J. Gwyther, MBBS, FRCS, FRCR

CONTENTS

INTRODUCTION
CONFIRMATION OF RESPONSE
COMPUTED TOMOGRAPHY IMAGING
MAGNETIC RESONANCE IMAGING
THE FUTURE
SUMMARY

1. INTRODUCTION

During the 1970s developments in technology, nursing techniques, and patient management led to a significant increase in the number of critically ill patients being successfully nursed back to health. This had ramifications for patients suffering from cancer. Prior to that time, the unwanted side effects associated with chemotherapy could not be adequately monitored nor patients satisfactorily managed. The number of chemotherapeutic agents available for use were therefore limited and aggressive treatment regimens could not be instituted. However, with technological advances the ability to treat and monitor tumors that previously could not be detected rose sharply. This, with intensive patient support, allowed aggressive chemotherapeutic regimes to be undertaken. Most chemotherapeutic agents currently on the market are cytotoxic, with a low therapeutic index, and act on rapidly dividing cells making no distinction between malignant cells and normal rapidly dividing cells such as the gastrointestinal tract and bone marrow.

Dose-limiting toxicity in the form of mucositis, nausea, vomiting, diarrhea, and bone marrow suppression is frequently encountered. Currently, one in three people will develop cancer at some time in their life and one in four will die from it *(1)*. In the year 2000, 10 million new cases of cancer were reported worldwide, which is expected to rise to 15 million by the year 2020, largely due to an aging population *(2)*. Conse-

From: *Cancer Drug Discovery and Development*
In Vivo Imaging of Cancer Therapy
Edited by: A.F. Shields and P. Price © Humana Press Inc., Totowa, NJ

quently, this has led to the search for new, active chemotherapeutic agents with different mechanisms of action, which will improve survival in patients with advanced cancer and enable the patient to have an enhanced quality of life (QOL).

Clinical trials are necessary to establish which potential agents are active and appropriate for use. The ultimate aim is to provide a "cure," or failing that a significant increase in survival with an improved QOL.

New drug development is a costly and time-consuming business. For every 10,000 drugs evaluated preclinically, five can be expected to reach clinical trials and only one will be approved for use on the market. The average time taken for a drug to pass from inception to market is about 15 years, of which 9 years are spent in clinical development (1). The cost of developing any given drug totals over $800 million and patency rights run for 20 years, so pharmaceutical companies have to recoup this outlay within a short time frame (1, 3). It is in everyone's interests to safely and thoroughly develop new agents in the shortest time and withdraw inactive agents as soon as possible. More importantly, it is unethical to subject large numbers of patients to inactive agents, or to those where the toxicity is so great that the drug cannot be used safely and reliably.

To reduce the number of patients involved in studies and to decrease the time taken to complete clinical trials, surrogates for survival have been established. One of the most common surrogates is tumor "response" to treatment. A tumor or the number of lesions is measured before treatment and then again during and after treatment. A decrease in size by a predetermined percentage of the before treatment (baseline) measurement is considered a "response." From this, "response rates" have been developed, where the proportion of patients "responding" to the agent under study in the clinical trial is recorded. Response rates have been developed to determine potential activity of cytotoxic agents, where the tumor would be expected to decrease in size during successful treatment. In solid tumors, it often takes two to four courses of treatment to demonstrate tumor shrinkage and some topoisomerase 1 inhibitors can take longer. It is unusual to see rapid and extensive tumor shrinkage within one or two courses of treatment, with a few exceptions, such as high-grade non-Hodgkins lymphoma and small cell lung cancer. Typically in single agent studies, active cytotoxic drugs have a response rate in the region of 15–40%. Two important points must be remembered. First, these studies are usually phase II studies. The primary aim of these studies is to establish whether the agent appears to have activity, as evidenced by response, and therefore whether the agent is potentially active. These studies are smaller than phase III studies, so if the agent proves to be inactive, as few patients as possible are exposed to it before it is discarded, but if it shows activity, it can be fast-tracked to phase III studies. Phase II studies may give an incomplete indication of toxicity and they give little information about QOL or long-term effects. Second, the duration of response is important; a drug that gives a high response rate that is short lived before progression ensues is of no value.

Response can be assessed by clinical means, but may suffer from subjectivity. The investigator may be biased toward a positive result and overestimate response, a relatively common problem in small single institution studies. To try and combat this, a second clinician may be asked to confirm the findings of the first, but this is not always appropriate. Moertel and Hanley demonstrated clinical subjectivity in a study in which a series of different sized steel spheres placed under a foam mattress to simulate subcutaneous metastases was assessed by 16 experienced clinicians. When a sphere

Table 1
Response Categories According to WHO Criteria

Complete response: Disappearance of all detectable disease, measurable and nonmeasurable
Partial response: A decrease in the product of bidimensionally measurable lesions by at least 50%, compared to the baseline examination, with no evidence of new lesions
Stable disease: A decrease in the product of bidimensionally measurable lesions by less than 50% and an increase in the product of any lesion by less than 25%, compared to that lesion's smallest measurement, *not* the baseline measurement
Progressive disease: The increase in product of any bidimensionally measurable lesion by at least 25%, the appearance of any new disease, or the increase in size of nonmeasurable disease

measuring $18.5\,cm^2$ was compared with a 7.3-cm^2 sphere [representing a greater than 50% decrease and therefore a partial response (PR)], 75% correctly recorded a PR. However, 16% recorded stable disease (SD) and 9% recorded progressive disease (PD) *(4)*!

To try and reduce measurement error and subjectivity, anatomical imaging has been used, so well defined lesions can be objectively measured, and in 1981 the WHO response criteria were introduced *(5)*. The WHO criteria required a lesion or number of lesions visible on the baseline examination to be measured, each in its longest diameter, with the greatest perpendicular diameter and the bidimensional product recorded. The sum of the bidimensional measurements for all lesions measured is recorded. During treatment, the same lesions are remeasured on subsequent examinations. The criteria recognize four responses: complete response (CR), PR, SD, and PD (Table 1). The WHO criteria make no imaging stipulations, because the only widely available imaging modality in 1981 was the plain chest radiograph (CXR). It was a simple matter to review the hard copy film on a viewing box, determine if one or more opacities could be seen clearly, and measure it/them with a ruler. A PR was defined as a 50% reduction in the product of the bidimensional disease. It must be remembered this is an arbitrary definition—there is nothing inherently special about the figure 50%. A PD could easily be determined using the CXR, either by the appearance of one or more new lesions or by an increase in bidimensional product of at least 25% in one or more lesions. To attain a PR, the sum of the bidimensional products must decrease by at least 50% compared to baseline. However, to develop PD, the size of preexisting lesions must increase by at least 25% compared with its smallest measurement, *not* the baseline measurement.

Since the early 1980s, other imaging modalities have become more widely available and have been introduced and have largely superseded the CXR in clinical trials. The three most widely used modalities in the clinical setting are all cross-sectional modalities, ultrasound (US), computed tomography (CT), and magnetic resonance imaging (MRI).

By the late 1980s, many clinical trials allowed the use of all the above imaging modalities (and clinical assessment). Response was determined by WHO criteria, by criteria developed by various cooperative groups, or further modifications to these criteria. All criteria used bidimensional measurements, though the definition of response and PD varied. The criteria did not provide any clear guidelines regarding minimum lesion size at baseline or imaging stipulations, which led to confusion and resulted in many clinical trials where the results from one study were not directly comparable to other studies.

During the early 1990s, it was recognised that US is a subjective examination and although of great value in the clinical setting, is not appropriate in clinical trials where lesions are required to be measured accurately in the same anatomical plane on successive examinations. Ultrasound is therefore no longer used as an imaging modality in clinical trials, except in a few specialized circumstances such as in the assessment of very superficial lesions, or superficial lymph nodes, as an alternative to clinical examination.

In 2000, the Response Evaluation Criteria In Solid Tumors (RECIST) criteria were published (6). The aim was to update the previous criteria and provide a single set of response criteria with imaging stipulations and minimum lesion size, thereby allowing a fair comparison between different clinical trials. The criteria are designed for CT and MRI, which are essentially the only anatomical imaging modalities used in clinical trials. The CXR is sometimes used, but most patients likely to have intrathoracic disease undergo CT in addition to CXR, and CT is the preferred modality because of its increased sensitivity and its ability to detect smaller lesions and to detect disease that cannot be assessed on the CXR, such as paratracheal lymphadenopathy.

Whatever imaging modality is used at the baseline examination, the same imaging modality using the same parameters must be used on subsequent examinations to ensure consistency. Any given lesion visible on one imaging modality, say CT, may appear to be a different size if different window settings are used or if a different imaging modality is used.

Exacting imaging stipulations are not prescribed by RECIST, because there is inevitably some variation in technique from one institution to another and if the stipulations are too "tight" there is the risk that many patients enrolled in clinical trials will become protocol violators and so will be excluded from the study. However, at the same time, the stipulations mandate that the examinations should be conducted in a similar manner.

RECIST also made one other significant change compared to previous imaging criteria. Unidimensional measurements are taken rather than bidimensional measurements. WHO used a 50% reduction in disease to achieve PR status. Using unidimensional measurements, this is equivalent to a 30% reduction in length (Table 2). WHO and RECIST therefore have similar definitions for achieving PR. This is true for spherical lesions that decrease in size uniformly. For other lesions that decrease in size eccen-

Table 2
Relationship between Change in Diameter and Bidimensional Product

	Diameter	*Bidimensional product*
Response	Decrease	Decrease
	30%	50%
Disease progression	Increase	Increase
	12%	25%
	20%	44%
	25%	56%

trically and become cylindrical in shape, because the longest diameter is measured, there is a greater likelihood of the lesion not decreasing by 30%, so it remains SD, even if the bidimensional product has clearly decreased by 50%.

WHO defined PD as a 25% increase in bidimensional product in one or more lesions, and with very small lesions there is a possibility of PD assignment, when there has simply been a measurement error. RECIST requires a 20% increase in the overall measurable disease, not just one lesion (or the appearance of new lesions) to be classified as PD. A 20% increase is the equivalent of a 44% increase in bidimensional disease, so there is less chance of a measurement error leading to PD assignment.

RECIST requires all lesions to be measured, up to a maximum of 10 in all and a maximum of five per organ. When the RECIST criteria are updated, it is likely the number of lesions required for measurement will be reduced to five, with a maximum of three per organ. Measuring the actual lesions is not difficult, but determining which image on subsequent examinations compares best with the corresponding baseline image can be very time consuming, particularly if many lesions have been measured and there are multiple subsequent examinations.

2. CONFIRMATION OF RESPONSE

This refers to a response being maintained for at least two successive examinations, not less than 28 days apart. If a response is attained only for one examination, then it is defined as an unconfirmed response.

Once PR or CR status is assigned, the patient cannot subsequently be assigned SD; it has to be PD, because the disease will have increased by more than 20%. Response is compared to the baseline measurements, but PD is compared to the smallest measurements.

The best response is the best response attained at any stage of the study, not the final response.

Whichever imaging modality is chosen, comparability is necessary, so the stipulations are designed to try and ensure consistency between examinations. Clinical trials used to support the application for a licence by regulatory authorities are (almost) always independently reviewed to ensure the data submitted are valid.

3. COMPUTED TOMOGRAPHY IMAGING

Even with cross-sectional imaging modalities, which are largely operator and patient independent, such as CT and MRI, for optimal objectivity and reproducibility, it is necessary to instigate certain protocols and stipulations. However, these stipulations need to take account of individual patient characteristics, such as cardiac output and the use and timing of scans after intravenous contrast agents and variations in practice from one center to another, while at the same time achieve broadly similar results, so a comparison can be made from one examination to the next for any given patient and also between patients in the study. A balance has to be struck between providing a window of acceptability that will enable most centers to enroll most patients using similar examinations, but without the stipulations being so "tight" that many patients enrolled in a study would be excluded due to protocol violation. To provide acceptable definitions is difficult. Add to this the constantly changing technology and difficulty predicting how it may change, criteria face the possibility of almost being out of date soon after publication. The imaging criteria set out in the RECIST paper were based largely on single and dual slice helical CT, but within a year of the publication, multislice CT (MSCT) was widely available with four slice scanners. At present, 16-slice scanners are the norm and within the last few years 64-slice scanners have become available, with 256-slice scanners now being tested. Most all CT scanners in use in the Western world are MSCT scanners.

To understand the need for certain stipulations, it is worth considering how a CT image is acquired. The original CT scanners were incremental scanners and it is easiest to describe the principles in a simplified manner using the original technology. An incremental scan means a "slice" of tissue of a certain thickness is imaged and detectors surrounding that volume of tissue sum the average attenuation (density) within the various voxels (small cubes of tissue) and a two-dimensional image is built up through a series of pixels using a gray scale corresponding to the voxels. The machine then moves a certain distance and repeats the process. Contiguous imaging means the slices are performed in continuity. Typically, in cancer imaging, contiguous imaging is performed using 10 mm slice thickness. This is a time-consuming process. Each slice takes 20–40 sec to acquire and the machine then has to move, which takes a few seconds longer. An examination of the thorax would take about 20 min. Further errors are introduced if the patient takes a different breath hold on each slice, which is difficult to correct.

3.1 Minimum Lesion Size at the Baseline Examination

Each "slice" has a certain thickness. The "slice" viewed is the sum of the attenuations between the two successive horizontal lines, not just the thickness of the line itself. Figure 1 illustrates the importance of minimum lesion size at baseline and why the minimum lesion size should be at least twice the slice thickness. Lesion (a) represents a lesion that is about twice the slice thickness. The apparent size of the lesion is the average of all the tissue in that volume, so in this case, on either of the slices it will be about the same size; although minimally smaller than in reality, this error is very small. However, lesion (b) is less than the slice thickness and when the other tissue is averaged with the tumor (partial volume effects) it will appear significantly smaller than it is in reality. Lesion (c) straddles two slices and so will appear to be even smaller than lesion (b), because of partial volume effects, even though it is the same size. This is important because if lesion (b) were seen at the baseline examination, then lesion (c) during treatment, this would appear to be a PR, even though it can be seen to be the same size. Equally importantly, if lesion (c) were seen at baseline and then (b) during treatment this would appear to be PD, even though this is not the case.

When incremental CT scanners are used, the usual slice thickness is 10 mm throughout the thorax, abdomen, and pelvis. The minimum lesion size at baseline therefore must be twice the slice thickness, so is 20 mm. For helical CT scanners, the mathematical algorithm used to reconstruct the slices is such that thinner slices can be obtained. Ideally, for the purpose of clinical trials a 5-mm slice thickness should be used, in which case the minimum lesion size is 10 mm, even though in clinical practice 7-mm slices are often used. However, with MSCT, yet thinner slices can be obtained, in the region of 1-mm slices for 16-slice machines. With such thin slices, the data can be reconstructed in different anatomical planes and a huge amount of data is potentially available. In practice, the policy is to "slice thin and image thick." Images can be acquired

Chapter 3 / Anatomical Measure of Tumor Growth with CT and MRI

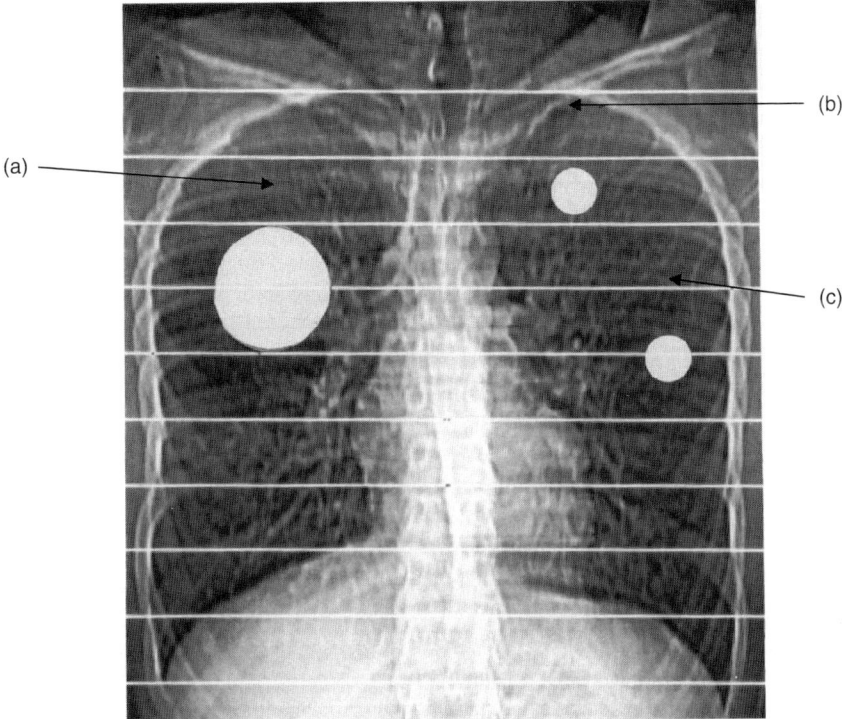

Fig. 1. A CT "Scanogram" of the thorax with the horizontal lines representing the boundaries of each "slice." The image generated for each slice is a two-dimensional representation of the volume between two horizontal lines, the slice thickness, represented as a gray scale in two-dimensional form. A simulated lesion (a) is of a diameter twice the slice thickness, so it will appear about the true size on each slice, though in reality it will be very slightly, but not significantly smaller. However, a simulated lesion (b) lies entirely within the slice thickness and will appear smaller than its real size. A simulated lesion (c) will appear to be even smaller, because the attenuation coefficient (density) averages "normal" tissue with the lesion, so it will appear smaller. This is important, because if lesion (c) is measured during treatment, after lesion (b) at baseline, it will appear to be smaller, though in reality it has not changed in size, and if lesion (c) were the baseline lesion and lesion (b) the lesion measured during treatment, it would appear to represent PD, even though we can see the lesion size has not actually changed.

at 1 mm intervals, but reconstructed in 5-mm slice thicknesses, to make reading the films manageable and without losing significant data. In practice, the images are reviewed on a work station, so it is possible to "scroll down" through the images, rather than study hard copy films, and the data can be reconstructed using an appropriate slice thickness. However, for any given patient, the slice thickness used at baseline should be used throughout subsequent examinations. Practically, lesions should not be less than 10 mm at the baseline examination, because of the problem with very small lesions and measurement errors. An error in measurement of 1 mm in a 5-mm lesion amounts to a 20% change in lesion measurement, which using RECIST criteria is enough to change the response to PD. Even when using electronic callipers on the machine and measuring the lesion on a large screen on a work station, measurement errors can occur.

One area not satisfactorily addressed is how to monitor lesions that become very small during treatment. One approach is to define lesions that decrease from a baseline measurement to less than 7 mm to nominally be ascribed a value of 7 mm, unless CR ensues. This acknowledges the continued presence of the lesion, but helps limit errors in the measurement of small lesions. If there is some doubt as to whether PD has occurred, all other things being equal, if the treatment continues, the next CT examination will determine if the patient does have PD or not. Phase II clinical trials are performed using experimental treatment when conventional treatment has failed, or there is no satisfactory treatment available, so further treatment options may not be available. It is therefore important to establish that PD is truly occurring before withdrawing the patient from a study.

With MSCT, it is possible to reconstruct the data set in different anatomical planes, so lesions can be measured. If this is undertaken, the same imaging plane and imaging parameters are required for subsequent examinations, though practically, response evaluation is usually performed in the axial plane.

3.2 Window Settings

When the CT examination is undertaken, the gray scale can be altered to demonstrate different structures to best effect. Manufacturers can preset different window levels and widths for different structures. Those most relevant in this context are soft tissue settings, to demonstrate the major viscera and soft tissues of the thorax, abdomen, and pelvis; lung windows do demonstrate the lung parenchyma, which detect small intraparenchymal metastases and bone windows. Whatever settings are used at the baseline examination must be used on subsequent examinations, as different window settings can make lesions "appear" to be a different size (Fig. 2). It is also important to review the entire examination on all window settings to ensure no new lesions have appeared (Fig. 3).

3.3 Contrast Agents

Oral and intravenous contrast agents contain iodine, and should be used except when contraindicated, such as iodine allergy, which can be life threatening. If no intravenous contrast agent is given at baseline, then it should not be used on subsequent examinations. Oral contrast agents delineate the bowel and IV contrast agents demonstrate the vessels and major viscera, so paraaortic lymphadenopathy and visceral metastases, particularly intrahepatic lesions, are more clearly defined. Most visceral metastases are hypointense compared to the adjacent normal tissue, though some metastases are hypervascular, e.g., carcinoid. The volume of contrast medium injected, whether it is injected by hand or by pump, and the concentration are all important factors. When incremental CT scanners were used, a contrast agent either was or was not administered. The time taken to image the viscera was such that several minutes elapsed before the whole organ could be scanned. However, with MSCT, the timing is very important. It allows the whole thorax, abdomen, and pelvis to be scanned in one breath hold and takes about 8 sec. Scans can therefore be performed through the liver during the arterial phase, where contrast is solely arriving from the hepatic artery, which occurs within about 20–30 sec after an upper limb venous injection, using a pump at a rate of 2–4 ml/sec. By 40–60 sec, there is additional input from the portal vein, a phase known as the equilibrium phase, and by 80–90 sec the true portal venous phase occurs. Delayed scans

Chapter 3 / Anatomical Measure of Tumor Growth with CT and MRI 41

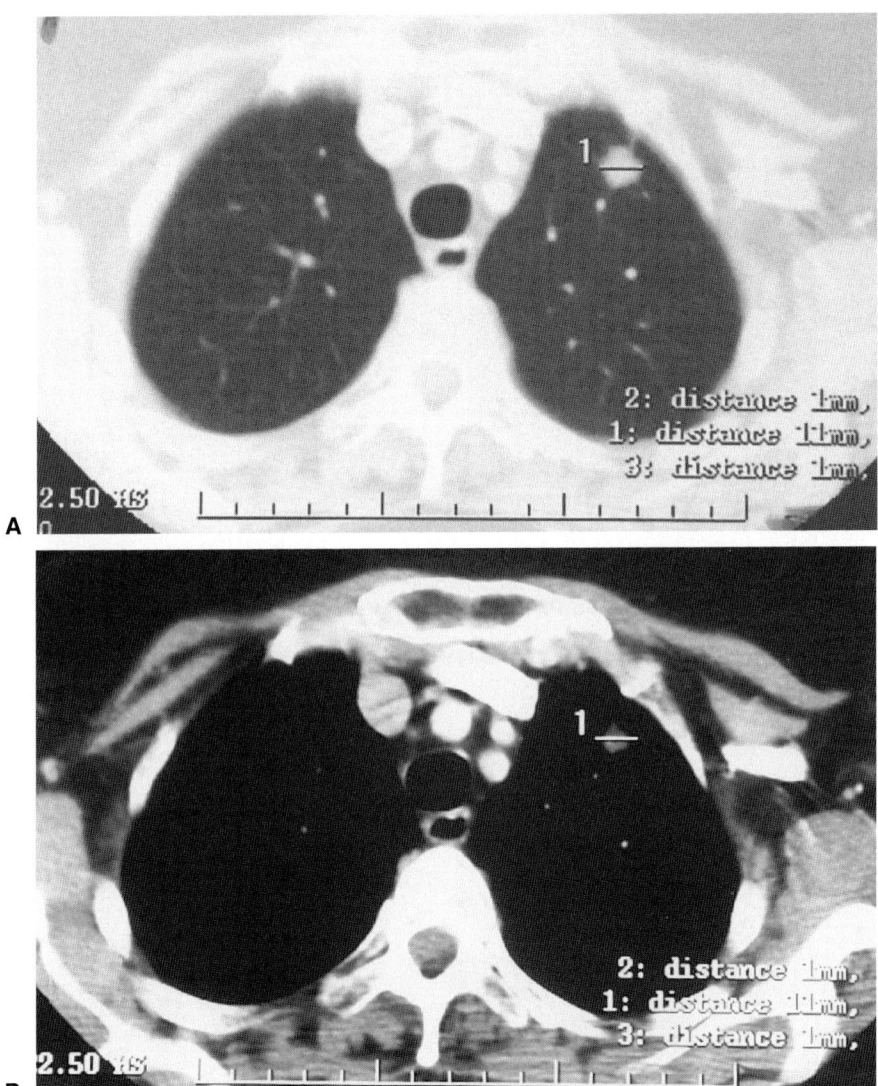

Fig. 2. A CT scan through the thorax at the level of the left brachiocephalic vein in a patient with colonic carcinoma with lung metastases. (A) Lung window settings with the electronic calliper accurately measuring the lesion in the left upper lobe at 11 mm. The same image on mediastinal window settings (B). The electronic calliper accurately measuring the lesion on lung windows remains and shows that the lesion "appears" to be a different size than when measured on lung window settings. The same window settings *must* be used on all examinations.

can be performed several minutes after injection, but this is usually performed only to demonstrate the characteristic "filling in" of a hemangioma. The actual timing varies from one patient to another and is dependent on cardiac output, volume injected, and rate of injection, among other factors. Although technically feasible, it is undesirable to perform scans during all these phases, due to the increased radiation dose. The apparent size of visceral lesions does appear to change with time, though for some lesions

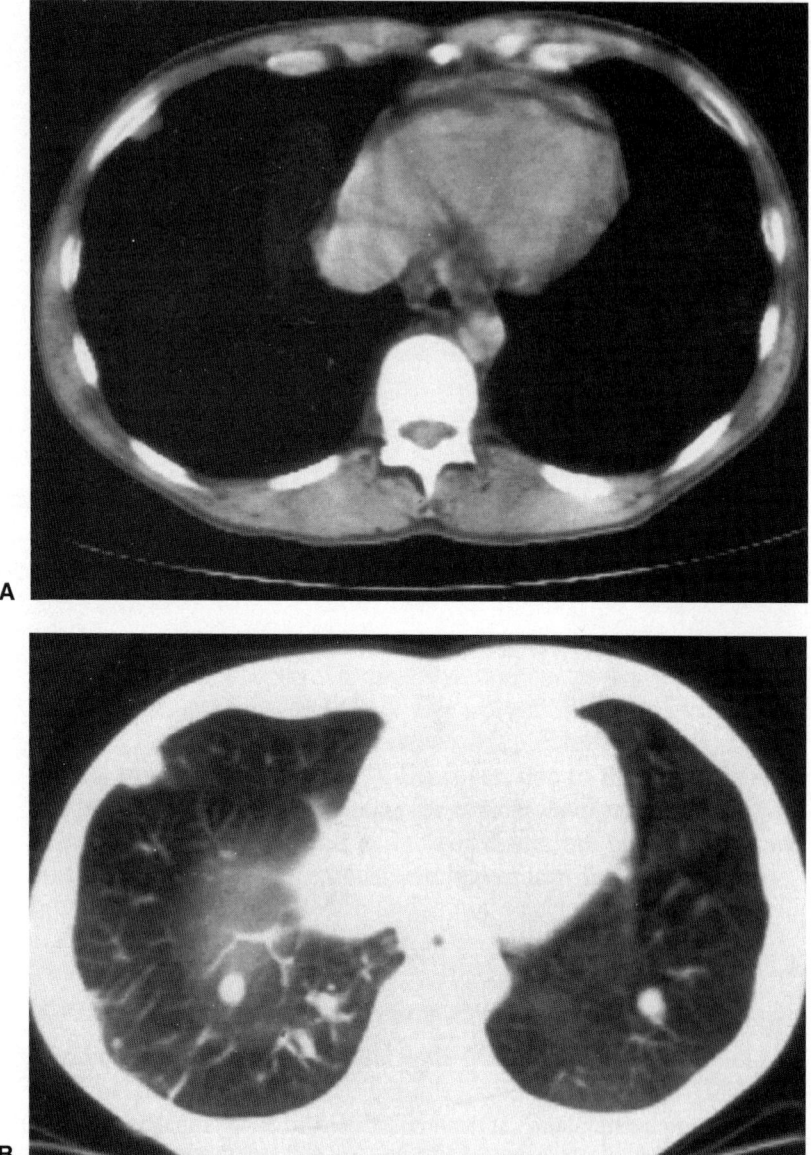

Fig. 3. A CT scan of the thorax at the level of the aortic root. (A) Mediastinal window settings showing no apparent abnormality. (B) The same image as (A), on lung window settings, showing several intraparenchymal lung metastases. It is important to review the entire examination on different window settings to ensure no evidence of new disease on subsequent examinations when the lung fields were initially clear, or to determine if nonmeasurable small metastases are resolving during treatment.

more than others even at the same examination (Fig. 4). When visceral metastases, particularly hepatic lesions are measured, it is important to ensure successive examinations are performed at approximately the same timing, preferably within about 10 sec. However, in reality, the volume of contrast injected and the rate and the timing of the

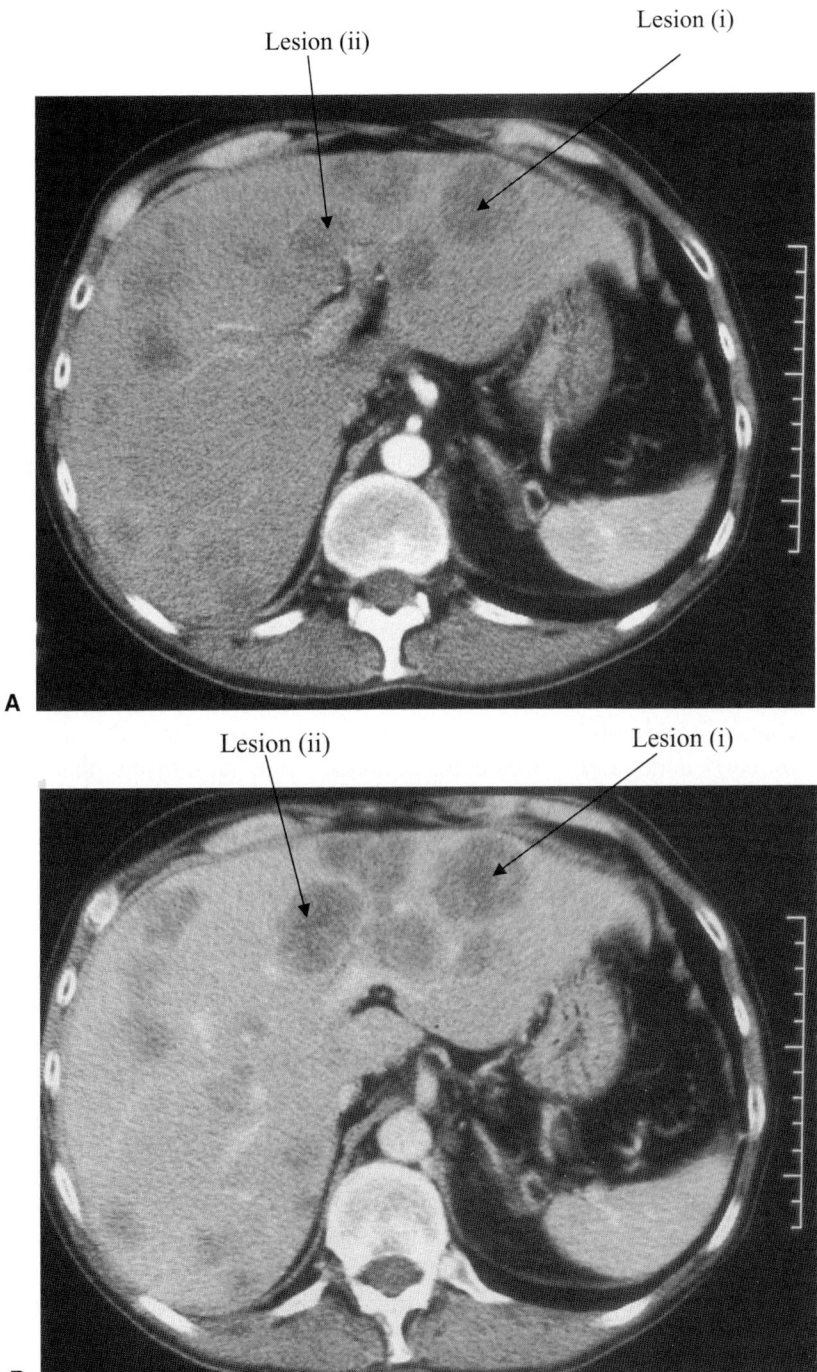

Fig. 4. Contrast-enhanced CT scan through the liver in a patient with colonic carcinoma, showing multiple intrahepatic metastases. (A) Arterial phase, about 30 sec after injection via a pump of 100 ml of a contrast agent containing 300 mg iodine per ml, at a rate of 3 ml/sec, showing several intrahepatic lesions. Two lesions have been arrowed: (i) in the left lobe and (ii) in the right lobe anteriorly and medially. (B) The same level performed during the portal venous phase about 80 sec after injection of the contrast agent. Lesion (i) appears the same size, but lesion (ii) appears much larger in size and other lesions are much more prominent. It is important, therefore, that lesions be measured at the same time after injection of the contrast agent on each examination. It may be at a different time for any individual patient, but it should be about the same time on successive patients for any given patient. This is usually relatively easy to arrange at any given institution, but may be a problem if different examinations are performed at different sites, with (slightly) different imaging protocols.

imaging are impossible to standardize between different institutions and patients, but wherever possible, for any given patient, the procedure should be standardized. Even this can be difficult, if the patient has the baseline examination at one center but is then referred to another for further treatment.

4. MAGNETIC RESONANCE IMAGING

Magnetic resonance imaging provides images in different anatomical planes and slice thickness is not such an issue. However, 10 mm should be the minimum lesion size, at the baseline examination, for the same reasons as given above. The physics behind acquiring images is complex and different sequences can be produced to highlight or suppress different tissue. Short duration scans acquired during one breath hold are necessary in the thorax, abdomen, and pelvis. The mainstay of imaging are the T1-weighted images where fluid appears black and T2-weighted images where fluid appears white. Most licensed contrast agents available are gadolinium based compounds, though some contain manganese, both of which are paramagnetic and induce T1 shortening effects, resulting in relative brightening of tissue, but are visible only on T1-weighted sequences. The timing of the injection of the agent is important and the capillary phase corresponds to the hepatic arterial phase on the CT scan, early hepatic venous (or early nonequilibrium) occurs at about 1 min, equilibrium phase between 1.5 and 5 min, and the wash out phase at 10 min or longer. If contrast-enhanced sequences are used for measurements, the timings must be standardized on successive examinations.

The images acquired are dependent on multiple factors, the most important of which are the strength of the magnet used, typically 1.5 T, the type of coil used, and the software package purchased with the scanner itself. For consistency, subsequent MRI scans should be performed ideally using the same scanner. It is necessary to use the same imaging sequences and in the same anatomical plane on subsequent examinations. It is important that the patient does not move during the examination, otherwise serious artifacts degrade the images. Magnetic resonance imaging can be a difficult examination for some patients with advanced cancer. Respiratory movement and normal bowel peristalsis can degrade the images significantly. It is vital to ensure patients have no ferrous material in their body, such as small metallic foreign bodies in the eyes, shrapnel, and some clips used in intracranial and cardiac surgery, as they can move while the patient is in the machine due to the high magnetic field and lead to serious injury. Most prosthetic cardiac valves, pacing wires, and intracranial and abdominal clips are nonferrous, but this must be established before scanning the patient. Fixed metallic prostheses, such as total hip replacements, do not move, but may heat up by 1–2°C during the examination, though this is not clinically relevant. However, these metallic foreign bodies can cause significant artifacts and degrade the images. Many MRI scanners have a narrow bore and many patients feel claustrophobic; approximately 2% of examinations are either not possible or have to be abandoned due to claustrophobia. The time taken to perform different sequences in different anatomical planes implies a much longer examination time, at least 30 min, compared to a scan time of a few seconds for MSCT. Magnetic resonance imaging scanners tend to have longer waiting times than CT and problems can be encountered when the scan has to be performed within a certain short time frame between treatments. However, having said this, MRI is perfectly acceptable, but the general availability of CT and the speed of the examination, particularly MSCT, implies this is the imaging modality of choice for clinical trials.

5. THE FUTURE

There has recently been a move away from response rates and to monitoring time to progression (TTP) or time to treatment failure. In part, this is to try and determine whether cytotoxic agents under review are providing patient benefit by stabilizing disease, without achieving a predefined tumor shrinkage. The opening paragraph of this chapter made reference to new classes of drugs under investigation, such as antiangiogenesis agents and intracellular or intramembrane receptor antagonists. Antiangiogenesis agents halt new vessel formation, preventing the tumor from growing, but tumor shrinkage would not be expected. These agents are not directly cytocidal, so it is inappropriate to measure response in the traditional manner, as tumor shrinkage may not occur, even though patient benefit is achieved. New methods of determining investigational agent activity are therefore necessary. Dynamic CT and MRI studies and PET can be used to assess blood flow, blood volume, and perfusion changes and tumor physiology and proliferation can be assessed. These surrogates predict agent activity in a much shorter time than tumor shrinkage, adding to patient benefit. However, standardized, validated, and reproducible criteria need to be devised to enable meaningful comparisons to be made with other agents. In the transition phase, anatomical imaging will continue to play a role, with increasing emphasis on the dynamic, functional aspects. However, further advances in technology and human genomics and proteonomics will undoubtedly influence further progress, with molecular and functional imaging playing a key role.

6. SUMMARY

Anatomical imaging in clinical trials uses CT and MRI to provide objective measurements of tumor size during treatment with potentially active new agents and acts as a surrogate for patient benefit. Classically, response rates have been used, which measure tumor shrinkage, but this is really applicable only for cytocidal agents. There are increasing numbers of trials where TTP or time to treatment failure is used as the main endpoint, partly due to the fact that patient benefit may occur with prolonged stabilization of disease, even with cytotoxic agent, and partly because new classes of drugs under investigation, such as antiangiogenesis agents, would not be expected to cause tumor shrinkage. For a comparison to be made, imaging stipulations are required to ensure consistency from one examination to the next, not only for the same patient, but between different patients within the same trial and from one clinical trial to another. Practically, CT is easier and quicker than MRI, though both modalities are perfectly acceptable. With the introduction of new classes of active agents and greater understanding of molecular biology, functional imaging using dynamic CT and MRI studies and PET imaging will play ever increasing roles. To allow consistency, validation of the methods and standardization are necessary, so anatomical imaging will remain in the short term.

REFERENCES

1. Seddon BM, Workman P. The role of functional and molecular imaging in cancer drug discovery and development. *Br J Radiol* 2003;76:S128–S138.
2. Stewart BW, Kleihuer P. World Cancer Report. World Health Organisation. International Agency for Research on Cancer, 2003.
3. DiMasi JA, Hansen RW, Grabowski HG. The price of innovation: New estimates of drug development costs. *J Health Econ* 2003;22:151–185.
4. Moertel CG, Hanley JA. The effect of measuring error on the results of therapeutic trials in advanced cancer. *Cancer* 1976;38(1):388–394.
5. Millar AB, Hogestraeten B, Staquet M, Winkler A. Reporting results of cancer treatment. *Cancer* 1981;47:207–214.
6. Therasse P, Arbuck SG, Eisenhauer EA, *et al*. New guidelines to evaluate the response to treatment in solid tumors. European Organisation for Research and Treatment of Cancer, National Cancer Institute of the United States, National Cancer Institute of Canada. *J Natl Cancer Inst* 2000;92:205–216.

4 Positron Emission Tomography Imaging of Blood Flow and Hypoxia in Tumors

Joseph G. Rajendran, MD, and
David A. Mankoff, MD, PhD

CONTENTS

INTRODUCTION
ANGIOGENESIS
TUMOR PERFUSION
TUMOR HYPOXIA
SUMMARY

1. INTRODUCTION

In this section, we summarize positron emission tomography (PET) imaging of tumor perfusion and hypoxia. We first summarize biological considerations, and then discuss the imaging approaches and results to date for PET imaging of tumor perfusion and tumor hypoxia. While we consider the importance of angiogenesis in the context of tumor hypoxia and tumor perfusion, we only briefly highlight recent PET imaging methods designed to specifically image angiogenesis and neovascularity. These topics are considered in more detail in other chapters in this text.

In the past two decades there has been a rapid growth in molecular imaging along with advances in morphological imaging providing a noninvasive tool to characterize and evaluate function and form in biological systems with the ability for serial imaging *(1–9)*. Intricacies of tumor biology can now be unraveled and answers provided to the complex clinical problems. In addition, combining anatomic and functional imaging provides the ability for image-guided therapy.

2. ANGIOGENESIS

Angiogenesis, the formation of new blood vessels, is essential for the delivery of nutrients needed for tumor growth, invasion, and metastatic spread. Angiogenesis in tumors is essentially a failure of the balance between proangiogenic and antiangiogenic

From: *Cancer Drug Discovery and Development*
In Vivo Imaging of Cancer Therapy
Edited by: A.F. Shields and P. Price © Humana Press Inc., Totowa, NJ

signals that are needed to maintain a balance for the animal or human to control the tumor. Tumors do not grow beyond a size of 1–2 mm without producing new blood vessels *(10)*.

Gene expression profiling has identified proteins that are selectively expressed by tumor endothelial cells, including a large class of integrins such as $\alpha_V\beta_3$ and $\alpha_V\beta_5$ *(11)* providing an opportunity for imaging as well as therapy *(12, 13)*. Angiogenesis, a frequent consequence of hypoxia, can develop in the absence of hypoxia and vice versa as a result of genetic abnormalities without always having a "cause and effect." In the example of *de novo* angiogenesis seen in Von Hippel–Lindau syndrome, spontaneous renal tumors develop due to the stabilization and overexpression of hypoxia-inducible factor (HIF1α) that results in widespread angiogenesis even in the absence of significant hypoxia. The relationship between hypoxia, vascularity, and prognosis has been found to be "U" shaped. This phenomenon was explained mechanistically; overall prognosis in a solid tumor is poor when there is insufficient vasculature, due to the presence of hypoxia, and at the other extreme, when there is increased vasculature as a result of profound angiogenesis, a poor prognosis is likely due to greater metastatic potential *(14)*. This is part of the reason that tumor hypoxia and tumor vascularity cannot be considered synonymous, and why the level of tumor vascularity and/or perfusion at the time of tumor detection is not always predictive of tumor response or prognosis.

3. TUMOR PERFUSION

3.1 Why Measure Perfusion?

Tumor blood flow, often referred to as tumor perfusion, has been measured by a variety of methods, including a number of different imaging modalities. The interest in quantitative measures of tissue perfusion stems from several factors. Angiogenesis is increasingly recognized as being fundamental to tumorigenesis and malignant progression *(15)*, and tumor blood flow is a readily quantifiable, though indirect, measure of angiogenesis. Second, tumor perfusion is important as a measure of the delivery of nutrients and systemic therapy to the tumor *(16)*, and measuring tumor perfusion may identify factors that affect the likelihood of delivery of systemic agents. Third, changes in perfusion may indicate the response to treatment, either targeted antiangiogenic therapy *(17)* or as a consequence of tumor response to nonspecific therapy *(18)*. Finally, measurement of tumor perfusion relative to metabolism may identify tumors under metabolic "stress" and may help elucidate factors relating to tumor hypoxia *(19, 20)*.

This section highlights PET methods to measure tumor perfusion and reviews approaches that have been used including experience in humans with PET tumor perfusion imaging and the relationship between perfusion and hypoxia. The reader is referred to comprehensive reviews of the approaches *(21)* for additional details on the subject.

3.2 Approaches to Measuring Tumor Perfusion

A variety of imaging modalities have been used to measure tumor perfusion, including computed tomography (CT) *(22)*, magnetic resonance imaging (MRI) *(23)*, ultrasound with Doppler measurements *(24)*, single-photon emission computed tomography

(SPECT), and PET. This section focuses on PET methods. Some other chapters in the text describe the other modalities in detail.

Relative to the other modalities, there are several advantages and disadvantages of PET measures of tumor perfusion. Of the imaging modalities used to measure tumor perfusion, PET is the most rigorously quantitative and thoroughly validated *(21)*. Validation of PET blood flow measures has been done for a variety of applications, including myocardial perfusion *(25)*, cerebral blood flow *(26)*, and tumor perfusion. These methods yield direct estimates of tumor perfusion in ml/min/g. Importantly, as a tracer method, PET does not perturb the system, as opposed to methods such as CT where the injected contrast material may lead to physiological effects. Since most PET methods of measuring tumor perfusion used radiopharmaceuticals with short-lived isotopes, early repeat measures to study the effect of interventions is possible *(27)*. Finally, PET imaging using highly permeable agents, such as $^{15}O[H_2O]$, require few assumptions in quantitative analysis and is therefore able to provide unbiased measures of tumor blood flow in a large variety of settings and is least likely to be affected by variations in tumor location, patient size, vascular permeability, and other anatomical or physiological factors *(21)*.

Positron emission tomography has some disadvantages over other methods. Its spatial resolution is limited compared to some of the other modalities such as CT and MRI. Furthermore, PET is a purely functional technique, sometimes making measures hard to relate to the structural features of the tumor. The recent advent of combined PET/CT devices *(28)* is likely to be quite advantageous in this regard. Since PET methods for measuring tumor perfusion use radiopharmaceuticals with short-lived isotopes, they require an on-site cyclotron. This limits research availability and makes PET perfusion assessment relatively expensive, especially compared to methods such as SPECT or Doppler ultrasound. The use of ^{62}Cu-pyruvaldehyde bis(*N*-4-methylthiosemicarbazone (^{62}Cu-PTSM) *(29)*, which uses an isotope that can be obtained from a radioisostope generator, may be advantageous in this regard; however, at present, copper radioisotope generators are not widely available.

Given these considerations, the choice of PET to measure tumor perfusion is appropriate for those applications requiring rigorous, robust, and precise quantitation in academic centers with the capability and expertise to analyze PET perfusion studies. These factors suggest the PET perfusion measures may be appropriate for studies focusing on preclinical drug development and testing and early (phase I or II) clinical therapy trials, especially of novel agents.

3.3 Approaches to Measuring Tumor Perfusion by Positron Emission Tomography

3.3.1 QUANTITATIVE APPROACHES

Positron emission tomography approaches to tumor perfusion methods can be broadly categorized by one of two approaches: (1) analogs of the Kety–Schmidt approach using freely permeable tracers such as $^{15}O[H_2O]$ or (2) analogs of microsphere approaches using "chemical microspheres", i/e., radiopharmaceuticals with high first-pass extraction such as $^{13}NH_3$ or ^{62}Cu-PTSM. The former approach requires high-speed dynamic imaging at high count rates and is the most technically challenging; however, it provides the most rigorous and direct measures of tumor blood flow with the fewest assumptions.

The use of highly extracted agents is less technically demanding and provides better qualitative images; however, since tracer extraction varies with blood flow, it is difficult to estimate blood flow directly without some bias, especially at higher flow rates. In addition, tracer extraction may be affected by the physiological state of the tumor cell (for example, membrane potential, the activity of membrane transporters), and measurements made pre- and posttherapy may be confounded by the cellular effects of therapy.

The freely permeable tracer approach for ^{15}O[H$_2$O] PET is described below followed by highlights of alternate approaches using highly extracted tracers.

3.3.2 Positron Emission Tomography Blood Flow Measured Using Freely Permeable Tracers: ^{15}O[H$_2$O]

^{15}O[H$_2$O] PET is performed either by a bolus injection of ^{15}O[H$_2$O] or by inhalation of C^{15}O$_2$, which is quickly converted into ^{15}O[H$_2$O] by pulmonary carbonic anhydrase. While the injection method is more technically challenging, it yields a tighter bolus and provides more precise estimates of tumor blood flow *(30)*. For the injection method, imaging generally involves a bolus injection, followed by 4–7 min of dynamic imaging, with early frames spaced at 2–3 sec per frame, lengthening to 10–15 seconds per frame by later studies *(19, 31)*. The blood clearance function, which serves as the input modeling, is obtained through arterial blood sampling or noninvasively from a large image blood pool structure such as the left atrium or aorta. Time–activity curves are shown in Fig. 1.

To estimate blood flow, the compartmental model illustrated in Fig. 2 is used. The time-varying blood clearance function, C_b (µCi/ml), serves as the input to a one-compartment model of tissue water space [C_t, (µCi/ml)] *(19, 31)*. The blood-to-tissue

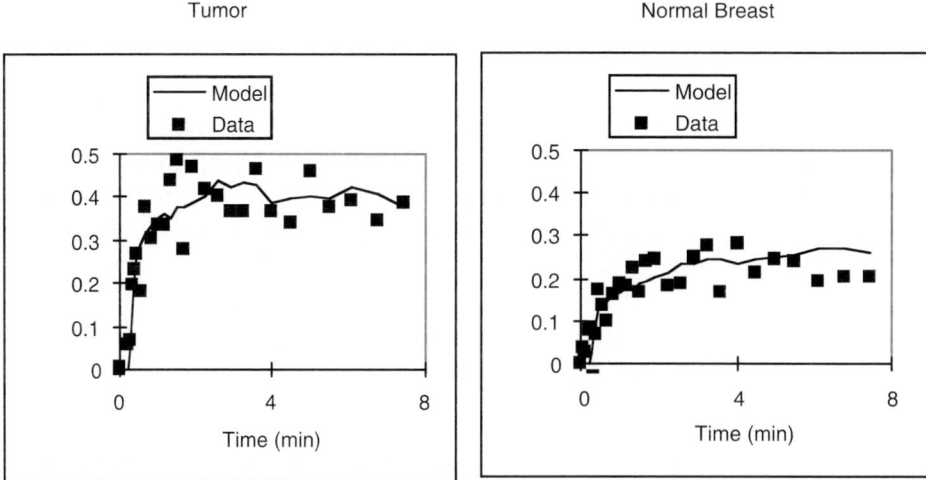

Fig. 1. Sample time–activity curves from ^{15}O[H$_2$O] PET study of breast cancer. Tissue time–activity curves following bolus water injection are shown for tumor (left) and normal breast (right). Model fits to data are also shown. Units are arbitrary but are consistent between the two graphs. The tumor curve rises more quickly, indicative of more rapid tracer delivery (i.e., higher blood flow), and plateaus at a higher value, indicating a higher water distribution volume compared to the relatively fatty normal breast.

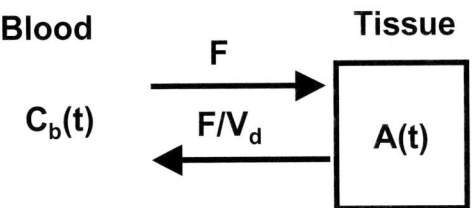

Fig. 2. Compartmental model of $^{15}O[H_2O]$ kinetics.

transport rate constant (K_1, ml/min/g) describes tracer movement into the tissue compartment and the parameter, k_2 (1/min), describes tracer efflux. For a highly diffusible tracer like water, tracer delivery is limited nearly entirely by blood flow, and K_1 can be taken to be equal to flow (F, ml/min/g). The components of k_2 can be inferred from the steady state (constant C_b), where water influx and efflux to the tissue must be the same. In steady state, the following formula applies:

$$K_1 C_b = k_2 C_t \tag{1}$$

therefore,

$$k_2 = K_1(C_t/C_b) = K_1 V_d \tag{2}$$

The steady-state ratio of tissue to plasma water (C_t/C_b) is the water volume of distribution [V_d, (ml/g)] and is analogous to the water partition coefficient. For most normal tissues, this value is close to 1; however, it can be more variable in tumors, depending upon their cellularity and the type of tissue. For example, in breast tumors, the normal breast tissue is rather fatty and has a low V_d; however, the tumor tissue has V_d ranging from close to normal breast to nearly 1, depending upon tumor tissue composition and cellularity *(19, 31)*.

With these considerations, and equating K_1 to flow (F), the compartmental model is governed by the following differential equation:

$$dC_t/dt = FC_b - (F/V_d)C_t - \lambda C_t \tag{3}$$

For water studies, with the short half-life of ^{15}O (~2 min), the tissue efflux rate and isotope decay rate [decay constant λ, (1/min)] are similar in magnitude, and the radioactive decay must be explicitly included in the model. Trying to fit the model using decay-corrected data without including the decay term will result in errors in the estimates of F and/or V_d.

Using Eq. (3) and the measured $C_b(t)$, the model parameters can be estimated by comparing them to the tissue uptake data measured by PET (A, µCi/g). Given

$$A = C_t + V_b C_b \tag{4}$$

V_b is the blood volume (ml/g) in the tissue region in the image and typically ranges from 0.03 to 0.20 ml/g. The combination of Eqs. (3) and (4) now provides a method for estimating model parameters from the best fit of the PET data. In practice, the blood volume term is difficult to estimate from typical PET data *(32)* and it is excluded from the formulation. The resulting formulation can be expressed simply by Eq. (4) with the goal of fitting to match the modeled $C_t(t)$ to the measured $A(t)$ *(31)*.

For a freely diffusible tracer such as $^{15}O[H_2O]$, tracer uptake and washout are rapid, and static images may not provide a good visual picture of regional blood flow. Lodge *(33)* reported on a parametric imaging approach using $^{15}O[H_2O]$, providing pixel-by-pixel images of estimated blood flow in ml/min/g. This provides the advantages of quantitative PET blood flow imaging, while also providing an accurate visual picture of regional blood flow.

3.3.3 OTHER POSITRON EMISSION TOMOGRAPHY TRACERS FOR TUMOR PERFUSION

Although $^{15}O[H_2O]$ is a robust and well-validated radiopharmaceutical for measuring tissue perfusion it has some practical disadvantages, which include a short half-life (approximately 2 min) and the need for high-count rate imaging, which is not feasible with all PET tomographs. In addition, for a freely diffusible tracer such as water, there is rapid uptake and washout resulting in modest qualitative image quality compared to radiopharmaceuticals for which longer periods of static imaging are possible. Arising from experience in myocardial perfusion imaging, several other tracers have been tested for tumor perfusion imaging. The alternate perfusion tracers share characteristics, such as a high first-pass extraction and high retention, giving them behavior close to microspheres. Tracer uptake after clearance from the blood is strongly dependent upon blood flow. Static images provide a relative indicator of perfusion and offer higher image quality compared to $^{15}O[H_2O]$. These highly extracted and retained radiopharmaceuticals have the disadvantage that their uptake is not always proportional to blood flow over the range of conditions encountered in tumor imaging. This stems from two issues: (1) the alternate tracers are less permeable to cell membranes than water; therefore they have lower extraction at higher flow rates. This creates a nonlinear relationship between blood-tissue transport of the tracers and blood flow that can lead to bias in the estimate of tumor perfusion, especially at higher flow rates. Their retention can be affected by cellular factors such as membrane potential and cellular metabolism; therefore the retention may vary with disease state and possibly with response to treatment.

^{62}Cu-pyruvaldehyde bis(N-4-methylthiosemicarbazone) is a highly extracted and retained tracer that has been tested for myocardial and cerebral perfusion, and preliminarily for tumor imaging *(29, 34)*. ^{62}Cu has a 10 min half-life and can be obtained from a radioisotope generator with a half-life sufficient for regional distribution, making it a potentially clinically feasible perfusion tracer. It has been used in a few settings in preliminary studies, including the perfusion of hepatic metastases under the effect of angiotensin II, used to increase tumor perfusion in an attempt to improve drug delivery *(35)*. ^{13}N-labeled ammonia is another highly extracted and retained PET perfusion tracer used widely in myocardial perfusion studies. It has also undergone preliminary testing in liver tumors *(36)*. Despite some promising preliminary studies, PTSM and ammonia have not seen wide use as tumor perfusion agents. Since the applications of PET tumor perfusion imaging have been largely scientific (versus clinical), the desire for unbiased estimates of tumor blood flow, independent of the chemical or metabolic state of the tumor cells, favors the use of $^{15}O[H_2O]$, given its mechanistic simplicity as a tracer of tumor perfusion. These agents may be desirable for small-animal imaging, where the use of $^{15}O[H_2O]$ is challenging due to logistic issues, including the difficulty of gaining venous access in animals as small as mice and the difficulty of dynamic blood sampling.

3.3.4 OTHER RADIOPHARMACEUTICALS

In some circumstances, it may be possible to infer tumor perfusion from the early delivery of radiopharmaceuticals designed for other purposes. For example, this was done by Cascari *(37)* in a kinetic model of [^{18}F]fluoromisonidazole (FMISO), where the blood-to-tissue transfer constant (K_1) provided a good indication of tumor blood flow for this highly lipophilic tumor. Recent analysis of blood flow and metabolism in breast cancer *(32, 38)* suggested that early delivery of FDG (given by K_1 in FDG compartmental models) may provide an approximate indication of tumor blood flow. Although FDG is not highly extracted, tumor FDG K_1 correlated with tumor blood flow measured by water PET with a correlation coefficient on the order of 0.7 *(32)*.

3.3.5 PRECISION OF THE MEASUREMENT

Knowledge of the precision (test/retest repeatability) of tumor perfusion measurements is important in interpreting the results from serial measurements of the course of treatment. This has been estimated for blood flow measured by ^{15}O[H_2O]. Using modeling simulations representative of conditions for breast tumor imaging, Mankoff and Tseng *(18, 32)* estimated a precision of 13% for blood flow measured by a ^{15}O[H_2O] bolus injection and found an 11% difference in a single patient undergoing repeat studies. Wells *(39)* measured a within-patient variability (CV) of 11% in five patients with abdominal tumors who were studied repeatedly using the $C_{15}O_2$ inhalation method. Using ^{62}Cu-PTSM PET, Flower *(40)* was able to achieve a precision of 10% or better for measurements of liver metastasis perfusion.

3.4 Experience with Tumor Perfusion Imaging in Cancer Patients

3.4.1 POSITRON EMISSION TOMOGRAPHY BLOOD FLOW IMAGING RESULTS IN VARIOUS TUMORS

Positron emission tomography imaging of tumor perfusion has been carried out in patients for a variety of tumors in a series of relatively small studies. Tumors that have been studied include brain *(41–43)*, breast *(19, 31, 32, 38)*, liver *(35, 44, 45)*, kidney *(46)*, cervical cancer *(47)*, head and neck cancers *(48–50)*, prostate *(51, 52)*, and lung metastases *(53)* (Table 1). These studies have found, in general, that blood flow is higher in tumors than in the surrounding normal tissues. An exception is renal cell cancer, which, although highly perfused, had lower average blood flow (0.87 ml/min/g) than the normal kidney (1.65 ml/min/g) *(46)*. Blood flow is highly variable both across and within tumor types, ranging from fairly modest flows as low as 0.1 ml/min/g in, for example, some breast tumors, to very high flows in some vascular tumors, such as renal cell cancer metastases, with blood flow as high as 4 ml/min/g, in the range of those found in stress myocardial perfusion studies. Some studies showed that tumor blood flow varied with histological tumor features for a particular type of cancer. For example, while low-grade brain tumors (oligodendrogliomas) had blood flow less than normal gray matter, high-grade tumors (glioblastoma multiforme) had blood flow higher than normal gray matter *(42)*. In a study of liver tumors, Fukudo *(45)* found that hepatocellular carcinomas had higher blood flow than colorectal cancer liver metastases. Yamaguchi *(44)* showed that blood flow measured by ^{15}O[H_2O] PET correlated with the degree of vascularity assessed by contrast CT in colorectal cancer liver metastases. Mankoff *(19)* showed that ER-expressing breast tumors had lower average blood flow

Table 1
Perfusion Measurements in Various Tumors

Tumor type	Study (reference) (type of tumors)	Number of patients (sites)	Tumor blood flow (ml/min/g)[a]	Normal tissue blood flow (ml/min/g)
Brain	Mineura (42) (oligodendroglioma)	5	0.24 [0.11–0.45]	0.40 [0.29–0.45]
Breast	Wilson (31)	20	0.30 [0.13–0.47]	0.05 [0.04–0.07]
	Mankoff (19)	37	0.32 [0.08–0.95]	0.06 [0.02–0.13]
	Zasadny (38)	9 (101)	0.15 [0.07–0.29]	—
Liver	Yamaguchi (44) (hepatocellular and metastases)	15 (22)	0.38 [0.32–0.53][b]	—
	Fukuda (45) [hepatocellular (HCC) and metastases (met)]	13	0.43 [0.15–1.06] 0.31 [0.15–0.44] (met) 0.57 [0.21–1.06] (HCC)	—
Prostate	Muramoto (51)	6	0.55 [0.28–0.99]	0.32 [0.23–0.38][c]
	Kurdziel (52) (mostly bone metastases)	6	0.78 [0.49–1.72]	—
Renal	Lodge (33)	5	[0.4–4.2]	—
	Anderson (46)	12	0.87 [0.33–1.67]	1.65 [1.16–2.88]
	Anderson (21)	13	0.46 [0.11–2.16]	1.32 [0.77–2.00]
Cervical	Ponto (47)	7	0.42 (0.24–0.58)	—
Lung	Logan (53) (metastases, various)	8	1.82 [0.70–3.44]	—
Head and neck	Lehtio (48)	21	0.30 [0.14–0.63]	[d]

[a] Parentheses indicate standard deviation; brackets indicate range of values.
[b] Range of means for different angiographic grades of tumor sites.
[c] Benign prostatic hypertrophy.
[d] Tumor to normal neck muscle blood flow ratio 9.1 from Lehtio et al. (50).

than ER-negative breast cancers. Lehtio (48) showed that patients with head and neck tumors with higher blood flow had poorer survival than those with low blood flow.

3.4.2 POSITRON EMISSION TOMOGRAPHY TUMOR PERFUSION IMAGING TO MEASURE RESPONSE TO THERAPY

Several studies have investigated the use of PET perfusion imaging to measure tumor response to therapy. This has been done both for nonspecific therapy, for example, chemotherapy, and for therapy specifically targeted to the vasculature. Mankoff (18) measured locally advanced breast cancer blood flow using $^{15}O[H_2O]$ PET in patients undergoing doxorubicin-based neoadjuvant chemotherapy. The change in blood flow after 2 months of treatment, midway through therapy, was highly predictive of pathological response to treatment, even more so than PET measures of glucose metabolism by FDG. Furthermore, the level of tumor blood flow after 2 months of treatment was predictive of survival, with patients having higher residual blood flow having significantly poorer survival.

Some studies have used PET perfusion imaging to investigate the response to targeted antiangiogenic therapy. Logan *(53)* measured the change in tumor blood flow by $^{15}O[H_2O]$ PET in eight patients undergoing interleukin (IL)-1 therapy as part of a phase I trial in lung cancer patients and showed significant decreases in tumor blood flow as early as 2 h after IL-1 infusion, returning to close to baseline by 24 h. Herbst *(54)* measured blood flow changes in 25 patients receiving endostatin therapy for a variety of tumors. A general decline in tumor blood flow was found at 8 weeks, with some association with tumor cell and endothelial cell apoptosis. Anderson *(46)* measured blood flow by $^{15}O[H_2O]$ in patients with primary and metastatic renal cell cancer treated with razoxane. No significant change in tumor blood flow was found in six patients scanned before and after drug administration. However, another study of 13 patients with a variety of solid tumors treated with combretastatin A4 phosphate performed by the same group *(46)* found a significant 49% decline in tumor perfusion as early as 30 min after the administration of the drug. These studies illustrate the valuable role played by quantitative tumor perfusion imaging in the evaluation of response to antiangiogenic drugs, especially in the early evaluation of new therapeutic agents.

Not all investigations of PET blood flow and antiangiogenic agents have supported the utility of blood flow measures. Kurdziel *(52)* used $^{15}O[H_2O]$ PET to investigate the response to thalidomide in six patients with androgen-refractory prostate cancer, largely in bone metastases. Changes in blood flow were lower than the variance in the blood flow measurements. In a follow-up study *(52)*, an inverse relationship between blood flow change and total prostate-specific antigen (PSA) change was found, as opposed to a positive correlation between the change in FDG uptake and PSA. These findings may be somewhat specific to measuring blood flow in prostate bone metastases due to the small blood flow in many bone metastases and artifacts from spillover from the highly vascular adjacent bone marrow. Nevertheless, they point out the need for more specific measures of angiogenesis to measure response to antiangiogenic treatments.

Other applications of PET tumor perfusion imaging in conjunction with drug therapy include studies using vasoactive agents to manipulate tumor blood flow relative to normal tissue. Flower *(40)* used ^{62}Cu-PTSM PET to look for changes in blood flow to colorectal cancer metastases associated with infusion of angiotensin II. The goal of such therapy is to increase the local delivery of therapeutic agents to the tumor sites while decreasing delivery to normal liver. No significant changes were found in tumor site perfusion in seven of nine patients studied. Further analysis was performed by Burke *(35)*, who found that relative tumor perfusion, assessed by the tumor-to-normal liver ratio (TNR), increased from a mean of 1.3 to 2.1 after angiotensin II infusion ($p < 0.01$). A similar study was performed by Koh *(27)* who used $^{15}O[H_2O]$ PET to measure blood flow changes with angiotensin II in patients ($N = 13$) with hepatocellular cancer or colorectal liver metastases. While tumor blood flow did not change, however, blood flow to normal liver and spleen declined. Furthermore, hepatic arterial blood flow did not change significantly, while portal blood flow did, indicating the mechanism of selectively enhancing blood flow to tumors, which are largely supplied by hepatic arterial flow.

3.4.3 Relationship of Tumor Perfusion to Metabolism and Hypoxia

The delivery of nutrients, such as glucose and oxygen, plays an important role in tumor perfusion. As such, PET imaging using multiple radiopharmaceuticals provides a method for assessing the relationship between tumor perfusion and tumor metabolism and hypoxia. Several smaller studies investigating these relationships have been conducted. Mineura *(42)* studied blood flow and metabolism in oligodendrogliomas using $^{15}O[H_2O]$, $^{15}O_2$, and FDG PET. In a study of five patients, tumor perfusion, oxygen consumption, and glucose metabolism were all found to be similarly lower than normal gray matter in these low-grade tumors. Fukuda *(45)* studied blood flow and glucose metabolism in 13 patients with liver tumors (7 with primary liver tumors and 6 with colorectal liver metastases) using $^{15}O[H_2O]$, $^{15}O_2$, and FDG PET. Hepatocellular cancers were found to have higher blood flow than colorectal metastases, but the hepatocelullar cancers had lower average glucose metabolism (FDG SUV) than colorectal metastases. As such an inverse correlation was found between blood flow and FDG uptake, although this may be related to the inclusion of two rather different tumor types. Mankoff *(19)* and Zasadny *(38)* examined blood flow and metabolism using $^{15}O[H_2O]$ and FDG PET in locally advanced breast cancer. While there was some correlation between tumor blood flow and metabolism, the relationship was not as closely seen as in studies of normal brain and myocardium. Results from one of the studies *(19)* suggested that an imbalance between blood flow and glucose metabolism, specifically a high glucose metabolism relative to blood flow, was predictive of poor response to subsequent chemotherapy and of poor disease-free survival (Fig. 3). These results were further analyzed by Tseng *(32)*. In untreated tumors, tumor blood flow and metabolism were only modestly correlated ($r = 0.34$, $p = 0.05$); however, blood flow and early FDG delivery

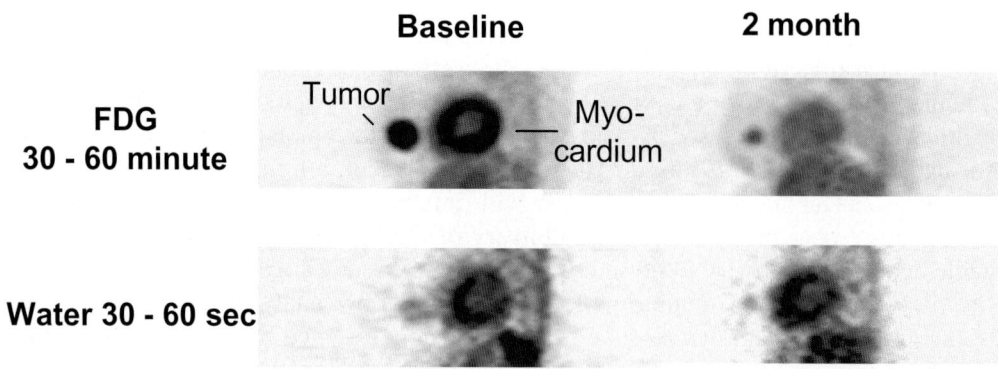

Fig. 3. Blood flow and metabolism in a patient with left locally advanced breast cancer before and after 2 months of chemotherapy. Thick sagittal images providing a lateral view of the breast are shown. Pretherapy, there is high FDG uptake, indicative of high glucose metabolism, with only modest blood flow. The central-most portion of the tumor has lower uptake in the early water scan, indicating less tumor perfusion in the center. Postchemotherapy, metabolism declined significantly; however, maximum tumor perfusion quantitatively increased slightly in the remnant tumor compared to pretherapy. Residual high-grade viable tumor was found at surgery, despite a significant reduction in tumor size. The patient had disease recurrence and death from disease with 2–3 years of treatment and surgery, despite an apparently good response by size reduction criteria.

(FDG K_1 in compartmental modeling) were well correlated ($r = 0.62$, $p < 0.01$). After chemotherapy, blood flow and glucose metabolism were more closely matched ($r = 0.76$, $p < 0.001$), suggesting a change in tumor metabolic phenotype posttherapy. These results point out the benefits of imaging studies examining multiple aspects of tumor biology, including tumor perfusion, and point out the potential of such studies to provide insight into tumor behavior that may have clinical relevance.

Tumor hypoxia reflects, in good part, a lack of oxygen delivery relative to oxygen need. As such, several studies have investigated the relationship between tumor perfusion and hypoxia directly using PET. Bruelheimer *(43)* measured tumor perfusion and hypoxia using $^{15}O[H_2O]$ and FMISO PET in 10 patients with glioblastoma multiforme or meningioma. There was a positive correlation between blood flow and early uptake of FMISO, as would be expected for a highly lipophilic tracer such as FMISO *(37)*. However, late FMISO retention was not correlated with blood flow and was associated with both hypo- and hyperperfusion on the tumors relative to normal brain. This also was expected, since while hypoperfusion may lead to hypoxia, hypoxia will also induce angiogenesis, ultimately leading to hyperperfusion, particularly at the tumor border. Importantly, this study showed that hypoxia could be measured with FMISO PET independent of tumor perfusion and blood–brain barrier disruption. Lehtio *(48)* also studied tumor perfusion and hypoxia in 21 patients with head and neck cancer using $^{15}O[H_2O]$ and [^{18}F]fluoroerythronitroimidazole (FTENIM) PET, a follow-up to an earlier study with 8 patients *(50)*. Both high tumor blood flow and high hypoxic volume by FTENIM PET portended poor survival, and higher blood flow was associated with poorer local control. These early studies indicate the utility of combined blood flow/hypoxia imaging studies and the potential to gain insight into factors associated with poor tumor response to treatment.

4. TUMOR HYPOXIA

4.1 Why Measure Tumor Hypoxia

During their evolution, many solid tumors develop chaotic and complex functions including altered metabolism, proliferation, invasiveness, and metastatic potential *(55)*. These differences separate the tumor microenvironment from the surrounding normal tissues and form the basis for many functional imaging techniques. The critical role of oxygen in cellular respiration makes it an essential metabolic substrate in normal tissues and tumors. The tissue oxygen levels, commonly reported as a partial pressure Po_2, can reach below 5 mm Hg and cancer cells can still survive and adapt to these circumstances. Tumor oxygenation is intimately related to the tumor vasculature and tumor perfusion.

Growth of a tumor is primarily a result of unregulated cellular growth, resulting in a greater demand on oxygen for energy metabolism *(56)*. Ischemia and hypoxia cannot be construed to be the same; hypoxia may not be evident until the late stages of ischemia and vice versa. The biological implications of hypoxia as a factor in treatment response were first explained by Thomlinson and Gray who, in studying lung cancer, showed that hypoxia develops beyond a distance of 120 µm from a capillary *(57)*. High interstitial pressure within a tumor may put additional stress on the already inefficient and often poorly organized tumor, and other factors such as low O_2 solubility (anemia) may contribute to tissue hypoxia in tumors *(58, 59)*.

4.2 Hypoxia-Induced Changes in Tumor Biology

Hypoxic cells attempt to adapt by using anaerobic glycolysis to maintain production of adequate amounts of ATP, resulting in accumulation of lactate in the cells, which changes the pH. If the poor delivery of oxygen and other nutrients to the tumor continues, the glycolytic activity itself can be shut down, in spite of continued hypoxia *(60)*. Hypoxia-induced homeostatic changes to maintain viability of the cell include more efficient extraction of oxygen from blood and induction of more aggressive survival traits through expression of new proteins. A number of hypoxia-related genes are responsible for these genomic changes that are mediated via downstream transcription factors *(61–64)*. These include expression of endothelial cytokines such as vascular endothelial growth factor (VEGF) and signaling molecules such as IL-1, tumor necrosis factor (TNF)-α, and tumor growth factor (TGF)-β and selection of cells with mutant p53 *(65, 66)*. Hypoxic cells do not readily undergo death by apoptosis *(67)* and may arrest in the G_1 phase of the cell cycle in response to sublethal DNA damage induced by radiation *(68, 69)*. Increased glucose transporter (GLUT) and hexokinase levels are responsible for much of the increased glucose uptake in hypoxia *(70–72)*.

4.3 Hypoxia-Inducible Factor (HIF)

The primary cellular oxygen-sensing mechanism appears to be mediated by a heme protein that uses O_2 as a substrate to catalyze hydroxylation of proline in a segment of HIF1α. This leads to rapid degradation of HIF1α by ubiquitination under normoxic conditions *(73)*. In the absence of O_2 HIF1α accumulates and forms a heterodimer with HIF1β that is transported to the nucleus and activates *hypoxia-responsive* genes, resulting in a cascade of genetic and metabolic events aimed at the effects of hypoxia on cellular energetics *(74, 75)*. In fact, overexpression of HIF1α has been seen even before the invasive stages or the development of frank hypoxic regions within a tumor *(76)*. Identification of overexpressed HIF1α in tissues by immunocytochemical (IHC) staining has been used as an indirect measure of hypoxia *(77–79)*, but its heterogeneous expression within a tumor and the nonspecific nature of HIF1α expression limit the prognostic utility of this method alone.

4.4 Tumor Hypoxia and Clinical Outcome: Current Understanding

It has long been known that hypoxia negatively impacts tumor biology and clinical outcome. Radiobiological experiments have overwhelmingly established that in the absence of oxygen, the free radicals formed by ionizing radiation recombine without producing the anticipated cellular damage *(80–82)*. Preclinical experience indicates that three times as much photon radiation dose is needed to cause the same lethality in hypoxic cells as compared to normoxic cells *(57, 82–85)*. Although these are established concepts, our understanding of the biological aspects of tumor hypoxia indicates that the development and selection of an aggressive phenotype would result in a poor response to treatment as well as a poor outcome due to increased metastatic potential *(67, 86–88)*. Hypoxia has also been known to promote resistance to chemotherapeutic agents by a number of mechanisms *(88, 89)* (Fig. 4).

In the past, many cancer treatment schemes that were introduced to overcome the cure-limiting consequences of hypoxia have not produced the expected results *(90)*.

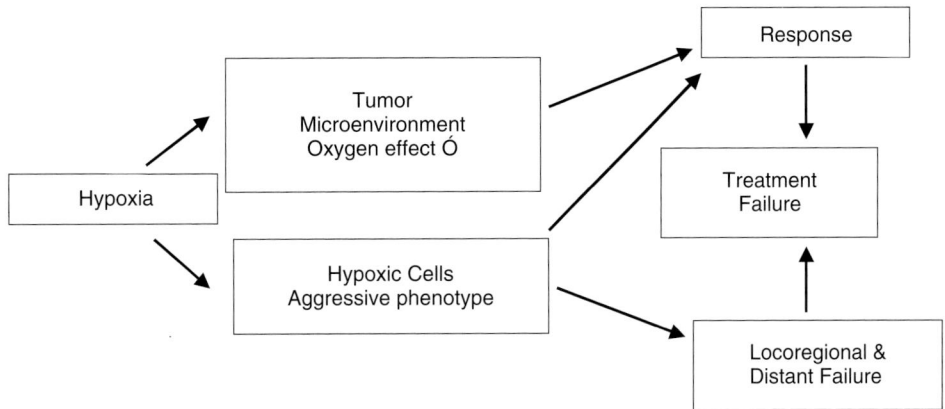

Fig. 4. The effect of hypoxia on cancer cells and the overall behavior and response of tumors as well as patient outcome.

They suffered from the lack of a noninvasive assay to identify patients with hypoxic tumors for rational patient selection.

It is logical to assume that the negative association of hypoxia with treatment response and patient outcome implies a role for evaluating hypoxia in a tumor that will help identify tumors with a high hypoxic fraction so that hypoxia-specific treatments can be successfully implemented. There is convincing evidence that tumor hypoxia does not correlate with tumor size, grade, and extent of necrosis or blood hemoglobin status *(91–96)*.

The very nature of hypoxic cells makes them attractive targets for hypoxia-activated prodrugs *(97, 98)*. While focal hypoxia in a tumor can be treated with a boost of radiation using intensity-modulation radiation therapy (IMRT) *(99, 100)*, more diffuse hypoxia will benefit from systemic administration of hypoxic cell toxins/sensitizers. Newer hypoxia-activated prodrugs *(101)* are less toxic and more effective than their predecessors *(102)*, e.g., tirapazamine (TPZ) (previously called SR 4233), and are being tested in a number of cancer types *(98, 103, 104)*. These agents, in addition to direct cytotoxic effects, have synergistic toxicity with radiation and chemotherapy. When some of the early results from these trials were analyzed *(105)*, it was obvious that TPZ was much more effective in the presence of hypoxia, indicating that identification of hypoxia prior to treatment would be beneficial in patient selection *(105, 106)*.

4.5 Evaluating Tumor Hypoxia

During the past several decades, tumor oxygenation and assays of tumor hypoxia have been evaluated to predict patient outcome in cancers of the uterine cervix *(107)*, lung *(93)*, head and neck *(99, 108–110)*, and glioma *(111, 112)*. These techniques have identified widespread heterogeneity in tumor hypoxia within a tumor, between tumors, and between patients with the same tumor type *(113)*.

Current hypoxia assays can be categorized as *in vivo* (both invasive and noninvasive) or *ex vivo* (invasive biopsy) *(5, 114, 115)*. A useful assay should distinguish normoxic regions from hypoxic regions at a level of oxygen relevant to cancer, P_{O_2} in the 3–5 mm Hg range.

4.6 Ideal Hypoxia Assay

Some of the desirable characteristics for an ideal clinical hypoxia assay include (1) a simple and noninvasive method, (2) nontoxic, (3) rapid and easy to perform with consistency between laboratories, and (4) the ability to quantify without the need for substantial calibration of the detection instrumentation. Location of the tumor in a patient should not be a limiting factor for the assay. The ideal assay must also be able to provide a complete locoregional evaluation of the tumor in view of the presence of spatial heterogeneity in the distribution of hypoxia within a tumor. To be maximally successful, hypoxia-directed imaging and treatment should target both chronic hypoxia as well as acute hypoxia resulting from transient interruption of blood flow *(116)*. The assay should reflect intracellular Po_2 rather than blood flow or some consequence of the O_2 level on downstream biochemical changes in, for example, thiols or NADH. All of these requirements suggest an important role for imaging in evaluating hypoxia.

4.7 Oxygen Electrode Measurements

Early measurements of oxygen levels in tumors were largely based on direct measurement of Po_2 levels using very fine polarographic electrodes considered as a *gold standard* for Po_2. Heterogeneity in hypoxia within a tumor presents a challenge for accurately mapping regional Po_2 *(92, 117)*. Interlaboratory variations in calibration of the electrodes further plague the results *(118)* and these measurements can be affected by the presence of blood in the interstitial or vascular spaces in tumors *(119)*. Adjuvant use of anatomic imaging, such as CT, to guide electrode deployment is plagued by the inability to differentiate viable tissue within a tumor *(119, 120)* as does choosing close entry points for the electrodes that will compromise patient comfort *(118)*. Other limitations of electrode measurements include the need for accessible tumor location and difficulties associated with serial measurements. An absolute Po_2 value may be less useful and less robust than accurate assessment of the volume or fraction of tumor cells that are hypoxic. The fraction of cells in the hypoxic peak may be much more important than absolute Po_2 values. Imaging methods for hypoxia, on the other hand, provide a complete map of relative oxygenation level in tumor regions with good spatial resolution in a microenvironment that tends to be highly heterogeneous.

4.8 Positron Emission Tomography Hypoxia Imaging

Hypoxia imaging presents the special challenge of making a positive image out of the relative absence of O_2. Chemists have developed two different classes of imaging agents to address this problem, bioreductive alkylating agents that are O_2 sensitive and metal chelates that are apparently sensitive to the intracellular redox state that develops as a consequence of hypoxia.

4.8.1 NITROIMIDAZOLE COMPOUNDS

Misonidazole, an azomycin-based hypoxic cell sensitizer introduced in clinical radiation oncology three decades ago, binds covalently to intracellular molecules at levels that are inversely proportional to intracellular oxygen concentration below about 10 mm Hg. It is a lipophilic 2-nitroimidazole derivative whose uptake in hypoxic cells is dependent on the sequential reduction of the nitro group on the imidazole ring *(121)* and the viability of cells with intact mitochondrial electron transport. In the presence of O_2, the nitroimidazole simply goes through a futile reduction cycle and is returned

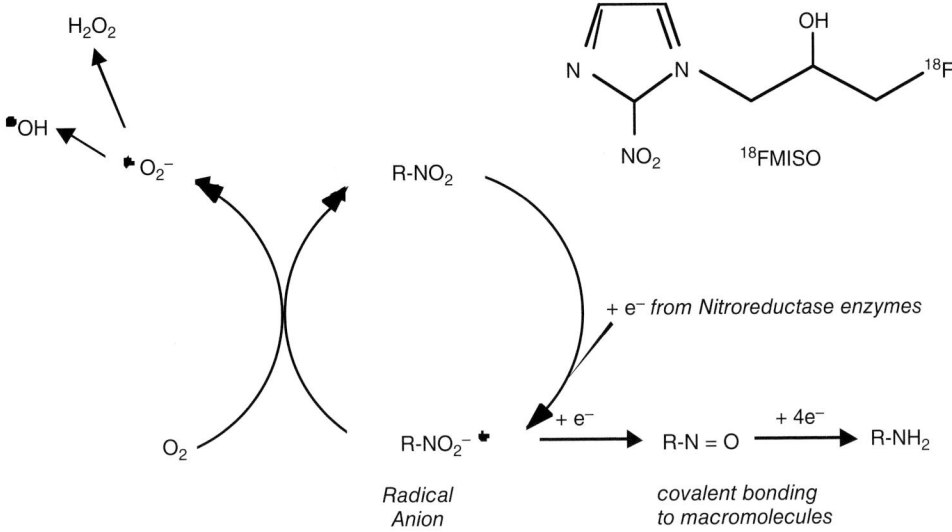

Fig. 5. Structure of misonidazole showing the mechanism of action in the presence and absence of oxygen.

to its initial nitroimidazole state. In the absence of a competitive electron acceptor, the nitroimidazole continues to accumulate electrons to form the hydroxylamine alkylating agent and becomes trapped within the viable but O_2-deficient cell (Fig. 5).

[^{18}F]Fluoromisonidazole is an imaging agent derived from misonidazole. It has a high *hypoxia-specific factor* (HSF) of 20–50, defined as the ratio of uptake in hypoxic cells compared to normoxic cells *(122)*. The uptake and retention of FMISO are inversely related to the instantaneous oxygen tension within the cell. *In vitro* studies have shown that reoxygenated cells exposed to a new batch of the tracer will not accumulate the 2-nitroimidazole compounds.

FMISO is a highly stable and robust radiopharmaceutical that can be used to quantify tissue hypoxia using PET imaging *(94, 123)*. Its easy synthesis and optimal safety profile led to its acceptance in the clinic. It is the most commonly used PET hypoxia tracer *(93, 94, 124–130)* and has biodistribution and dosimetry characteristics ideal for PET imaging *(131)*. The partition coefficient of FMISO is 0.41 *(132)*, and after about an hour the distribution reflects its partition coefficient *(133)* (Figs. 6 and 7).

The narrow distribution of pixel uptake values after about 90 min prompted a simple analysis of FMISO PET images by scaling the pixel uptake to plasma concentration. The mean value for this ratio in all tissues is close to unity and almost all normoxic pixels have a value of less than 1.2. The optimum time for imaging appears to be between 90 and 150 min and can be adjusted to fit the clinic schedule and has logistical similarity to the ubiquitous methylene diphosphonate (MDP) bone scan. FMISO images can be interpreted by either qualitative *(105)* or quantitative methods. Extensive validation studies have confirmed the simple but accurate quantitative method of using a venous blood sample to calculate a tissue:blood ratio *(4, 129, 134)*.

The use of a tumor hypoxic volume (HV) parameter, which is the total number of pixels with a T:B ≥1.2 expressed in milliliters *(4, 130)*, obviates the need for accurate delineation of tumor margins in order to define the denominator in calculating fractional

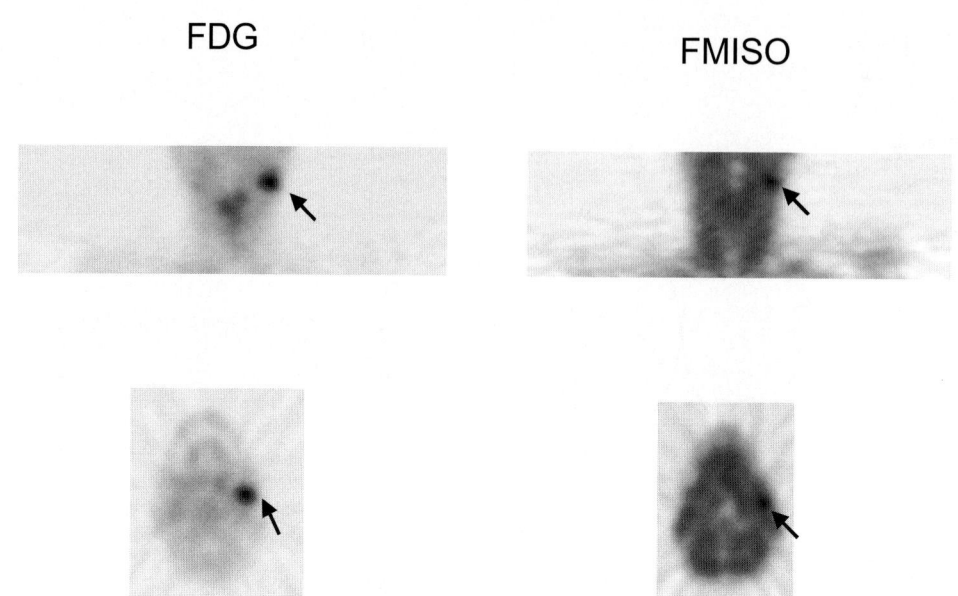

Fig. 6. Patient with T3N2M0 of the tonsil. Coronal (top) and transaxial (bottom) slices of FDG and FMISO showing the uptake in the left lymph node (arrows). FMISO T:B_{max} = 1.92 and HV = 51.1 ml and FDG SUV_{max} = 7.25.

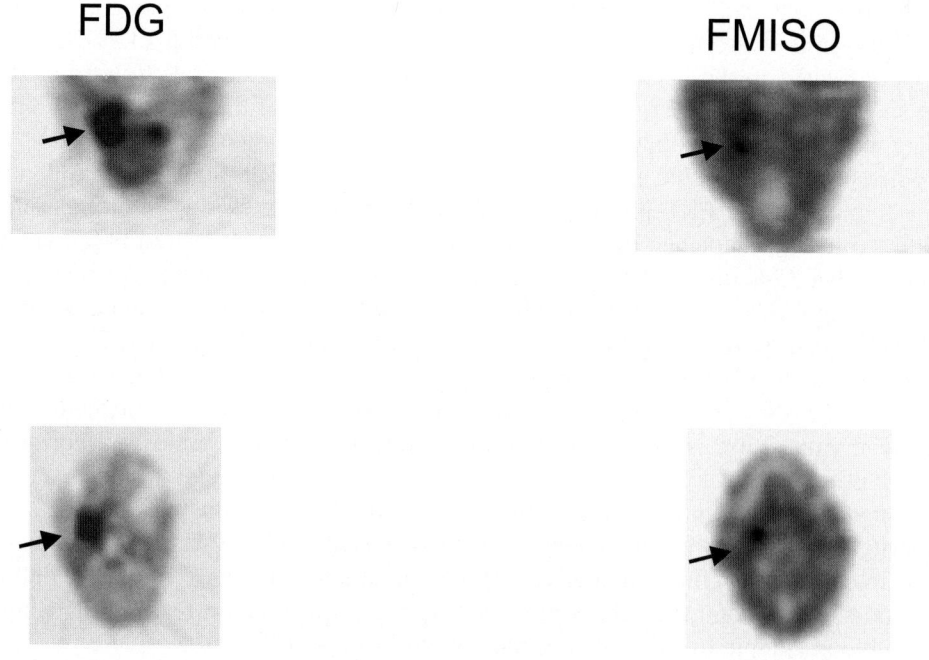

Fig. 7. Patient with T3N2M0 cancer of the tongue. Coronal (top) and transaxial slices (bottom) of FDG and FMISO images showing the uptake in the primary tumor (arrows). FMISO T:B = 1.63 and HV = 16.6 ml and FDGSUV_{max} = 6.

hypoxic volume (FHV) *(124)*. Although more detailed approaches to quantifying FMISO uptake and kinetics have been pursued *(37)*, static measures provide most of the information regarding oxygenation status, and it is not likely that a detailed mathematical modeling for image analysis would play a role in the clinic.

A typical protocol for PET scanning with FMISO uses an intravenous administration of a dose of 3.7 MBq (0.1 mCi)/kg, which results in an effective total body dose equivalent of 0.0126 mGy/MBq *(131)*. Scanning typically begins at about 120 min and lasts for 20 min with blood sampling during the scan. A transmission scan is used for attenuation correction of emission data. Typically one axial field of view (AFOV) of 15-cm in the craniocaudal dimension is acquired. An FDG PET scan of the entire torso including the region in question is obtained, taking care to reposition the patient between images. Use of immobilization devices such as radiation treatment masks would be helpful to maintain accuracy in image fusion. Addition of FDG imaging data increases the sensitivity of FMISO imaging by indicating the full extent of the tumor and helps in correlating metabolic activity and hypoxia in the tumor as well as in staging *(60)*.

4.8.2 OTHER AZOMYCIN-BASED IMAGING AGENTS

Some research groups have developed alternative azomycin (nitroimidazole) radiopharmaceuticals for hypoxia imaging by attempting to manipulate the rate of blood clearance in order to improve image contrast *(135–137)*. These include EF-1, initially developed because of the availability of an antibody stain to verify the distribution in tissue samples *(138)*. Fluoroerythronitroimidazole (FETNIM), a more hydrophilic derivative than fluoroetanidazole, shows less retention in liver and fewer metabolites in animals *(139)*.

A number of SPECT-based hypoxia imaging compounds have been introduced with the hope of taking advantage of gamma camera imaging *(140)*, e.g., BMS181321, BMS194796, and HL91 *(135, 141, 142)*. The main drawbacks with the SPECT radiopharmaceuticals, both the iodinated compounds [e.g., [^{123}I]IAZA *(143)*] and the technetium-based agents, are the lower image contrast and less potential for quantification than the PET agents *(136)*.

OTHER HYPOXIA IMAGING AGENTS

Copper bis(thiosemicarbazones) are a class of molecules evaluated as freely diffusible blood flow tracers that are retained once they enter cells. The resulting images have a higher contrast because of altered redox environment associated with hypoxia. The longer half-life of the ^{64}Cu-labeled acetyl derivative of pyruvaldehyde-bis[*N*4-methylthiosemicarbazonato] copper (II) complex, Cu-ATSM, is potentially advantageous in the clinic *(144–146)* although the mechanism of retention is less well validated than FMISO. Retention of Cu-ATSM in hypoxic regions and rapid washout from normal regions have been documented *(147)*, although diffusion of NADH and other related reducing equivalents might make Cu-ATSM less reflective of the spatial heterogeneity of hypoxia. *(145, 148)*.

5. SUMMARY

Hypoxia, a significant problem in solid tumors, can now be clinically evaluated with modern imaging techniques and tackled with effective treatments to specifically overcome the cure-limiting effects of hypoxia. Tumor perfusion can also be measured quantitatively and accurately by PET and may play a role, especially in evaluating systemic therapy, in both the delivery and effect of new treatment agents. Angiogenesis-specific imaging approaches are being developed that will be useful in monitoring specific antiangiogenic therapy. Technological advances in the field of cancer imaging make PET imaging ideal for evaluating the entire tumor and regional lymph nodes noninvasively in a snapshot-repeated manner *(149)*. The explosive growth in the availability of PET scanners and PET/CT scanners and the greater distribution of ^{18}F tracers in the community will make most PET imaging procedures within reach of community nuclear medicine and radiation oncology centers. Clinical perfusion, hypoxia, and possibly angiogenesis imaging can help in several ways, both in guiding therapy selection and evaluating its efficacy.

The combined use of perfusion, hypoxia, and specific angiogenesis imaging in a single patient is feasible, may offer unique biologic insights, and may be an effective tool for guiding patient-specific cancer therapy. In addition, PET/CT scanners will facilitate the incorporation of quantitative, functional PET imaging into radiation treatment plans that will explore the role of IMRT-based boosts to target subvolumes that may be resistant on the basis of hypoxia or other tumor biological factors *(99, 100, 150–153)*. Also, the ability to detect alterations in tumor perfusion and tumor hypoxia could guide the use of a systemic and specific hypoxic cell cytotoxin *(154)*. In this way, assessing hypoxia and perfusion will also help in developing and evaluating novel hypoxia-directed and/or antiangiogenesis drugs *(97, 155–157)*.

As cancer treatment becomes more sophisticated, noninvasive molecular imaging methods will play a pivotal role in characterizing the tumor and its microenvironment and in guiding treatment decisions for the individual patient. There is a need for large-scale multicenter trials on the utility of hypoxia and other specific imaging agents in patient selection and guiding treatment.

ACKNOWLEDGMENTS

We thank the following individuals for the help they provided: Eric Ford, PhD, and Kristi Hendrickson, PhD, for help with IMRT planning and Lanell M. Peterson and Holly Pike for help with the manuscript preparation. This work was supported in part by NIH Grants P01 CA42045, CA72064, and S10RR17229, and a Pilot grant from the Seattle Cancer Consortium.

REFERENCES

1. Wahl RL. Anatomolecular imaging with 2-deoxy-2-[^{18}F]fluoro-D-glucose: Bench to outpatient center. *Mol Imaging Biol* 2003;5:49–56.
2. Herschman HR. Molecular imaging: Looking at problems, seeing solutions. *Science* 2003;302:605–608.
3. Chapman JD, Bradley JD, Eary JF, Haubner R, Larson SM, Michalski JM, Okunieff PG, Strauss HW, Ung YC, Welch MJ. Molecular (functional) imaging for radiotherapy applications: An RTOG symposium. *Int J Radiat Oncol Biol Phys* 2003;55:294–301.
4. Rajendran J, Muzi M, Peterson LM, Diaz AZ, Spence AM, Schwartz DS, Krohn KA. Analyzing the results of [F-18] FMISO PET hypoxia imaging: What is the best way to quantify hypoxia? *J Nucl Med* 2002;43:102P.
5. Peters L, McKay M. Predictive assays: Will they ever have a role in the clinic? *Int J Radiat Oncol Biol Phys* 2001;49:501–504.

6. Rowland DJ, Lewis JS, Welch MJ. Molecular imaging: The application of small animal positron emission tomography. *J Cell Biochem Suppl* 2002;39:110–115.
7. Maclean D, Northrop JP, Padgett HC, Walsh JC. Drugs and probes: The symbiotic relationship between pharmaceutical discovery and imaging science. *Mol Imaging Biol* 2003;5:304–311.
8. Collier TL, Lecomte R, McCarthy TJ, Meikle S, Ruth TJ, Scopinaro F, Signore A, VanBrocklin H, Van De Wiele C, Waterhouse RN. Assessment of cancer-associated biomarkers by positron emission tomography: Advances and challenges. *Dis Markers* 2002;18:211–247.
9. Gambhir SS. Molecular imaging of cancer with positron emission tomography. *Nat Rev Cancer* 2002;2:683–693.
10. Folkman J. Tumor angiogenesis: Therapeutic implications. *N Engl J Med* 1971;285:1182–1186.
11. McDonald DM, Teicher BA, Stetler-Stevenson W, Ng SS, Figg WD, Folkman J, Hanahan D, Auerbach R, O'Reilly M, Herbst R, Cheresh D, Gordon M, Eggermont A, Libutti SK. Report from the Society for Biological Therapy and Vascular Biology Faculty of the NCI Workshop on Angiogenesis Monitoring. *J Immunother* 2004;27:161–175.
12. Costouros NG, Diehn FE, Libutti SK. Molecular imaging of tumor angiogenesis. *J Cell Biochem Suppl* 2002;39:72–78.
13. Weber WA, Haubner R, Vabuliene E, Kuhnast B, Wester HJ, Schwaiger M. Tumor angiogenesis targeting using imaging agents. *Q J Nucl Med* 2001;45:179–182.
14. Koukourakis MI, Giatromanolaki A, Sivridis E, Fezoulidis I. Cancer vascularization: Implications in radiotherapy? *Int J Radiat Oncol Biol Phys* 2000;48:545–553.
15. Folkman J. Role of angiogenesis in tumor growth and metastasis. *Semin Oncol* 2002;29:15–18.
16. Jain RK. Haemodynamic and transport barriers to the treatment of solid tumors. *Int J Radiat Biol* 1991;60:85–100.
17. Herbst RS, Hidalgo M, Pierson AS, Holden SN, Bergen M, Eckhardt SG. Angiogenesis inhibitors in clinical development for lung cancer. *Semin Oncol* 2002;29:66–77.
18. Mankoff DA, Dunnwald LK, Gralow JR, Ellis GK, Schubert EK, Tseng, Lawton TJ, Linden HM, Livingston RB. Changes in blood flow and metabolism in locally advanced breast cancer treated with neoadjuvant chemotherapy. *J Nucl Med* 2003;44:1806–1814.
19. Mankoff DA, Dunnwald LK, Gralow JR, Ellis GK, Charlop A, Lawton TJ, Schubert EK, Tseng J, Livingston RB. Blood flow and metabolism in locally advanced breast cancer: Relationship to response to therapy. *J Nucl Med* 2002;43:500–9.
20. Rajendran JG, Krohn KA. Imaging hypoxia and angiogenesis in tumors. *Radiol Clin North Am* 2005;43:169–187.
21. Anderson H, and Price P. Clinical measurement of blood flow in tumours using positron emission tomography: A review. *Nucl Med Commun* 2002;23:131–138.
22. Lee TY, Purdie TG, Stewart E. CT imaging of angiogenesis. *Q J Nucl Med* 2003;47:171–87.
23. Padhani AR. MRI for assessing antivascular cancer treatments. *Br J Radiol* 2003;76(Spec No 1):S60–S80.
24. Cosgrove D. Angiogenesis imaging—ultrasound. *Br J Radiol* 2003;76(Spec No 1):S43–S49.
25. Schelbert HR. Cardiac PET: Microcirculation and substrate transport in normal and diseased human myocardium. *Ann Nucl Med* 1994;8:91–100.
26. Raichle ME, Martin WR, Herscovitch P, Mintun MA, Markham J. Brain blood flow measured with intravenous H2(15)O. II. Implementation and validation. *J Nucl Med* 1983;24:790–798.
27. Koh T, Taniguchi H, Yamagishi H. Oxygen-15 positron-emission tomography for predicting selective delivery of a chemotherapeutic agent to hepatic cancers during angiotensin II-induced hypertension. *Cancer Chemother Pharmacol* 2003;51:349–358.
28. Alessio AM, Kinahan PE, Cheng PM, Vesselle H, Karp JS. PET/CT scanner instrumentation, challenges, and solutions. *Radiol Clin North Am* 2004;42:1017–1032.
29. Mathias CJ, Welch MJ, Perry DJ, McGuire AH, Zhu X, Connett JM, Green MA. Investigation of copper-PTSM as a PET tracer for tumor blood flow. *Int J Rad Appl Instrum B* 1991;18:807–811.
30. Schmidt KC, Turkheimer FE. Kinetic modeling in positron emission tomography. *Q J Nucl Med* 2002;46:70–85.
31. Wilson CBJH, Lammertsma AA, McKenzie CG, Sikora K, Jones T. Measurements of blood flow and exchanging water space in breast tumors using positron emission tomography: A rapid and non-invasive dynamic method. *Cancer Res* 1992;52:1592–1597.

32. Tseng J, Dunnwald LK, Schubert EK, Link JM, Minoshima S, Muzi M, Mankoff DA. 18F-FDG kinetics in locally advanced breast cancer: Correlation with tumor blood flow and changes in response to neoadjuvant chemotherapy. *J Nucl Med* 2004;45:1829–1837.
33. Lodge MA, Carson RE, Carrasquillo JA, Whatley M, Libutti SK, Bacharach SL. Parametric images of blood flow in oncology PET studies using [^{15}O]water. *J Nucl Med* 2000;41:1784–1792.
34. Mathias CJ, Green MA, Morrison WB, Knapp DW. Evaluation of Cu-PTSM as a tracer of tumor perfusion: Comparison with labeled microspheres in spontaneous canine neoplasms. *Nucl Med Biol* 1994;21:83–87.
35. Burke D, Davies MM, Zweit J, Flower MA, Ott RJ, Dworkin MJ, Glover C, McCready VR, Carnochan P, Allen-Mersh TG. Continuous angiotensin II infusion increases tumour: Normal blood flow ratio in colo-rectal liver metastases. *Br J Cancer* 2001;85:1640–1645.
36. Shibata T, Yamamoto K, Hayashi N, Yonekura Y, Nagara T, Saji H, Mukai T, Konishi J. Dynamic positron emission tomography with 13N-ammonia in liver tumors. *Eur J Nucl Med* 1998; 14:607–611.
37. Casciari JJ, Graham MM, Rasey JS. A modeling approach for quantifying tumor hypoxia with [F-18]fluoromisonidazole PET time-activity data. *Med Phys* 1995;22:1127–1139.
38. Zasadny KR, Tatsumi M, Wahl RL. FDG metabolism and uptake versus blood flow in women with untreated primary breast cancers. *Eur J Nucl Med Mol Imaging* 2003;30:274–280.
39. Wells P, Jones T, Price P. Assessment of inter- and intrapatient variability in $C^{15}O_2$ positron emission tomography measurements of blood flow in patients with intra-abdominal cancers. *Clin Cancer Res* 2003;9:6350–6356.
40. Flower MA, Zweit J, Hall AD, Burke D, Davies MM, Dworkin MJ, Young HE, Mundy J, Ott RJ, McCready VR, Carnochan P, Allen-Mersh TG. ^{62}Cu-PTSM and PET used for the assessment of angiotensin II-induced blood flow changes in patients with colorectal liver metastases. *Eur J Nucl Med* 2001;28:99–103.
41. Leenders KL. PET: Blood flow and oxygen consumption in brain tumors. *J Neurooncol* 1994; 22:269–273.
42. Mineura K, Shioya H, Kowada M, Ogawa T, Hatazawa J, Uemura K. Blood flow and metabolism of oligodendrogliomas: A positron emission tomography study with kinetic analysis of ^{18}F-fluorodeoxyglucose. *J Neurooncol* 1999;43:49–57.
43. Bruehlmeier M, Roelcke U, Schubiger PA, Ametamey SM. Assessment of hypoxia and perfusion in human brain tumors using PET with ^{18}F-fluoromisonidazole and ^{15}O-H$_2$O. *J Nucl Med* 2004;45: 1851–1859.
44. Yamaguchi A, Taniguchi H, Kunishima S, Koh T, Yamagishi H. Correlation between angiographically assessed vascularity and blood flow in hepatic metastases in patients with colorectal carcinoma. *Cancer* 2000;89:1236–1244.
45. Fukuda K, Taniguchi H, Koh T, Kunishima S, Yamagishi H. Relationships between oxygen and glucose metabolism in human liver tumours: Positron emission tomography using (15)O and (18)F-deoxyglucose. *Nucl Med Commun* 2004;25:577–583.
46. Anderson H, Yap JT, Wells P, Miller MP, Propper D, Price P, Harris AL. Measurement of renal tumour and normal tissue perfusion using positron emission tomography in a phase II clinical trial of razoxane. *Br J Cancer* 2003;89:262–267.
47. Ponto LL, Madsen MT, Hichwa RD, Mayr N, Yuh WT, Magnotta VA, Watkins GL, Ehrhardt JC. Assessment of blood flow in solid tumors using PET. *Clin Positron Imaging* 1998;1:117–121.
48. Lehtio K, Eskola O, Viljanen T, Oikonen V, Gronroos T, Sillanmaki L, Grenman R, Minn H. Imaging perfusion and hypoxia with PET to predict radiotherapy response in head-and-neck cancer. *Int J Radiat Oncol Biol Phys* 2004;59:971–982.
49. Lehtio K, Oikonen V, Nyman S, Gronroos T, Roivainen A, Eskola O, Minn H. Quantifying tumour hypoxia with fluorine-18 fluoroerythronitroimidazole ([^{18}F]FETNIM) and PET using the tumour to plasma ratio. *Eur J Nucl Med Mol Imaging* 2003;30:101–108.
50. Lehtio K, Oikonen V, Gronroos T, Eskola O, Kalliokoski K, Bergman J, Solin O, Grenman R, Nuutila P, Minn H. Imaging of blood flow and hypoxia in head and neck cancer: Initial evaluation with [(15)O]H(2)O and [(18)F]fluoroerythronitroimidazole PET. *J Nucl Med* 2001;42:1643–1652.
51. Muramoto S, Uematsu H, Sadato N, Tsuchida T, Matsuda T, Hatabu H, Yonekura Y, Itoh H. H(2)(15)0 positron emission tomography validation of semiquantitative prostate blood flow determined by double-echo dynamic MRI: A preliminary study. *J Comput Assist Tomogr* 2002;26:510–514.

52. Kurdziel KA, Figg WD, Carrasquillo JA, Huebsch S, Whatley M, Sellers D, Libutti SK, Pluda JM, Dahut W, Reed E, Bacharach SL. Using positron emission tomography 2-deoxy-2-[^{18}F]fluoro-D-glucose, 11CO, and ^{15}O-water for monitoring androgen independent prostate cancer. *Mol Imaging Biol* 2003;5:86–93.
53. Logan TF, Jadali F, Egorin MJ, Mintun M, Sashin D, Gooding WE, Choi Y, Bishop H, Trump DL, Gardner D, Kirkwood J, Vlock D, Johnson C. Decreased tumor blood flow as measured by positron emission tomography in cancer patients treated with interleukin-1 and carboplatin on a phase I trial. *Cancer Chemother Pharmacol* 2002;50:433–444.
54. Herbst RS, Mullani NA, Davis DW, Hess KR, McConkey DJ, Charnsangavej C, O'Reilly MS, Kim HW, Baker C, Roach J, Ellis LM, Rashid A, Pluda J, Bucana C, Madden TL, Tran HT, Abbruzzese JL. Development of biologic markers of response and assessment of antiangiogenic activity in a clinical trial of human recombinant endostatin. *J Clin Oncol* 2002;20 3804–3814.
55. Hanahan D, Weinberg RA. The hallmarks of cancer. *Cell* 2000;100:57–70.
56. Simon LM, Robin ED, Theodore J. Differences in oxygen-dependent regulation of enzymes between tumor and normal cell systems in culture. *J Cell Physiol* 1981;108:393–400.
57. Thomlinson RH, Gray LH. The histological structure of some human lung cancers and the possible implications for radiotherapy. *Br J Cancer* 1955;9:537–549.
58. Bhujwalla ZM, Artemov D, Aboagye E, Ackerstaff E, Gillies RJ, Natarajan K, Solaiyappan M. The physiological environment in cancer vascularization, invasion and metastasis. *Novartis Found Symp* 2001;240:23–38; discussion 38–45, 152–153.
59. Folkman J. Tumor angiogenesis. *Adv Cancer Res* 1974;19:331–358.
60. Rajendran JG, O'Sullivan F, Peterson LM, Schwartz DL, Conrad EU, Spence AM, Muzi M, Farwell DG, Krohn K. Hypoxia and glucose metabolism in malignant tumors: Evaluation by FMISO and FDG PET imaging. *Clin Cancer Res* 2004;10:2245–2252.
61. Scanduro AB, Weldon CW, Figueroa YG, Alam J, Beckman BS. Gene microarray analysis reveals a novel hypoxia signal transduction pathway in human hepatocellular carcinoma cells. *Int J Oncol* 2001;19:129–135.
62. Villaret DB, Wang T, Dillon D, Xu J, Sivam D, Cheever MA, Reed SG. Identification of genes overexpressed in head and neck squamous cell carcinoma using a combination of complementary DNA subtraction and microarray analysis. *Laryngoscope* 2000;110:374–381.
63. Agani F, Semenza GL. Mersalyl is a novel inducer of vascular endothelial growth factor gene expression and hypoxia-inducible factor 1 activity. *Mol Pharmacol* 1998;54:49–54.
64. Bae MK, Kwon YW, Kim MS, Bae SK, Bae MH, Lee YM, Kim YJ, Kim KW. Identification of genes differentially expressed by hypoxia in hepatocellular carcinoma cells. *Biochem Biophys Res Commun* 1998;243:158–162.
65. Dachs GU, Tozer GM. Hypoxia modulated gene expression: Angiogenesis, metastasis and therapeutic exploitation. *Eur J Cancer* 2000;36:1649–1660.
66. Eisma RJ, Spiro JD, Kreutzer DL. Vascular endothelial growth factor expression in head and neck squamous cell carcinoma. *Am J Surg* 1997;174:513–517.
67. Hockel M, Schlenger K, Hockel S, Vaupel P. Hypoxic cervical cancers with low apoptotic index are highly aggressive. *Cancer Res* 1999;59:4525–4528.
68. Guillemin K, Krasnoq MA. The hypoxic response: Huffing and HIFing. *Cell* 1997;89:9–12.
69. Jiang BH, Semenza GL, Bauer C, Marti HH. Hypoxia-inducible factor 1 levels vary exponentially over a physiologically relevant range of O_2 tension. *Am J Physiol* 1996;271:C1172–C1180.
70. Clavo AC, Wahl RL. Effects of hypoxia on the uptake of tritiated thymidine, L-leucine, L-methionine and FDG in cultured cancer cells. *J Nucl Med* 1996;37:502–506.
71. Burgman P, Odonoghue JA, Humm JL, Ling CC. Hypoxia-induced increase in FDG uptake in MCF7 cells. *J Nucl Med* 2001;42:170–175.
72. Hwang DY, Ismail-Beigi F. Glucose uptake and lactate production in cells exposed to CoCl(2) and in cells overexpressing the Glut-1 glucose transporter. *Arch Biochem Biophys* 2002;399:206–211.
73. Ivan M, Kondo K, Yang H, Kim W, Valiando J, Ohh M, Salic A, Asara JM, Lane WS, Kaelin WG Jr. HIFalpha targeted for VHL-mediated destruction by proline hydroxylation: Implications for O_2 sensing. *Science* 2001;292:464–468.
74. Huang LE, Arany Z, Livingston D.M, Bunn HF. Activation of hypoxia-inducible transcription factor depends primarily upon redox-sensitive stabilization of its alpha subunit. *J Biol Chem* 1996; 271:32253–32259.

75. Guillemin K, Krasnow MA. The hypoxic response: Huffing and HIFing. *Cell* 1997;89:9–12.
76. Bos R, Zhong H, Hanrahan CF, Mommers EC, Semenza GL, Pinedo HM, Abeloff MD, Simons JW, van Diest PJ, van der Wall E. Levels of hypoxia-inducible factor-1 alpha during breast carcinogenesis. *J Natl Cancer Inst* 2001;93:309–314.
77. Zhong H, De Marzo AM, Laughner E, Lim M, Hilton DA, Zagzag D, Buechler P, Isaacs WB, Semenza GL, Simons JW. Overexpression of hypoxia-inducible factor 1alpha in common human cancers and their metastases. *Cancer Res* 1999;59:5830–5835.
78. Marxsen JH, Schmitt O, Metzen E, Jelkmann W, Hellwig-Burgel T. Vascular endothelial growth factor gene expression in the human breast cancer cell line MX-1 is controlled by O_2 availability in vitro and in vivo. *Ann Anat* 2001;183:243–249.
79. Yaziji H, Gown AM. Immunohistochemical analysis of gynecologic tumors. *Int J Gynecol Pathol* 2001;20:64–78.
80. Hall EJ. Radiobiology for the Radiologist. Philadelphia, PA: Lippincott Williams & Wilkins, 2000.
81. Marples B, Greco O, Joiner MC, Scott SD. Molecular approaches to chemo-radiotherapy. *Eur J Cancer* 2002;38:231–239.
82. Overgaard J, Horsman MR. Modification of hypoxia-induced radioresistance in tumors by the use of oxygen and sensitizers. *Semin Radiat Oncol* 1996;6:10–21.
83. Fowler JF. Eighth annual Juan del Regato lecture. Chemical modifiers of radiosensitivity—theory and reality: a review. *Int J Radiat Oncol Biol Phys* 1985;11:665–674.
84. Frommhold H, Guttenberger R, Henke M. The impact of blood hemoglobin content on the outcome of radiotherapy. The Freiburg experience. *Strahlenther Onkol* 1998;174(Suppl 4):31–34.
85. Evans SM, Koch CJ. Prognostic significance of tumor oxygenation in humans. *Cancer Lett* 2003; 195:1–16.
86. Koong AC, Denk NC, Hudson KM, Schindler C, Swiersz L, Koch C, Evans S, Ibrahim H. Le QT, Terris DJ, Giaccia AJ. Candidate genes for the hypoxic tumor phenotype. *Cancer Res* 2000; 60:883–887.
87. Blancher C, Moore JW, Talks KL, Houlbrook S, Harris AL. Relationship of hypoxia-inducible factor (HIF)-1alpha and HIF-2alpha expression to vascular endothelial growth factor induction and hypoxia survival in human breast cancer cell lines. *Cancer Res* 2000;60:7106–7113.
88. Sutherland RM. Tumor hypoxia and gene expression—implications for malignant progression and therapy. *Acta Oncol* 1998;37:567–574.
89. Amellem O, Pettersen EO. Cell inactivation and cell cycle inhibition as induced by extreme hypoxia: The possible role of cell cycle arrest as a protection against hypoxia-induced lethal damage. *Cell Prolif* 1991;24:127–141.
90. Moulder JE, Rockwell S. Tumor hypoxia: Its impact on cancer therapy. *Cancer Metastasis Rev* 1987; 5:313–341.
91. Brown MJ. The hypoxic cell: A target for selective cancer therapy—Eighteenth Bruce F. Cain memorial award lecture. *Cancer Res* 1999;59:5863–70.
92. Hockel M, Schlenger K, Knoop C, Vaupel P. Oxygenation of carcinoma of the uterine cervix: Evaluation by computerized oxygen tension measurements. *Cancer Res* 1991;51:6098–6102.
93. Koh WJ, Bergman KS, Rasey JS, Peterson LM, Evans ML, Graham MM, Grierson JR, Lindsley KL, Lewellen TK, Krohn KA, et al. Evaluation of oxygenation status during fractionated radiotherapy in human nonsmall cell lung cancers using [F-18]fluoromisonidazole positron emission tomography. *Int J Radiat Oncol Biol Phys* 1995;33:391–398.
94. Rajendran JG, Wilson D, Conrad EU, Peterson LM, Bruckner JD, Rasey JS, Chin LK, Hofstrand PD, Grierson JR, Eary JF, Krohn KA. F-18 FMISO and F-18 FDG PET imaging in soft tissue sarcomas: Correlation of hypoxia, metabolism and VEGF expression. *Eur J Nuc Med* 2003; 30:695–704.
95. Rajendran JGNP, Peterson LM, Schwartz DL, Scharnhrost J, Conrad EU, Grierson JR, Krohn KA. F-18 FMISO PET tumor hypoxia imaging: Investigating the tumor volume-hypoxia connection. *J Nucl Med* 2003;44:1340, 1376P.
96. Adam M, Gabalski EC, Bloch DA, Ochlert JW, Brown JM, Elsaid AA, Pinto HA, Terris DJ. Tissue oxygen distribution in head and neck cancer patients. *Head Neck* 1999;21:146–153.
97. Blancher C, Harris AL. The molecular basis of the hypoxia response pathway: Tumour hypoxia as a therapy target. *Cancer Metastasis Rev* 1998;17:187–194.
98. Brown JM. Exploiting the hypoxic cancer cell: Mechanisms and therapeutic strategies. *Mol Med Today* 2000;6:157–162.

99. Rajendran JGMJ, Schwartz DL, Kinahan PE, Cheng P, Hummel SM, Lewellen B, Philips M, Krohn KA. Imaging with F-18 FMISO-PET permits hypoxia directed radiotherapy dose escalation for head and neck cancer. *J Nucl Med* 2003;44:415, 127P.
100. Chao KS, Bosch WR, Mutic S, Lewis JS, Dehdashti F, Mintun MA, Dempsey JF, Perez CA, Purdy JA, Welch MJ. A novel approach to overcome hypoxic tumor resistance: Cu-ATSM-guided intensity-modulated radiation therapy. *Int J Radiat Oncol Biol Phys* 2001;49:1171–1182.
101. Lee DJ, Moini M, Giuliano J, Westra WH. Hypoxic sensitizer and cytotoxin for head and neck cancer. *Ann Acad Med Singapore* 1996;25:397–404.
102. Sartorelli AC, Hodnick WF. Mitomycin C: A prototype bioreductive agent. *Oncol Res* 1994;6:501–508.
103. Denny WA, Wilson WR. Tirapazamine: A bioreductive anticancer drug that exploits tumour hypoxia. *Expert Opin Investig Drugs* 2000;9:2889–2901.
104. von Pawel J, von Roemeling R, Gatzemeier U, Boyer M, Elisson LO, Clark P, Talbot D, Rey A, Butler TW, Hirsh V, Olver I, Bergman B, Ayoub J, Richardson G, Dunlop D, Arcenas A, Vescio R, Viallet J, Treat J. Tirapazamine plus cisplatin versus cisplatin in advanced non-small-cell lung cancer: A report of the international CATAPULT I study group. Cisplatin and Tirapazamine in Subjects with Advanced Previously Untreated Non-Small-Cell Lung Tumors. *J Clin Oncol* 2000;18:1351–1359.
105. Rischin D, Peters L, Hicks R, Hughes P, Fisher R, Hart R, Sexton M, D'Costa I, von Roemeling R. Phase I trial of concurrent tirapazamine, cisplatin, and radiotherapy in patients with advanced head and neck cancer. *J Clin Oncol* 2001;19:535–542.
106. Vordermark D, Brown JM. Endogenous markers of tumor hypoxia predictors of clinical radiation resistance? *Strahlenther Onkol* 2003;179:801–811.
107. Hockel M, Schlenger K, Knoop C, Vaupel P. Oxygenation of carcinomas of the uterine cervix: Evaluation by computerized O_2 tension measurments. *Cancer Res* 1991;51:6098–6102.
108. Brizel DM, Sibley GS, Prosnitz LR, Scher RL, Dewhirst MW. Tumor hypoxia adversely affects the prognosis of carcinoma of the head and neck. *Int J Radat Oncol Biol Phys* 1997;38:285–289.
109. Lartigau E, Lusinchi A, Weeger P, Wibault P, Luboinski B, Eschwege F, Guichard M. Variations in tumour oxygen tension (pO_2) during accelerated radiotherapy of head and neck carcinoma. *Eur J Cancer* 1998;34:856–861.
110. Ng PRJ, Peterson LM, Schwartz DL, Scharnhrost J, Krohn KA. Can F-18 fluoromisonidazole PET imaging predict treatment response in head and neck cancer? *J Nucl Med* 2003;44:416, 128P.
111. Muzi M, Spence AM, Rajendran JG, Grierson JR, Krohn KA. Glioma patients assessed with FMISO and FDG: Two tracers provide different information. *J Nucl Med* 2003;44:878, 243P.
112. Valk P, Mathis C, Prados M, Gilbert J, Budinger T. Hypoxia in human gliomas: Demonstration by PET with flouorine-18-fluoromisonidazole. *J Nucl Med* 1992;33:2133–2137.
113. Rajendran J, Peterson L, Schwartz DS, Muzi M, Scharnhorst JD, Eary JF, Krohn KA. [F-18] FMISO PET hypoxia imaging in head and neck cancer: Heterogeneity in hypoxia—primary tumor vs lymph nodal metastases. *J Nucl Med* 2002;43:73P.
114. Stone HB, Brown JM, Phillips TL, Sutherland RM. Oxygen in human tumors: Correlations between methods of measurement and response to therapy. Summary of a workshop held November 19–20, 1992, at the National Cancer Institute, Bethesda, Maryland. *Radiat Res* 1993;136:422–434.
115. Hockel M, Vaupel, P. Tumor hypoxia: Definitions and current clinical, biologic, and molecular aspects. *J Natl Cancer Inst* 2001;93:266–276.
116. Rasey JS, Casciari JJ, Hofstrand PD, Muzi M, Graham MM, Chin LK. Determining hypoxic fraction in a rat glioma by uptake of radiolabeled fluoromisonidazole. *Radiat Res* 2000;153:84–92.
117. Vaupel P, Kelleher DK, Hockel M. Oxygen status of malignant tumors: Pathogenesis of hypoxia and significance for tumor therapy. *Semin Oncol* 2001;28:29–35.
118. Nozue M, Lee I, Yuan F, *et al*. Interlaboratory variation in oxygen tension measurement by Eppendorf "histograph" and comparision withhypoxic marker. *J Surg Oncol* 1997;66:30–38.
119. Lartigau E, Le Ridant AM, Lambin P, Weeger P, Martin L, Sigal R, Lusinchi A, Luboinski B, Eschwege F, Guichard M. Oxygenation of head and neck tumors. *Cancer* 1993;71:2319–2325.
120. Brizel DM, Rosner GL, Harrelson J, Prosnitz LR, Dewhirst MW. Pretreatment oxygenation profiles of human soft tissue sarcomas. *Int J Radiation Oncol Biol Phys* 1994;30:635–642.
121. Prekeges JL, Rasey JS, Grunbaum Z, Krohn KH. Reduction of fluoromisonidazole, a new imaging agent for hypoxia. *Biochem Pharmacol* 1991;42:2387–2395.
122. Chapman JD, Engelhardt EL, Stobbe CC, Schneider RF, Hanks GE. Measuring hypoxia and predicting tumor radioresistance with nuclear medicine assays. *Radiother Oncol* 1998;46:229–237.

123. Grierson JR, Link JM, Mathis CA, Rasey JS, Krohn KA. Radiosynthesis of of fluorine-18 fluoromisonidazole. *J Nucl Med* 1989;30:343–350.
124. Rasey JS, Koh WJ, Evans ML, Peterson LM, Lewellen TK, Graham MM, Krohn KA. Quantifying regional hypoxia in human tumors with positron emission tomography of [^{18}F]fluoromisonidazole: A pretherapy study of 37 patients. *Int J Radiat Oncol Biol Phys* 1996;36:417–428.
125. Rajendran JG, Mankoff DA, O'Sullivan F, Peterson LM, Schwartz DL, Conrad EU, Spence AM, Muzi M, Farwell DG, Krohn KA. Hypoxia and glucose metabolism in malignant tumors: Evaluation by [(18)f]fluoromisonidazole and [(18)f]fluorodeoxyglucose positron emission tomography imaging. *Clin Cancer Res* 2004;10:2245–2252.
126. Liu RS, Chu LS, Yen SH, Chang CP, Chou KL, Wu LC, Chang CW, Lui MT, Chen KY, Yeh SH. Detection of anaerobic odontogenic infections by fluorine-18 fluoromisonidazole. *Eur J Nucl Med* 1996;23:1384–1387.
127. Bentzen L, Keiding S, Horsman MR, Falborg L, Hansen SB, Overgaard J. Feasibility of detecting hypoxia in experimental mouse tumours with 18F-fluorinated tracers and positron emission tomography—a study evaluating [18F]fluoro-2-deoxy-D-glucose. *Acta Oncol* 2000;39:629–637.
128. Read SJ, Hirano T, Abbott DF, Sachinidis JI, Tochon-Danguy HJ, Chan JG, Egan GF, Scott AM, Bladin CF, McKay WJ, Donnan GA. Identifying hypoxic tissue after acute ischemic stroke using PET and 18F-fluoromisonidazole. *Neurology* 1998;51:1617–1621.
129. Yeh SH, Liu RS, Wu LC, Yang DJ, Yen SH, Chang CW, Yu TW, Chou KL, Chen KY. Fluorine-18 fluoromisonidazole tumour to muscle retention ratio for the detection of hypoxia in nasopharyngeal carcinoma. *Eur J Nucl Med* 1996;23:1378–1383.
130. Dubois L, Landuyt W, Haustermans K, Dupont P, Bormans G, Vermaelen P, Flamen P, Verbeken E, Mortelmans L. Evaluation of hypoxia in an experimental rat tumour model by [(18)F]fluoromisonidazole PET and immunohistochemistry. *Br J Cancer* 2004;91:1947–1954.
131. Graham MM, Peterson LM, Link JM, Evans ML, Rasey JS, Koh WJ, Caldwell JH, Krohn KA. Fluorine-18-fluoromisonidazole radiation dosimetry in imaging studies. *J Nucl Med* 1997;38:1631–1636.
132. Rasey JS, Koh WJ, Grierson JR, Grunbaum Z, Krohn KA. Radiolabelled fluoromisonidazole as an imaging agent for tumor hypoxia. *Int J Radiat Oncol Biol Phys* 1989;17:985–991.
133. Martin GV, Caldwell JH, Graham MM, Grierson JR, Kroll K, Cowan MJ, Lewellen TK, Rasey JS, Casciari JJ, Krohn KA. Noninvasive detection of hypoxic myocardium using fluorine-18-fluoromisonidazole and positron emission tomography. *J Nucl Med* 1992;33:2202–2208.
134. Koh WJ, Rasey JS, Evans ML, Grierson JR, Lewellen TK, Graham MM, Krohn KA, Griffin TW. Imaging of hypoxia in human tumors with [F-18]fluoromisonidazole. *Int J Radiat Oncol Biol Phys* 1992;22:199–212.
135. Chapman JD, Schneider RF, Urbain JL, Hanks GE. Single-photon emission computed tomography and positron-emission tomography assays for tissue oxygenation. *Semin Radiat Oncol* 2001;11:47–57.
136. Nunn A, Linder K, Strauss HW. Nitroimidazoles and imaging hypoxia. *Eur J Nucl Med* 1995;22:265–280.
137. Biskupiak JE, Krohn KA. Second generation hypoxia imaging agents [editorial; comment]. *J Nucl Med* 1993;34:411–413.
138. Kachur AV, Dolbier WR Jr, Evans SM, Shiue CY, Shiue GG, Skov KA, Baird IR, James BR, Li AR, Roche A, Koch CJ. Synthesis of new hypoxia markers EF1 and [^{18}F]-EF1. *Appl Radiat Isot* 1999;51:643–650.
139. Tewson TJ. Synthesis of [^{18}F]fluoroetanidazole: A potential new tracer for imaging hypoxia. *Nucl Med Biol* 1997;24:755–760.
140. Wiebe LI, Stypinski D. Pharmacokinetics of SPECT radiopharmaceuticals for imaging hypoxic tissues. *Q J Nucl Med* 1996;40:270–284.
141. Siim BG, Laux WT, Rutland MD, Palmer BN, Wilson WR. Scintigraphic imaging of the hypoxia marker (99m)technetium-labeled 2,2'-(1,4-diaminobutane)bis(2-methyl-3-butanone) dioxime (99mTc-labeled HL-91; prognox): Noninvasive detection of tumor response to the antivascular agent 5,6-dimethylxanthenone-4-acetic acid. *Cancer Res* 2000;60:4582–4588.
142. Rumsey WL, Kuczynski B, Patel B, Bauer A, Narra R.K, Eaton SM, Nunn AD, Strauss HW. SPECT imaging of ischemic myocardium using a technetium-99m-nitroimidazole ligand. *J Nucl Med* 1995;36:1445–1450.

143. Stypinski D, Wiebe LI, McEwan AJ, Schmidt RP, Tam YK, Mercer JR. Clinical pharmacokinetics of ^{123}I-IAZA in healthy volunteers. *Nucl Med Commun* 1999;20:559–667.
144. Shelton ME, Green MA, Mathias CJ, Welch MJ, Bergmann SR. Assessment of regional myocardial and renal blood flow with copper-PTSM and positron emission tomography. *Circulation* 1990; 82:990–997.
145. Lewis JS, McCarthy DW, McCarthy TJ, Fujibayashi Y, Welch MJ. Evaluation of Cu-64-ATSM in vitro and in vivo in a hypoxic model. *J Nucl Med* 1999;40:177–183.
146. Dehdashti F, Mintun MA, Lewis JS, Bradley J, Govindan R, Laforest R, Welch MJ, Siegel BA. In vivo assessment of tumor hypoxia in lung cancer with 60Cu-ATSM. *Eur J Nucl Med Mol Imaging* 2003;30:844–850.
147. Fujibayashi Y, Taniuchi H, Yonekura Y, Ohtani H, Konishi J, Yokoyama A. Copper-62-ATSM: A new hypoxia imaging agent with high membrane permeability and low redox potential. *J Nucl Med* 1997;38:1155–1160.
148. Ballinger JR. Imaging hypoxia in tumors. *Semin Nucl Med* 2001;31:321–329.
149. Gabalski EC, Adam M, Pinto H, Brown JM, Bloch DA, Terris DJ. Pretreatment and midtreatment measurement of oxygen tension levels in head and neck cancers. *Laryngoscope* 1998;108: 1856–1860.
150. Klabbers BM, Lammertsma AA, Slotman BJ. The value of positron emission tomography for monitoring response to radiotherapy in head and neck cancer. *Mol Imaging Biol* 2003;5:257–270.
151. Alber M, Paulsen F, Eschmann SM, Machulla HJ. On biologically conformal boost dose optimization. *Phys Med Biol* 2003;48:N31–N35.
152. Buatti J, Yao M, Dornfeld K, Skwarchuk M, Hoffman HT, Funk GF, Smith RB, Graham SM, Menda Y, Graham MM. Efficacy of IMRT in head and neck cancer as monitored by post-RT PET scans. *Int J Radiat Oncol Biol Phys* 2003;57:S305.
153. Ling CC, Humm J, Larson S, Amols H, Fuks Z, Leibel S, Koutcher JA. Towards multidimensional radiotherapy (MD-CRT): Biological imaging and biological conformality. *Int J Radiat Oncol Biol Phys* 2000;47:551–60.
154. Peters LJ. Targeting hypoxia in head and neck cancer. *Acta Oncol* 2001;40:937–940.
155. Solomon B, McArthur G, Cullinane C, Zalcberg J, Hicks R. Applications of positron emission tomography in the development of molecular targeted cancer therapeutics. *BioDrugs* 2003; 17:339–354.
156. Klimas MT. Positron emission tomography and drug discovery: Contributions to the understanding of pharmacokinetics, mechanism of action and disease state characterization. *Mol Imaging Biol* 2002;4:311–337.
157. Hammond LA, Denis L, Salman U, Jerabek P, Thomas CR Jr, Kuhn JG. Positron emission tomography (PET): Expanding the horizons of oncology drug development. *Invest New Drugs* 2003;21:309–340.

5 Magnetic Resonance Measurement of Tumor Perfusion and Vascularity

Jeffrey L. Evelhoch, PhD

CONTENTS

INTRODUCTION
DEUTERIUM MAGNETIC RESONANCE IMAGING
CONTRAST AGENT-BASED MAGNETIC RESONANCE

1. INTRODUCTION

Several approaches to magnetic resonance (MR) measurements of tumor perfusion (i.e., the nutritive blood flux through tissues at the capillary level, alternatively termed tumor blood flow) and other properties of the tumor vasculature have been used in both preclinical and clinical studies. This chapter will first describe the principal approaches that have been used for measuring tumor perfusion and vascularity, including the data analysis methods used to extract quantitative information relating to the underlying tumor physiology. The remainder of the chapter will focus on dynamic contrast-enhanced MRI (DCE-MRI), which is currently the most widely used of these approaches. The methodological considerations for data acquisition, consensus approaches for data analysis, potential advances in DCE-MRI, and applications representative of how it is being used in drug development will be considered.

2. DEUTERIUM MAGNETIC RESONANCE IMAGING

2.1 General Approaches

In the late 1980s, deuterium MR spectroscopy (MRS) or imaging (MRI) was used to follow the clearance of deuterium-enriched water (D_2O) after direct injection into rodent tumors *(1)*. Outside of the brain, where the blood–brain barrier limits the exchange of most diffusible tracers between blood and tissue, the tissue–blood exchange of water is limited only by its supply to the tissue via perfusion (flow limited), so the injected D_2O is cleared from the tumor at a rate determined by the tumor perfusion. Since the MR signal observed is directly proportional to the concentration of HDO (formed by proton-deuteron exchange with water), the principles developed for external

From: *Cancer Drug Discovery and Development
In Vivo Imaging of Cancer Therapy*
Edited by: A.F. Shields and P. Price © Humana Press Inc., Totowa, NJ

residue detection *(2, 3)* can be applied to determine perfusion directly *(4)*. However, the data fitted to these models must be limited to the earliest times after injection (i.e., prior to HDO recirculation) or fit to a two-compartment model accounting for recirculation from the body *(1)*. In addition to perturbing the vasculature when the water is injected, these perfusion measurements reflect only the local region surrounding the injection site *(5)*.

To address these limitations, an alternate "uptake" approach using deuterium MRS or MRI to follow the increase in HDO in the tumor after intravenous D_2O injection was introduced in 1991 *(6, 7)*. Due to the difficulty in obtaining a pure blood signal via deuterium MRI, the initial area under the curve (IAUC) method introduced for positron emission tomography (PET) measurements of perfusion using $H_2^{15}O$ *(8)* was adapted to measure relative tumor blood flow *(6)*. Tumor perfusion estimated with this technique using an appropriate common arterial input function correlates highly with that measured by the microsphere method *(9, 10)*, yielding no significant differences *(11)*.

2.2 Applications

Both the clearance and uptake approaches have been used in a variety of preclinical studies. For example, the uptake approach was used to provide the first evidence that flavone acetic, a predecessor to 5,6-dimethylxanthenone-4-acetic acid [DMXAA, studied in the clinic using DCE-MRI *(12)*] with a broad spectrum of preclinical antitumor efficacy, but a narrow therapeutic window that precluded its use clinically, acted by destroying the tumor vasculature *(13)*. However, due to the low MR sensitivity of deuterium relative to protons, its potential for toxicity with accumulating HDO after multiple perfusion measurements, and its lack of deuterium observation capability on standard clinical scanners, these methods were never translated into humans.

3. CONTRAST AGENT-BASED MAGNETIC RESONANCE

3.1 Effects on Magnetic Resonance Signal

Characterization of tumor vasculature with MR contrast agents most commonly uses low-molecular-weight (<1000 g) paramagnetic gadolinium (III) chelates that extravasate in the absence of a blood–brain barrier, but cannot permeate viable cell membranes *(14)*. These contrast agents, which are extensively used in clinical radiology, alter the MR signal due to their effect on the relaxation processes of tissue water protons. The unpaired electrons in these contrast agents provide an efficient mechanism for spin-lattice relaxation of water protons when the water molecule binds in the first or second coordination sphere of the contrast agent complex *(15)*. As a consequence, the spin-lattice relaxation rate (R_1, the reciprocal of the first-order time constant for spin-lattice relaxation, T_1) is decreased in proportion to the contrast agent concentration *(16)*. The decreased R_1 leads to an increase in MRI signal intensity, which, if the MRI acquisition parameters are selected judiciously (see Fig. 1), increases linearly in proportion to the contrast agent concentration. This effect of low-molecular-weight Gd(III)-based contrast agents on R_1 is the basis for DCE-MRI, the most commonly used method for clinical assessment of the effects of anticancer treatment on tumor vasculature.

Chapter 5 / MR Measurement of Tumor Perfusion and Vascularity

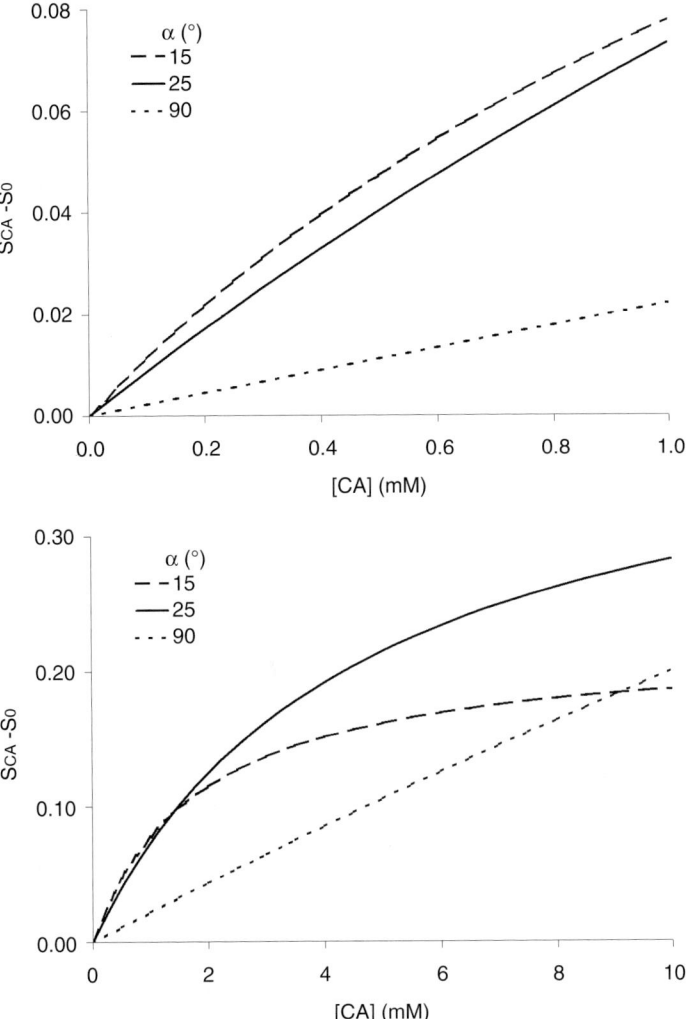

Fig. 1. Impact of acquisition parameters on the relationship between contrast agent concentration ([CA]) and increase in signal due to contrast agent ($S_{CA} - S_0$). Plots show relationships for a 5 msec repetition time, 750 msec T_1, and three flip angles (α). A 15° flip angle provides the greatest sensitivity over the range of [CA] likely to be found in tissues (top plot), but a 90° flip angle provides a linear relationship between [CA] and signal increase to much higher [CA], including that likely to be observed in blood (bottom plot). Note, a 25° flip angle results in a small loss in signal increase at [CA] < 1 mM, and a nearly linear relationship up to 4 mM [CA], thus providing a reasonable compromise.

If the MR contrast agent remains concentrated within the vasculature, the magnetic susceptibility of the blood is increased relative to the surrounding tissue leading to a local loss of signal, commonly referred to as T_2^* relaxation. The concentration difference between blood and surrounding tissue resulting in substantial T_2^* relaxation is seldom observed in tumors with low-molecular-weight Gd chelates. However, it is evident in regions with an intact blood–brain barrier and for either high-molecular-weight Gd chelates or another class of contrast agents known as superparamagnetic iron oxide nonoparticles. While this effect can be used to characterize vasculature using an approach known as dynamic susceptibility contrast MRI *(17)*, the contrast agents required are not readily available for clinical use and this approach is not commonly used outside the brain. Hence, the remainder of this chapter will focus on DCE-MRI.

3.2 Dynamic Contrast-Enhanced Magnetic Resonance Imaging Protocol

Dynamic contrast-enhanced MRS involves acquisition of a series of T_1-weighted images before, during, and after bolus intravenous injection of a of low-molecular-weight Gd(III)-based contrast agent. The oncology DCE-MRI community has established and updated consensus recommendations for acquisition and analysis of DCE-MRI data for oncology applications in general *(18)*, and more recently for early clinical trials of anticancer therapeutics affecting tumor vascular function *(19, 20)*. Specific recommendations have been made for the type of measurement, images to be acquired before contrast injection, requirements for contrast agent injection, the dynamic acquisition protocol, primary endpoints, measurement requirements for the primary and secondary end points, trial design, nomenclature, image analysis, data reduction, and the definition of region of interest. The most recent recommendations are available at the National Cancer Institute Cancer Imaging Program website *(21)* and will be published in greater detail in the magnetic resonance literature in the near future. Since these recommendations provide sufficient guidance to the practical aspects of successfully implementing DCE-MRI to measure the effects of anticancer treatment on tumor vasculature, the remainder of this section will provide some background relevant to understanding both the basis for these recommendations and how ongoing research may impact this approach in the future.

3.3 Dynamic Contrast-Enhanced Magnetic Resonance Imaging Background

3.3.1 Relation to Physiology

The change in signal over time measured by DCE-MRI reflects the exchange of contrast agent between vascular space and, since the contrast agent does not penetrate viable cells, extravascular–extracellular space. That exchange depends upon the capillary blood flow (F), capillary permeability-surface area product (PS), contrast agent distribution volume [V_d, which is commonly assumed to equal the fractional volume of extravascular–extracellular space, V_e *(22)*] and the blood contrast agent concentration as a function of time *(23)*. The tumor (and blood) contrast agent concentration is inferred from the magnitude of the signal change (see Section 3.1) and parameters reflecting the underlying vascular physiology are derived using various analytical approaches *(20)*. The two primary endpoints recommended for early phase trials of anticancer therapeutics *(20)* are the transfer constant [K^{trans}, *(22)*] and the IAUC (contrast agent concentration–time curve) *(24)*. K^{trans}, which requires fitting the contrast–time curve to a two-compartment model, reflects contrast delivery (F) and transport across the vascular endothelium (PS). The relative impact of F and PS depends on the specific values of F and PS unless F is much greater than PS (tissue–blood exchange is permeability limited, K^{trans} reflects PS only) or vice versa (tissue–blood exchange is flow limited, K^{trans} reflects only F; see Fig. 2). Fitting the contrast concentration time

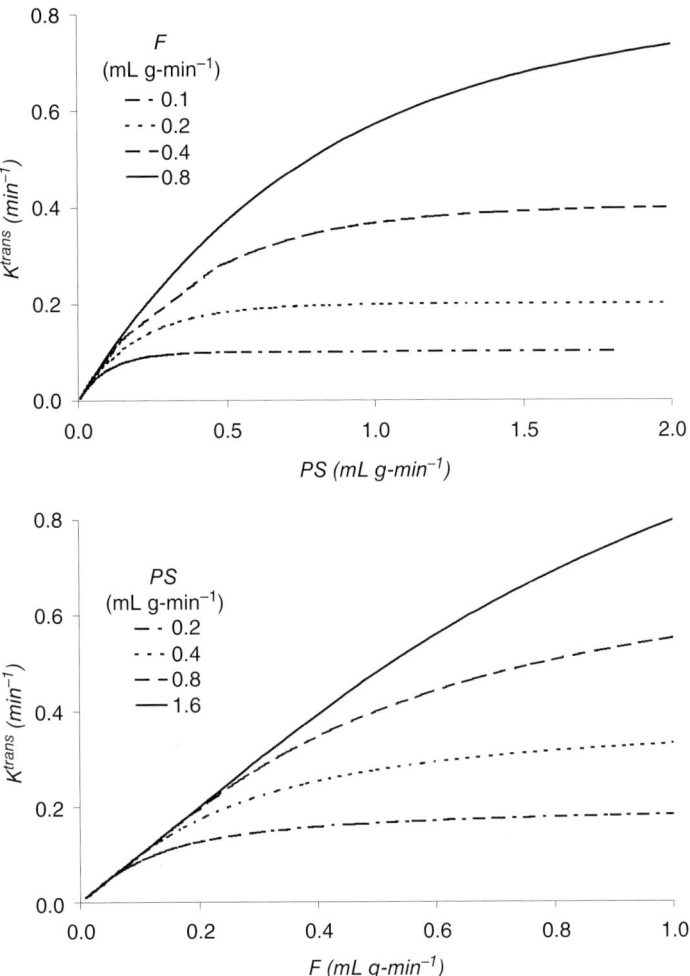

Fig. 2. Relationships among K^{trans}, permeability-surface area product (PS) and flow (F) based on a two-compartment model [tissue and blood *(22, 23)*]. The top figure shows dependence of K^{trans} on PS for fixed F and the bottom figure shows dependence of K^{trans} on F for fixed PS. Note that K^{trans} is limited by the fixed variable and is linearly related to the nonfixed variable at low K^{trans}. This corresponds to a flow-limited exchange of contrast agent between blood and tissue when $PS/F \gg 1$ and permeability-limited exchange when $PS/F \ll 1$.

curve also provides a measure of V_d; *IAUC*, which does not require a model, reflects V_d in addition to F and PS (see Fig. 3).

It should be noted that the assumption that V_d is equivalent to V_e has not been tested. For measurements of V_e with radiolabeled EDTA (e.g., ^{51}Cr-EDTA, note that the extravascular–extracellular space is also referred to as interstitial space in the physiology literature), at least 30–60 min are allowed for the EDTA to distribute throughout interstitial space *(25)*. Moreover, additional procedures such as constant infusion *(26)* or, in animals, renal ligature *(27)* are often used to ensure that radiolabeled EDTA distributes throughout the interstitial space. Given the similarity of the chelating agents EDTA and DTPA, the contrast agent may reach tumor extravascular–extracellular space in close

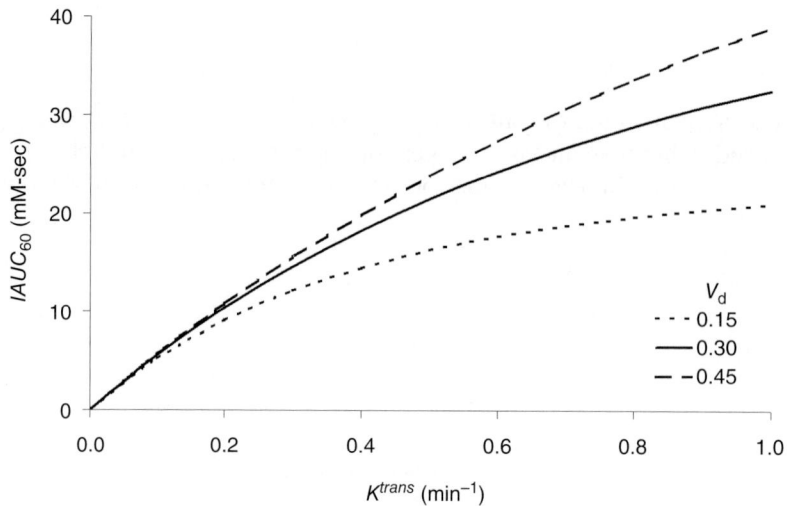

Fig. 3. The relationship between *IAUC* and K^{trans} also depends on the volume of contrast agent distribution (V_d). The initial area under the contrast–time curve for the first 60 sec after bolus arrival ($IAUC_{60}$) increases with K^{trans} over the range likely to be observed in tumors. However, that relationship also depends on V_d, which is particularly evident at low V_d.

proximity to the vasculature during data acquisition only in typical DCE-MRI experiments (<10 min). Hence, in regions with low vascular density, V_d may underestimate the true V_e. This is consistent with the 2- to 3-fold lower V_e reported for rodent tumor core than in the (better perfused) rim *(28)*.

3.3.2 Change Measurement

In consideration of the relation to physiology discussed above, treatment-induced changes in K^{trans} can reflect changes in *F* and/or *PS*, while changes in *IAUC* can reflect changes in V_d as well as *F* and/or *PS*. As illustrated in Fig. 4, unless contrast agent exchange is flow or permeability limited, a 50% reduction in K^{trans} requires either a greater than 50% reduction in one of the variables or a change in both *F* and *PS*. A comparison of the time- and dose-dependent changes in K^{trans}, *IAUC*, and *F* [measured using the freely diffusible radiotracer, iodoantipyrene *(29)*] induced by the vascular targeting agent combretastatin A-4 3-O-phosphate (CA-4-P) investigated the relationship to *F* in rodent tumors *(30)*. Dose- and time-dependent changes in both K^{trans} and *IAUC* were very similar to those measured in independent animals for *F*, but as expected by the simulations summarized in Fig. 4, the magnitudes of the changes were greater for *F*. A sense of the relative importance of changes in V_d for antiangiogenic therapy can be gained by comparing treatment-induced changes in K^{trans} and *IAUC* observed in phase 1 patients 2 days after starting treatment with the novel multityrosine kinase inhibitor, AG-013736 *(31)*. As evident in Fig. 5, there is a strong one-to-one relationship between the changes in K^{trans} and *IAUC* suggesting that there is little contribution from altered V_d for this agent shortly after the start of treatment.

3.3.3 Input Function

The importance of the accounting for differences in the blood contrast concentration–time curve (commonly referred to as the input function) between DCE-MRI measurements is widely recognized *(24)*. In 2001, an approach to identify pixels within the imaged volume reflecting the input function was used to demonstrate its impact experimentally *(32)*. Test–retest data from 11 patients with different types of tumor demonstrated a clear improvement in the reproducibility when individual input functions were used rather than an assumed general input function. Although the test–retest data were not reported in terms of the root mean square coefficient of variability (rms CV), extracted data from the figures suggest a 3-fold improvement [from 25% rms CV with a general input function, which is comparable to other reports where individual input functions were not measured *(33)*, to 8% rms CV with individual input functions]. Also, it should be noted that normalization of the tumor *IAUC* with a reference tissue *(24)*, preferably blood *(34)*, also accounts for variations in the input function.

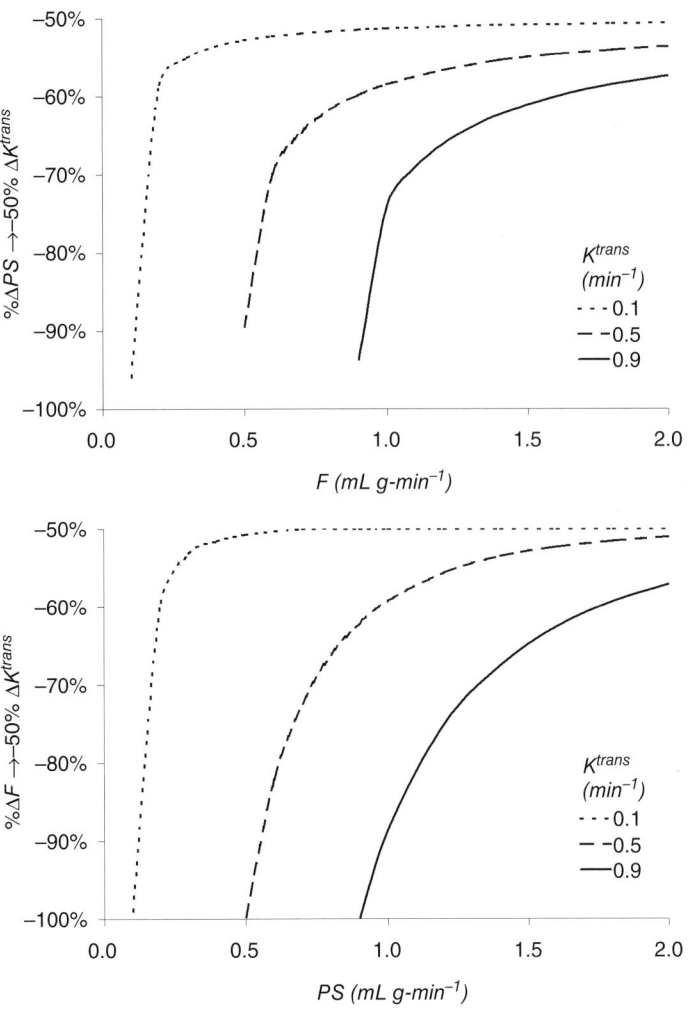

Fig. 4. Relationships among change in *PS* or *F* required for a 50% reduction in K^{trans} as a function of *F* or *PS* for $0.1 \, \text{min}^{-1} < $ initial $K^{trans} < 0.9 \, \text{min}^{-1}$. The top figure shows the change in *F* as a function of *PS* and the bottom figure shows a change in *PS* as a function of *F*. Unless contrast agent exchange is flow or permeability limited, a 50% reduction in K^{trans} requires either a greater than 50% reduction in one of the variables or a change in both *F* and *PS*.

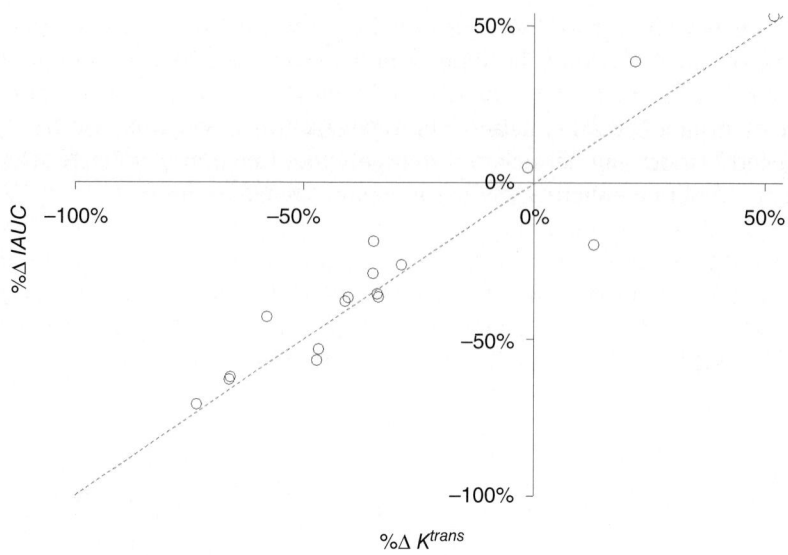

Fig. 5. The relationship between changes measured by *IAUC* and K^{trans} in response to a multityrosine kinase inhibitor and the relationship between the change in *IAUC* and K^{trans} 2 days after treatment with AG-013736 ($N = 17$; Pearson product–moment correlation coefficient = 0.943; two-tailed paired Student's *t* test = 0.6). The dashed line corresponds to a 1:1 relationship.

3.4 Potential Advances in Dynamic Contrast-Enhanced Magnetic Resonance Imaging

3.4.1 Transcytolemmal Water Exchange

With respect to the relationship between signal change and contrast agent concentration, it is commonly assumed that the linear relationship observed between R_1 and contrast agent concentration in homogeneous solutions also applies to biological tissues. However, since contrast agent does not enter viable cells, most tissue water is intracellular, and water molecules must be in direct contact with the contrast agent to alter R_1, this assumption may not be valid *(35)*. The exchange between intracellular and extracellular water would have to be much faster than the difference in R_1 in the presence and absence of contrast agent for all water molecules in the tissue to have equal access to the contrast agent (i.e., equivalent to a homogeneous solution) *(35)*. This is generally not the case after a bolus injection of contrast agent *(36)* resulting in underestimation of contrast agent concentration, which is greatest at highest concentrations *(37)*. As a result, there is a K^{trans}-dependent underestimation of K^{trans} if the rate of exchange between intra- and extracellular spaces is not taken into account. A "shutter-speed" model to account for the effect of transcytolemmal water exchange was introduced in 1999 *(35)* and extended to include a blood compartment in 2005 *(38)*. Of particular interest, when the "shutter-speed" model is applied to DCE-MRI data from patients with breast lesions *(39)*, K^{trans} in an invasive ductal carcinoma increased 3-fold compared to the standard model (from $0.41 \, \text{min}^{-1}$ to $1.22 \, \text{min}^{-1}$), while K^{trans} in a fibroadenoma remained constant ($0.023 \, \text{min}^{-1}$ and $0.024 \, \text{min}^{-1}$). Thus, use of the "shutter-speed" model appears to increase the dynamic range of DCE-MRI considerably.

It should be noted that this approach has been used almost exclusively by the investigators who have developed this model and has not, to the author's knowledge, been applied to data acquired in the context of treatment monitoring. If the data from such studies are of sufficient quality to account for transcytolemmal water exchange and the "shutter-speed" model can be included routinely, the sensitivity of DCE-MRI to treatment effects should be enhanced by the increased dynamic range.

3.4.2 Improved Acquisition Methods

Acquisition of DCE-MRI data requires a tradeoff among spatial resolution (needed to characterize heterogeneous tumor vasculature), temporal resolution [needed to characterize the input function and allow use of sophisticated analytical models *(40, 41)*], and field of view (needed to sample entire tumor or multiple tumors) *(42)*. Over a decade ago, the "keyhole" approach *(43, 44)* was introduced to increase the temporal resolution by dynamically sampling only the center of k-space [an array representing the spatial frequency content of the imaged object into which the MR signals are collected prior to image reconstruction *(45)*]. However, use of the keyhole technique distorts the contrast time course, especially for smaller lesions *(46, 47)*, so its use to assess treatment effects has been limited. A number of alternate approaches for sampling k-space that provide a better compromise between temporal and spatial resolution have been developed *(48–55)*. Some of these approaches [e.g., k-space weighted image contrast or KWIC *(53, 56)*] provide k-space data that can be reconstructed with high temporal resolution or high spatial resolution, thereby maximizing the information content. However, these acquisition and reconstruction methods are not widely available, so their use has been limited to the groups developing these methods thus far.

3.5 Dynamic Contrast-Enhanced Magnetic Resonance Imaging Applications

There are multiple reviews of the applications of DCE-MRI to measure tumor perfusion and vascularity *(57–62)*. Hence, the following is a brief summary of the results from phase 1 clinical trials evaluating the impact of vascular targeted therapies *(63)* on tumor perfusion and vascularity. For VEGF-targeted agents, it appears that a substantial decrease in *F* and/or *PS* is necessary, but not sufficient for a significant reduction in tumor size *(31, 64)*. Interestingly, for vascular disrupting agents, a similar reduction in *F* and/or *PS* is not associated with a reduction in tumor size *(12, 65–67)*. It is also worth noting that initial use of DCE-MRI in phase I studies involved single center studies, at sites with considerable DCE-MRI expertise, raising concern about the ability to use this approach more generally *(68)*. However, one recent study included three centers, without specific DCE-MRI expertise at all sites, demonstrating that the methodology can be standardized to yield consistent results in an early clinical trial at multiple institutions *(69)*.

REFERENCES

1. Kim SG, Ackerman JJ. Multicompartment analysis of blood flow and tissue perfusion employing D2O as a freely diffusible tracer: A novel deuterium NMR technique demonstrated via application with murine RIF-1 tumors. *Magn Reson Med* 1988;8:410–426.
2. Kety SS. Measurement of regional circulation by the local clearance of radioactive sodium. *Am Heart J* 1949;38:321–328.

3. Zierler KL. Equations for measuring blood flow by external monitoring of radioisotopes. *Circ Res* 1965;16:309–321.
4. Ackerman JJ, *et al.* Deuterium nuclear magnetic resonance measurements of blood flow and tissue perfusion employing 2H2O as a freely diffusible tracer. *Proc Natl Acad Sci USA* 1987;84: 4099–4102.
5. Larcombe McDouall JB, Evelhoch JL. Deuterium nuclear magnetic resonance imaging of tracer distribution in D2O clearance measurements of tumor blood flow in mice. *Cancer Res* 1990;50: 363–369.
6. Mattiello J, Evelhoch JL. Relative volume-average murine tumor blood flow measurement via deuterium nuclear magnetic resonance spectroscopy. *Magnet Reson Med* 1991;18:320–334.
7. Evelhoch JL, *et al.* Measurement of relative regional tumor blood flow in mice by deuterium NMR imaging. *Magnet Reson Med* 1992;24:42–52.
8. Herscovitch P, *et al.* Brain blood flow measured with intravenous H2150. I. Theory and error analysis. *J Nucl Med* 1983;24:782–789.
9. Abel FL, *et al.* Use of fluorescent latex microspheres to measure coronary blood flow distribution. *Circ Shock* 1993;41:156–161.
10. Heymann MA, *et al.* Blood flow measurements with radionuclide-labeled particles. *Progr Cardiovasc Dis* 1977;20:55–79.
11. Simpson NE, Evelhoch JL. Deuterium NMR tissue perfusion measurements using the tracer uptake approach: II. Comparison with microspheres in tumors. *Magn Reson Med* 1999;42:240–247.
12. Galbraith SM, *et al.* Effects of 5,6-dimethylxanthenone-4-acetic acid on human tumor microcirculation assessed by dynamic contrast-enhanced magnetic resonance imaging. *J Clin Oncol* 2002;20:3826–3840.
13. Evelhoch JL, *et al.* Flavone acetic acid (NSC 347512)-induced modulation of murine tumor physiology monitored by *in vivo* nuclear magnetic resonance spectroscopy. *Cancer Res* 1988;48: 4749–4755.
14. Mitchell DG. MR imaging contrast agents–what's in a name? *J Magn Reson Imaging* 1997;7:1–4.
15. Springer CS Jr. Physico-chemical principles influencing magnetopharmaceuticals. In: Gillies RJ, ed. NMR in Physiology and Biomedicine. Orlando, FL: Academic Press, Inc., 1994:75–99.
16. Donahue KMB, *et al.* Studies of Gd-DTPA relaxivity and proton exchange rates in tissue. *Magn Reson Med* 1994;32:66–76.
17. Cha S, *et al.* Intracranial mass lesions: Dynamic contrast-enhanced susceptibility-weighted echo-planar perfusion MR imaging. *Radiology* 2002;223:11–29.
18. Evelhoch J. Consensus recommendation for acquisition of dynamic contrasted-enhanced MRI data in oncology. In: Dynamic Contrast-Enhanced Magnetic Resonance Imaging in Oncology. Berlin: Springer, 2005:109–114.
19. Evelhoch J, *et al.* Expanding the use of magnetic resonance in the assessment of tumor response to therapy: Workshop report. *Cancer Res* 2005;65:7041–7044.
20. Leach MO, *et al.* The assessment of antiangiogenic and antivascular therapies in early-stage clinical trials using magnetic resonance imaging: Issues and recommendations. *Br J Cancer* 2005;92: 1599–1610.
21. Recommendations for MR measurement methods at 1.5-Tesla and endpoints for use in phase 1/2a trials of anti-cancer therapeutics affecting tumor vascular function, 2004.
22. Tofts PS, *et al.* Estimating kinetic parameters from dynamic contrast-enhanced T(1)-weighted MRI of a diffusable tracer: Standardized quantities and symbols. *J Magn Reson Imaging* 1999;10:223–32.
23. Kety SS. Theory and application of the exchange of inert gas at the lungs and tissues. *Pharmacol Rev* 1951;3:1–41.
24. Evelhoch JL. Key factors in the acquisition of contrast kinetic data for oncology. *J Magn Reson Imaging* 1999;10:254–259.
25. Levitt DG. The pharmacokinetics of the interstitial space in humans. *BMC Clin Pharmacol* 2003;3.
26. Larsson M, *et al.* Plasma water and 51Cr EDTA equilibration volumes of different tissues in the rat. *Acta Physiol Scand* 1980;110:53–57.
27. Reed RK, *et al.* Interstitial exclusion of albumin in rat dermis and subcutis in over- and dehydration. *Am J Physiol* 1989;257:H1819–H1827.
28. Zhou R, *et al.* Simultaneous measurement of arterial input function and tumor pharmacokinetics in mice by dynamic contrast enhanced imaging: Effects of transcytolemmal water exchange. *Magn Reson Med* 2004;52:248–257.

29. Sakurada O, et al. Measurement of local cerebral blood flow with iodo[14C]antipyrine. *Am J Physiol* 1978;234:H59–H66.
30. Maxwell RJ, et al. Evaluation of the anti-vascular effects of combretastatin in rodent tumours by dynamic contrast enhanced MRI. *NMR Biomed* 2002;15:89–98.
31. Liu G, et al. Dynamic contrast-enhanced magnetic resonance imaging as a pharmacodynamic measure of response after acute dosing of AG-013736, an oral angiogenesis inhibitor, in patients with advanced solid tumors: Results from a phase I study. *J Clin Oncol* 2005;23:5464–5473.
32. Rijpkema M, et al. Method for quantitative mapping of dynamic MRI contrast agent uptake in human tumors. *J Magn Reson Imaging* 2001;14:457–463.
33. Galbraith SM, et al. Reproducibility of dynamic contrast-enhanced MRI in human muscle and tumours: Comparison of quantitative and semi-quantitative analysis. *NMR Biomed* 2002;15:132–142.
34. Redman BG, et al. Phase II trial of tetrathiomolybdate in patients with advanced kidney cancer. *Clin Cancer Res* 2003;9:1666–1672.
35. Landis CS, et al. Equilibrium transcytolemmal water-exchange kinetics in skeletal muscle in vivo. *Magn Reson Med* 1999;42:467–478.
36. Landis CS, et al. Determination of the MRI contrast agent concentration time course in vivo following bolus injection: Effect of equilibrium transcytolemmal water exchange. *Magn Reson Med* 2000;44:563–574.
37. Yankeelov TE, et al. Evidence for shutter-speed variation in CR bolus-tracking studies of human pathology. *NMR Biomed* 2005;18:173–185.
38. Li X, et al. A unified magnetic resonance imaging pharmacokinetic theory: Intravascular and extracellular contrast reagents. *Magn Reson Med* 2005;54:1351–1359.
39. Li X, et al. Shutter-speed analysis of contrast reagent bolus-tracking data: Preliminary observations in benign and malignant breast disease. *Magn Reson Med* 2005;53:724–729.
40. Henderson E, et al. Temporal sampling requirements for the tracer kinetics modeling of breast disease. *Magn Reson Imaging* 1998;16:1057–1073.
41. Jackson A, et al. Breath-hold perfusion and permeability mapping of hepatic malignancies using magnetic resonance imaging and a first-pass leakage profile model. *NMR Biomed* 2002;15:164–173.
42. Krishnan S, Chenevert TL. Spatio-temporal bandwidth-based acquisition for dynamic contrast-enhanced magnetic resonance imaging. *J Magn Reson Imaging* 2004;20:129–137.
43. Jones RA, et al. K-space substitution: A novel dynamic imaging technique. *Magn Reson Med* 1993;29:830–834.
44. van Vaals, JJ, et al. "Keyhole" method for accelerating imaging of contrast agent uptake. *J Magn Reson Imaging* 1993;3:671–675.
45. Paschal CB, Morris HD. K-space in the clinic. *J Magn Reson Imaging* 2004;19:145–159.
46. Bishop JE, et al. Limitations of the keyhole technique for quantitative dynamic contrast-enhanced breast MRI. *J Magn Reson Imaging* 1997;7:716–723.
47. Plewes DB, et al. Errors in quantitative dynamic three-dimensional keyhole MR imaging of the breast. *J Magn Reson Imaging* 1995;5:361–364.
48. Daniel BL, et al. Breast disease: Dynamic spiral MR imaging. *Radiology* 1998;209:499–509.
49. Korosec FR, et al. Time-resolved contrast-enhanced 3D MR angiography. *Magn Reson Med* 1996;36:345–351.
50. Parrish T, Hu X. Continuous update with random encoding (CURE): A new strategy for dynamic imaging. *Magn Reson Med* 1995;33:326–336.
51. Pipe JG. Motion correction with PROPELLER MRI: Application to head motion and free-breathing cardiac imaging. *Magn Reson Med* 1999;42:963–969.
52. Shimizu K, et al. Partial wavelet encoding: A new approach for accelerating temporal resolution in contrast-enhanced MR imaging. *J Magn Reson Imaging* 1999;9:717–724.
53. Song HK, et al. Simultaneous acquisition of multiple resolution images for dynamic contrast enhanced imaging of the breast. *Magn Reson Med* 2001;46:503–509.
54. Tsao J, et al. k-t BLAST and k-t SENSE: Dynamic MRI with high frame rate exploiting spatiotemporal correlations. *Magn Reson Med* 2003;50:1031–1042.
55. d'Arcy JA, et al. Applications of sliding window reconstruction with cartesian sampling for dynamic contrast enhanced MRI. *NMR Biomed* 2002;15:174–183.
56. Song HK, Dougherty L. Dynamic MRI with projection reconstruction and KWIC processing for simultaneous high spatial and temporal resolution. *Magn Reson Med* 2004;52:815–824.

57. Hylton N. Dynamic contrast-enhanced magnetic resonance imaging as an imaging biomarker. *J Clin Oncol* 2006;24:3293–3298.
58. Padhani AR, Leach MO. Antivascular cancer treatments: Functional assessments by dynamic contrast-enhanced magnetic resonance imaging. *Abdom Imaging* 2005;30:324–341.
59. Martincich L, *et al.* Monitoring response to primary chemotherapy in breast cancer using dynamic contrast-enhanced magnetic resonance imaging. *Breast Cancer Res Treat* 2004;83:67–76.
60. Padhani AR. MRI for assessing antivascular cancer treatments. *Br J Radiol* 2003;76(Spec No 1): S60–S80.
61. Choyke PL, *et al.* Functional tumor imaging with dynamic contrast-enhanced magnetic resonance imaging. *J Magn Reson Imaging* 2003;17:509–520.
62. Padhani AR. Functional MRI for anticancer therapy assessment. *Eur J Cancer* 2002;38:2116–2127.
63. Siemann DW, *et al.* Differentiation and definition of vascular-targeted therapies. *Clin Cancer Res* 2005;11:416–420.
64. Morgan B, *et al.* Dynamic contrast-enhanced magnetic resonance imaging as a biomarker for the pharmacological response of PTK787/ZK 222584, an inhibitor of the vascular endothelial growth factor receptor tyrosine kinases, in patients with advanced colorectal cancer and liver metastases: Results from two phase I studies. *J Clin Oncol* 2003;21:3955–3964.
65. Evelhoch JL, *et al.* Magnetic resonance imaging measurements of the response of murine and human tumors to the vascular-targeting agent ZD6126. *Clin Cancer Res* 2004;10:3650–3657.
66. Galbraith SM, *et al.* Combretastatin A4 phosphate has tumor antivascular activity in rat and man as demonstrated by dynamic magnetic resonance imaging. *J Clin Oncol* 2003;21:2831–2842.
67. Stevenson JP, *et al.* Phase I trial of the antivascular agent combretastatin A4 phosphate on a 5-day schedule to patients with cancer: Magnetic resonance imaging evidence for altered tumor blood flow. *J Clin Oncol* 2003;21:4428–4438.
68. Collins JM. Functional imaging in phase I studies: Decorations or decision making? *J Clin Oncol* 2003;21:2807–2809.
69. Collins JM. Imaging and other biomarkers in early clinical studies: One step at a time or re-engineering drug development? *J Clin Oncol* 2005;23:5417–5419.

Color Plate 1

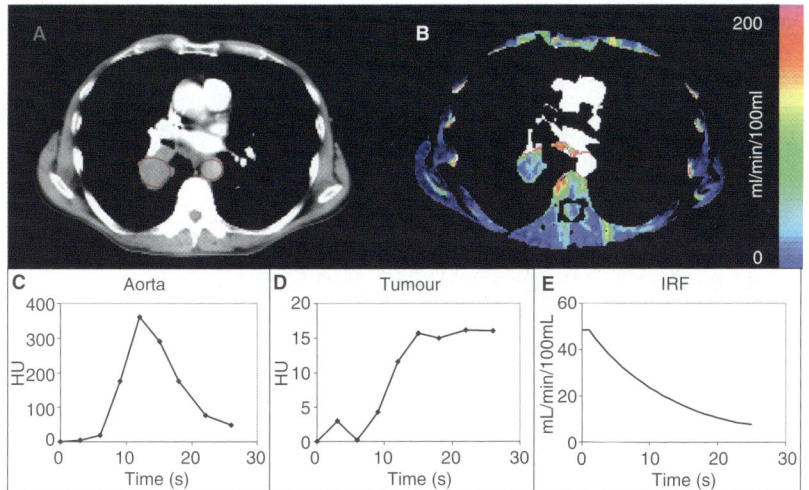

Fig. 6.1. For the figure legend, see page 87.

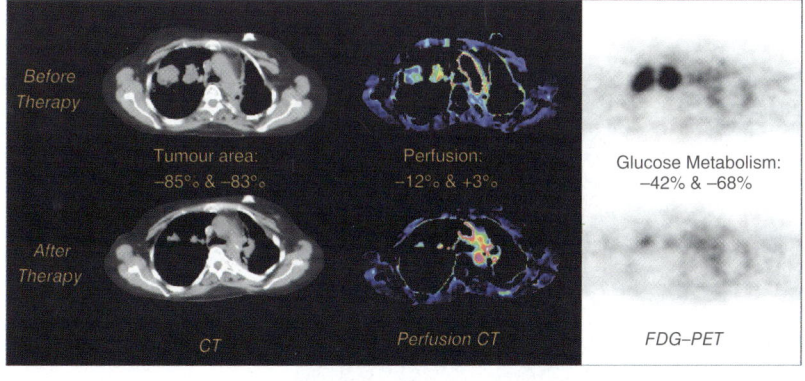

Fig. 6.2. For the figure legend, see page 99.

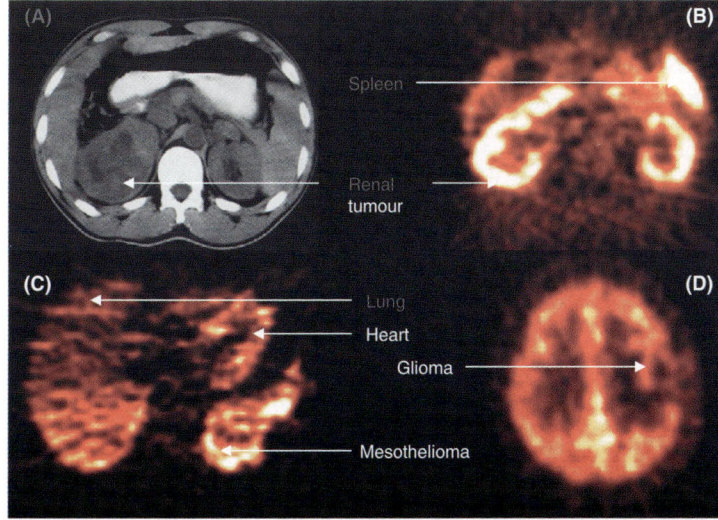

Fig. 11.3. For the figure legend, see page 183.

Color Plate 2

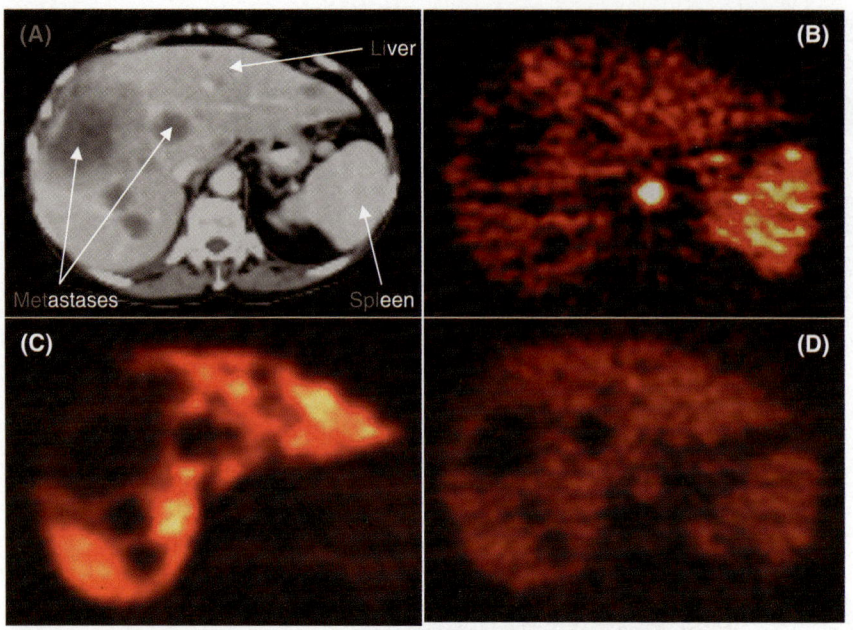

Fig. 11.6. For the figure legend, see page 189.

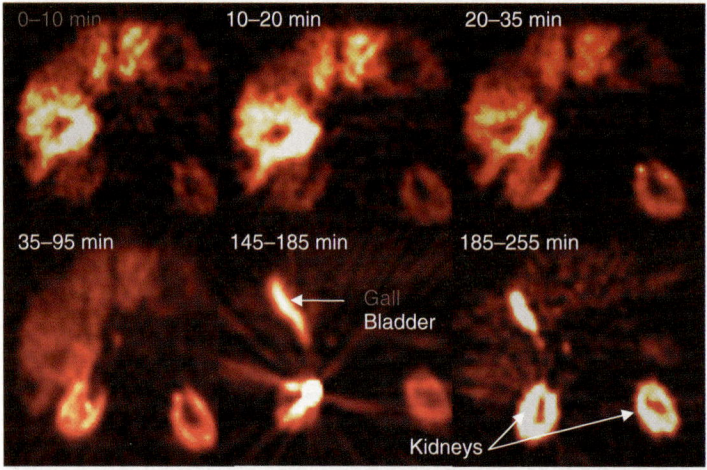

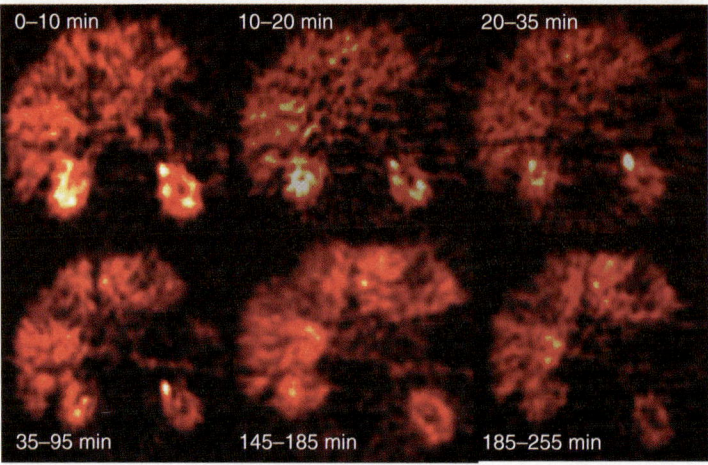

Fig. 11.7. For the figure legend, see page 190.

Color Plate 3

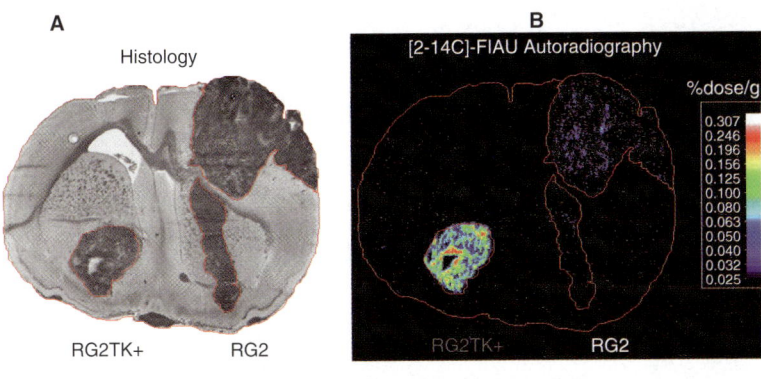

Fig. 12.3. For the figure legend, see page 211.

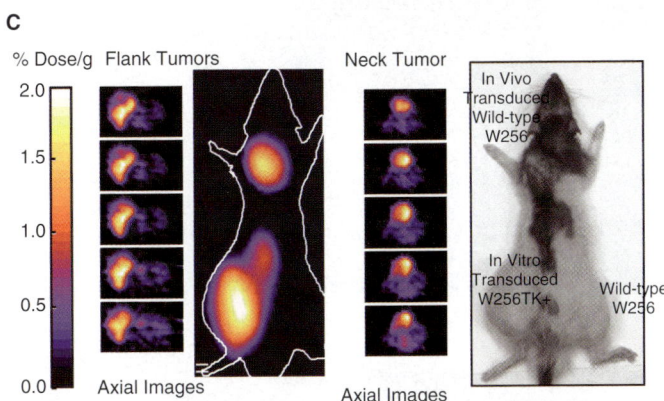

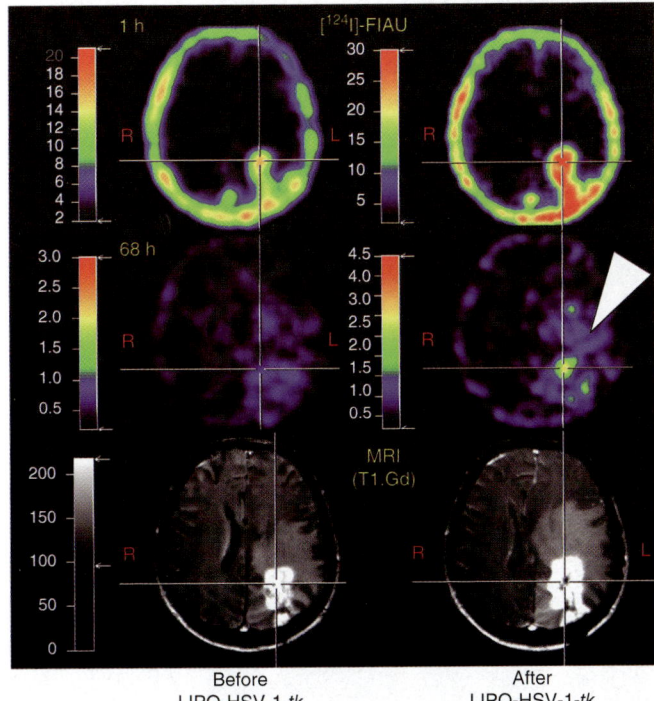

Fig. 12.4. For the figure legend, see page 212.

Color Plate 4

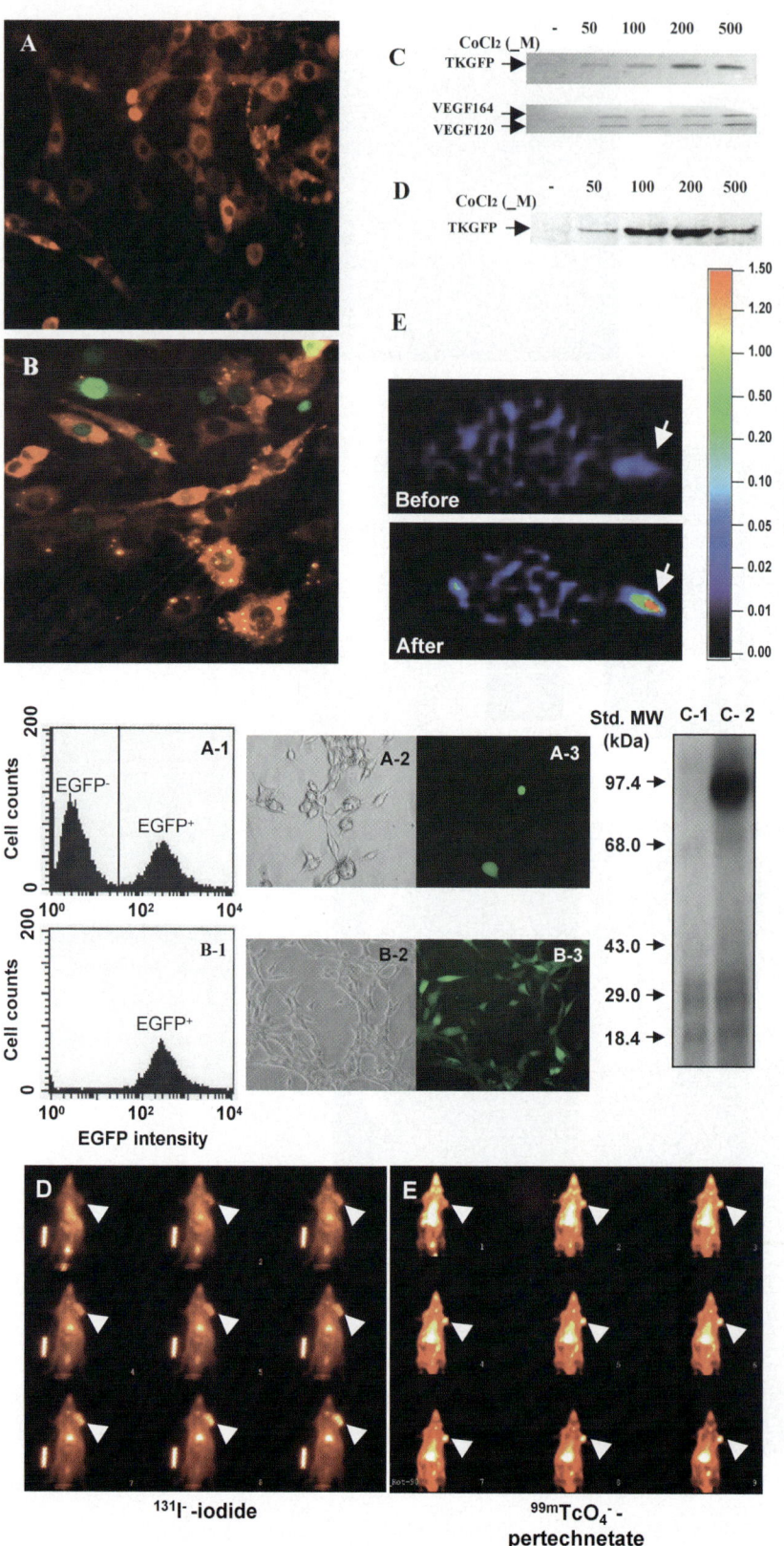

Fig. 12.5. For the figure legend, see page 213.

Fig. 12.6. For the figure legend, see page 217.

Color Plate 5

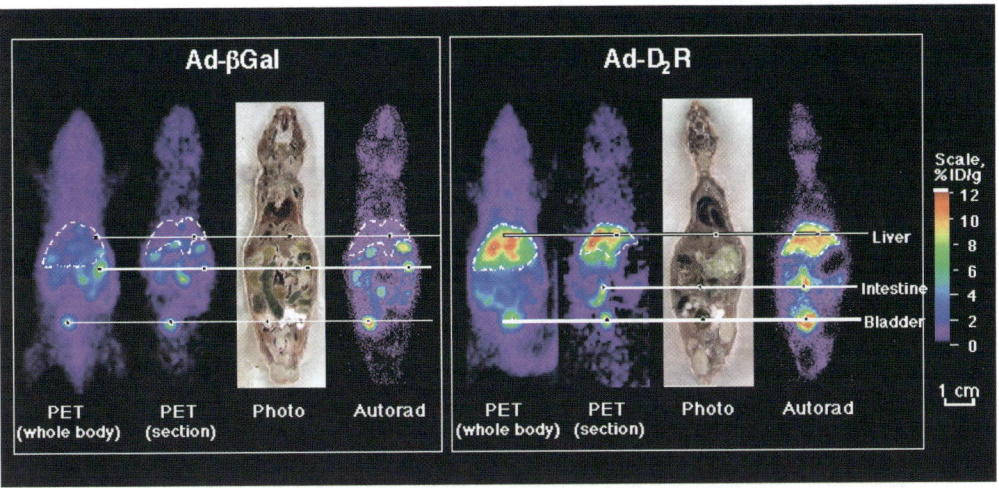

Fig. 12.7. For the figure legend, see page 219.

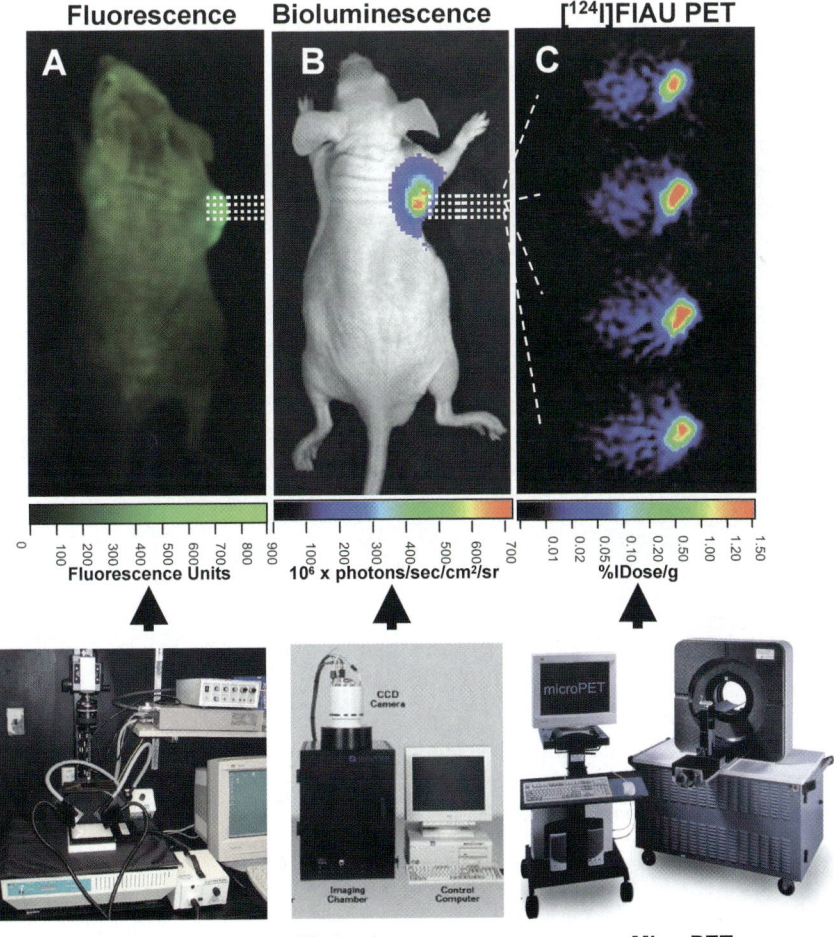

Fig. 12.8. For the figure legend, see page 220.

Color Plate 6

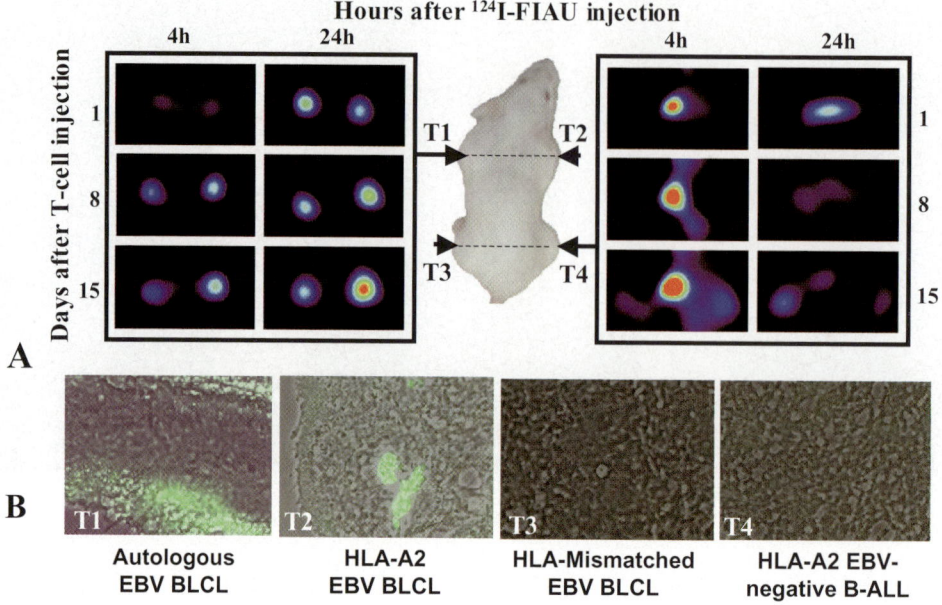

Fig. 12.10. For the figure legend, see page 227.

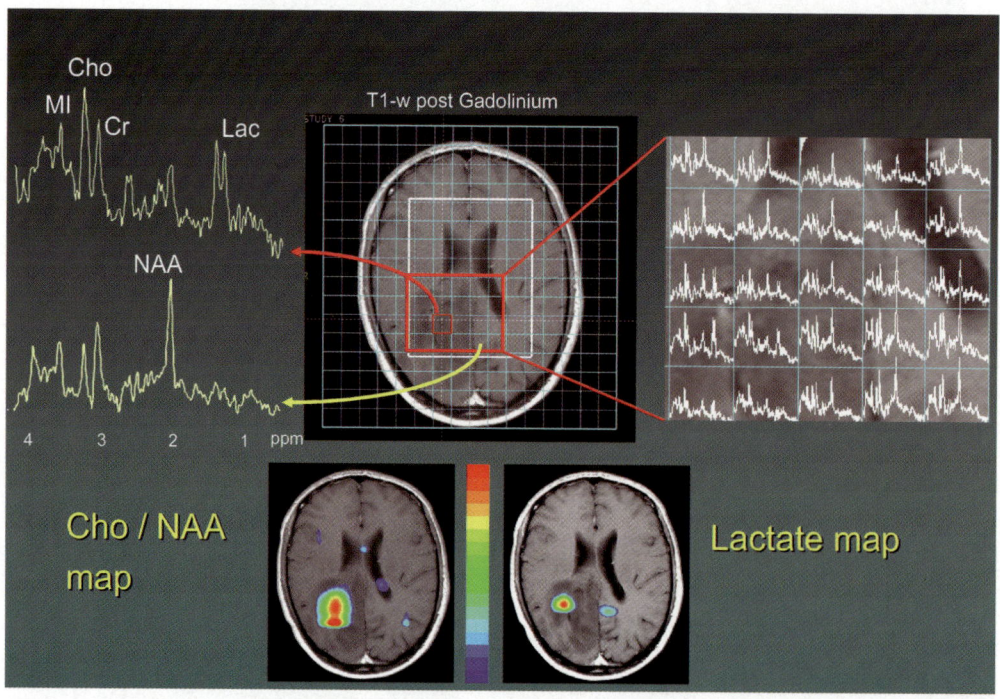

Fig. 13.2. For the figure legend, see page 245.

Color Plate 7

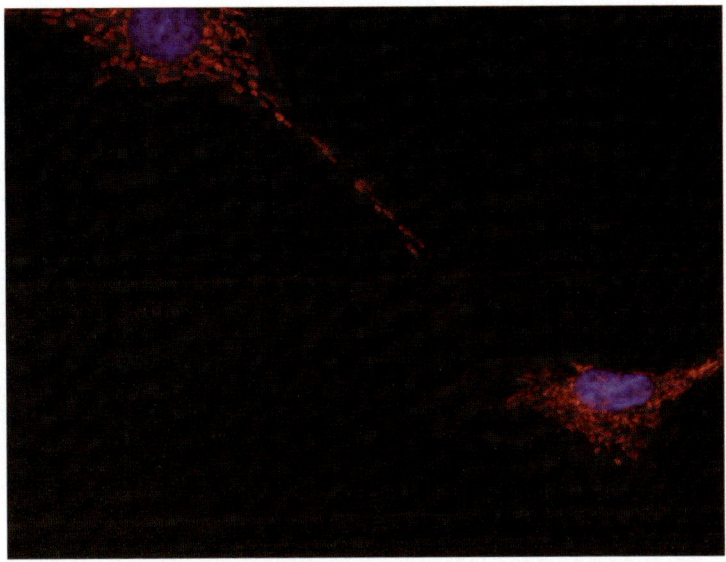

Fig. 15.4. For the figure legend, see page 287.

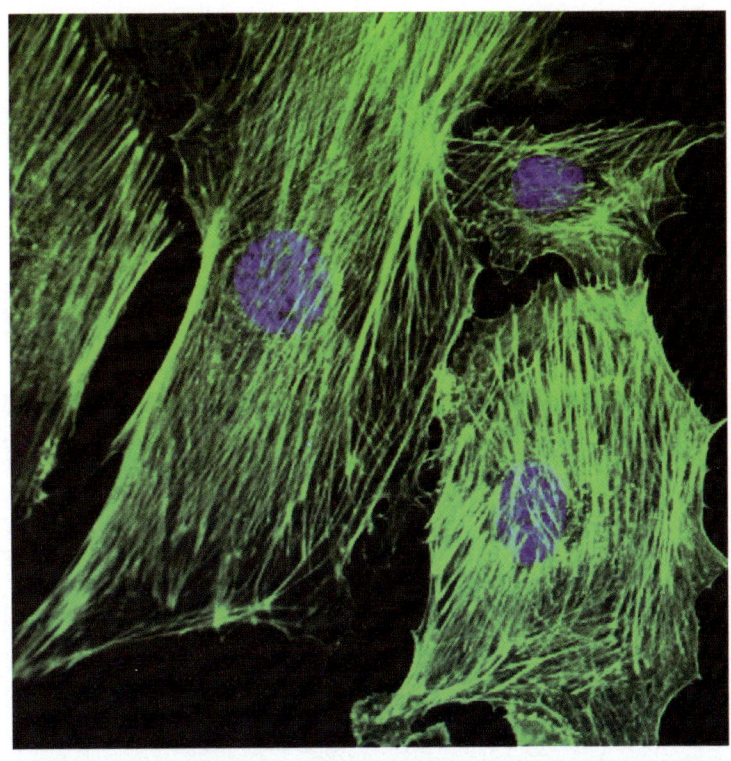

Fig. 15.5. For the figure legend, see page 288.

Color Plate 8

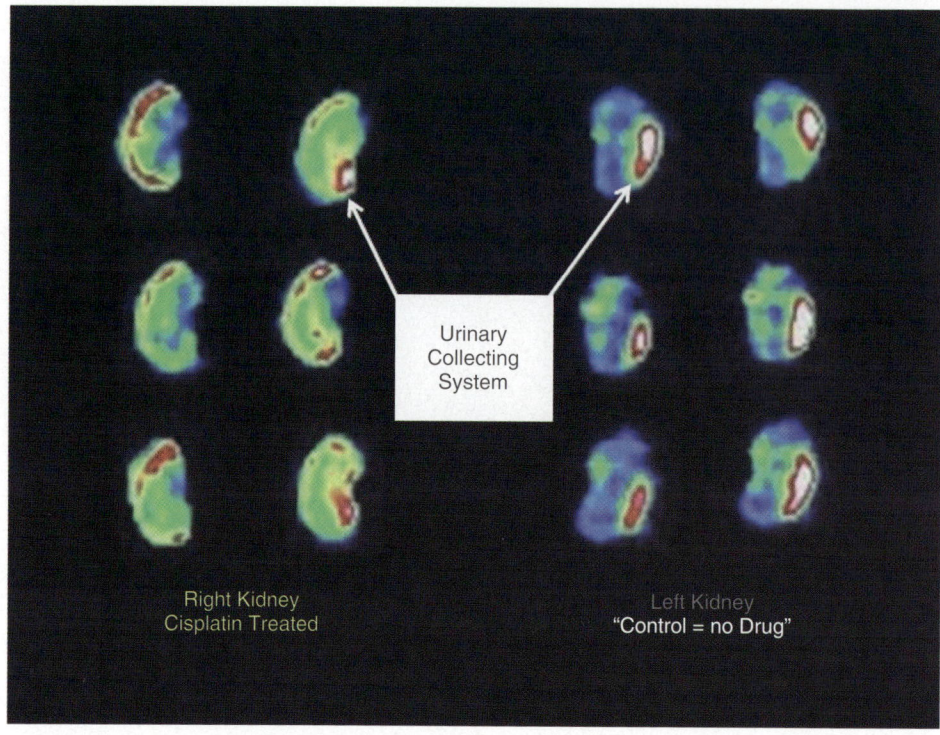

Fig. 16.1. For the figure legend, see page 310.

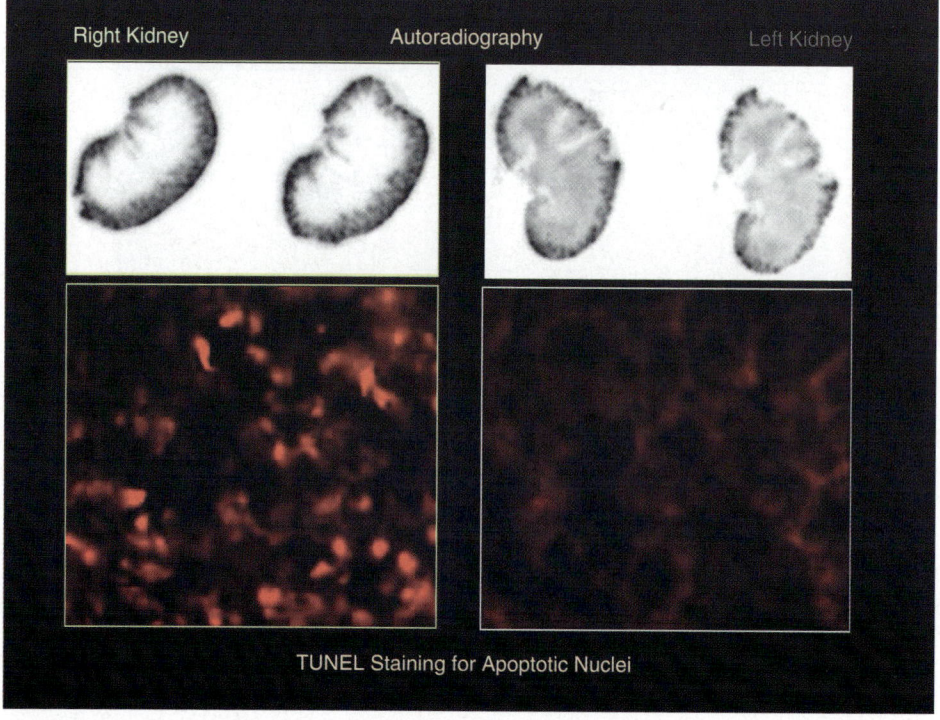

Fig. 16.2. For the figure legend, see page 311.

6 Computed Tomography Measurements of Perfusion in Cancer Therapy

Ken Miles, MD

CONTENTS

    INTRODUCTION
    DETERMINANTS OF CONTRAST ENHANCEMENT OF TUMORS
      ON COMPUTED TOMOGRAPHY
    IMAGE ACQUISITION
    DATA PROCESSING
    TECHNICAL VALIDATION AND REPRODUCIBILITY
    TECHNICAL LIMITATIONS AND ADVANTAGES
    TUMOR RESPONSE EVALUATION WITH PERFUSION
      COMPUTED TOMOGRAPHY
    PERFUSION COMPUTED TOMOGRAPHY/POSITRON
      EMISSION TOMOGRAPHY
    SUMMARY

1. INTRODUCTION

Computed tomography (CT) remains one of the mainstay techniques for anatomical evaluation of tumor growth and response to therapy, both in clinical practice and drug trials (see Chapter 3). Computed tomography measurements of perfusion can be added to a conventional CT examination to provide a functional response assessment within the same examination. This combined approach can overcome some of the limitations of a purely structural evaluation, such as slow response to therapy and residual nonmalignant masses, while avoiding the inconvenience to the patient and additional cost of further examinations using different imaging modalities. Furthermore, as positron emission tomography (PET) systems are now commonly integrated with CT, functional CT techniques can be combined with PET evaluations of tumor physiology using a single imaging device.

From: *Cancer Drug Discovery and Development*
In Vivo Imaging of Cancer Therapy
Edited by: A.F. Shields and P. Price © Humana Press Inc., Totowa, NJ

The use of CT for measuring perfusion was proposed within a decade of the modality's introduction by Hounsfield and Ambrose, when Axel published a methodology for determination of cerebral blood flow by rapid-sequence contrast-enhanced CT *(1)*. However, the slow speed of image acquisition and data processing of conventional CT systems at that time limited initial application of the technique to research studies of myocardial and renal blood flow using electron beam CT systems *(2, 3)*. The ability to perform perfusion CT on more widely available conventional systems came in the 1990s with the advent of spiral CT *(4)*. The subsequent development of multidetector CT (MDCT) and the release of commercial perfusion CT software have now moved perfusion CT into the clinical arena. The first reported measurement of tumor perfusion using conventional spiral CT was a study of hepatic perfusion, including patients with metastases, in 1993 *(5)* with the first reports of the technique's use in measuring tumor response to drug therapy published one year later *(6, 7)*. This chapter describes the use of CT in the assessment of tumor vascular physiology and illustrates how the technique can offer a widely available, low-cost adjunct to existing methods for evaluating treatment response in a broad range of tumors.

2. DETERMINANTS OF CONTRAST ENHANCEMENT OF TUMORS ON COMPUTED TOMOGRAPHY

CT measurements of perfusion and other aspects of tumor vascular physiology are based upon the use of conventional contrast medium as a physiological indicator. The iodine component of CT contrast media is attenuating to X-rays and causes a local increase in the X-ray attenuation within the organs and blood vessels to which it is distributed following administration. A CT image displays the measured X-ray attenuation of each volume element (voxel) within the anatomical slice studied and, by acquiring CT images before and after the administration of contrast medium, it is possible to quantify the increase in attenuation produced by contrast medium. If a series of images is obtained, the temporal changes in attenuation, and hence iodine concentration, can be displayed as a time–attenuation curve (Fig. 1C and D). The increase in attenuation is linearly proportional to the iodine concentration with a concentration of 1 mg/ml producing an increase in attenuation typically between 20 and 30 Hounsfield units (HU), depending upon the tube current selected and the CT system used. Selecting a lower tube current results in a greater increase in attenuation for a given iodine concentration but increases image noise. The precise relationship between measured attenuation change and iodine concentration for particular image parameters on an individual system can be determined by using a simple phantom that contains solutions of contrast medium at different concentrations. The phantom can be left empty or filled with water to replicate examinations of the chest and abdomen or head, respectively. Greater beam hardening from surrounding tissues in the abdomen and head result in a higher mean energy of the X-ray beam and reduces the increase attenuation for a given iodine concentration *(8)*. The differences in enhancement for a particular concentration of contrast material can vary on a single CT system over time, and between different CT systems, by up to 20% *(9)*.

Following intravenous administration, the distribution of CT contrast media within the body approximates a two-compartment model, with intravascular and extravascular

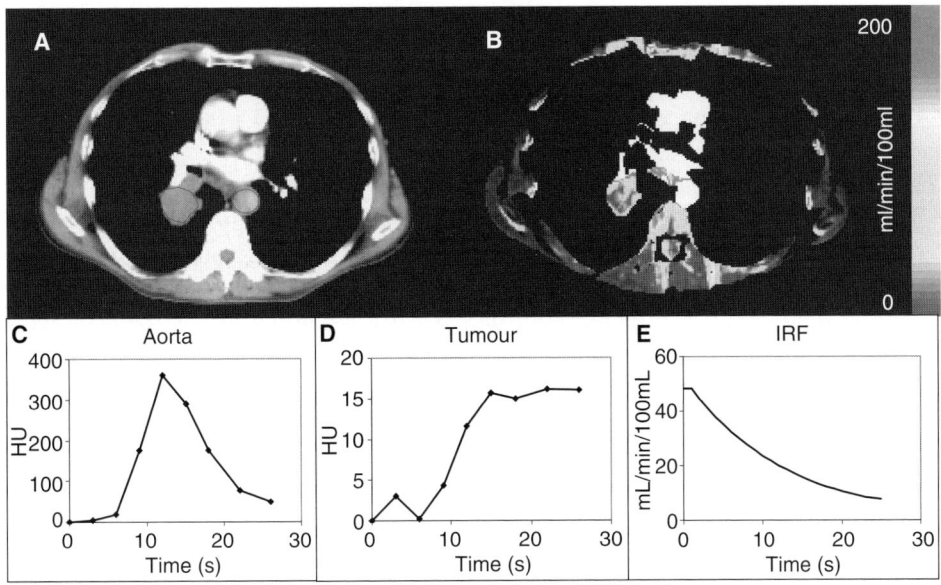

Fig. 1. Conventional CT (A) and perfusion CT images (B) of right lung carcinoma. Time–attenuation curves (TAC) have been derived from the regions of interest over the aorta (C) and tumor (D). Tumor perfusion can be calculated from the maximal slope of the tumor TAC divided by the peak value of the aortic TDC (slope method) to give 40 ml/min/100 ml. Tumor perfusion can also be determined from the flow-corrected impulse residue function (IR)F, calculated by deconvolution, giving 48 ml/min/100 ml (E). (*See* color plate.)

components. These pharmacokinetic properties are reflected in the pattern of contrast enhancement within a particular tissue over time. Initially, contrast medium is predominantly intravascular but subsequently a proportion of the contrast medium passes into the extravascular space. Thus, the temporal changes in contrast enhancement depend upon tissue perfusion, the relative size of the vascular space, i.e., relative blood volume, the rate of leakage into the extravascular space reflecting vascular permeability, and relative size of the extravascular space (Table 1). It is possible to quantify each of these

Table 1
Physiological Parameters Quantifiable by Functional Computed Tomography and Corresponding Features in the Tumor Time–Attenuation Curve and Impulse Residue Function following Deconvolution[a]

Physiological parameter	*Corresponding feature of tumor time–attenuation curve*	*Corresponding feature of impulse residue function*
Perfusion	Maximum enhancement rate during first pass Peak enhancement	Initial height
Blood volume	Area under first pass curve Initial slope of delayed phase	Area under curve
Capillary permeability	Slope of delayed phase	Height of second component

[a] See Section 4.2.

parameters in tumors and other tissues by applying physiological models to enhancement data from an appropriate series of images *(10)*. However, as the pattern of enhancement within the supplying blood vessel, i.e., the input function, is also a major determinant of the tissue enhancement pattern, it is essential to obtain enhancement data from a major vessel as well as from the tissue of interest.

The processes of angiogenesis, by which tumors develop the blood supply needed for growth and metastasis, result in changes in vascular physiology and hence determine the manner in which tumors enhance on CT following intravenous administration of contrast medium. The increased density of tumor microvessels associated with angiogenesis translates *in vivo* to increased tumor perfusion and blood volume. The incomplete basement membranes exhibited by tumor microvessels result in increased permeability and increased size of the extravascular space. Tumor enhancement has been shown to correlate with histological measurements of angiogenesis, such as microvascular density (MVD), in lung and renal cancer *(11–15)*, and with the expression of vascular endothelial growth factor (VEGF) in lung cancer *(12, 15)*. These findings verify the ability for contrast enhancement on CT to provide an *in vivo* correlate for the microvascular changes of angiogenesis that is also confirmed by clinical use of perfusion CT *(16)*. For example, by signifying differences in levels of angiogenesis in benign and malignant tissues, quantification of contrast enhancement and perfusion has been advocated for the characterization of pulmonary nodules, potentially reducing health care expenditure *(17–19)*. Furthermore, the recognized association between high levels of angiogenesis and an aggressive tumor phenotype with poor survival is mirrored by the ability of perfusion CT to estimate tumor grade in cerebral glioma and lymphoma *(20, 21)* and to stratify risk for patients with hepatic metastases *(22)*.

The emergence of antiangiogenesis treatment strategies for cancer has produced an interest in imaging techniques that reflect angiogenesis as *in vivo* markers of tumor response. Indeed, some studies have suggested that perfusion imaging may have advantages over other functional response markers, such as glucose metabolism, in the evaluation of response to antiangiogenesis agents *(23, 24)*. However, a reduction in perfusion has been observed in response to cancer treatments not primarily directed at the vascular system, again in some instances predicting response better than changes in glucose metabolism *(25)*. On the other hand, the hyperemia associated with radiotherapy can cause a temporary increase in tumor perfusion and vascular permeability that may not reflect ultimate response *(26)*. A similar difficulty can arise with other functional response markers such as glucose metabolism. Correspondingly, these factors will impact the changes in tumor enhancement following therapy and the use of perfusion CT for tumor response evaluation.

3. IMAGE ACQUISITION

The acquisition parameters to be considered are (1) the overall length of time of the image series, (2) the number and frequency of images, (3) the number and thickness of CT slices, (4) the X-ray exposure factors, (5) the volume and concentration of contrast medium injected, and (6) the phase of respiration. The organ of interest, the physiological parameters to be studied, and the data processing method used by the analysis software all impact upon the precise protocol adopted. The protocol will also determine the radiation dose to the patient. Although in the context of oncology, the radiation exposure associated with perfusion CT is small compared to the radiotherapy dose that many patients will receive, there remains a need to limit the radiation burden associated with perfusion CT studies. All protocols require a baseline image acquisition without intravenous contrast enhancement to enable baseline attenuation values to be subtracted from subsequent contrast-enhanced images.

3.1 Overall Length of Time of the Image Series

The overall length of the series determines which physiological parameters can be determined. Perfusion and blood volume can be assessed during the first pass of contrast material through the vascular system at which time the contrast material is predominantly intravascular. The length of the first pass depends upon an individual cardiac output and circulating blood volume, but typically comprises the first 45–60 sec immediately after intravenous injection. Assessments of vascular permeability and relative volume of the extravascular space require longer series to allow for sufficient passage of contrast material passes into the extravascular space. In tumors, the increased permeability of the vascular endothelium means that leakage of contrast medium sufficient for reliable measurements occurs within 2–10 min of the injection of contrast medium. Blood volume can also be estimated from such image series (see the Patlak analysis below). Vascular permeability studies may be particularly appropriate for the study of brain tumors where the differences in permeability between tumor vessels and the normal blood–brain barrier are considerably greater than the differences between tumor perfusion and cerebral cortical perfusion.

3.2 The Number and Frequency of Images

The number and frequency of images obtained will be a balance between the quality of the data and the radiation dose for the patient. A high image frequency will be required for reliable measurements from first pass data. Although modern CT systems can acquire images with a frequency of less than one image every second, image frequency can be reduced to every 2–3 sec without adversely affecting the perfusion values obtained *(27)*. After the first pass, images can be acquired less frequently (every 5–10 sec) as changes in contrast enhancement become less rapid. A protocol that aims to use a single administration of contrast material to assess not only perfusion and blood volume but also vascular permeability will usually involve an initially rapid sequence of images during the first pass with less frequent images later.

3.3 The Number and Thickness of Computed Tomography Slices

Acquiring images at a frequency close to the time taken for the CT system to rotate the X-ray tube around the patient (typically 0.5–1 sec) does not allow sufficient time for table top movement during the study. Thus, the volume of tissue examined is constrained in the craniocaudal direction by the width of the CT detector, typically 2 to 4 cm for current MDCT systems. The detector can be divided so that a number of slices are obtained simultaneously, e.g., four slices 5 mm thick. Although slices as thin as 0.5 mm can be obtained, reducing slice thickness increases image noise, which can be remedied only by increasing the radiation exposure.

Greater volumes of tissue can be examined at lower frequency by using helical (spiral) acquisitions that incorporate movement of the imaging table through the gantry during the acquisition. Such protocols can be used to measure tumor vascular permeability but are associated with an increased radiation burden to the patient. By focusing on a particular moment in the first pass, for example, the time of peak tumor enhancement measurement, a combined technique is feasible in which a timing sequence of frequent images using a small test bolus of contrast medium is performed without table movement to determine the time of peak *tissue* enhancement (analogous to the timing sequences often used during CT angiography to determine the time of peak *vascular* enhancement). A larger bolus of contrast medium (given over the same time as the test bolus) is then used for a volume acquisition that has been programmed to occur at the moment of peak tissue enhancement.

3.4 X-Ray Exposure Factors

The tube voltage (kVp), tube current (mA), and exposure time used for each image will determine the amount of noise in the image and the radiation dose to the patient. Higher values for each of these parameters reduce noise but increase radiation dose. Typical exposure times for current CT scanners are 1 sec or less. Selecting a tube voltage lower than that typically used for diagnostic studies (e.g., 80–100 kVp instead of 120–140 kVp) increases the amount of attenuation produced by a given concentration of contrast medium but increases image noise. Image noise can be reduced by selecting a smoother construction filter (e.g., soft tissue).

Analysis methods that use deconvolution to determine perfusion values (see below) are less sensitive to noise in individual images and can therefore tolerate a lower tube current (allowing a higher image frequency). However, with compartment analysis (see below), image noise can result in overestimation of tissue enhancement rates and miscalculation of perfusion values. Thus, time–attenuation data from protocols that adopt a higher tube current (with a lower image frequency to minimize radiation dose) are appropriate for compartmental analysis methods. Such data sets can also be successfully processed using deconvolution analysis (M.R. Griffiths, 2001, personal communication), as illustrated in Fig. 1.

3.5 Volume and Concentration of Contrast Medium

Maximizing contrast enhancement in blood vessels and tissues improves the signal-to-noise ratios for time–attenuation data for perfusion measurement and can be achieved by a rapid injection rate (at least 4 ml/sec) and by using contrast media with a high iodine concentration (i.e., 350–400 mg iodine/ml). A short sharp bolus is particularly important when using compartmental analysis to obtain perfusion values (see below), because the validity of the method requires that peak arterial concentration occurs prior to the time of maximal increase in tissue enhancement. Typical protocols use a relative small bolus (40–50 ml) administered with higher injection rates of between 5 and 10 ml/sec.

3.6 Phase of Respiration

As discussed above, measurements of enhancement on CT required subtraction of baseline attenuation values. Any change in position of the patient will result in misregistration between the unenhanced baseline image and subsequent contrast-enhanced images. Respiratory motion is a major cause of such misregistration, leading to errors in perfusion values and artifacts on parametric images. Many patients will be unable to suspend respiration adequately for image series longer than 45–60 sec unless acquisition pauses are created to allow the patient to take a breath. Even with shorter series when it is possible to suspend respiration, patients will often slowly exhale during the image series leading to motion artifacts. If images are acquired during quiet breathing, the patient must be warned to avoid the temptation to take a deep breath when experiencing the "hot flush" commonly associated with a rapid bolus of contrast medium. With such precautions, it is usually possible to obtain reliable perfusion data during quiet respiration. Quiet respiration will also be appropriate when using a combined PET/CT system to coregister CT perfusion and PET images (see below), as suspended respiration is not possible for the PET images that take several minutes.

4. DATA PROCESSING

Ease of processing is a particular advantage for perfusion CT over other functional imaging methods. The linear relationship between enhancement and concentration of contrast medium, the ability to obtain an arterial input function directly from images, and the commercial availability of validated analysis software all contribute to the simplicity of the technique while avoiding the pitfalls associated with semiquantitative analyses that overlook the importance of the arterial input. Software packages support region of interest analysis as well as pixel-by-pixel analysis to generate quantified parametric images, often color coded, that display intratumoral variations in perfusion and other physiological aspects (Fig. 1B). The methods most commonly used for functional CT measurements have been developed from compartmental analysis and linear systems theory (deconvolution). Commercial software has adopted both methods; Siemens and Picker use compartmental analysis while General Electric has implemented a linear systems approach. Detailed descriptions of these approaches are available elsewhere *(10, 16)*.

4.1 Compartmental Analysis

A single compartmental model is used for measurement of tumor perfusion while a two-compartmental analysis allows determination of vascular permeability and leakage space. Blood volume measurements can be derived from both models.

The single compartmental model applies the Fick principle to data obtained during the first pass of contrast. If the organ concentration of contrast material is measured before any contrast agent has left the organ of interest, then tissue blood flow per unit volume (*F/V*), i.e., perfusion, can be determined by

$$F/V = [dCt/dt(\max)]/Ca(\max) \qquad (1)$$

or

$$F/V = Ct(\max)/\int_0^t Ca(t)\,dt \qquad (2)$$

where *Ct* and *Ca* are the tissue and arterial concentrations of contrast material at any time (*t*). For Eq. (1), *dCt/dt*(max) is derived from the maximal slope of the tissue concentration–time curve and *Ca*(max) the peak height of the arterial curve (Fig. 1C and D). This technique, sometimes known as the "slope method," was first applied to CT by Miles *(28)*. For Eq. (2), *Ct*(max) is the peak height of the tissue curve and $_0\!\int^t Ca(t)\,dt$ is the area under the arterial curve corrected for recirculation using a gamma variate fit. This implementation is also known as the Mullani–Gould method *(29)*. (Note that for both these methods, knowledge of the precise relationship between enhancement and iodine concentration is not required as the conversion factor relating these parameters would cancel above and below the line.)

Relative blood volume within the tumor describes the fraction of tumor volume occupied by the blood space and can be estimated from first pass data in two ways: (1) from the ratio of the areas under the tissue and arterial time–attenuation curves, or (2) from parameters reflecting the mean transit time (MTT) of contrast medium through the tumor, for example, estimated from the full-width half-maximum value of the tissue time–attenuation curve. Relative blood volume is then calculated from the MTT and the perfusion value using

$$\text{Relative blood volume} = \text{Perfusion} \times \text{MTT} \qquad (3)$$

A recent development of the Mullani–Gould method derives the standardized perfusion value (SPV) representing the ratio of the perfusion in the tissue of interest to mean whole body perfusion *(8)*. Mean whole body perfusion is defined by the cardiac output divided by the patient's weight (W):

$$\text{SPV} = Ct(\max)/[\text{iodine dose}/W] \qquad (4)$$

The iodine dose needs to be expressed in HUs and therefore determination of SPV requires calibration of the individual CT scanner using appropriate image acquisition parameters as described in Section 2 above. Note also that the SPV is closely related to peak enhancement as long as the contrast medium is administered on a dose-by-weight basis.

The normalization of tumor perfusion to the patient's cardiac output and weight afforded by the SPV means that this parameter will be unchanged in the presence of any alteration in cardiac output. On the other hand, tumor perfusion will fall in the presence of reduced cardiac output despite a lack of change in tumor vascularity or MVD. Thus SPV is likely to be more closely related to tumor vascularity than is absolute tumor perfusion, a fact that offers an explanation for the observed correlation between peak tumor enhancement and tumor MVD. Similarly, SPV measurements may be particularly useful in monitoring anticancer drugs known to alter cardiac output. By incorporating fewer calculation steps, peak enhancement and, therefore, SPV measurements are also less prone to interobserver error than the more complex perfusion analyses. In addition, the SPV benefits from a derivation analogous to that of the standardized uptake value (SUV) widely used in PET, facilitating comparison between the two measurements.

An important limitation to single-compartment models for calculating perfusion is the assumption that no contrast medium has left the tissue of interest at the time of measurement. In some instances, the transit time through certain tissues may not be sufficiently long to allow this assumption to be met, leading to an underestimation of the perfusion value, particularly for the Mullani–Gould method. There are few data available to indicate the likelihood or magnitude of such errors. However, there is a theoretical possibility that the presence and size of such errors could change following treatment.

The two-compartment model can be described mathematically by

$$Q(t) = V_b Ca(t) + K^{trans} \int_0^t Ca(u) e^{-[Ktrans/Ve](t-u)} du \qquad (5)$$

where $Q(t)$ is the quantity of contrast material in the tissue of interest, V_b is the relative blood volume, $Ca(t)$ is the arterial concentration at time (t) K^{trans} is the capillary permeability, and V_e is the relative volume of the extravascular space or leakage space. $Q(t)$ and $Ca(t)$ are derived from tissue and arterial time–attenuation curves, respectively. To determine values for all three physiological parameters, the equation must be solved iteratively. However, a simplified method assumes that back flux of contrast medium from extravascular to intravascular compartments is negligible for the first 60–120 sec after contrast medium administration, such that Patlak analysis *(30)* can be used to measure capillary permeability and relative blood volume from

$$Q(t)/Ca(t) = V_b \times K^{trans} \int_0^t Ca(u)du / Ca(t) \qquad (6)$$

A graph plotting $Q(t)/Ca(t)$ (y-axis) against $\int_0^t Ca(u)\,du/Ca(t)$ (x-axis) yields a straight line portion with slope K^{trans} and intercept V_b.

4.2 Linear Systems Approach (Deconvolution)

The mathematical process of deconvolution uses the concept of the impulse residue function (IRF) for the tissue of interest, where the IRF is a theoretical tissue curve that would be obtained from an instantaneous arterial input (Fig. 1E). Using the arterial and tissue time–attenuation curves to obtain $Ct(t)$ and $Ca(t)$ [i.e., the concentration of contrast medium in tissue and artery at any time (t)] is given by

$$Ct(t) = F/V\,[Ca(t) * R(t)] = Ca(t) * F/V\,R(t) \qquad (7)$$

where $R(t)$ is the IRF and $*$ denotes the convolution operator (other symbols are as for the equations described above). For ease of calculation, the shape of the IRF is usually constrained to comprise a plateau followed by a single exponential decay. The height of the flow-corrected IRF will give the tissue perfusion (F/V) and the area under the curve will determine the relative blood volume (Table 1). Measurement of capillary permeability is achieved by modelling the decay of the IRF with two components, a rapid component determined by blood flow and a slower component reflecting exchange with the extracellular space. Although appropriate for tumors, such IRF models may not be valid for organs with complex circulations (e.g., liver, spleen, and kidney).

5. TECHNICAL VALIDATION AND REPRODUCIBILITY

Perfusion CT methods have been extensively validated in a range of tissues using reference standards such as microspheres in animal studies or stable xenon washout and [^{15}O]H$_2$O PET in humans *(16)*. Specific validation studies in tumors are summarized in Table 2. The three animal studies used VX2 tumors or rat-derived mammary adenocarcinoma implanted into the thigh or VX2 tumors implanted into brain. A strong correlation between functional CT and microsphere perfusion values was obtained in all studies (r values: 0.83–0.96) *(31–33)*. The animal study by Pollard *et al.* also validated Patlak analysis of functional CT data for evaluation of tumor capillary permeability by comparison with the Evan's Blue dye technique, finding a strong correlation between the two methods for viable tumor (r value: 0.930) *(33)*. Validation of perfusion CT using the slope method in human tumors has been performed by Hattori *et al.* who reported good correlations between perfusion CT and the results of thermal clearance and PET techniques (r values: 0.873 and 0.791, respectively) *(34)*.

Table 2
Validation of Perfusion Computed Tomography in Tumors

Study	Subjects	Tumor type	CT analysis method	Reference standard
Cenic et al. (31)	NZ white rabbits	VX2 in brain	Deconvolution	Microspheres
Purdie et al. (32)	NZ white rabbits	VX2 in thigh	Deconvolution	Microspheres
Pollard et al. (33)	Fischer 344 rats	Rat-derived mammary adenoma	Mullani–Gould Patlak	Microspheres Evan's Blue Dye
Hatorri et al. (33)	Humans (n = 27)	Various superficial tumors	Slope	Thermal clearance PET

High levels of reproducibility are essential for imaging techniques used for evaluating response to therapy. The tumor validation studies of Cenic and Purdie in animals also evaluated reproducibility using a test–retest protocol, finding low variability for measurements of perfusion (13–14%), relative blood volume (7–20%), and capillary permeability (18%) *(31, 32)*. The requirement for repeated irradiation has meant that test–retest studies in humans are uncommon. Using the slope method to measure normal cerebral perfusion in humans, Gillard et al. *(35)* showed little variability in repeated CT studies in seven patients 24 h apart ($r = 0.88$). These data produced a variability of 13% when reanalyzed using the GE deconvolution software (M.R. Griffiths, 2002, personal communication). The variability values above compare to reductions in perfusion due to antiangiogenesis drug therapy of between 30% and greater than 90% *(23, 24, 36)*.

Interoperator variability is low (8%) for measurements of normal splenic perfusion (M.R. Griffiths, unpublished observations, 1999), peak aortic CT number ($r^2 = 0.99$), and maximal slope of liver time–attenuation curves ($r^2 = 0.83$) *(37)*. Interoperator reproducibility deteriorates significantly for more complex techniques such as Patlak analysis (Student Selected Component, Brighton & Sussex Medical School, 2004). A preliminary investigation into the comparability of perfusion values derived using slope and deconvolution methods in 16 lung nodules has demonstrated good correlations ($r = 0.86$) (M.R. Griffiths, personal communication, 2001).

6. TECHNICAL LIMITATIONS AND ADVANTAGES

The limited anatomical coverage afforded by the detector design of current CT systems confers a significant constraint upon the application of functional perfusion. Until recently, the maximum axial field of view on current machines has been of the order of 20 mm, but as CT detector tracks have become wider, greater volumes of tissue can be evaluated. Sixty-four-slice systems are now available with z-axis coverage of 48 mm and future developments are likely to advance this coverage further.

Motion artifacts resulting from movement of the patient during image acquisition can create significant problems for functional CT, particularly for those organs that are subject to respiratory motion, such as the lung or liver. Careful instruction of the patients helps to minimize these difficulties *(16)*. Motion within the image plane can be corrected to some extent during image processing. Respiratory gating techniques are under development but may increase the time between image acquisitions.

Compared to imaging techniques that do not use ionizing radiation such as ultrasound and MRI, the radiation exposure associated with functional CT is a disadvantage. Typical whole-body equivalent doses range between 1 and 10 mSv depending upon the protocol and body region examined and are therefore comparable to many examinations in routine clinical use. Improvements in detector design that allow selection of a lower tube current without substantial loss of image quality may reduce radiation doses in the future.

The major advantages of functional CT are the technique's simplicity, wide availability, and low cost. Simplicity is afforded by the similarity of image acquisition protocols to other CT and angiographic techniques, the ease of quantification, and the availability of commercial software for analysis and display. The reproducibility is similar to that of other techniques for imaging perfusion. The wide availability and low cost result from the use of conventional CT systems and standard contrast agents.

7. TUMOR RESPONSE EVALUATION WITH PERFUSION COMPUTED TOMOGRAPHY

7.1 Predicting Response

An adequate tumor blood supply is essential for the effective delivery of chemotherapeutic drugs to tumor tissue. Furthermore, the heterogeneous vascular networks typical of tumors result in an imbalance between oxygen supply and consumption and areas of tumor hypoxia. Hypoxia is known to confer resistance not only to chemotherapy but also to radiotherapy. Thus, functional CT measurements would be expected to predict tumor response to chemotherapy or radiotherapy with low and/or heterogeneous contrast enhancement and perfusion implying a likelihood of an unfavorable outcome. Preliminary studies have confirmed this expectation.

A CT perfusion study by Hermans *et al.* stratified 105 patients with head and neck cancer undergoing radiotherapy with curative intent, according to the median perfusion value of 83.5 ml/min/100 g *(38)*. In multivariate analysis, low perfusion (along with T stage) was an independent predictor of local control but not of regional control or cause-specific survival. Perfusion values could stratify patients within T stages 3 and 4; among 34 patients with T4 tumors, the likelihood of local control at 18 months was less than 10% if tumor perfusion was less than 83.5 ml/min/100 g. Choi *et al.* *(39)* determined peak contrast enhancement in small cell lung cancers from spiral CT acquisitions performed at 40 sec and 2–3 min after a 120 ml bolus of contrast medium (300 mg/ml). Peak tumor enhancement correlated with the subsequent reduction in tumor volume following chemotherapy ($r = 0.57$, $p < 0.002$). Ten of 11 (91%) patients with tumor enhancement less than 30 HU failed to achieve a reduction in tumor volume of 70% or more. Sommerfield *et al.* *(40)* used perfusion CT to make separate measurements of hepatic arterial and portal perfusion in a group of patients with colon cancer. Of 22 patients subsequently undergoing chemotherapy, those whose disease progressed despite treatment exhibited significantly lower levels of portal perfusion (29 versus 42 ml/min/100 ml, $p < 0.05$). A portal perfusion value of 30 ml/min/100 ml had a predictive value for progression despite treatment of 80%.

The use of imaging to identify those unlikely to respond to cancer therapy has the potential to save the morbidity and cost of futile treatment. However, the specificity of the test must be sufficiently high to ensure that treatment is not withheld from potential responders in error. The predictive values for poor response of above 90%, as found in T4 head and neck cancer and small cell lung cancer, emphasize the potential role for perfusion CT in patient selection. By reflecting the vascular heterogeneity that leads to hypoxia, the development of parameters that simultaneously encapsulate both the intensity and heterogeneity of contrast enhancement and/or perfusion may be able to improve these predictive values further.

7.2 Measuring Response

7.2.1 Chemotherapy

Functional CT has been used to demonstrate the physiological effects of a range of pharmacological interventions for cancer. One of the first of such studies was reported in 1994 by Yeung *et al.* who used two-compartmental modeling of contrast enhancement in the brain to demonstrate the effect of dexamethasone on the vascular permeability of cerebral tumors in 10 patients *(7)*. After 7 days of treatment (4×4 mg), permeability fell by a mean of 32% and relative blood volume by 10% ($p < 0.01$ and $p < 0.09$, respectively). A simplified two-compartmental model was used by Ford *et al.* to study the effect of a bradykinin analogue, RMP-7, upon the permeability of cerebral gliomas *(41)*. The mode of action of RMP-7 is to increase the vascular permeability of tumors and so increase the delivery of chemotherapeutic agents given in conjunction. The principle was confirmed by increases in median permeability in tumor from 41 µl/min/ml to 74 µl/min/ml while normal brain permeability was unchanged.

Two studies have used perfusion CT to study pharmacological interventions in colorectal cancer. Falk *et al.* used perfusion CT as one of a range of techniques to assess the impact on tumor perfusion produced by BW12C, an agent that aimed to increase the efficacy of bioreductive chemotherapy by increasing tissue hypoxia through modulation hemoglobin oxygen affinity *(8)*. The study group was composed of patients with metastatic colon cancer. Marked reductions in perfusion were seen in some tumors, particularly if perfusion levels were high prior to treatment. The study concluded that the reduction in perfusion produced would reduce delivery of the agent and so reduce efficacy. More recently, perfusion CT has been used in patients with rectal cancer to confirm the antivascular effects of bevacizumab, a VEGF-specific antibody *(24)*. With bevacizumab monotherapy, perfusion and relative blood volume fell by means of 34.6% and 26.5%, respectively, in line with a 47% reduction in microvascular density on tumor biopsy. Changes in permeability were highly variable. There was no significant reduction in fluorodeoxyglucose (FDG) uptake on PET during monotherapy, but FDG uptake did fall when the agent was used in combination with chemoradiation.

The potential for functional CT to assess the activity of lymphoma was studied by Dugdale *et al. (21)*. Perfusion values were found to be higher in masses containing active disease, with values below 20 ml/min/100 ml being found only in inactive disease. Serial perfusion measurements were made in two patients. In one, perfusion fell from 70 ml/min/100 ml to 18 ml/min/100 ml in parallel with the change from active to inactive disease by retrospective clinical assessment. In another, persistently active disease was accompanied by persistently raised perfusion (56 and 46 ml/min/100 ml). Permeability measurements did not appear to correlate with disease activity in group studies while serial studies found variable changes in permeability in association with therapeutic response.

The potential for perfusion CT to evaluate treatment response in lung cancer has been emphasized by two recent studies. Choi *et al.* describe seven patients who underwent follow-up measurements of peak tumor enhancement in residual masses of small cell cancer following chemotherapy *(39)*. Peak enhancement values increased in four, decreased in one, and were unchanged in two. All four patients showing an increase in enhancement were reported to demonstrate improvement. As part of a larger study, Kiessling *et al.* present a single case of non-small-cell lung cancer in which a partial response on size criteria was associated with a reduction in perfusion *(42)*.

The above studies suggest that CT measurements of capillary permeability may have value for assessing pharmacological response in brain tumors. However, the data from rectal cancer and lymphoma raise questions about the value of permeability measurements in extracranial tumors. The data on changes in perfusion and peak enhancement following therapy are encouraging, but more studies are needed to address unanswered questions concerning the meaning of perfusion changes after therapy. For drug treatments that target the tumor vasculature, in many cases a reduction in perfusion appears to indicate efficacy. However, more studies are required to determine whether this case will hold for other drug classes and tumor types.

7.2.2 RADIOTHERAPY

The feasibility of using functional CT for demonstrating the physiological effects of radiotherapy was first demonstrated by Harvey *et al. (26, 43)*. Within the prostate gland, measurements within 1–2 weeks of radiotherapy demonstrated increases in perfusion, blood volume, and permeability of 116%, 35%, and 33%, respectively. All three parameters remained elevated at 6–12 weeks. However, the regions of interest for analysis may have encompassed tumor and normal prostate gland and therefore it is possible that a differential response between tumor and prostate tissue may have masked any therapeutic response. Bondestam *et al.* subsequently used perfusion CT to monitor the effect of iodine-125 brachytherapy on the perfusion of cerebral meningioma in six patients *(44)*. At 3 months following therapy, mean perfusion within the center of the tumors had fallen by 41% (from 231 to 224 ml/min/100 g) with a further reduction to 68.7 ml/min/100 g at 1 year.

7.2.3 OTHER THERAPIES

Perfusion CT has also been used to evaluate changes in hepatic perfusion following transcatheter arterial chemoembolization of liver tumors using adriamycin and lipiodol *(45)*. Mean arterial values in four tumors fell from 90 ml/min/100 ml to 28 ml/min/ml. The potential utility of perfusion CT for monitoring laser thermal therapy of tumors has been demonstrated by a recent animal study *(46)*. The mean decrease in tumor perfusion was $41 \pm 14\%$. Hypocapnia produced an even greater reduction in tumor perfusion ($64 \pm 10\%$, $p < 0.001$) thereby minimizing heat dissipation through blood flow and producing a significantly larger thermal lesion.

8. PERFUSION COMPUTED TOMOGRAPHY/POSITRON EMISSION TOMOGRAPHY

Although introduced only recently, technologies that integrate CT and PET within a single imaging device are fast becoming the standard for delivery of clinical PET services. The CT component of these combined examinations generally involves an examination for attenuation correction and anatomical assignment of abnormalities identified on PET and is therefore performed without contrast medium. However, there is a growing interest in the use of intravenous contrast media during PET/CT *(47)*. Extending these applications for contrast media to include perfusion CT would enable anatomical information about tumors to be coregistered with perfusion data and metabolic information, such as glucose metabolism, in a single examination. The use of CT to assess perfusion as opposed to administration of a second PET tracer, such as [^{15}O]H$_2$O, avoids the need for an on-site cyclotron and depicts the perfusion data with higher spatial resolution. The analogous derivations of the SPV for CT contrast enhancement and the SUV for FDG uptake facilitate comparisons between these parameters and development of combined indices. Such combined data have the potential for improved prediction and subsequent measurement of therapeutic response. However, experience of performing perfusion CT during PET/CT is limited and there is a need for further development work to optimise protocols.

8.1 Perfusion Computed Tomography/Positron Emission Tomography and Prediction of Response

The separate applications of perfusion CT and FDG-PET to prediction of outcome in head and neck cancer illustrate the synergies that could be obtained by combining the techniques into a single examination. As discussed above, low perfusion as assessed by CT was found to be an independent predictor for poor local control following treatment *(38)*. In a separate study, Allal *et al.* demonstrated that high FDG uptake in head and neck cancer pretreatment was also an independent predictor for poor local control and reduced disease-free survival *(48)*. Tumor adaptation to hypoxia provides an explanatory link between these findings.

The reduced delivery of oxygen associated with poor tumor vascularization and low perfusion results in hypoxia. Hypoxia-inducible factors (HIFs), such as HIF-1α and HIF-2α, are important mediators of the tumor metabolic response to hypoxia. They increase the transcription of several molecules that adapt the tumor to its hypoxic environment, simultaneously promoting tumor aggression and resistance to chemotherapy and radiotherapy *(49)*. The degree of adaptation to hypoxia is likely to be of greater prognostic significance than the presence of hypoxia itself. Although the demonstration of reduced tumor perfusion may imply tumor hypoxia, perfusion measurements alone cannot assess the level of adaptation to hypoxia.

Increased HIF activity also increases expression of glucose transporters and promotes anaerobic glycolysis *(49)*. However, increased HIF activity can also occur as a consequence of oncogene mutations, resulting in not only increased glucose metabolism but also increased angiogenesis and perfusion *(49)*. Hence increased glucose metabolism in a tumor may reflect hypoxia, oncogene mutation, or both and FDG-PET alone will be unable to distinguish between these possible tumor phenotypes.

The balance between glucose metabolism and perfusion will more closely reflect tumor adaptation to hypoxia, and hence the likely resistance to treatment, than either alone. High FDG uptake with high perfusion would therefore represent a different biological status of the tumor than high FDG uptake with low perfusion, the latter indicating adaptation to hypoxia. Perfusion CT with FDG-PET would enable this balance to be assessed using techniques available in routine clinical practice. Perfusion

CT with PET measurements of hypoxia could also be combined using tracers such as [^{18}F]fluoromisonidazole (as discussed in Chapter 4).

8.2 Perfusion Computed Tomography/Positron Emission Tomography and Tumor Response

Measurements of perfusion and glucose metabolism have each been advocated as techniques for evaluation of the functional response of tumors to treatment. However, studies in which both parameters have been measured before and after treatment show that perfusion and glucose metabolism may not change in parallel in response to therapy *(23–25, 50)* (Fig. 2). In three of these four studies, the alterations in perfusion were of greater magnitude than the change in glucose metabolism. Although performed on separate imaging systems, the study of Willett *et al.* demonstrating differential perfusion CT and FDG-PET responses to the VEGF-antibody bevacizumab emphasizes the benefits of combining perfusion CT with FDG-PET *(24)*. Uncoupling of flow and metabolism appears to be particularly likely following antivascular therapy, probably reflecting drug-induced hypoxia and secondary stimulation of glucose metabolism (see Section 8.1). In a study of locally advanced breast cancer treated with neoadjuvant chemotherapy, perfusion increased in tumors failing to respond to treatment but decreased in tumors that subsequently proceeded to partial or complete response *(25)*. On the other hand, a study of androgen-independent prostate cancer treated with thalidomide demonstrated a negative correlation between PSA response and change in perfusion *(50)*. Thus, the relative magnitude of changes in tumor perfusion and glucose metabolism in response to therapy may depend upon both tumor type and treatment regime. By implementing perfusion CT on integrated PET/CT systems, it will be possible to monitor changes in both functional parameters, as well as any morphological change, in a single examination.

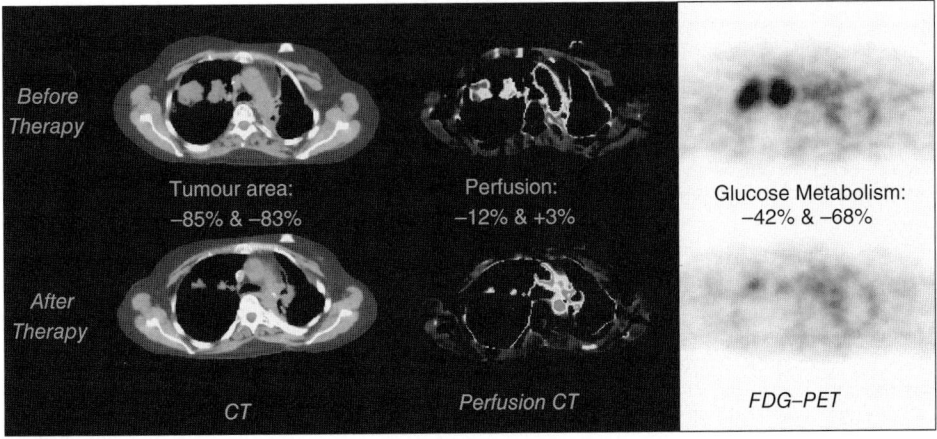

Fig. 2. Conventional CT, perfusion CT, and FDG-PET studies before and after therapy from a patient with two tumors in the right leg. There are differential morphological and physiological responses to therapy. Tumor areas have reduced by 85% and 83% respectively whereas tumor perfusion has changed little (−12% and +3%). There have been moderate reductions in glucose metabolism (42% and 62%), possibly exaggerated by partial volume effects. (*See* color plate.)

Table 3
Capabilities of Perfusion Computed Tomography (CT) as a Tumor Response Marker

Criterion	Capabilities of perfusion CT
Accurately and reproducibly distinguish responding patients from those demonstrating no response or progressive disease	Accurate and reproducible measurements of perfusion, blood volume, and capillary permeability reflecting angiogenesis *in vivo*
Identify nonresponders either before treatment or early in their course of treatment	Predicts response to treatment in head and neck cancer, small cell lung cancer, and colorectal cancer
	Demonstrates physiological changes in response to chemotherapy, radiotherapy, chemoembolization, and hyperthemia
Produce sufficient benefit at low cost	Wide availability at low cost
	Technical simplicity
	Can be performed in combination with other techniques, i.e., conventional CT and PET

9. SUMMARY

An ideal marker of tumor response to therapy would (1) accurately and reproducibly distinguish responding patients from those demonstrating no response or progressive disease, (2) identify nonresponders either before treatment or early in their course of treatment, so that the morbidity of ineffective therapy can be avoided, and (3) produce sufficient benefit at low cost. The capabilities of perfusion CT as outlined in Table 3 indicate that perfusion CT could fulfill many of these requirements, offering a widely available, low-cost adjunct to existing methods for evaluating treatment response in a broad range of tumors.

REFERENCES

1. Axel L. Cerebral blood flow determination by rapid-sequence computed tomography; theoretical analysis. *Radiology* 1980;137:679.
2. Jaschke W, Sievers RS, Lipton MJ, Cogan MG. Cine-CT computed tomographic assessment of regional renal blood flow. *Acta Radiol* 1989;31:77–81.
3. Wolfkiel CJ, Ferguson JL, Chomka EV, Law WR, Labin IN, Tenzer ML, Booker M, Brundage BH. Measurement of myocardial blood flow by ultrafast computed tomography. *Circulation* 1987;76:1262–1273.
4. Miles KA, Hayball MP, Dixon AK. Colour perfusion imaging: A new application of computed tomography. *Lancet* 1991;337:643–645.
5. Miles KA, Hayball MP, Dixon AK. Functional images of hepatic perfusion obtained with dynamic computed tomography. *Radiology* 1993;188:405–411.
6. Falk SJ, Ramsay JR, Ward R, Miles K, Dixon AK, Bleehen NM. BW12C perturbs normal and tumour tissue oxygenation and blood flow in man. *Radiother Oncol* 1994;32:210–217.
7. Yeung WT, Lee TY, Del Maestro RF, Kozak R, Bennett J, Brown T. Effect of steroids on iopamidol blood-brain transfer constant and plasma volume in brain tumors measured with X-ray computed tomography. *J Neurooncol* 1994;18:53–60.
8. Miles KA, Griffiths MR, Fuentes MA. Standardized perfusion value: Universal CT contrast enhancement scale that correlates with FDG PET in lung nodules. *Radiology* 2001;220:548–553.
9. Miles KA, Young H, Chica SL, Esser PD. Quantitative contrast-enhanced computed tomography: Is there a need for system calibration? *Eur Radiol* 2007;17:919–926.

10. Miles KA, Charnsangavej C, Lee F, Fishman E, Horton K, Lee T-Y. Application of CT in the investigation of angiogenesis in oncology. *Acad Radiol* 2000;7:840–850.
11. Swensen SJ, Brown LR, Colby TV, Weaver AL, Midthun DE. Lung nodule enhancement at CT: Prospective findings. *Radiology* 1996;201:447–455.
12. Tateishi U, Nishihara H, Watanabe S, Morikawa T, Abe K, Miyasaka K. Tumor angiogenesis and dynamic CT in lung adenocarcinoma: Radiologic-pathologic correlation. *J Comput Assist Tomogr* 2001;25:23–27.
13. Jinzaki M, Tanimoto A, Mukai M, Ikeda E, Kobayashi S, Yuasa Y, Narimatsu Y, Murai M. Double-phase helical CT of small renal parenchymal neoplasms: Correlation with pathologic findings and tumor angiogenesis. *J Comput Assist Tomogr* 2000;24:835–842.
14. Tateishi U, Nishihara H, Tsukamoto E, Morikawa T, Tamaki N, Miyasaka K. Lung tumors evaluated with FDG-PET and dynamic CT: The relationship between vascular density and glucose metabolism. *J Comput Assist Tomogr* 2002;26:185–190.
15. Yi CA, Lee KS, Kim EA, Han J, Kim H, Kwon OJ, Jeong YJ, Kim S. Solitary pulmonary nodules: Dynamic enhanced multi-detector row CT study and comparison with vascular endothelial growth factor and microvessel density. *Radiology* 2004;233:191–199.
16. Miles KA, Griffiths M. CT Perfusion: A worthwhile enhancement? *Br J Radiol* 2003;76(904): 220–231.
17. Swensen SJ, Viggiano RW, Midthun DE, Muller NL, Sherrick A, Yamashita K, Naidich DP, Patz EF, Hartman TE, Muhm JR, Weaver AL. Lung nodule enhancement at CT: Multicenter study. *Radiology* 2000;214:73–80.
18. Pastorino U, Bellomi M, Landoni C, De Fiori E, Arnaldi P, Picchio M, Pelosi G, Boyle P, Fazio F. Early lung-cancer detection with spiral CT and positron emission tomography in heavy smokers: 2-year results. *Lancet* 2003;362:593–597.
19. Comber LA, Keith CJ, Griffiths MR, Miles KA. Solitary pulmonary nodules: Impact of quantitative contrast enhanced CT on the cost-effectiveness of FDG-PET. *Clin Radiol* 2003;58:706–711.
20. Leggett DA, Miles KA, Kelley BB. Blood-brain barrier and blood volume imaging of cerebral glioma using functional CT: A pictorial review. *Australasian Radiol* 1998;42(4):335–340.
21. Dugdale PE, Miles KA, Kelley BB, Bunce IH, Leggett DAC. CT measurements of perfusion and permeability within lymphoma masses: Relationship to grade, activity and chemotherapeutic response. *J Comput Tomogr* 1999;23:540–547.
22. Dugdale PE, Miles KA. Hepatic metastases: The value of quantitative assessment of contrast enhancement on computed tomography. *Eur J Radiol* 1999;30:206–213.
23. Mullani N, Herbst R, Abbruzzese J, Charnsangavej C, Kim E, Tran H, Barron B, Lamki L, Gould K. Antiangiogenic treatment with endostatin results in uncoupling of blood flow and glucose metabolism in human tumors. *Clin Positron Imaging* 2000;3:151.
24. Willett CG, Boucher Y, di Tomaso E, Duda DG, Munn LL, Tong RT, Chung DC, Sahani DV, Kalva SP, Kozin SV, Mino M, Cohen KS, Scadden DT, Hartford AC, Fischman AJ, Clark JW, Ryan DP, Zhu AX, Blaszkowsky LS, Chen HX, Shellito PC, Lauwers GY, Jain RK. Direct evidence that the VEGF-specific antibody bevacizumab has antivascular effects in human rectal cancer. *Nat Med* 2004;10: 145–147.
25. Mankoff DA, Dunnwald LK, Gralow JR, Ellis GK, Schubert EK, Tseng J, Lawton TJ, Linden HM, Livingston RB. Changes in blood flow and metabolism in locally advanced breast cancer treated with neoadjuvant chemotherapy. *J Nucl Med* 2003;44:1806–1814.
26. Harvey CJ, Blomley MJ, Dawson P Morgan JA, Dooher A, Deponte J, Vernon CC, Price P. Functional CT imaging of the acute hyperemic response to radiation therapy of the prostate gland: Early experience. *J Comput Assist Tomogr* 2001;25:43–49.
27. Wintermark M, Smith WS, Ko NU, et al. Dynamic perfusion CT: Optimizing the temporal resolution and contrast volume for calculation of perfusion CT parameters in stroke patients. *Am J Neuroradiol* 2004;25:720–729.
28. Miles KA. Measurement of tissue perfusion by dynamic computed tomography. *Br J Radiol* 1991; 64:409–412.
29. Mullani N, Gould KL. First pass measurements of regional blood flow using external detectors. *J Nucl Med* 1983;24:577–581.
30. Patlak CS, Blasberg RG, Fenstermacher JD. Graphical evaluation of blood-to-brain transfer constants from multiple-time uptake data. *J Cereb Blood Flow Metab* 1983;3(1):1–7.

31. Cenic A, Nabavi DG, Craen RA, Gelb AW, Lee TY. A CT method to measure hemodynamics in brain tumors: Validation and application to cerebral blood flow maps. *Am J Neuroradiol* 2000;21:462–470.
32. Purdie TG, Henderson E, Lee TY. Functional CT imaging of angiogenesis in rabbit VX2 soft-tissue tumour. *Phys Med Biol* 2001;46:3161–3175.
33. Pollard RE, Garcia TC, Stieger SM, Ferrara KW, Sadlowski AR, Wisner ER. Quantitative evaluation of perfusion and permeability of peripheral tumours using contrast-enhanced computed tomography. *Invest Radiol* 2004;39:340–349.
34. Hattori H, Miyoshi T, Okada J, Yoshikawa K, Arimizu N, Hattori N. Tumor blood flow measured using dynamic computed tomography. *Invest Radiol* 1994;29:873–876.
35. Gillard JH, Antoun NM, Burnet NG, Pickard JD. Reproducibility of quantitative CT perfusion imaging. *Br J Radiol* 2001;74:552–555.
36. Maxwell RJ, Wilson J, Prise VE, Vojnovic B, Rustin GJ, Lodge MA, Tozer GM. Evaluation of the anti-vascular effects of combretastatin in rodent tumours by dynamic contrast enhanced MRI. *NMR Biomed* 2002;15:89–98.
37. Blomley MJ, Coulden R, Dawson P, Kormano M, Donlan P, Bufkin C, et al. Liver perfusion studied with ultrafast CT. *J Comput Assist Tomogr* 1995;19(3):424–433.
38. Hermans R, Meijerink M, Van den Bogaert W, Rijnders A, Weltens C, Lambin P. Tumor perfusion rate determined noninvasively by dynamic computed tomography predicts outcome in head-and-neck cancer after radiotherapy. *Int J Radiat Oncol Biol Phys* 2003;57:1351–1356.
39. Choi J-B, Park C-K, Park DW, Kim Y, Kim Y-S, Choi YW, Jeon SC. Does contrast enhancement on CT suggest tumor response for chemotherapy in small cell carcinoma of the lung? *J Comput Assist Tomogr* 2002;26(5):797–800.
40. Sommerfeld NWB, Miles KA, Dugdale P, Leggett DAC, Bunce IH. Colorectal cancer: Progressive disease is associated with altered liver perfusion on functional CT. 50th Annual Meeting of the Royal Australia & New Zealand College of Radiologists, 1999. Abstract No. 56.
41. Ford J, Miles K, Hayball M, Bearcroft P, Bleehan N, Osborn C. A simplified method for measurement of blood-brain barrier permeability using CT: Preliminary results and the effect of RMP-7. In: Faulkner K, et al., eds. Quantitative Imaging in Oncology. London: British Institute of Radiology, 1996:1–5.
42. Kiessling F, Boese J, Corvinus C, Ederle JR, Zuna I, et al. Perfusion CT in patients with advanced bronchial carcinomas: A novel chance for characterisation and treatment monitoring? *Eur Radiol* 2004;14:1226–1233.
43. Harvey C, Dooher A, Morgan J, Blomley M, Dawson P. Imaging of tumour therapy responses by dynamic CT. *Eur J Radiol* 1999;30:221–226.
44. Bondestam S, Halavaara JT, JAaskelainen JE, Kinnunen JJ, Hamberg LM. Perfusion CT of the brain in the assessment of flow alterations during brachytherapy of meningioma. *Acta Radiol* 1999;40:469–473.
45. Tsushima Y, Funabasama S, Aoki J, Sanada S, Endo K. Quantitative perfusion map of malignant liver tumors created from dynamic computed tomography data. *Acad Radiol* 2004;11:215–223.
46. Purdie TG, Sherar MD, Lee TY. The use of CT perfusion to monitor the effect of hypocapnia during laser thermal therapy in a rabbit model. *Int J Hypertherm* 2003;19:461–479.
47. Antoch G, Freudenberg LS, Beyer T, Bockisch A, Debatin JF. To enhance or not to enhance? 18F-FDG and CT contrast agents in dual-modality 18F-FDG PET/CT. *J Nucl Med* 2004;45(Suppl 1):56S–65S.
48. Allal AS, Slosman DO, Kebdani T, Allaoua M, Lehmann W, Dulguerov P. Prediction of outcome in head-and-neck cancer patients using the standardized uptake value of 2-[^{18}F]fluoro-2-deoxy-D-glucose. *Int J Radiat Oncol Biol Phys* 2004;5:1295–1300.
49. Semenza GL. HIF-1 and tumor progression: Pathophysiology and therapeutics. *Trends Mol Med* 2002;8(4 Suppl):S62–S67.
50. Kurdziel KA, Figg WD, Carrasquillo JA, Huebsch S, Whatley M, Sellers D, Libutti SK, Pluda JM, Dahut W, Reed E, Bacharach SL. Using positron emission tomography 2-deoxy-2-[18F]fluoro-D-glucose, 11CO, and 15O-water for monitoring androgen independent prostate cancer. *Mol Imaging Biol* 2003;5:86–93.

7 [^{18}F]Fluorodeoxyglucose Positron Emission Tomography Assessment of Response

Wolfgang A. Weber, MD

CONTENTS

INTRODUCTION
LIMITATIONS OF CURRENT TECHNIQUES TO MONITOR
   ANTICANCER THERAPY
MONITORING OF TUMOR RESPONSE BY
   [^{18}F]FLUORODEOXYGLUCOSE POSITRON EMISSION
   TOMOGRAPHY: METHODOLOGICAL CONSIDERATIONS
CLINICAL STUDIES ON TREATMENT MONITORING WITH
   [^{18}F]FLUORODEOXYGLUCOSE POSITRON EMISSION
   TOMOGRAPHY
SUMMARY AND OUTLOOK

1. INTRODUCTION

During the past 10 years, positron emission tomography with the glucose analog fluorodeoxyglucose (FDG PET) has evolved from a research tool to a clinical test that is used for diagnosis and staging of a variety of malignant tumors. More recently FDG PET has been evaluated for monitoring tumor response to therapy. Most of these studies have used FDG PET after completion of therapy in order to differentiate between viable tumor and therapy-induced fibrosis. However, there are also encouraging data that FDG PET may be used to predict tumor response during therapy. This chapter summarizes the results of recent studies on treatment monitoring by FDG PET and discusses potential clinical applications. Different approaches for quantitative analysis of FDG PET studies are also reviewed, since monitoring tumor response by FDG PET frequently relies on quantifying tumor metabolic activity over time. To put the results achieved by FDG PET in a more general context, the current clinical practice of assessing tumor response and its scientific background are briefly discussed.

From: *Cancer Drug Discovery and Development*
In Vivo Imaging of Cancer Therapy
Edited by: A.F. Shields and P. Price © Humana Press Inc., Totowa, NJ

2. LIMITATIONS OF CURRENT TECHNIQUES TO MONITOR ANTICANCER THERAPY

Conventional criteria for monitoring cytotoxic therapy of malignant tumors are defined by therapy-induced reduction of tumor size, generally measured by radiological techniques. The World Health Organization (WHO) has defined standardized criteria for assessment of tumor response. These criteria request that the size of the tumor has to be measured in two perpendicular diameters. Tumor response was defined as a therapy-induced reduction of the product of these two diameters by at least 50% *(1)*.

Given the broad acceptance of the WHO response criteria it is interesting to look at the data that formed the basis for their definition. In the publication of the response criteria in 1981 *(1)*, the major reference for justifying a 50% decrease in tumor size as a criterion for tumor response is a study performed by Moertel and Hanley in 1976 *(2)*. In this study wooden spheres were placed on a soft mattress and covered with a layer of rubber foam. Then 16 experienced oncologists measured the diameters of these spheres in random order using rulers or calipers. In a detailed analysis Moertel and Hanley point out that due to measurement errors the size of *identical* spheres differed by at least 25% in 25% of the measurements but by at least 50% in only 6.8% of the measurements. Thus, using a 25% decrease of lesion size as a criterion for tumor response would bear the risk of an unacceptable high rate of "responses" (25%) when the tumor was in fact unchanged in size. The false-positive rate would only be 6.8% when a decrease of lesion size by 50% was used as a criterion. This false-positive rate was considered acceptable and a 50% decrease of tumor size was recommended as a criterion for response in clinical studies.

This recommendation has been accepted by the panel defining the WHO criteria and has then been translated without further evaluation to all modern imaging techniques. More recently new "Response Evaluation Criteria for Solid Tumors" (RECIST) have been introduced by the National Cancer Institute (NCI) and the European Association for Research and Treatment of Cancer (EORTC). It includes requirements for measuring lesion size in clinical trials for different imaging techniques (e.g., minimum lesion size). However, the criteria for a tumor response have been essentially unchanged. The only major change is that that the bidimensional measurements required by the WHO criteria have been replaced by unidimensional measurements *(3)*. The new criteria define response as a 30% decrease of the largest diameter of the tumor. For a spherical lesion this is equivalent to a 50% decrease of the product of two diameters. Thus, when tumors are currently evaluated after therapy by magnetic resonance imaging (MRI) or multislice computed tomography (CT) the criteria for response stem from an experiment performed more than 25 years ago, which determined the accuracy by which physicians could measure tumor size by palpation.

In addition to radiological criteria tumor response can also be evaluated histopathologically. A histopathological response is commonly defined by the percentage of viable tumor relative to therapy-induced fibrosis. This percentage is expressed as a regression score. The most commonly used histopathological regression score is probably the Salzer–Kuntschik score for osteosarcomas *(4)*. Similar scoring systems of tumor response have been established for other tumor types such as non-small-cell lung cancer *(5)*, esophageal cancer *(6)*, and gastric cancer *(7)*. Histopathological regression scores have shown a close correlation with survival. In particular, patients with no or only minimal (less than 10%) residual tumor have been found to have a markedly improved prognosis *(5–8)*. Therefore, a histopathological response is often used as the gold standard for the evaluation of imaging techniques. However, complete resection of the tumor is necessary for a valid histopathological response evaluation. Thus, histopathological response can be determined only at the end of therapy and cannot be used to modify treatment. For these reasons there is a clear need for techniques that allow noninvasive monitoring of tumor response early in the course of therapy.

3. MONITORING OF TUMOR RESPONSE BY [^{18}F]FLUORODEOXYGLUCOSE POSITRON EMISSION TOMOGRAPHY: METHODOLOGICAL CONSIDERATIONS

3.1 Visual Interpretations versus Quantitative Measurements of Tumor Glucose Utilization

For staging of malignant tumors FDG PET scans are assessed visually, and focally increased FDG uptake not explained by the normal biodistribution of FDG is considered to be suspicious for metastatic disease. In a similar way PET scans may also be read *after completion* of chemotherapy or radiotherapy. Uptake of FDG should have normalized at this time and focal FDG uptake generally indicates residual viable tumor tissue. As described in Section 4.1 there are now numerous studies in malignant lymphoma as well as several solid tumors indicating that focal FDG uptake after therapy is a relatively specific sign for viable tumor tissue and is associated with a poor prognosis. Quantitative analysis is frequently not required at this time to make the diagnosis of residual tumor tissue. However, quantitative assessment of tumor metabolism is frequently necessary when FDG PET scans are performed during treatment in order to *predict* subsequent tumor response. At this time the metabolic activity of the tumor tissue has decreased in responders, but generally there will still be considerable residual FDG uptake (Fig. 1). In a recent study Wieder *et al. (9)* evaluated the time course of changes in tumor FDG uptake in patients with locally advanced esophageal cancer treated with chemoradiotherapy followed by surgical resection; FDG PET was performed prior to chemoradiotherapy, 2 weeks after initiation of therapy, and 3–4 weeks after completion of chemoradiotherapy. After the third PET scans the tumors were resected and tumor response was assessed histopathologically. In the baseline scan there was no significant differences between the FDG uptake of responding and nonresponding tumors. At the time of the first follow-up scan (at a radiation dose of 15–20 Gy) FDG uptake of responding tumors had significantly decreased ($p < 0.001$). However, most of the tumors still showed marked focal FDG uptake at this time. The intensity of tumor FDG uptake in histopathological responders (SUV 5.3 ± 2.1) was not significantly different from histopathological nonresponders (SUV 6.7 ± 2.1, $p = 0.11$). In contrast, the *relative decrease* in FDG uptake from the baseline scan to the first follow-up scan was more than two times larger for histopathological responders than for nonresponders (44% versus 20%, $p = 0.0055$). At the time of the third, preoperative scan FDG uptake of the histopathologically responding tumors had almost decreased to background levels [standardized uptake value (SUV) 2.7 ± 0.8].

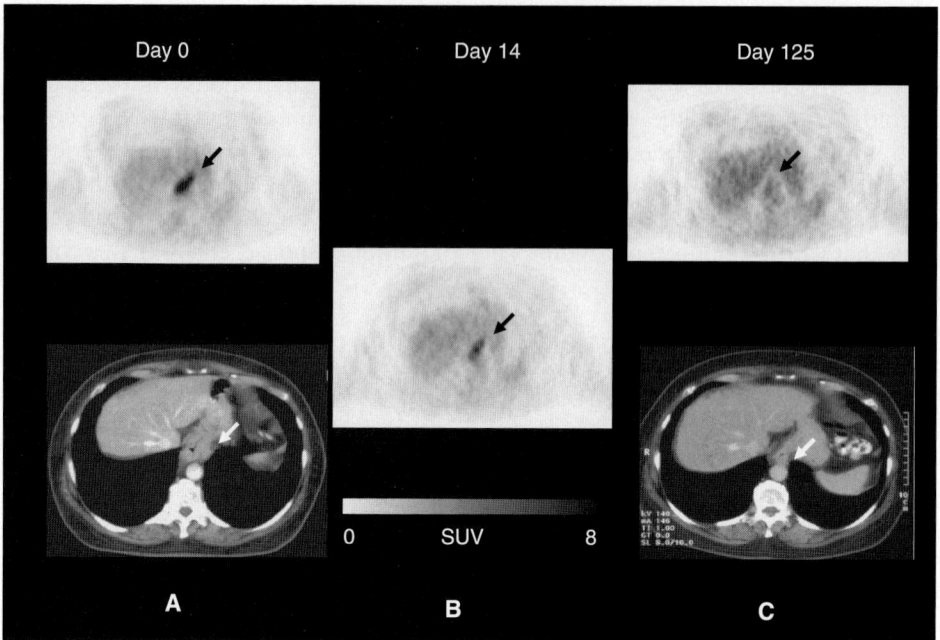

Fig. 1. Changes in tumor FDG uptake in a patient with distal esophageal cancer and histopathological complete response after 3 months of chemotherapy. In the baseline PET scan the tumor (arrow) demonstrates marked FDG uptake. (A) Fourteen days after initiation of therapy there is a marked reduction of FDG uptake. (B) However, the tumor still demonstrates increased metabolic activity when compared to surrounding normal tissues. After completion of chemotherapy the tumor shows no focal FDG uptake and the wall thickness of the distal esophagus has almost normalized (C).

3.2 Factors Influencing Quantitative Measurements of Tumor Glucose Use by [^{18}F]Fluorodeoxyglucose Positron Emission Tomography

Quantification of tumor metabolic activity by FDG PET is complicated by the fact that several factors *(10)* other than tumor glucose use have an impact on the FDG signal. Partial volume effects can cause a marked underestimation of the true activity concentration within smaller tumors *(11)*. Of note, the activity concentration may be considerably underestimated even in large tumors due to heterogeneous FDG uptake. It is also necessary to consider that FDG uptake of malignant tumors is time dependent. Thus SUVs will generally be considerably higher at later than at earlier time points. For example, the SUV of gastric cancers has been shown to increase by 50% between 40 min and 90 min postinjection *(12)*. Plasma glucose levels have a significant influence on tumor FDG uptake, since FDG and glucose compete for glucose transport and phosphorylation by hexokinase *(13)*. Considering all these factors it becomes clear that it is challenging to quantify tumor glucose utilization by FDG PET in a clinical setting. Therefore, quantitative measurements of tumor FDG uptake have been criticized and it has been suggested that SUV stands for "silly useless value" *(14)* and not standardized uptake value. However, this does not mean that it is equally difficult to measure

Table 1
Common Sources of Errors in the Measurement of Standardized Uptake Values (SUVs)

Error	Effect on tumor SUV
Paravenous FDG injection, residual activity in the syringe	Incorrectly low SUV because the area under the plasma time activity curve is lower
No decay correction of the injected activity	Incorrectly low SUV
Incorrect cross-calibration of scanner and dose calibrator	Incorrectly low or high SUV, depending on the error of the calibration factor
Variable uptake period (time between injection and imaging)	The longer the uptake period, the higher the SUV

relative *changes* in tumor glucose utilization over time. In this case only an intraindividual comparison of two studies is performed. This significantly reduces the number of factors that may confound the FDG signal *(15)*. Several recent studies have shown that changes in FDG uptake during chemotherapy or chemoradiotherapy are significantly correlated with patient survival (see Section 4.2).

Although calculation of SUVs is straightforward, it is necessary to follow a strict protocol for data acquisition and analysis and to check the calculated values for consistency. Frequent sources of error in calculating SUVs are listed in Table 1. To check for errors in the calculation of SUVs changes in FDG uptake should also be evaluated visually. For this it is helpful to review the baseline and the follow-up study side by side and to normalize the display of both studies to the same maximum. If there are marked differences in the FDG uptake of normal organs an error in the calculation of the SUVs in one of the studies is very likely. For comparison of the baseline and the follow-up study the intensity of liver FDG uptake can provide helpful orientation, since the SUVs of normal liver show only a very low variation over time *(16)*.

3.3 Which Degree of Change in Tumor Metabolic Activity Is "Significant"?

Unfortunately there are currently no generally accepted criteria for a "metabolic response" in FDG PET. The EORTC published preliminary criteria for assessment of tumor response in 1999 *(17)*. However, at that time only a limited amount of data on the use of FDG PET for treatment monitoring was available. Since then numerous studies on treatment monitoring with FDG PET have been published and there is now a great need to standardize the criteria used for monitoring anticancer therapy with FDG PET.

Based on the reproducibility of the FDG signal in untreated tumors relative changes of approximately 20% are very unlikely to be due to measurement errors or spontaneous fluctuations of tumor metabolic activity *(18, 19)*. This applies to measurements of SUVs as well as to measurements of FDG flux (K_i) by Patlak–Gjedde analysis. However, it is important to note that this criterion is only valid for tumors with sufficient baseline metabolic activity. In our study evaluating 50 lesions in 16 patients the 95% normal range for these differences in SUV was ± 0.9. According to these data a change in SUV can be considered to be significant only when the difference between the baseline and the follow-up scan is more than 0.9 (baseline SUV approximately 5) *(19)*.

These data establish the minimal effect of treatment on tumor metabolic activity that can be assessed by FDG PET. However, a measurable change in metabolic activity does not necessarily imply that treatment has a beneficial effect for the patient. We have therefore recently evaluated the prognostic implications of a measurable change in tumor glucose utilization in patients with advanced non-small-cell lung cancer who were treated with palliative platinum-based chemotherapy. A "metabolic response" in PET was prospectively defined as a decrease of the SUV of the primary tumor by at least 20%. A total of 57 patients were included in the study and 28 tumors showed a metabolic response after the first chemotherapy cycle. Median progression-free survival of metabolic nonresponders was only 1.8 months versus 5.9 months for metabolic responders. Median overall survival of metabolic responders was 8.4 months and only 5.0 months for metabolic nonresponders *(20)*. These data indicate that a measurable change in tumor FDG uptake after the first cycle of chemotherapy is associated with a palliative effect of therapy.

Other threshold values for definition of a metabolic response are necessary when chemotherapy is used with a curative intent. For example, in patients with high grade malignant lymphomas a mean decrease of FDG uptake by more than 45% has been observed within 24 h after the administration of the first dose of chemotherapy *(21)*. In patients with solid tumors treated by preoperative chemotherapy a change in FDG uptake of 35–50% *(9, 20, 22–25)* within the first weeks of chemotherapy has been found to provide the highest accuracy for prediction of histopathologically complete or subtotal tumor regression (see Table 2). These differences in the changes of tumor FDG uptake in different clinical situations are not unexpected since the degree of tumor response to treatment is also clearly different. While chemotherapy induces only a minor reduction of tumor size in palliative treatment of non-small-cell lung

Table 2
Prognostic Relevance of Quantitative Changes in Tumor Fluorodeoxyglucose Uptake during Chemotherapy or Chemoradiotherapy

Tumor	Reference	Year	N	Criteria	Median survival		p value
					Responder	Nonresponder	
Lymphoma	Kostagoglu (22)	2002	30	visual	>24	5	<0.001[a]
Esophagus	Weber (72)	2001	37	−35%	>48	20	0.04
	Wieder (9)	2004	22[b]	−30%	>38	18	0.011
Gastric	Ott (24)	2002	35	−35%	>48	17	0.001
Head and neck	Brun (25)	2002	47	−50%	>120	40	0.004
Lung	Weber (20)	2003	57	−20%	9	5	0.005

[a] Progression-free survival; otherwise overall survival.
[b] Chemoradiotherapy; otherwise chemotherapy.

cancer it reduces the viable tumor cell mass by more than 90% in patients with a histopathological response to preoperative therapy and it cures many patients with high-grade malignant lymphomas (i.e., it eliminates 100% of the tumor cells). Thus, the interpretation of a metabolic response in FDG PET will necessarily depend on the clinical context.

3.4 When Should [^{18}F]Fluorodeoxyglucose Positron Emission Tomography Scans Be Performed to Assess or Predict Treatment Response?

When FDG PET is performed after completion of potentially curative chemotherapy or radiotherapy only small amounts of residual viable tumor may be present. In this situation differentiation between "responders" and "nonresponders" by FDG PET can be challenging. To achieve the highest sensitivity for detection of residual tumor tissue FDG PET should therefore be performed as late as possible after completion of therapy in order to enhance the detection of residual tumor tissue. In our experience, a waiting period of 4–6 weeks after completion of therapy is a reasonable compromise. Imaging at later time points would probably improve the accuracy of FDG PET for detection of residual tumor tissue, but is frequently of limited clinical relevance.

In vitro studies have suggested that chemotherapy and radiotherapy may cause a "metabolic flare phenomenon" *(26, 27)*. In these *in vitro* studies, however, FDG uptake was measured per *surviving* cells after chemotherapy or radiation therapy. This differs from the clinical situation, where the change in the PET signal is determined by a combination of decreased FDG uptake due to cancer cell death plus potentially increased FDG uptake by surviving tumor cells. In clinical studies a mild to moderate increase in tumor FDG uptake has been observed only in the first hours after high-dose radiotherapy of brain tumors *(28, 29)*. A "metabolic flare" phenomenon has also been observed in metastatic breast cancer treated with tamoxifen and was associated with a good response to therapy. This initial increase in tumor metabolic activity is likely due to the partial estrogen-like stimulatory activity of this antiestrogen, which may be particularly apparent during the initial days of treatment when its levels are still low *(30)*.

3.5 Monitoring Radiotherapy or Chemoradiotherapy with [^{18}F]Fluorodeoxyglucose Positron Emission Tomography

Radiotherapy often causes inflammatory reactions, which has raised concerns about using FDG PET for assessment of tumor response to radiotherapy or chemoradiotherapy. It has frequently been recommended that FDG PET should not be performed until several months after completion of radiotherapy. However, there is a surprising lack of data to support this recommendation. Although there is no doubt that radiation-induced inflammation accumulates FDG, the intensity of FDG uptake is often considerably lower than in untreated primary tumors. Furthermore, the configuration of increased FDG uptake in radiation-induced inflammation is often markedly different from a malignant tumor. It is therefore frequently possible to differentiate between radiation-induced inflammation and residual tumor tissue *(9, 31)*, especially when comparing a pretreatment with a posttreatment PET scan (Fig. 2).

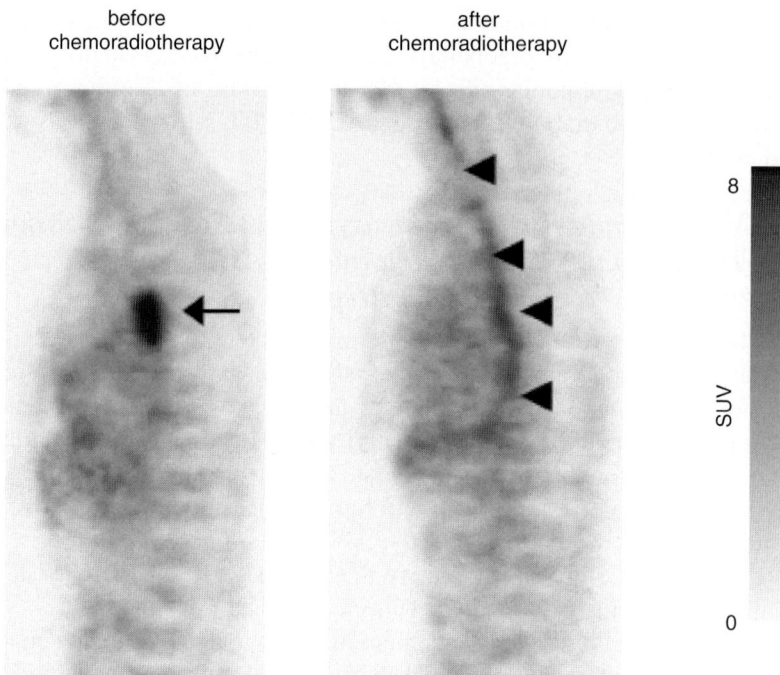

Fig. 2. By comparing the baseline and the follow-up scan radiation-induced inflammation can frequently be differentiated from viable tumor tissue. This patient with esophageal cancer (arrow) was studied by FDG PET prior to and after completion of chemoradiotherapy. In the posttherapeutic scan there is linear uptake along the esophagus (arrowheads). The pattern of FDG uptake allows differentiation between residual tumor and esophagitis.

4. CLINICAL STUDIES ON TREATMENT MONITORING WITH [^{18}F]FLUORODEOXYGLUCOSE POSITRON EMISSION TOMOGRAPHY

4.1 Assessment of Tumor Response after Completion of Therapy

4.1.1 MALIGNANT LYMPHOMA

Anatomic imaging modalities often reveal residual masses after completion of therapy for lymphoma. It is very difficult to assess whether this represents viable tumor or fibrotic scar tissue. Even biopsy may be inaccurate because residual masses frequently contain a mixture of viable tumor cells and fibrosis, which may cause false-negative results. The clinical value of FDG PET in detecting residual viable tumor tissue has been demonstrated for Hodgkin's disease and high-grade non-Hodgkin's lymphoma. Jerusalem *et al.* were the first to demonstrate in a larger series of patients that focal FDG uptake in a residual mass is associated with a poor outcome *(32)*. These findings have been confirmed by several studies published in the past 5 years (Table 3). In one of the largest series Zinzani *et al.* report on 75 patients with Hodgkin's disease or aggressive non-Hodgkin's lymphoma who were studied after chemotherapy *(33)*. Four out of five (80%) patients who were positive in PET, but negative in CT, relapsed, as compared with 0 out of 29 patients who were negative in PET, but positive in CT. Among the 41 patients with a residual mass in CT, 10 out of 11 (91%) who were PET positive relapsed, as compared with 0 out of 30 who were PET negative. The relapse-free 1-year survival rates were 9% and 100% for patients with and without metabolically active lesions in PET.

The treatment and prognosis of Hodgkin's disease and non-Hodgkin's lymphoma are clearly different, and recently PET studies have been published taking these differences into account. De Wit et al. (34) compared PET with CT in 37 patients after treatment for Hodgkin's lymphoma. The sensitivity of FDG PET to predict disease-free survival was 91%. Surprisingly the specificity of FDG PET was only 69%. However, six patients underwent additional radiotherapy after the PET scan. These patients might have had residual disease at the time of the PET scan that was controlled by radiotherapy. Another study focusing on Hodgkin's disease included 28 patients with a residual mediastinal mass of at least 2 cm after initial therapy or after salvage chemotherapy (35). A PET-negative mediastinal tumor was observed in 19 patients, of whom 16 remained in remission and 3 patients relapsed. In 6 out of 10 patients with a positive PET, progression of disease or relapse occurred, whereas 4 patients remained in remission.

Several studies also addressed the role of FDG PET for treatment evaluation in high-grade non-Hodgkin's lymphoma (NHL). Mikhaeel et al. (36) reported on 49 patients with aggressive NHL. The results of posttreatment PET were well correlated with patient outcome, with relapse rates of 100% (9 of 9) for positive PET scans and only 17% (6 of 36) when the PET was negative. The relapse rate was 100% for positive PET and only 18% for negative PET, compared with 41% and 25% for patients with

Table 3
Prognostic Relevance of Residual Fluorodeoxyglucose Uptake after Completion of Chemotherapy or Chemoradiotherapy

Tumor	Reference	Year	N	Median survival		p value
				Responder	Nonresponder	
Lymphoma	Spaepen (37)	2001	93	>46	7	<0.001[a]
	Weihrauch (35)	2001	28	>50	3	0.004
	Spaepen (38)	2003	60	>60	30	<0.001
	Schot (39)	2003	46	>30	8	0.048
	Kumar (56)	2004	19	>30	9	<0.001[a]
	Zinzani (33)	2004	75	>15	9	<0.001[a]
Esophagus	Flamen (41)	2002	36[b]	>34	7	0.005
	Swisher (44)	2004	103[b]	>24	15	0.01
Lung	Mac Manus (45)	2003	73[b]	>36	12	0.001
	Hellwig (46)	2004	47[b]	56	19	<0.001
Head/Neck	Kunkel (55)	2003	35[b]	>60	18	0.002[a]
Cervix	Grigsby (51)	2003	152[b]	>60	30 (persistent FDG uptake) 7 (new lesions)	<0.001
Soft tissue sarcomas	Schuetze (52)	2005	47	>100	40	0.02

[a] Progression free survival; otherwise overall survival.
[b] Chemoradiotherapy; otherwise chemotherapy.

positive and negative CT, respectively. In a larger series, including 93 patients with non-Hodgkin's lymphoma, Spaepen et al. *(37)* evaluated PET in predicting relapse after first-line treatment. A normal FDG PET scan was found in 67 patients; within a median follow-up of 22 months, 56 out of 67 remained in complete remission and 11 of 67 patients relapsed with a median progression-free survival of 13 months. Persistent abnormal FDG uptake was seen in 26 patients, and all of them relapsed with a median progression-free survival of only 2 months.

[^{18}F]Fluorodeoxyglucose positron emission tomography also appears to be helpful in the evaluation of patients prior to high-dose chemotherapy and stem cell transplantation *(38)*. In a retrospective study of 60 patients with induction failure or relapsing chemosensitive lymphoma the findings in FDG PET were significantly correlated with progression-free and overall survival. Thirty patients showed a negative FDG PET scan before high-dose chemotherapy; 25 of those remained in complete remission, with a median follow-up of 50 months. Only 3 patients had a relapse after a negative FDG PET scan. Persistent abnormal FDG uptake was seen in 30 patients and 26 progressed; of these 26, 16 died from progressive disease. Schot et al. *(39)* studied 46 patients with Hodgkin's disease and NHL prior to stem cell transplantation. Progression-free survival at 2 years was 62% for PET-negative patients versus 32% for PET-positive patients.

In summary, persistent increased FDG uptake in initially involved tumor sites in patients with Hodgkin's disease or non-Hodgkin's lymphoma is highly predictive for residual or recurrent disease. If PET shows areas of increased FDG outside the initially involved sites the differential diagnosis includes inflammation, bone marrow stimulation, or thymic hyperplasia. Minimal residual disease can still be present in patients with a negative PET scan and result in subsequent late relapses.

4.1.2 Esophageal Cancer

In patients with esophageal cancer residual FDG uptake after chemoradiotherapy appears to be a specific marker for viable residual tumor tissue and is associated with a poor prognosis. Brucher et al. *(40)* studied 27 patients with locally advanced squamous cell carcinomas of the esophagus before neoadjuvant chemoradiotherapy and 3–4 weeks after completion of therapy. Therapy-induced reduction of tumor FDG uptake was 72% for histopathological responders compared to 42% for nonresponders. Using a threshold of 51% SUV decrease of baseline resulted in a sensitivity of 100% and a specificity of 52% for PET assessment of tumor response. Tumor response assessed by PET was also a strong prognostic factor. Median survival of PET responders was 23 months compared with just 9 months in PET nonresponders. The prognostic relevance of FDG PET has been confirmed in three recent clinical trials. Flamen et al. studied 36 patients with esophageal cancer before and 3–4 weeks after completion of preoperative chemoradiotherapy *(41)*. Using visual analysis of FDG PET scans this group obtained a sensitivity of 71% and specificity of 81% for PET assessment of histopathological response. Patients classified as nonresponders in FDG PET had a median survival of only 8 months compared with more than 24 months for PET responders. In a relatively small group of 17 patients studied before and after neoadjuvant chemoradiotherapy the 2-year survival rate of PET responders, defined as a greater than 60% decrease in FDG uptake, was 63% compared with 38% in PET nonresponders *(42)*. In the largest study published so far Swisher et al. *(43)* evaluated 103 patients treated by preoperative chemoradiotherapy followed by surgical resection. The accuracy of FDG PET to predict histopathological response was compared with CT and endoscopic ultrasound. Postchemoradiotherapy PET SUV equal to or greater than 4 had the highest accuracy for pathological response (76%). Univariate and multivariate Cox regression analysis demonstrated that a postchemoradiotherapy SUV equal to or greater than 4 was an independent predictor of survival (hazard ratio 3.5, $p = 0.04$). This group has also studied the relationship between the amount of residual tumor tissue and the intensity of FDG uptake. Mean FDG uptake in the tumor bed was not different for patients with no residual viable tumor cells and patients with up to 10% viable tumor cells *(44)*. Thus FDG PET cannot rule out residual microscopic disease after chemoradiotherapy of esophageal cancer.

4.1.3 LUNG CANCER

MacManus *et al.* studied the use of FDG PET after chemoradiotherapy in patients with locally advanced non-small-cell lung cancer. Seventy-three patients were prospectively evaluated for tumor response to chemoradiotherapy by CT and FDG PET *(45)*. Complete response in FDG PET was defined as normalization of all sites with abnormal FDG uptake and partial response as a significant reduction in FDG uptake of all known lesions without the appearance of new lesions. Tumor response assessed by FDG PET predicted better patient survival than response by CT criteria, the pretreatment tumor stage, or patient performance status. The correlation between tumor FDG uptake after chemoradiotherapy and patient outcome was confirmed in a recent study by Hellwig *et al. (46)*. These investigators studied 47 patients after preoperative chemoradiotherapy. Patients were classified as responders if the SUV of the primary tumor was less than 4. Median survival after resection was greater than 56 months for PET responders and 19 months for PET nonresponders ($p < 0.001$). In several studies FDG uptake after chemoradiotherapy and or changes during chemoradiotherapy have been correlated with histopathological tumor regression *(47–50)*. All these studies report a significant correlation between the findings in FDG PET and histopathological tumor regression. The individual values for sensitivity and specificity, however, vary widely (58–100%). This is likely due to the fact that different criteria for a histopathological response were used in this study (no viable tumor cells, less than 10% viable tumor cells). Furthermore, the number of patients with a histopathological response was generally small in these studies; as a consequence, the values for the specificity of FDG PET to detect residual tumor tissue (nonresponders) must be interpreted with caution.

4.1.4 OTHER TUMORS

The prognostic relevance of FDG PET after chemotherapy or chemoradiotherapy has been evaluated in several other tumor types. Grigsby *et al. (51)* retrospectively evaluated the FDG PET scans of 152 patients with carcinoma of the cervix. Positron emission tomography imaging was performed before and after chemoradiotherapy. Patients with a normal FDG PET scan after therapy were characterized by an excellent prognosis with a 5-year survival rate of 90%. In contrast, 5-year survival was only 45% in patients with persistent FDG uptake at the site of the primary tumors. If the posttherapeutic PET scan demonstrated new metastatic lesions, the prognosis of the patients was poor (5-year survival of 15%).

Schuetze *et al.* studied 46 patients with high-grade soft tissue sarcomas before neoadjuvant chemotherapy and again before surgery. Patients with a decrease of FDG uptake by less than 40% were characterized by a poor prognosis. In 90% of these patients recurrent disease was diagnosed within 4 years. The 2-year overall survival rate was 80% for the 17 patients with a decrease in FDG uptake of at least 40%, but only 40% for patients with a decrease in FDG uptake of less than 40% *(52)*. In patients with osteosarcoma and Ewing's sarcoma changes in FDG uptake after neoadjuvant chemotherapy have been shown to be significantly correlated with histological tumor regression, which is one of the most important prognostic factors *(53, 54)*.

4.2 Prediction of Tumor Response during Therapy

Several studies have indicated that measurements of changes in tumor SUVs during chemotherapy allow prediction of subsequent reduction of the tumor mass as well as of patient survival. The use of quantitative changes in tumor metabolism to predict the outcome of therapy goes back to a pioneering study by Wahl *et al.* in 1993 that evaluated tumor glucose utilization during chemohormonotherapy of breast cancer *(57)*. The results of this study indicated that in responding tumor metabolic activity markedly changes within the first weeks of therapy. Subsequent studies by Jansson *et al.* *(58)* in breast cancer and by Findlay *et al.* in colorectal cancer *(59)* have also suggested that tumor glucose utilization is rapidly decreased by effective therapy. More recently the accuracy of FDG PET to predict response and patient survival has been evaluated in larger studies and other tumor types. The results of these trials are summarized in Table 2. In these studies FDG PET generally had a high negative predictive value for response and patients who did not show a significant decrease in FDG uptake early in the course of treatment were unlikely to benefit from continued therapy. Early identification of nonresponding patients is of great clinical importance since the response rates of common malignant tumors to chemotherapy are in the range of only 20–30% *(60)*. This means that the majority of patients will be treated without significant benefit. Response rates to targeted therapy, e.g., EGFR kinase inhibitors, are even lower, in the range of 10–20% *(61, 62)*. Early identification of nonresponding patients by PET imaging therefore has the potential to significantly reduce side effects and costs of ineffective therapy.

4.2.1 BREAST CANCER

Neoadjuvant chemotherapy is increasingly used to treat patients with locally advanced breast cancer in order to increase the rate of curative resections. Additionally, patients with a histopathological response have significantly higher disease-free and overall survival rates than nonresponders *(63)*.

Smith *et al.* evaluated the accuracy of FDG PET to predict histopathological response in 30 patients with locally advanced breast cancer undergoing preoperative chemotherapy *(64)*. After a single cycle of chemotherapy, PET predicted complete pathological response with a sensitivity of 90% and specificity of 74%. In another study, Schelling *et al.* compared results from PET imaging with pathological response *(65)*. After the first course of therapy, responding and nonresponding tumors could be differentiated by PET. In contrast, Mankoff *et al.* *(66)* found a large overlap between changes in metabolic activity in histopathological responders and nonresponders. This discrepant finding may be explained by the different timing of the PET scans. In the study by Mankoff *et al.* the follow-up PET scan was performed after 2 months of chemotherapy. After that period of time histopathological nonresponding tumors may demonstrate a relatively large decrease in tumor size and FDG PET may be unable to differentiate between small absolute differences in the amount of viable tumor cells. Consistent with this explanation, Smith et al. *(64)* also observed that the accuracy of FDG PET for prediction of tumor response was higher after the first cycle of chemotherapy than at later points in time. A similar trend has been observed by Wieder et al. in esophageal cancer *(9)*.

4.2.2 ESOPHAGEAL AND GASTRIC CANCER

Most patients with gastric or esophageal cancer present with locally advanced disease. To improve the rate of curative surgical resections, preoperative (neoadjuvant) chemotherapy or chemoradiotherapy has been evaluated over many years. There is still no consensus, however, as to whether neoadjuvant therapy improves patient survival *(67, 68)*. Nevertheless, data suggest that in patients responding to preoperative chemotherapy or chemoradiotherapy survival is significantly improved compared with surgical treatment alone. This beneficial effect appears to be outweighed by the poor prognosis of nonresponding patients *(69–71)*. Therefore, early prediction of tumor response is of particular importance in patients with esophageal and gastric cancer. We have studied 40 patients with locally advanced adenocarcinomas of the esophagogastric junction who underwent preoperative (neoadjuvant) chemotherapy. [^{18}F]Fluorodeoxyglucose positron emission tomography imaging was performed at baseline and on day 14 of the first cycle of chemotherapy. Changes in tumor FDG uptake were correlated with histopathological response after 3 months of chemotherapy. Using a threshold of 35% decrease of baseline metabolic activity histopathological response could be predicted with a sensitivity and specificity of 89% and 75%, respectively. The 2-year survival of patients responding to FDG PET imaging was 49%, compared with only 9% for PET nonresponders *(72)*. In a more recent study we prospectively applied the threshold of 35% SUV decrease from baseline in patients with gastric cancer *(24)*. Forty-four patients with locally advanced gastric cancer underwent serial FDG PET imaging; nine patients were excluded from further analysis because of low tumor FDG uptake in the baseline scan. In the remaining 35 patients the sensitivity and specificity of FDG PET for prediction of histopathological response were 77% and 86%, respectively. The 2-year survival was 90% for PET responders compared to 25% for PET nonresponders. These data suggest that changes in tumor metabolic activity may be used to individualize the use of chemotherapy in patients with esophageal and gastric cancer. Positron emission tomography nonresponders may undergo salvage therapy; alternative therapeutic options include chemoradiotherapy or immediate surgical resection. Individualization of preoperative chemotherapy for esophageal cancer is currently being evaluated in the MUNICON trial. An interim analysis of this study has confirmed that FDG PET allows selection of patients with a high probability of a histopathological response *(73)*. As an increasing number of second- and third-line chemotherapy regimens and targeted anticancer treatments are emerging it will also become more and more feasible to perform early treatment adjustments in patients who are identified as nonresponders in FDG PET.

4.3 Monitoring Treatment with Protein Kinase Inhibitors

Protein kinases are enzymes that catalyze the transfer of a phosphate group to amino acid residues of proteins. This phosphorylation activates or inhibits the functional activity of the target protein. Protein kinases play an essential role in cellular signaling in response to growth factors and other stimuli. Activating mutations of protein kinases regulating cellular proliferation and apoptosis have been observed in a large number of tumor types and are considered to be a key factor for the uncontrolled growth of cancer cells. Inhibition of protein kinases has therefore been extensively studied as an approach for "targeted" anticancer therapy. Landmark clinical trials of the protein kinase inhibitor imatinib in patients with chronic myeloid leukemia and gastrointestinal stromal tumors (GIST) *(36)* have proven the feasibility of this approach for treatment of cancer *(74)*.

[^{18}F]Fluorodeoxyglucose positron emission tomography is particularly attractive for monitoring treatment with protein kinase inhibitors, since many signaling pathways targeted by protein kinase inhibitors also have a well-established role in regulating tumor glucose metabolism *(75, 76)*. New techniques to monitor treatment with protein kinase inhibitors are urgently needed, since response rates, as assessed by routine anatomic measurements, to protein kinase inhibitors in the treatment of common solid tumors are low (10–20%). However, patients who do respond appear to benefit markedly from therapy with kinase inhibitors. For the further development and clinical application of protein inhibitors it will therefore be imperative to develop tests that allow prediction of tumor response to the inhibition of a particular kinase or to monitor the effectiveness of therapy early in the course of therapy.

[^{18}F]Fluorodeoxyglucose positron emission tomography has already been used in clinical studies to monitor the response of gastrointestinal stromal tumors to treatment with imatinib *(77–79)*. Gastrointestinal stromal tumors are characterized by a mutationally activated KIT receptor tyrosine kinase, which is inhibited by imatinib *(80)*. A marked reduction of tumor metabolic activity was noted as early as 24 h after the first dose *(77, 81)*. Moreover, extensive anatomical abnormalities observed by CT persisted at a time when metabolic alterations had already resolved. In a study of 21 patients with GIST or other soft tissue sarcomas *(81)*, the decrease in FDG uptake after only 1 week of treatment with imatinib was closely correlated with patient outcome. Progression free survival at 1 year was 92% in patients who were classified as responders in PET ($N = 13$, decrease in FDG uptake by more than 25%). In contrast, progression free survival at 1 year was only 12% for PET nonresponders ($N = 8$, $p < 0.005$). These data suggest that FDG PET may become a valuable tool to monitor treatment with imatinib and potentially other protein kinase inhibitors.

5. SUMMARY AND OUTLOOK

[^{18}F]Fluorodeoxyglucose positron emission tomography has been evaluated in numerous studies to monitor tumor response in patients undergoing chemotherapy and chemoradiotherapy. Its clinical value for differentiation of residual or recurrent viable tumor and therapy-induced fibrosis or scar tissue has been well documented for malignant lymphomas and various solid tumors. Furthermore, there are now several reports suggesting that quantitative assessment of therapy-induced changes in tumor FDG uptake may allow prediction of tumor response and patient outcome very early in the course of therapy. In nonresponding patients treatment may be adjusted according to the individual chemosensitivity and radiosensitivity of the tumor tissue. This indicates that FDG PET has an enormous potential to "personalize" treatment and to reduce the side effects and costs of ineffective therapy. Since new "targeted" forms of anticancer therapy (e.g., protein kinase inhibitors) are expected to be effective only in a relatively small subset of patients, early prediction of tumor response by FDG PET is expected to become even more important for clinical trials and patient management in the future.

REFERENCES

1. Miller AB, Hoogstraten B, Staquet M, Winkler A. Reporting results of cancer treatment. *Cancer* 1981;47:207–214.
2. Moertel CG, Hanley JA. The effect of measuring error on the results of therapeutic trials in advanced cancer. *Cancer* 1976;38:388–394.
3. Therasse P, Arbuck SG, Eisenhauer EA, et al. New guidelines to evaluate the response to treatment in solid tumors. European Organization for Research and Treatment of Cancer, National Cancer Institute of the United States, National Cancer Institute of Canada. *J Natl Cancer Inst* 2000;92: 205–216.
4. Salzer-Kuntschik M, Delling G, Beron G, Sigmund R. Morphological grades of regression in osteosarcoma after polychemotherapy—-study COSS 80. *J Cancer Res Clin Oncol* 1983;106(Suppl):21–24.
5. Junker K, Langner K, Klinke F, Bosse U, Thomas M. Grading of tumor regression in non-small cell lung cancer: Morphology and prognosis. *Chest* 2001;120:1584–1591.
6. Mandard A, Dalibard F, Mandard J, et al. Pathologic assessment of tumor regression after preoperative chemoradiotherapy of esophageal carcinoma. Clinicopathologic correlations. *Cancer* 1994;73:2680–2686.
7. Becker K, Mueller JD, Schulmacher C, et al. Histomorphology and grading of regression in gastric carcinoma treated with neoadjuvant chemotherapy. *Cancer* 2003;98:1521–1530.
8. Bielack SS, Kempf-Bielack B, Delling G, et al. Prognostic factors in high-grade osteosarcoma of the extremities or trunk: An analysis of 1,702 patients treated on neoadjuvant cooperative osteosarcoma study group protocols. *J Clin Oncol* 2002;20:776–790.
9. Wieder HA, Brucher BL, Zimmermann F, et al. Time course of tumor metabolic activity during chemoradiotherapy of esophageal squamous cell carcinoma and response to treatment. *J Clin Oncol* 2004;22:900–908.
10. Thie JA. Understanding the standardized uptake value, its methods, and implications for usage. *J Nucl Med* 2004;45:1431–1434.
11. Geworski L, Knoop BO, de Cabrejas ML, Knapp WH, Munz DL. Recovery correction for quantitation in emission tomography: A feasibility study. *Eur J Nucl Med* 2000;27:161–169.
12. Stahl A, Ott K, Schwaiger M, Weber WA. Comparison of different SUV-based methods for monitoring cytotoxic therapy with FDG PET. *Eur J Nucl Med Mol Imaging* 2004;31:1471–1478.
13. Torizuka T, Clavo AC, Wahl RL. Effect of hyperglycemia on in vitro tumor uptake of tritiated FDG, thymidine, L-methionine and L-leucine. *J Nucl Med* 1997;38:382–386.
14. Keyes JW Jr. SUV: Standard uptake or silly useless value? *J Nucl Med* 1995;36:1836–1839.
15. Boellaard R, Krak NC, Hoekstra OS, Lammertsma AA. Effects of noise, image resolution, and ROI definition on the accuracy of standard uptake values: A simulation study. *J Nucl Med* 2004;45: 1519–1527.
16. Paquet N, Albert A, Foidart J, Hustinx R. Within-patient variability of (18)F-FDG: Standardized uptake values in normal tissues. *J Nucl Med* 2004;45:784–788.
17. Young H, Baum R, Cremerius U, et al. Measurement of clinical and sublinical tumour response using F-18-fluorodeoxyglucose and positron emission tomography: Review and 1999 EORTC recommendations. *Eur J Cancer* 1999;35:1773–1782.
18. Minn H, Zasadny KR, Quint LE, Wahl RL. Lung cancer: Reproducibility of quantitative measurements for evaluating 2-[F-18]-fluoro-2-deoxy-D-glucose uptake at PET. *Radiology* 1995;196:167–173.
19. Weber WA, Ziegler SI, Thodtmann R, Hanauske AR, Schwaiger M. Reproducibility of metabolic measurements in malignant tumors using FDG PET. *J Nucl Med* 1999;40:1771–1777.

20. Weber WA, Petersen V, Schmidt B, et al. Positron emission tomography in non-small-cell lung cancer: Prediction of response to chemotherapy by quantitative assessment of glucose use. *J Clin Oncol* 2003;21:2651–2657.
21. Yamane T, Daimaru O, Ito S, Yoshiya K, Nagata T, Uchida H. Decreased 18F-FDG uptake 1 day after initiation of chemotherapy for malignant lymphomas. *J Nucl Med* 2004;45:1838–1842.
22. Kostakoglu L, Coleman M, Leonard JP, Kuji I, Zoe H, Goldsmith SJ. PET predicts prognosis after 1 cycle of chemotherapy in aggressive lymphoma and Hodgkin's disease. *J Nucl Med* 2002;43:1018–1027.
23. Weber W, Dick S, Reidl G, et al. Correlation between postoperative 123I-alpha-methyl-L-tyrosine uptake and survival in patients with gliomas. *J Nucl Med* 2001;42:1144–1150.
24. Ott K, Fink U, Becker K, et al. Prediction of response to preoperative chemotherapy in gastric carcinoma by metabolic imaging: Results of a prospective trial. *J Clin Oncol* 2003;21:4604–4610.
25. Brun E, Kjellen E, Tennvall J, et al. FDG PET studies during treatment: Prediction of therapy outcome in head and neck squamous cell carcinoma. *Head Neck* 2002;24:127–135.
26. Haberkorn U, Morr I, Oberdorfer F, et al. Fluorodeoxyglucose uptake in vitro: Aspects of method and effects of treatment with gemcitabine. *J Nucl Med* 1994;35:1842–1850.
27. Higashi K, Clavo AC, Wahl RL. In vitro assessment of 2-fluoro-2-deoxy-D-glucose, L-methionine and thymidine as agents to monitor the early response of a human adenocarcinoma cell line to radiotherapy [see comments]. *J Nucl Med* 1993;34:773–779.
28. Rozental JM, Levine RL, Nickles RJ, Dobkin JA. Glucose uptake by gliomas after treatment. A positron emission tomographic study [see comments]. *Arch Neurol* 1989;46:1302–1307.
29. Maruyama I, Sadato N, Waki A, et al. Hyperacute changes in glucose metabolism of brain tumors after stereotactic radiosurgery: A PET study. *J Nucl Med* 1999;40:1085–1090.
30. Mortimer JE, Dehdashti F, Siegel BA, Trinkaus K, Katzenellenbogen JA, Welch MJ. Metabolic flare: Indicator of hormone responsiveness in advanced breast cancer. *J Clin Oncol* 2001;19:2797–2803.
31. Hicks RJ, Mac Manus MP, Matthews JP, et al. Early FDG PET imaging after radical radiotherapy for non-small-cell lung cancer: Inflammatory changes in normal tissues correlate with tumor response and do not confound therapeutic response evaluation. *Int J Radiat Oncol Biol Phys* 2004;60:412–418.
32. Jerusalem G, Beguin Y, Fassotte MF, et al. Whole-body positron emission tomography using 18F-fluorodeoxyglucose for posttreatment evaluation in Hodgkin's disease and non-Hodgkin's lymphoma has higher diagnostic and prognostic value than classical computed tomography scan imaging. *Blood* 1999;94:429–433.
33. Zinzani PL, Fanti S, Battista G, et al. Predictive role of positron emission tomography (PET) in the outcome of lymphoma patients. *Br J Cancer* 2004;91:850–854.
34. de Wit M, Bohuslavizki KH, Buchert R, Bumann D, Clausen M, Hossfeld DK. 18FDG PET following treatment as valid predictor for disease-free survival in Hodgkin's lymphoma. *Ann Oncol* 2001;12:29–37.
35. Weihrauch MR, Re D, Scheidhauer K, et al. Thoracic positron emission tomography using 18F-fluorodeoxyglucose for the evaluation of residual mediastinal Hodgkin disease. *Blood* 2001;98:2930–2934.
36. Mikhaeel NG, Timothy AR, O'Doherty MJ, Hain S, Maisey MN. 18-FDG PET as a prognostic indicator in the treatment of aggressive non-Hodgkin's lymphoma–comparison with CT. *Leuk Lymphoma* 2000;39:543–553.
37. Spaepen K, Stroobants S, Dupont P, et al. Prognostic value of positron emission tomography (PET) with fluorine-18 fluorodeoxyglucose ([18F]FDG) after first-line chemotherapy in non-Hodgkin's lymphoma: Is [18F]FDG PET a valid alternative to conventional diagnostic methods? *J Clin Oncol* 2001;19:414–419.
38. Spaepen K, Stroobants S, Dupont P, et al. Prognostic value of pretransplantation positron emission tomography using fluorine 18-fluorodeoxyglucose in patients with aggressive lymphoma treated with high-dose chemotherapy and stem cell transplantation. *Blood* 2003;102:53–59.
39. Schot B, van Imhoff G, Pruim J, Sluiter W, Vaalburg W, Vellenga E. Predictive value of early 18F-fluoro-deoxyglucose positron emission tomography in chemosensitive relapsed lymphoma. *Br J Haematol* 2003;123:282–287.
40. Brucher BL, Weber W, Bauer M, et al. Neoadjuvant therapy of esophageal squamous cell carcinoma: Response evaluation by positron emission tomography. *Ann Surg* 2001;233:300–309.
41. Flamen P, Van Cutsem E, Lerut A, et al. Positron emission tomography for assessment of the response to induction chemotherapy in locally advanced esophageal cancer. *Ann Oncol* 2002;13:361–368.

42. Downey RJ, Akhurst T, Ilson D, et al. Whole body 18FDG PET and the response of esophageal cancer to induction therapy: Results of a prospective trial. *J Clin Oncol* 2003;21:428–432.
43. Swisher SG, Maish M, Erasmus JJ, et al. Utility of PET, CT, and EUS to identify pathologic responders in esophageal cancer. *Ann Thorac Surg* 2004;78:1152–1160; discussion 1152–1160.
44. Swisher SG, Erasmus J, Maish M, et al. 2-Fluoro-2-deoxy-D-glucose positron emission tomography imaging is predictive of pathologic response and survival after preoperative chemoradiation in patients with esophageal carcinoma. *Cancer* 2004;101:1776–1785.
45. Mac Manus MP, Hicks RJ, Matthews JP, et al. Positron emission tomography is superior to computed tomography scanning for response-assessment after radical radiotherapy or chemoradiotherapy in patients with non-small-cell lung cancer. *J Clin Oncol* 2003;21:1285–1292.
46. Hellwig D, Graeter TP, Ukena D, Georg T, Kirsch CM, Schafers HJ. Value of F-18-fluorodeoxyglucose positron emission tomography after induction therapy of locally advanced bronchogenic carcinoma. *J Thorac Cardiovasc Surg* 2004;128:892–899.
47. Akhurst T, Downey RJ, Ginsberg MS, et al. An initial experience with FDG PET in the imaging of residual disease after induction therapy for lung cancer. *Ann Thorac Surg* 2002;73:259–264; discussion 264–266.
48. Ryu JS, Choi NC, Fischman AJ, Lynch TJ, Mathisen DJ. FDG PET in staging and restaging non-small cell lung cancer after neoadjuvant chemoradiotherapy: Correlation with histopathology. *Lung Cancer* 2002;35:179–187.
49. Cerfolio RJ, Bryant AS, Winokur TS, Ohja B, Bartolucci AA. Repeat FDG PET after neoadjuvant therapy is a predictor of pathologic response in patients with non-small cell lung cancer. *Ann Thorac Surg* 2004;78:1903–1909; discussion 1909.
50. Port JL, Kent MS, Korst RJ, Keresztes R, Levin MA, Altorki NK. Positron emission tomography scanning poorly predicts response to preoperative chemotherapy in non-small cell lung cancer. *Ann Thorac Surg* 2004;77:254–259; discussion 259.
51. Grigsby PW, Siegel BA, Dehdashti F, Rader J, Zoberi I. Posttherapy [18F] fluorodeoxyglucose positron emission tomography in carcinoma of the cervix: Response and outcome. *J Clin Oncol* 2004;22:2167–2171.
52. Schuetze SM, Rubin BP, Vernon C, et al. Use of positron emission tomography in localized extremity soft tissue sarcoma treated with neoadjuvant chemotherapy. *Cancer* 2005;103:339–348.
53. Schulte M, Brecht-Krauss D, Werner M, et al. Evaluation of neoadjuvant therapy response of osteogenic sarcoma using FDG PET. *J Nucl Med* 1999;40:1637–1643.
54. Hawkins DS, Rajendran JG, Conrad EU 3rd, Bruckner JD, Eary JF. Evaluation of chemotherapy response in pediatric bone sarcomas by [F-18]-fluorodeoxy-D-glucose positron emission tomography. *Cancer* 2002;94:3277–3284.
55. Kunkel M, Forster GJ, Reichert TE, et al. Radiation response non-invasively imaged by [18F]FDG PET predicts local tumor control and survival in advanced oral squamous cell carcinoma. *Oral Oncol* 2003;39:170–177.
56. Kumar R, Xiu Y, Potenta S, et al. 18F-FDG PET for evaluation of the treatment response in patients with gastrointestinal tract lymphomas. *J Nucl Med* 2004;45:1796–1803.
57. Wahl RL, Zasadny K, Helvie M, Hutchins GD, Weber B, Cody R. Metabolic monitoring of breast cancer chemohormonotherapy using positron emission tomography: Initial evaluation. *J Clin Oncol* 1993;11:2101–2111.
58. Jansson T, Westlin JE, Ahlstrom H, Lilja A, Langstrom B, Bergh J. Positron emission tomography studies in patients with locally advanced and/or metastatic breast cancer: A method for early therapy evaluation? *J Clin Oncol* 1995;13:1470–1477.
59. Findlay M, Young H, Cunningham D, et al. Noninvasive monitoring of tumor metabolism using fluorodeoxyglucose and positron emission tomography in colorectal cancer liver metastases: Correlation with tumor response to fluorouracil. *J Clin Oncol* 1996;14:700–708.
60. Schiller JH, Harrington D, Belani CP, et al. Comparison of four chemotherapy regimens for advanced non-small-cell lung cancer. *N Engl J Med* 2002;346:92–98.
61. Haringhuizen A, van Tinteren H, Vaessen HF, Baas P, van Zandwijk N. Gefitinib as a last treatment option for non-small-cell lung cancer: Durable disease control in a subset of patients. *Ann Oncol* 2004;15:786–792.
62. Fukuoka M, Yano S, Giaccone G, et al. Multi-institutional randomized phase II trial of gefitinib for previously treated patients with advanced non-small-cell lung cancer. *J Clin Oncol* 2003;21: 2237–2246.

63. Honkoop AH, van Diest PJ, de Jong JS, *et al*. Prognostic role of clinical, pathological and biological characteristics in patients with locally advanced breast cancer. *Br J Cancer* 1998;77:621–626.
64. Smith IC, Welch AE, Hutcheon AW, *et al*. Positron emission tomography using [(18)F]-fluorodeoxy-D-glucose to predict the pathologic response of breast cancer to primary chemotherapy. *J Clin Oncol* 2000;18:1676–1688.
65. Schelling M, Avril N, Nahrig J, *et al*. Positron emission tomography using [(18)F]fluorodeoxyglucose for monitoring primary chemotherapy in breast cancer. *J Clin Oncol* 2000;18:1689–1695.
66. Mankoff DA, Dunnwald LK, Gralow JR, *et al*. Changes in blood flow and metabolism in locally advanced breast cancer treated with neoadjuvant chemotherapy. *J Nucl Med* 2003;44:1806–1814.
67. Kelsen DP, Minsky B, Smith M, *et al*. Preoperative therapy for esophageal cancer: A randomized comparison of chemotherapy versus radiation therapy. *J Clin Oncol* 1990;8:1352–1361.
68. Medical_Research_Council. Surgical resection with or without preoperative chemotherapy in oesophageal cancer: A randomised controlled trial. *Lancet* 2002;359:1727–1733.
69. Kelsen D. Preoperative chemoradiotherapy for esophageal cancer. *J Clin Oncol* 2001;19:283–285.
70. Urba SG, Orringer MB, Turrisi A, Iannettoni M, Forastiere A, Strawderman M. Randomized trial of preoperative chemoradiation versus surgery alone in patients with locoregional esophageal carcinoma. *J Clin Oncol* 2001;19:305–313.
71. Ajani JA, Mansfield PF, Lynch PM, *et al*. Enhanced staging and all chemotherapy preoperatively in patients with potentially resectable gastric carcinoma. *J Clin Oncol* 1999;17:2403–2411.
72. Weber WA, Ott K, Becker K, *et al*. Prediction of response to preoperative chemotherapy in adenocarcinomas of the esophagogastric junction by metabolic imaging. *J Clin Oncol* 2001;19:3058–3065.
73. Lordick F, Weber WA, Stein HJ, *et al*. Individualized neoadjuvant treatment strategy in adenocarcinoma of the esophago-gastric junction (AEG): Interim report on the MUNICON trial. *J Clin Oncol* 2004;22:328S.
74. Sawyers C. Targeted cancer therapy. *Nature* 2004;432:294–297.
75. Whiteman EL, Cho H, Birnbaum MJ. Role of Akt/protein kinase B in metabolism. *Trends Endocrinol Metab* 2002;13:444–451.
76. Blume-Jensen P, Hunter T. Oncogenic kinase signalling. *Nature* 2001;411:355–365.
77. Van den Abbeele AD, Badawi RD. Use of positron emission tomography in oncology and its potential role to assess response to imatinib mesylate therapy in gastrointestinal stromal tumors (GISTs). *Eur J Cancer* 2002;38(Suppl 5):S60–S65.
78. Antoch G, Kanja J, Bauer S, *et al*. Comparison of PET, CT, and dual-modality PET/CT imaging for monitoring of imatinib (STI571) therapy in patients with gastrointestinal stromal tumors. *J Nucl Med* 2004;45:357–365.
79. Gayed I, Vu T, Iyer R, *et al*. The role of 18F-FDG PET in staging and early prediction of response to therapy of recurrent gastrointestinal stromal tumors. *J Nucl Med* 2004;45:17–21.
80. Demetri GD, von Mehren M, Blanke CD, *et al*. Efficacy and safety of imatinib mesylate in advanced gastrointestinal stromal tumors. *N Engl J Med* 2002;347:472–480.
81. Stroobants S, Goeminne J, Seegers M, *et al*. 18FDG-Positron emission tomography for the early prediction of response in advanced soft tissue sarcoma treated with imatinib mesylate (Glivec). *Eur J Cancer* 2003;39:2012–2020.

8 Measurement of Tumor Proliferation with Positron Emission Tomography and Treatment Response

Anthony F. Shields, MD, PhD

CONTENTS

    INTRODUCTION
    CELL CYCLE AND EXPERIMENTAL MEASUREMENTS OF DNA
       SYNTHESIS AND PROLIFERATION
    IMAGING TUMOR GROWTH
    THYMIDINE IMAGING OF TUMOR PROLIFERATION
    THYMIDINE IMAGING AND THE ASSESSMENT OF
       TREATMENT RESPONSE
    IODINATED AND BROMINATED PYRIMIDINES
    FLUORINATED PYRIMIDINE ANALOGS
    3′-FLUORO-3′-DEOXYTHYMIDINE
    1-(2′-DEOXY-2′-FLUORO-β-D-ARABINOFURANOSYL)THYMINE
    CONCLUSIONS

1. INTRODUCTION

While the ultimate goal of cancer treatment is to eliminate all evidence of the tumor's presence, the more immediate goal of treatment with chemotherapy, radiation, and biological agents is to decrease the tumor's ability to replicate and increase the death rate of cancer cells. This basis has inspired researchers to design and develop imaging approaches to assess tumor proliferation and, more importantly, a tumor's response to new treatments. Such approaches, while still in development, may complement the routine imaging of tumor size now done as part of standard clinical care. In general, successful therapy should lead to declines in the size of tumors as reflected by techniques such as computed tomography (CT) and magnetic resonance imaging (MRI) *(1, 2)*. While anatomic imaging is relatively straightforward and readily available, it has a number of limitations. First, it measures the size of the mass, but does not determine the cellularity or growth rate of the tumor. Second, after treatment, the tumor may

From: *Cancer Drug Discovery and Development*
In Vivo Imaging of Cancer Therapy
Edited by: A.F. Shields and P. Price © Humana Press Inc., Totowa, NJ

be left with a fibrotic mass that can persist even after successful treatment. While eventually a mass may decline in size after therapy, this can take many weeks to months for the cells to lyse and finally to be absorbed. Finally, when therapy is unsuccessful, it may take months for the failure of treatment to become apparent, since tumors may grow very slowly. In fact, the doubling time of most tumors is generally from 1 to 3 months *(3)*. It is for these reasons that imaging cell proliferation is attractive to assess treatment response and for potential use to steer or change a course of therapy. This approach to positron emission tomography (PET) imaging may also complement imaging other aspects of tumor metabolism, such as energetics, protein and membrane synthesis, and apoptosis. Energetics imaging is most readily and widely done using 3′-fluorodeoxyglucose (FDG), yet other measures of metabolism may provide more rapid measurements of response in some situations *(4, 5)*.

The best way to image response after therapy may depend on the treatment employed and the timing of the answer desired. The gamut ranges from simple anatomic imaging to determine if a patient has had a complete response to treatment with all visual disappearance of tumor as an indicator to complex kinetic modeling and agent fractional analysis to determine if a new targeted agent has simply blocked the main proliferation pathway.

One of the hallmarks of cancer is uncontrolled proliferation of cells. Over the years different approaches to measuring cell growth have been developed for *in vitro* and *in vivo* use. Each has its own benefits and limitations, with variations in the accuracy of providing a reflection of cell growth and the ease of conducting the measurement. When cells are grown in tissue culture, the simplest measure of growth is the quantitation of cell number over time; this can be done using a microscope or a flow cytometer. This type of measurement is analogous to measuring the size of a lesion using anatomic imaging techniques and is subject to many of the limitations, as discussed below. This constraint has led to more sophisticated and accurate biochemical and physiological approaches to the measurement of cell proliferation. Often the fraction of viable cells is measured using techniques such as staining with the tetrazolium dye MTT (3-[4,5-dimethylthiazol-2-yl]2,5-diphenyltetrazolium bromide) *(6)*. Cells that take up and retain MTT must have an intact mitochondrial reduction system.

Once DNA synthesis was determined to be an essential part of cell growth and division, techniques for measuring DNA replication were developed. Radioactively labeled nucleosides were studied to better understand the biochemical pathways involved in DNA replication and these approaches were found to also provide a measurement of cellular proliferation *(7)*. While DNA synthesis is restricted to proliferating cells, RNA synthesis is a continual process, driving the design of a probe that reflects the former without interference from the latter. The cytidine, adenine, and guanine nucleotides can be incorporated into RNA or DNA, while uracil and thymine are restricted and uniquely incorporated into either RNA or DNA, respectively *(8)*. This cellular distinction has led to the consistent use of thymidine, the nucleoside produced from thymine, as a routine measure of DNA synthesis in the laboratory. Thymidine can be labeled with ^{3}H or ^{14}C and most of the label retained in the cell is present in DNA. While thymidine is rapidly catabolized *(8)*, as discussed below, this is not a major issue in tissue culture where the metabolites are biologically removed leaving predominate activity in DNA. Translating knowledge and applications using labeled pyrimidines from the laboratory in tissue culture and animals for use in patients requires a thorough understanding of the pharmacokinetics of the tracer and its retention in normal and tumor tissues. Studies by a number of investigators throughout the world have explored the promises and limitations of a number of tracers for DNA synthesis.

2. CELL CYCLE AND EXPERIMENTAL MEASUREMENTS OF DNA SYNTHESIS AND PROLIFERATION

As cells replicate they proceed through an orderly cycle through a DNA synthetic phase (S portion of the cycle) on to mitosis (M phase). These are separated by two gaps (G_1 and G_2, while G_0 represents a noncycling phase) (Fig. 1). In the clinic one of simplest measures of the aggressiveness of a tumor is the mitotic index (MI), the fraction of cells undergoing mitosis in a histological section. A limitation of this approach, like a number of the measures of cell growth, is that it requires a tissue specimen for evaluation. Tissue is regularly obtained as part of the initial diagnosis of a tumor, but infrequently repeated during the course of therapy. Common to other measurements based on biopsies, MI does not provide a measure of the variability of tumor growth from lesion to lesion in patients with metastatic disease. The small specimen used for histological analysis may not even provide an accurate sample from a large tumor mass.

Flow cytometry provides more quantitative information about the distribution of cells through the cycle by staining the cells and measuring the amount of DNA within each cell (Fig. 2) *(9)*. This allows more precise measurement of the distribution of cells within the phases of the cell cycle and is most useful in measuring the percentage of cells in S and G_2 phases. The limitation of this approach is that the speed with which

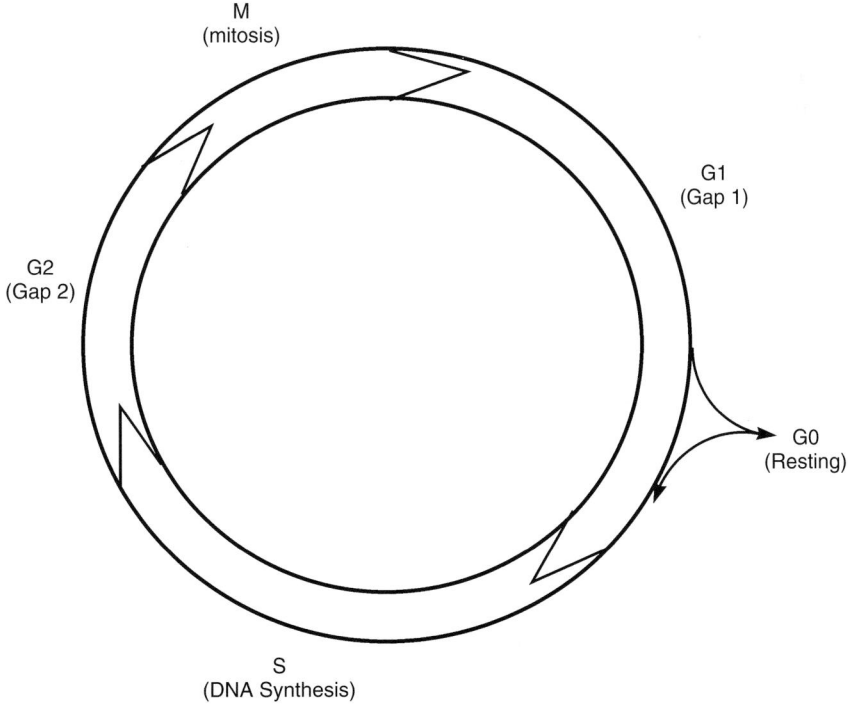

Fig. 1. Cell cycle.

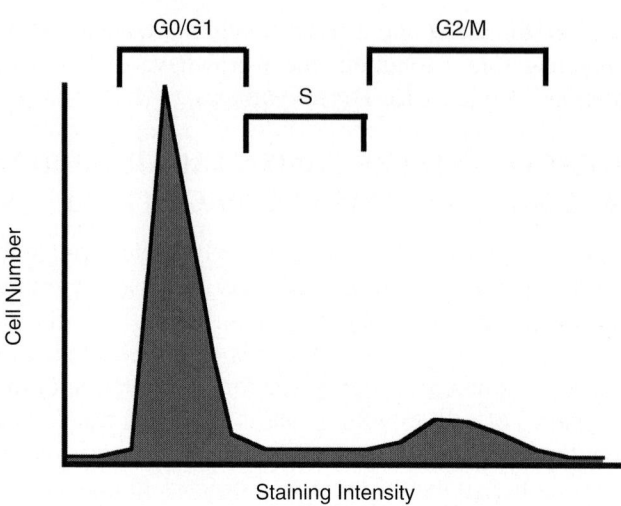

Fig. 2. Flow cytometry schematic of cycling cells.

cells can transverse these different phases of the cell cycle can vary greatly, therefore providing more limited information on the overall doubling time of the cells. Furthermore, cells that are noncycling (G_0) are not differentiated from cells that are preparing to replicate (G_1), but still have the usual complement of diploid DNA.

The advent of tritium-labeled thymidine provided an approach to measuring cell growth that offers a more direct measure of the rate of replication of cells in culture *in vivo* *(7)*. In tissue culture the incorporation of labeled thymidine is a simple approach to measuring cell growth. Cells are exposed to the labeled nucleoside for a short period of time, the unincorporated tracer and metabolites are removed, and the activity trapped in DNA is determined. In culture, most of the activity retained in growing cells is present as DNA, which can be validated by various extraction techniques. *In vivo* studies have been conducted with [^{3}H]thymidine in animal systems and occasionally in patients *(10)*. One major limitation of this technique is the need to obtain tissue samples. Monitoring treatment response requires repeated biopsies and small biopsies may not be representative of the bulk of the tumor or multiple metastatic sites. Another major limitation, discussed below, is the catabolism of thymidine. While rapid catabolism may limit the tracer available to the tumor for labeling, the presence of metabolites is not a major problem, since it is possible to remove those with extraction or from histological specimens. In patients the amount of [^{3}H]thymidine that can be injected is a significant limitation, providing levels of tracer too low for simple scintillation counting on a regular basis. This has led to the establishment of the labeling index (LI), an indicator that measures the fraction of cells in S phase *(7)*. Injection of labeled thymidine, biopsy of the tumor, preparation of histological sections, and then placement of photographic emulsion on the slide are procedural steps to determine LI. After exposure it is possible to measure the fraction of cells that displays grains of photographic emulsion from radioactive decay. This technique is laborious, measures a limited area of the tumor, and simply quantitates the fraction of cells in S phase and not the speed of replication.

Probably the most accurate and complete picture of cellular proliferation is obtained after the injection of unlabeled 5-bromodeoxyuridine (BUdR) (Fig. 3). The bromine in the 5-position has almost the same van der Waals radius as thymidine, so that the compound is readily taken up and incorporated into DNA using the thymidine pathways. Techniques have been developed to measure the presence of BUdR in DNA in fixed histological specimens or dispersed cells using appropriate antibodies and microscopy or flow cytometry *(11)*. At first impression, this would simply provide another way to measure the LI, since it is possible to measure the fraction of cells in S phase. The innovation in using BUdR is that the compound is injected a number of hours before the planned biopsy or surgery to sample the tumor. Using flow cytometry, the place in the cell cycle and the presence of BUdR in each cell from the tumor can then be determined. Cells that have taken up BUdR were by definition in the S phase at the time of injection, but several hours later some of these cells may have moved into G_2 or G_1. It is possible to quantitate the cells in each phase of the cell cycle that began in S phase. Thus BUdR staining provides information about the fraction of cells in S phase (like the LI and standard flow cytometry) and dynamic information about the rate of movement of cells through S phase. While theoretically this provides superior information, this approach has a number of practical limitations. It requires the injection of unlabeled BUdR a few hours before a biopsy is done. The difficulties of obtaining biopsies and the problem with their limited sampling all have led to limited adoption of this technique.

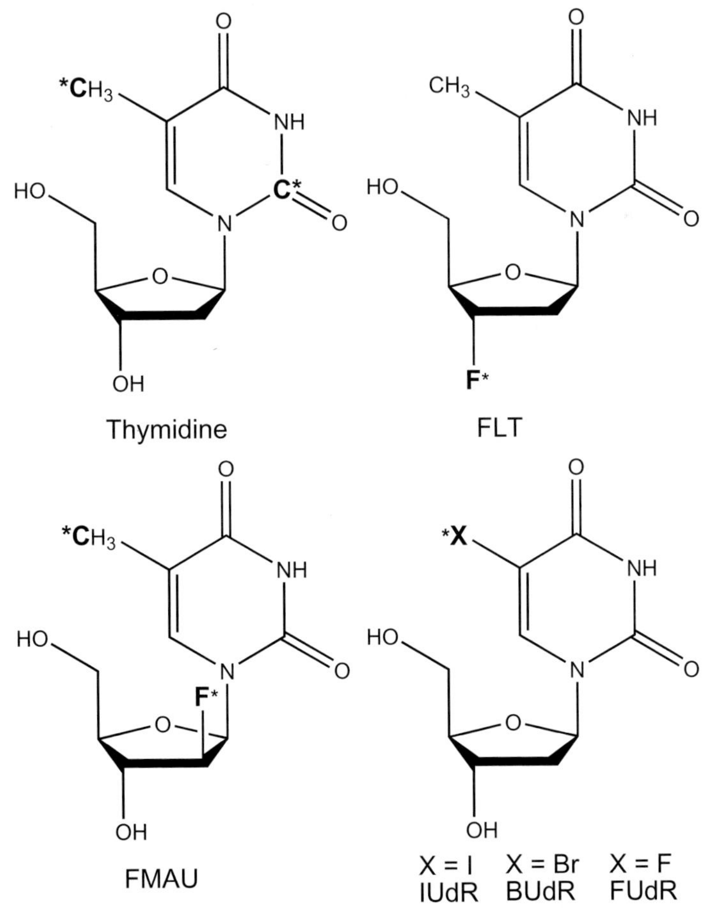

Fig. 3. Structures of thymidine and its analogs: FLT, FMAU, and 5'-halogenated analogs.

While unlabeled BUdR is a superb, although difficult, method for assessing tumor proliferation, labeled BUdR has not been found to be generally useful for imaging proliferation. BUdR can be labeled with ^{76}Br, with a 16 h half-life, and ^{77}Br, with a 56 h half-life. The former can be used for PET imaging and the latter for single-photon emission computed tomography (SPECT). The major problem is the rapid dehalogenation of BUdR, obscuring tumor uptake *(12, 13)*.

Today, the most commonly used approach to measure proliferation on biopsies is to assess the level of Ki-67, an antigen present in proliferative cells. While the exact function of Ki-67 remains to be determined, it is clear that it is expressed in cells with proliferative capacity during any point of the cell cycle *(14)*. Thus cells that are cycling but are presently in G_1 are differentiated from cells not undergoing replication (G_0). Staining for Ki-67 can be done in fixed tissues using the MIB-1 antibody. Increased expression of Ki-67 has been shown to predict poor survival in a number of cancers, including lung, breast, and prostate *(14, 15)*. While Ki-67 measurements obtained from biopsy specimens have the same sampling problems discussed above, this approach is now being used for comparison with noninvasive imaging approaches as will be discussed below.

3. IMAGING TUMOR GROWTH

Imaging tumor growth and response to therapy is the ultimate goal for many clinicians and investigators and a number of different approaches have been developed and tested to address this issue. Measurements of DNA synthesis using labeled thymidine and its analogs have provided the most promising approach, but other measurements of tumor metabolism may also provide indirect assessments of tumor proliferation. For example, some, but not all, studies using FDG have found that the level of activity in the glycolytic pathway correlated with proliferation, measured on biopsy specimens. This is not surprising since tumors that are more rapidly growing might also be more metabolically active. For example, in a small series of patients with gliomas PET imaging with FDG did correlate with proliferation *(16)*. It is notable that a larger study by the same group did not find FDG uptake correlated with proliferation, while imaging with [^{11}C]methionine did correlate with Ki-67 staining *(17)*. On the other hand, in pediatric brain tumors neither methionine nor FDG uptake correlated with measurements of Ki-67 proliferation *(18)*. In some lung cancer studies, FDG uptake did correlate with proliferation *(19)*, but not in others *(16, 20)*. It is likely that general measures of tumor metabolism, such as those obtained with FDG and methionine, provide a gauge of tumor well being and thus correlate with proliferation in some but not all situations. Clearly a more direct measure of tumor growth is needed to obtain a more accurate measure of proliferation.

4. THYMIDINE IMAGING OF TUMOR PROLIFERATION

Given the large number of studies using labeled thymidine in the laboratory to assess cell proliferation it was appropriate to try and translate such measurements to the clinic. This led to developing approaches to labeling thymidine with ^{11}C. The initial synthesis, done at the Brookhaven National Laboratory (Upton, NY), placed the label in the methyl position *(21)*. Studies in mice demonstrated high retention in organs, such as the spleen, with rapid cellular proliferation. Subsequent studies in mice and dogs with tumors demonstrated increased retention of labeled thymidine *(22, 23)*. Thymidine was found to be rapidly taken up into the cells and incorporated into DNA. Since thymidine is rapidly cleared from the circulation there initially was concern that its distribution would reflect blood flow. Studies in mice demonstrated that after the first minutes, metabolism and DNA incorporation were the primary determinants of thymidine retention *(23)*. Thymidine has been labeled with ^{11}C in both the methyl and ring-2 positions *(24–26)*. Despite the 20 min half-life of *(27)* thymidine, the synthesis can be reasonably accomplished in about 1 h and produce enough tracer to image one patient. While the short half-life limits the commercial utility of labeled thymidine, it has the advantage of being the natural compound and it is not necessary to worry about differences noted in transport and enzymatic activity seen with all the analogs. For this reason labeled thymidine has served as the standard agent with which all the other analogs in development should be compared.

Thymidine labeled with ^{11}C has a number of limitations, however, in addition to its challenging synthesis and short half-life. Thymidine is rapidly catabolized in both animals and humans *(28, 29)*. Within a couple of minutes the glycosidic bond is broken and thymine is released, followed by cleavage of the pyrimidine ring (Fig. 4). The metabolic products differ depending on the site labeled within the molecule.

Methyl-labeled thymidine results in the production of a number of varying metabolites once the pyrimidine ring is cleaved *(8, 28)*. Labeling in the ring-2 position has the advantage that after a few minutes the principal catabolite is carbon dioxide *(30)*. While this is still excreted relatively slowly, it is possible to measure its presence in the blood and take this into account when producing kinetic models of thymidine retention

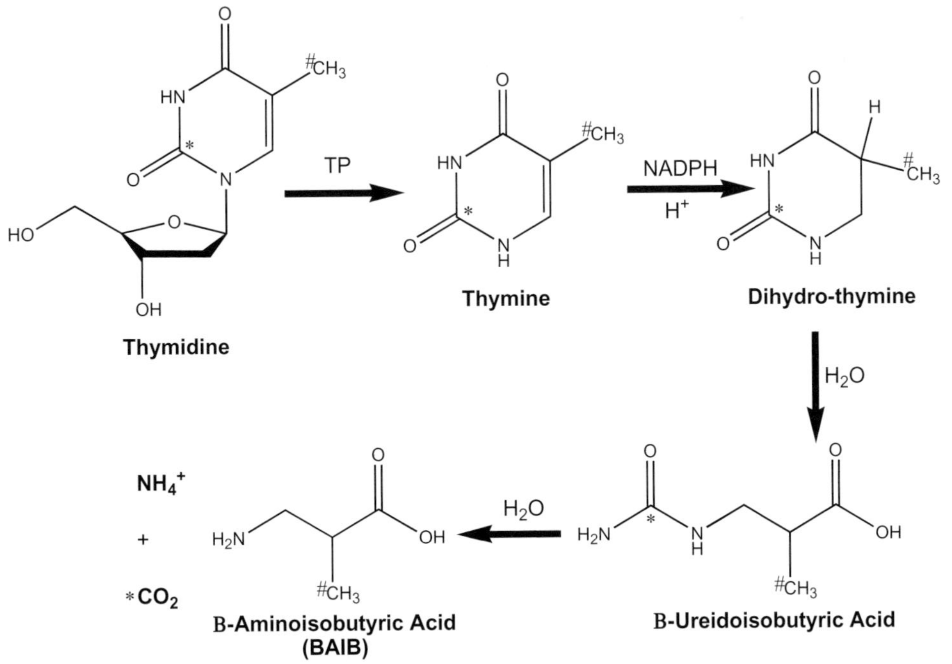

Fig. 4. Catabolism of thymidine. Breakdown products from label placed in the 5-methyl position (#) and ring-2 position (*).

(31–33). The most accurate way to account for the distribution and clearance of the labeled carbon dioxide is to obtain a second scan and measurements after injection of labeled carbon dioxide *(34)*. It is possible to combine the blood activity curves of thymidine and its metabolites with the tumor time–activity curves (TAC) to measure the flux of thymidine into DNA. It should be noted that such kinetic models are always a simplification of the complex mechanisms of thymidine delivery, transport, catabolism, and DNA incorporation. It is necessary to make a number of simplifying assumptions. For example, most cellular thymidine is actually synthesized intracellularly from deoxyuridine monophosphate. Thymidine used in tracer studies utilizes the exogenous or salvage pathway that involves uptake and phosphorylation of extracellular thymidine. The kinetic models assume that transport is a simple process that is included in the delivery of thymidine to the cell. In reality uptake appears to involve a number of facilitated and active transporters *(35, 36)*. Once thymidine is intracellular it is phosphorylated by thymidine kinase (TK1). This cytosolic enzyme is closely controlled by the cell and its activity increases several-fold as the cell enters the S or DNA synthetic phase *(37)*. At this point thymidine from the endogenous and exogenous pathways mix as thymidine monophosphate (TMP). One concern was that these two pathways would be treated differently and that both sources would not freely mix. Another possibility was that the relative levels of endogenous synthesis and exogenous thymidine utilization might vary greatly from tissue to tissue, tumor to tumor, or time to time. This has been studied in cell lines, tissues, and tumors and it was found that all utilized exogenous thymidine to the same extent, which was dependent on the level of exogenous thymidine in the incubation medium *(38)*. Based on these results it is reasonable to assume that the uptake and retention of labeled thymidine provide an overall reflection of the cellular level of DNA synthesis.

The greatest issue in dealing with labeled thymidine, as noted above, is that it is rapidly cleaved and the contribution of metabolites to the images obtained with PET must be understood. This is difficult to do with thymidine labeled in the methyl position, given the large number of varied metabolites (Fig. 4), but with ring-2 labeled thymidine the only significant metabolite after a few minutes is labeled CO_2. Compartmental models have been developed that use information from PET and measurements of labeled thymidine, thymine, and CO_2 in the blood *(31, 39)*. Because of the large number of variables that are measured and the parameters that could be fit, it is necessary to constrain the model and realize that individual parameters, such as the incorporation rate of thymidine triphosphate into DNA, will be difficult to accurately determine. The main parameter of interest, the overall uptake and incorporation into DNA or DNA flux, can be measured with reliability.

In one imaging study, 17 patients with intraabdominal tumors were imaged with [^{11}C]thymidine and the fractional retention of thymidine was calculated using kinetic models and compared to the assessment of proliferation based on measurement of the Ki-67 index using the MIB1 antibody *(33)*. It was found that these two measurements correlated ($r = 0.58$; $p = 0.01$), but there was no correlation with measurement of thymidine standardized uptake values (SUV) or area under the tissue activity curve. This was also the first study to actually compare thymidine retention and tumor perfusion in patients, using inhaled [^{15}O]CO_2. There was no correlation between thymidine retention and perfusion, consistent with the data obtained previously in mice.

5. THYMIDINE IMAGING AND THE ASSESSMENT OF TREATMENT RESPONSE

Labeled thymidine has been used to image a number of different tumor types including brain, head and neck, lung, lymphoma, lung, sarcomas, stomach, and colon tumors *(5, 40–44)*.

Since thymidine does not readily cross the blood–brain barrier, there is little uptake in the normal brain, unlike the high levels seen with FDG. Thus patients with brain tumors have lesions seen above background in most cases, whether imaged with either ring-2 or methyl-labeled thymidine *(40, 43, 45)*. With [2-^{11}C]thymidine the presence of CO_2 contributes to the background activity, but this can be removed by appropriate kinetic modeling *(40)*. Elsewhere in the body thymidine retention is seen in the normal myocardium as the result of thymidine kinase 2 (TK2) present within the mitochondria and kidneys *(42)*. When imaging was done with [*methyl*-^{11}C]thymidine retention within the liver is seen due to the retention of metabolites, but this is not seen with ring-2-labeled thymidine where the primary metabolite is CO_2.

A limited number of studies have evaluated PET imaging with [2-^{11}C]thymidine in the assessment of treatment response. In one study, six patients with either small cell lung cancer or high grade sarcoma were imaged before and about 1 week after the start of therapy *(5)*. Patients also had FDG imaging performed on the same day. In four patients with clinical response to therapy thymidine retention, as measured by SUV and metabolic rate, declined by an average of 65% and 84%, respectively. In these same patients FDG retention also declined, but not as dramatically, with mean decreases of 51% and 63% for SUV and metabolic rates, respectively. In the two patients who subsequently progressed there was no change in thymidine retention.

PET has also been used in a phase I study of a protein kinase C inhibitor (*N*-benzoyl staurosporine, PKC412) *(46)*. Patients were imaged with [2-^{11}C]thymidine at baseline and after the first cycle of treatment and changes in the thymidine area under the curve (AUC) of the tissues and tumors were compared *(47)*. In a series of seven patients imaged without treatment the average change in thymidine retention was 1% (range –5% to +10%). In this pilot study four treated patients had an average decline in thymidine retention of 10% (the four patients had actual declines of 1, 5, 14, and 21%). This type of study demonstrates the possible utility of thymidine imaging for testing new drug therapies and gauging their effectiveness.

One of the most exciting uses of PET imaging is in the evaluation of new therapeutic agents. One study used imaging of abdominal tumors to assess metabolic changes after treatment with a new thymidylate synthase inhibitor (nolatrexed, AG337) *(48)*. It is notable that in this study seven patients were imaged 1 week apart to assess the reproducibility of the technique and the difference in SUV and fractional retention of thymidine was –7% (range –14 to 0%) and 3% (range –11 to 17%), respectively *(44)*. Since nolatrexed would inhibit endogenous thymidine synthesis, tumor cells might be expected to compensate by increased utilization of the exogenous pathway and hence increase uptake and retention of labeled thymidine. In fact, when another five patients were imaged 3 days after the start of treatment with nolatrexed they noted an increase in SUV and fractional retention of thymidine of 43% (range 24–62%) and 38% (range 8–68%), respectively. In this study, thymidine is not being used to measure proliferation, but rather the effect of nolatrexed on the thymidine synthetic pathway. While this study does demonstrate a pharmacological effect of nolatrexed, it must be understood that the mechanism of increased retention of thymidine is complex. For example, the cell may increase TK in order to compensate for declines in TS. On the other hand, there may actually be declines in overall DNA synthesis because thymidine is limiting and at some point the cell may alter TK activity to reflect this decline. In any case, the use of thymidine imaging is very helpful in documenting a pharmacological effect and may help in understanding the pharmacodynamics of the drugs.

6. IODINATED AND BROMINATED PYRIMIDINES

Since the initial development of 5-fluorouracil by Dr. Charles Heidelberger in 1957 *(49)* numerous pyrimidine analogs have been developed as possible antineoplastic and antiviral agents. Many of these have been developed and tested as possible tracers to track proliferation of tumors *in vivo*. Among the first was 5-iododeoxyuridine (IUdR), which has been studied since 1959 *(50)*. It can be labeled with ^{131}I for SPECT imaging or ^{124}I for use with PET. It is readily incorporated into DNA, but also undergoes substantial dehalogenation. It is possible to limit the contribution of the labeled free iodine to the images by waiting for over 12 h for washout of the catabolites *(51, 52)*. While this approach has been demonstrated to produce imaging with a low level of background activity, the extent of dehalogenation, time needed for washout, and longer half-lives needed for the tracers limit the number of counts available at the time of imaging. This would be a problem even if ^{123}I for SPECT (half-life 13 h) or ^{124}I for PET (half-life 4.2 days) was used. This approach, therefore, is not routinely used at present.

Another halogenated pyrimidine of note is BUdR. As previously discussed, unlabeled BUdR provides an excellent measure of cell proliferation by using antibody to detect cells in S phase. In such a staining technique dehalogenation is not an issue, since free bromine is cleared in fixation and is not detected by the antibody. Bromine has appropriate isotopes for use with SPECT (^{77}Br, half-life 56 h) or PET (^{76}Br, half-life 16 h). As with IUdR, rapid dehalogenation results in the release of 90% of the label within minutes of injection *(53)*. Studies in animals suggested that this problem could be overcome by either a separate imaging study after the injection of free bromide or by the induction of diuresis *(54)*. In another study patients with brain tumors were imaged with [^{76}Br]BUdR immediately after injection and then a few hours later and the next day *(55)*. The patients also underwent diuresis and then had surgery on the second day. The specimens taken at surgery were analyzed for their radioactive content and only 9% activity was present in DNA. Furthermore, there was only a 5% decline in the level of free bromide in the plasma, despite the diuresis. The authors concluded that labeled BUdR was not a promising tracer for imaging proliferation.

7. FLUORINATED PYRIMIDINE ANALOGS

5-Fluorouracil (5-FU) was the first fluorinated analog synthesized as an inhibitor of cellular pyrimidine metabolism *(49)*. It was subsequently labeled for study with ^{18}F *(56)*. This tracer has found use in assessing the retention of this antineoplastic drug in patients with advanced colon cancer who were to undergo therapy with unlabeled drug *(57)*. While such a use may be appropriate, the ability to measure tumor growth is limited because 5-FU can be catabolized or conjugated with either ribose sugar as fluorouridine (FUR) or deoxyribose sugar as FUdR. These nucleosides can be incorporated into either RNA or DNA, resulting in relatively poor imaging properties *(58, 59)*. Similarly, labeled FUR has also been examined on its own, but it is primarily incorporated into RNA *(58, 60)*. Of these tracers FUdR had the most promise, since it is primarily incorporated into DNA, has demonstrated improved tumor to background ratios *(58)*, and its retention is correlated with proliferation in animal studies *(61)*. Studies in patients by the same investigators have found that [^{18}F]FUdR did not provide high contrast images in most tumors and its retention did not correlate with proliferation as measured by Ki-67 *(62)*. The major limitation of FUdR may be attributed to its metabolism and cleavage of the glycosidic bond.

One of the primary limitations of many of these tracers discussed above has been in the *in vivo* catabolism of the tracers including dehalogenation or cleavage of the glycosidic bond. This has led to the development and testing of nucleosides that were resistant to degradation (Fig. 5). As before, a number of appropriate compounds have been developed as antiviral and antineoplastic agents and have been further tested as imaging agents. These have included a number of tracers with fluorine placed in the 2′- and 3′-position of the deoxyribose including FLT (3′-fluoro-3′-deoxythymidine), FMAU [(1-(2′-deoxy-2′-fluoro-β-D-arabinofuranosyl)thymine], FBAU [1-(2′-deoxy-2′-fluoro-1-β-D-arabinofuranosyl)-5-bromouracil], and related compounds *(63–67)*. All of these compounds are resistant to degradation greatly simplifying their use in imaging.

Of these compounds, FBAU takes advantage of the good incorporation found with BUdR, but improves upon this molecule by limiting its degradation. The presence of fluorine in the 2′-sugar has been shown to result in negligible degradation in mouse and dog studies *(64, 65)*. This compound can be labeled with ^{77}Br and ^{76}Br for SPECT and PET and recent work has also produced this as a ^{18}F-labeled compound for PET *(64, 68)*. There are relative advantages to both PET tracers in that the longer lived ^{76}Br (16h half-life) allows for easy distribution of the compound, but this isotope is not available in most centers and the long lived results in dosimetry require a lower injected dose. These studies have demonstrated that most of the activity is in proliferative tissues and tumors, it is incorporated into DNA, and that there is good contrast with nonproliferative tissues that would include the background. Further studies of FBAU are indicated and should be compared to FMAU and FLT.

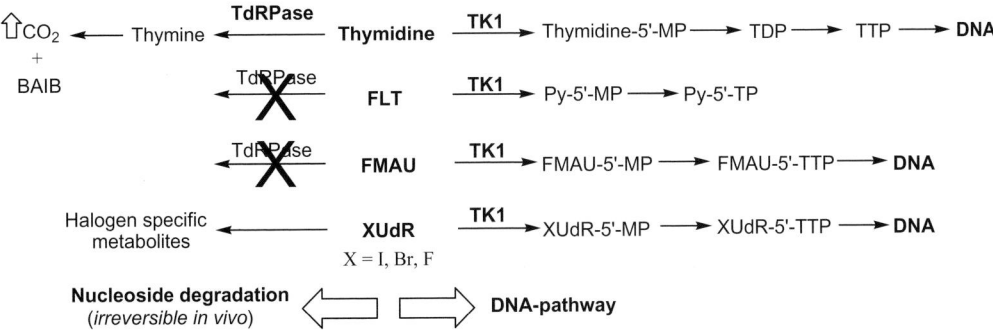

Fig. 5. Pathways of retention and excretion of thymidine and its analogs.

8. 3'-FLUORO-3'-DEOXYTHYMIDINE

The tracer that has undergone the most extensive recent exploration is FLT. This compound was originally synthesized as a possible antineoplastic compound *(69)* and subsequently studied as an agent to treat HIV *(70)* once the activity of the related compound, 3'-azidothymidine (AZT) was noted. It was thought to be a very promising agent based in part on its slower clearance from the blood and its minimal binding to plasma proteins *(71)*. A number of laboratory and animal studies led to a phase I trial in HIV patients *(72)*, which noted increased marrow and hepatic toxicity from FLT, and further clinical development of this agent was discontinued. While this toxicity precluded use of FLT as a therapeutic compound, at the miniscule doses used for imaging such toxicity was not considered to be an issue when used for PET. Thus FLT was labeled with ^{18}F *(73)* and a number of synthetic routes have since been developed that produce high yields, with good specific activity, in techniques that can be automated *(74–76)*. This has led to the commercial availability of a number of possible precursors and the sale of automated synthetic boxes for shape parameter recovery from images.

The first study of FLT imaging was done in dogs and patients and it demonstrated that FLT produced high contrast images of proliferative tissues, such as the bone marrow, as well as in tumors *(66)* (Fig. 6). While there was no breakdown of FLT in either species, in humans there is significant glucuronidation of FLT that needs to be taken into account when kinetic models are being developed and tested *(77, 78)*. FLT is retained in tissues by the action of TK1, which traps the tracer intracellularly as FLT-monophosphate *(79, 80)*. A small amount of FLT is incorporated into DNA (<2%), which primarily acts as a chain terminator as DNA is synthesized *(81)*. TK1 is cytosolic and increases several-fold as cells enter their S phase *(37)*. Also present within mitochondria is thymidine kinase 2 (TK2), and FLT is not a substrate for TK2 *(82)*. Therefore FLT demonstrates no visible uptake within the heart, unlike labeled thymidine, which demonstrates increased cardiac retention *(83)*.

In general it is possible to model the retention of FLT using a three-compartment model analogous to that utilized for FDG *(84, 85)* (Fig. 7). Over a 1-h period of imaging, dephosphorylation (k4) appears to be negligible, although it can be detected by careful analysis if imaging is conducted for 2 h *(77)*. A comparison of the estimates of the overall flux of FLT using the three-parameter fit obtained for 60 min compared to the four-parameter fit over 120 min correlated well ($r = 0.95$), yet the actual value was consistently underestimated with the shorter imaging time *(86)*. It is necessary to

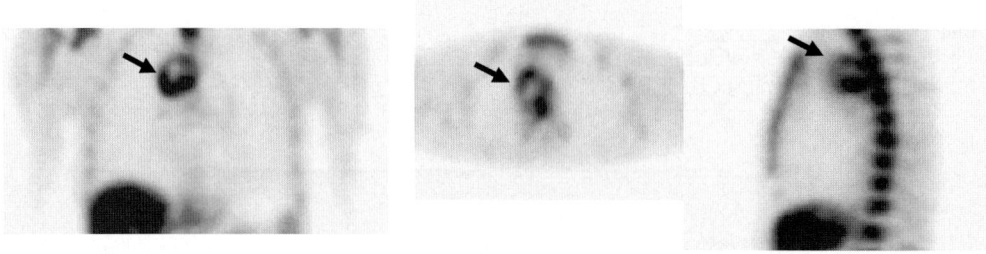

Fig. 6. Image of a patient with lung cancer imaged with FLT PET. Activity is seen in the tumor (arrow), bone marrow of the ribs, sternum, and vertebrae, and in the liver.

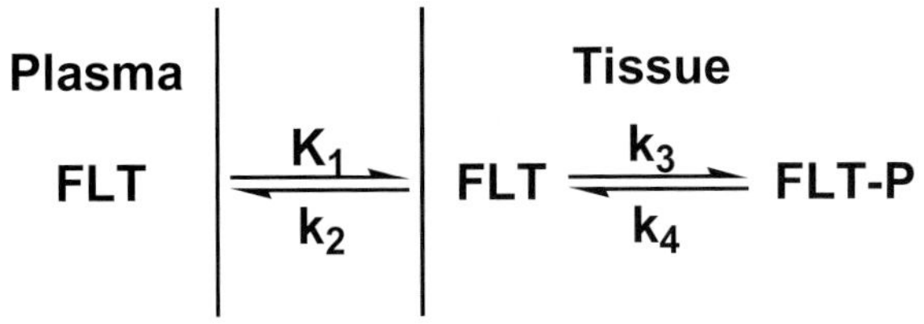

$$\text{Plasma} \quad | \quad \text{Tissue}$$
$$\text{FLT} \underset{k_2}{\overset{K_1}{\rightleftharpoons}} \text{FLT} \underset{k_4}{\overset{k_3}{\rightleftharpoons}} \text{FLT-P}$$

Fig. 7. Kinetic model of FLT uptake and retention.

take into account the activity in the blood that is present in FLT and its glucuronide, which can be done with analysis of a single blood sample done at the end of the imaging period *(78)*. On average, over the period of 60 min, 25% of the FLT is converted to the glucuronide, but this ranged from 57% to 87% in a series of 19 patients *(77, 78, 87)*. The dynamic uptake of FLT can also be measured using the graphic analysis approach developed by Patlak and Gjedde for use with FDG *(88, 89)*. In patients with untreated breast cancer, both compartmental and graphic approaches give comparable results ($r^2 = 0.98$, $p < 0.0001$) and the graphic approach is computationally simpler to perform *(78)*. Even simpler is just to measure SUV in patients with breast cancer. There was a significant correlation with FLT flux ($r^2 = 0.85$, $p = 0.0002$). It was also found that SUV correlated well with net influx constant in patients with colon cancer ($r^2 = 0.84$) *(85)*. In measuring treatment response, although it would certainly be simpler just to measure SUV, this would not take into account differences in the clearance and delivery of FLT to the tumor, which might change during the course of therapy. Future studies need to determine if kinetic measurements are necessary for accurate measurement of FLT retention or if SUV measurements are sufficient. Another issue that needs careful consideration is the reproducibility of the FLT measurements. Only limited studies of reproducibility have been done with FDG, which have demonstrated errors of less than about 20% *(90, 91)*, similar to preliminary studies with FLT *(92)*. A study in mice with tumor xenographs, where two scans were done on the same day 6 h apart, demonstrated a coefficient of variation of 14% ± 10% when the data were expressed as %ID/g *(93)*. It should be noted that mice have native thymidine levels about 10-fold higher than humans (about 10 µM in mice). Since thymidine may compete for FLT uptake, high thymidine levels in rodents may decrease FLT uptake. In fact, this competition has been demonstrated in tissue culture and mice and may vary with mouse strain *(93, 94)*.

3′-Fluoro-3′-deoxythymidine is retained in the DNA incorporation pathway, but not in DNA itself. To demonstrate that FLT does correlate with tumor growth in patients, a number of studies have compared FLT retention to proliferative activity as measured on biopsy specimens to assess Ki-67 *(79, 87, 95–98)* (Table 1). In general, FLT SUV has correlated nicely with Ki-67 in lung, colorectal, and breast cancers, sarcomas, and lymphoma. For example, in the study of Buck *et al.* FLT and Ki-67 significantly correlated ($r = 0.92$, $p < 0.0001$) in patients with untreated lung cancer, while the correlation was not as robust with FDG ($r = 0.59$, $p < 0.001$) (Fig. 8). In one study of breast cancer, FLT retention did not correlate with Ki-67 *(99)*, and in a study of esophageal cancer there was actually a negative correlation *(100)*. Overall, all of these studies had relatively small numbers of patients.

Table 1
Correlation of 3'-Fluoro-3'-deoxythymidine Retention, Measured as Standardized Uptake Values, and Biopsy Measurements of Proliferation Made by Staining for the Ki-67 Proliferation Antigen

Tumor type	Patient number	Correlation (r)	p value	Reference
Lung	26	0.92	<0.000	Buck, 2003 (95)
Lung	11	0.84	0.0011	Vesselle, 2002 (98)
Colorectal	10	0.8	<0.01	Francis, 2003 (97)
Breast	12	0.14	NS	Smyczek-Gargya, 2004 (99)
Breast	15	0.92	<0.0001	Kenny, 2005 (87)
Sarcoma	19	0.652	<0.005	Cobben, 2004 (96)
Lymphoma	10	0.95	<0.005	Wagner, 2003 (79)
Esophageal	8	−0.74	0.034	van Westreenen, 2005 (100)

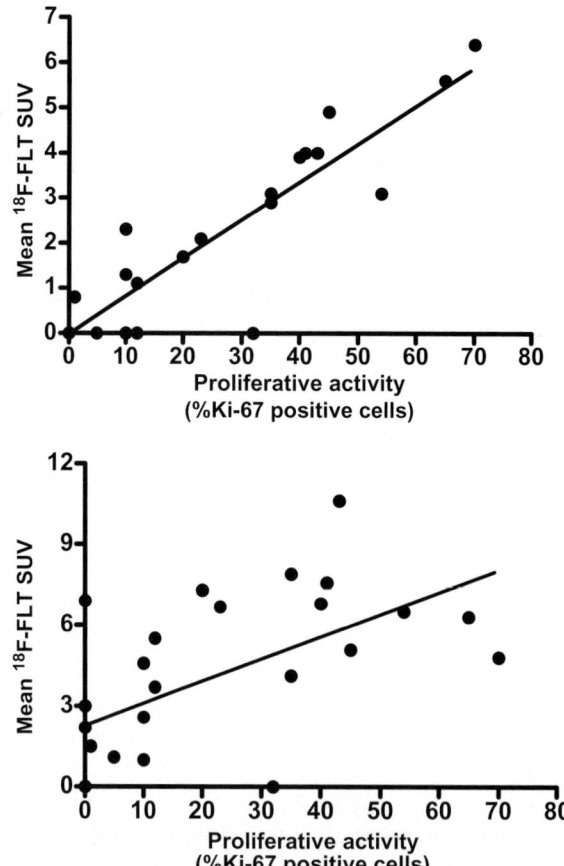

Fig. 8. Comparison of tumor proliferative activity, as measured by Ki-67 level, compared to retention of FLT and FDG, as mean SUV, in patients with untreated lung cancer. [Redrawn from data of Buck et al. (95).]

8.1 Use of 3′-Fluoro-3′-deoxythymidine to Detect Cancer

3′-Fluoro-3′-deoxythymidine imaging can also be employed to detect, stage, and assess prognosis in patients with cancer. In patients with lung lesions FLT was more specific than FDG in determining if a lesion was malignant, in that four of eight benign lesions demonstrated increased activity with FDG, while FLT was negative in all eight *(95)*. On the other hand, FDG was more sensitive, missing only 1/18 malignant lesions versus 3/18 with FLT. The mean SUV was also higher with FDG than FLT, 4.1 and 1.8, respectively. FLT can also readily detect esophageal cancer, which is aided, in part, by the low retention of FLT in the normal organs of the thorax *(101)*. In colon cancer, FLT and FDG did almost equally well in detecting extrahepatic disease despite the higher SUVs seen with FDG *(102)*. Within the liver, however, FDG had a much higher sensitivity than FLT, 97% and 34%, respectively. This is partly attributable to the high background uptake of FLT in the normal liver due to metabolism. One area in the body with very low background uptake of FLT and other pyrimidines is the brain. The blood–brain barrier makes it possible to obtain high contrast images of rapidly proliferating tumors, both with FLT and agents such as FMAU *(103–105)*.

8.2 3′-Fluoro-3′-deoxythymidine Use in Assessing Treatment

A number of recent studies in both tissue culture and rodents have used FLT to assess response to chemotherapy, endocrine treatment, or radiation. In mice implanted with an androgen-dependent prostate cancer FLT could be readily used to image the tumors *(106)*. Furthermore, there was a rapid decrease in FLT retention in mice treated by castration or with diethylstilbestrol.

In a study of mice with an implanted fibrosarcoma treated with cisplatin, declines in FLT retention were noted at 24 and 48 h of 25% and 50%, respectively *(107)*. The changes in FLT retention reflected the declines in TK1 levels. In mice implanted with a murine squamous cell cancer treated with a single dose of 20 Gy of radiation FLT retention decreased by 39% at 6 h, while a significant decline in FDG retention was not seen until 3 days *(108)*. These investigators also examined the use of photodynamic therapy in nude mice implanted with HeLa cells. By 24 h there was a 64% decline in FLT retention, but not a significant decrease in FDG uptake.

In another study, mice with a human epidermoid carcinoma were treated with a tyrosine kinase inhibitor directed at ErbB *(109)*. FLT retention declined by over 50% at 48 h and by almost 80% at 7 days. In this particular study FDG uptake also declined almost as much and the retention of both tracers correlated with tumor measurements of proliferation by staining for proliferating cell nuclear antigen. Thus it is necessary to determine whether FLT or FDG is needed, depending on the tumor being imaged and treatment employed.

It is necessary to be careful when using FLT to monitor response after the use of antimetabolites. Since these drugs inhibit the synthesis of endogenous thymidine, the cell may compensate by increasing activity within the salvage pathway. In cell lines this resulted in a several-fold increase in FLT retention with 5-FU and methotrexate within 24 h, while FLT retention declined after treatment with cisplatin *(110)*. In contrast, mice bearing an implanted firbrosarcoma and treated with 5FU had decreased retention of FLT at 24 and 48 h *(4)*. This decline correlated with a decrease in tumor proliferating cell nuclear antigen staining. The difference between these results may reflect differences in the tumor type studied, sensitivity to 5-FU, and cell culture versus *in vivo*. Nevertheless, it serves to caution investigators about the interpretation of FLT imaging soon after treatment with antimetabolites.

In summary, a number of studies have now demonstrated in culture and in mice that treatment with chemotherapy, radiation, hormonal manipulation, and targeted drugs can result in rapid declines in FLT retention. In many cases, the decline in FLT uptake precedes changes seen in FDG retention. Pilot studies using FLT in assessing treatment response in patients are now just being completed and will need to be expanded if FLT is going to find routine clinical use to assess treatment response.

9. 1-(2′-DEOXY-2′-FLUORO-β-D-ARABINOFURANOSYL)THYMINE

1-(2′-Deoxy-2′-fluoro-D-arabinofuranosyl)thymine (FMAU) has a number of differences compared to FLT in its metabolism and imaging characteristics. Both tracers are stabilized by the presence of fluoride on the sugar resulting in similar stability for FMAU over the course of imaging in animals and humans *(105, 111, 112)*. One significant factor in imaging with FMAU is its rapid clearance from the blood in humans, primarily into the liver, with over 90% of the tracer cleared within about 10 min *(105)*. Unlike FLT, FMAU is readily incorporated into DNA, with the level of incorporation reflective of the proliferative rate *(113)*. In animal studies, the activity present in proliferating tissues, such as bone marrow and intestine, was primarily present in DNA (87% and 64%, respectively) *(112)*. Less activity was present in most nonproliferating tissues in dogs, such as the lung and heart, and less than 10% was in DNA. It is necessary to acknowledge that high FMAU uptake is seen in the heart in humans, which has a high concentration of TK2. As previously noted, thymidine is also retained in the heart, while FLT, which has a low affinity for TK2, has minimal cardiac retention.

In patients, FMAU imaging may have limited use in the lower thorax and upper abdomen because of high physiological retention in the normal heart, liver, and kidney *(105)*. On the other hand, the rapid clearance and retention in these organs result in relatively less bladder activity, improving imaging in the pelvis (Fig. 9). Work in evaluating FMAU to assess treatment response is now needed.

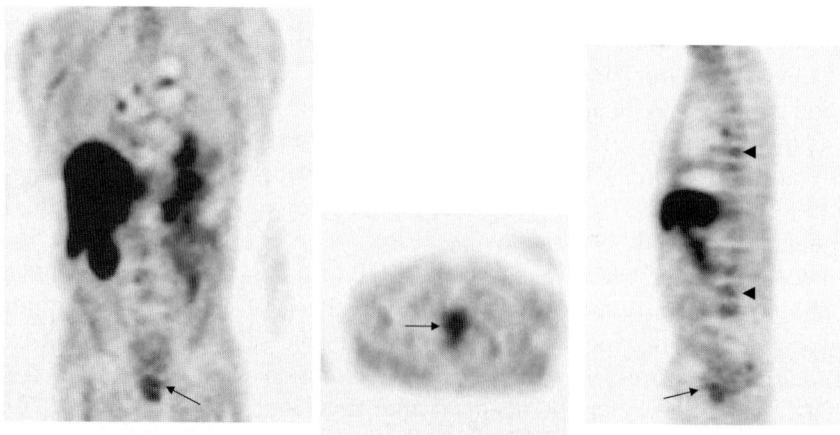

Fig. 9. Image of a prostate cancer patient with FMAU PET. Activity is seen in the prostate (arrow) and bone metastases (arrowheads). Physiological retention is also seen in the liver and kidneys.

10. CONCLUSIONS

A critical measurement in the assessment of tumor response is the measurement of proliferation. While a number of laboratory measures have been developed to measure DNA synthesis and tumor growth rates, each has its limitations. When applying such techniques to clinical studies and care, the greatest challenge is the requirement for processing of tissue samples. The heterogeneity of tumors is also problematic when analyzing biopsies from a single area. The design and validation of new imaging methods to evaluate proliferation using nuclear techniques offer noninvasive assessment options. A number of tracers have been developed for use with PET. Thymidine labeled with ^{11}C is the standard agent, but it is difficult to use in practice because of its short physical and biological half-life. The use of FLT and FMAU offers good opportunities to image tumor proliferation with practical tracers. Further work in cancer patients is needed to demonstrate that such tracers can be used to rapidly and accurately to predict treatment response for use in optimizing routine care and enhancing drug development.

REFERENCES

1. Miller AB, Hoogstraten B, Staquet M, Winkler A. Reporting results of cancer treatment. *Cancer* 1981;47:207–214.
2. Therasse P, Arbuck SG, Eisenhauer EA, Wanders J, Kaplan RS, Rubinstein L, *et al*. New guidelines to evaluate the response to treatment in solid tumors. European Organization for Research and Treatment of Cancer, National Cancer Institute of the United States, National Cancer Institute of Canada. *J Natl Cancer Inst* 2000;92(3):205–216.
3. Skehan P. On the normality of growth dynamics of neoplasms in vivo: A data base analysis. *Growth* 1986;50(4):496–515.
4. Barthel H, Cleij MC, Collingridge DR, Hutchinson OC, Osman S, He Q, *et al*. 3′-Deoxy-3′-[18F]fluorothymidine as a new marker for monitoring tumor response to antiproliferative therapy in vivo with positron emission tomography. *Cancer Res* 2003;63(13):3791–3798.
5. Shields AF, Mankoff DA, Link JM, Graham MM, Eary JF, Kozawa M, *et al*. [11C]Thymidine and FDG to measure therapy response. *J Nucl Med* 1998;39:1757–1762.
6. Mossman PB, Young LL, 3rd. Testing for degrees of color blindness. *Occup Health Saf* 1983;52(8):49–53, 55.
7. Tannock I. Cell kinetics and chemotherapy: A critical review. *Cancer Treat Rep* 1978;62(8):1117–1133.
8. Cleaver JE. Thymidine metabolism and cell kinetics. *Frontiers Biol* 1967;6:43–100.
9. Reid BJ, Haggitt RC, Rubin CE, Rabinovitch PS. Barrett's esophagus. Correlation between flow cytometry and histology in detection of patients at risk for adenocarcinoma. *Gastroenterology* 1987;93(1):1–11.
10. Livingston RB, Sulkes A, Thirwell MP, Murphy WK, Hart JS. Cell kinetic parameters: Correlation with clinical response. In: Drewinko B, Humphrey RM, eds. Growth Kinetics and Biochemical Regulation of Normal and Malignant Cells. Baltimore: Williams & Wilkins, 1977:767–785.
11. Wilson GD. Assessment of human tumour proliferation using bromodeoxyuridine–current status. *Acta Oncol* 1991;30(8):903–910.
12. Gardelle O, Roelcke U, Vontobel P, Crompton NE, Guenther I, Blauenstein P, *et al*. [76Br]Bromodeoxyuridine PET in tumor-bearing animals. *Nucl Med Biol* 2001;28(1):51–57.
13. Ryser JE, Blauenstein P, Remy N, Weinreich R, Hasler PH, Novak-Hofer I, *et al*. [76Br]Bromodeoxyuridine, a potential tracer for the measurement of cell proliferation by positron emission tomography, in vitro and in vivo studies in mice. *Nucl Med Biol* 1999;26(6):673–679.
14. Scholzen T, Gerdes J. The Ki-67 protein: From the known and the unknown. *J Cell Physiol* 2000;182(3):311–322.
15. Pugsley JM, Schmidt RA, Vesselle H. The Ki-67 index and survival in non-small cell lung cancer: A review and relevance to positron emission tomography. *Cancer J* 2002;8(3):222–233.

16. Chung JK, Lee YJ, Kim SK, Jeong JM, Lee DS, Lee MC. Comparison of [18F]fluorodeoxyglucose uptake with glucose transporter-1 expression and proliferation rate in human glioma and non-small-cell lung cancer. *Nucl Med Commun* 2004;25(1):11–17.
17. Kim S, Chung JK, Im SH, Jeong JM, Lee DS, Kim DG, et al. 11C-Methionine PET as a prognostic marker in patients with glioma: Comparison with 18F-FDG PET. *Eur J Nucl Med Mol Imaging* 2005;32(1):52–59.
18. Utriainen M, Metsahonkala L, Salmi TT, Utriainen T, Kalimo H, Pihko H, et al. Metabolic characterization of childhood brain tumors: Comparison of 18F-fluorodeoxyglucose and 11C-methionine positron emission tomography. *Cancer* 2002;95(6):1376–1386.
19. Higashi K, Ueda Y, Yagishita M, Arisaka Y, Sakurai A, Oguchi M, et al. FDG PET measurement of the proliferative potential of non-small cell lung cancer. *J Nucl Med* 2000;41(1):85–92.
20. Brown RS, Leung JY, Kison PV, Zasadny KR, Flint A, Wahl RL. Glucose transporters and FDG uptake in untreated primary human non-small cell lung cancer. *J Nucl Med* 1999;40(4):556–565.
21. Christman D, Crawford EJ, Friedkin M, Wolf AP. Detection of DNA synthesis in intact organisms with positron-emitting [methyl-^{11}C]thymidine. *Proc Natl Acad Sci USA* 1972;69(4).
22. Larson SM, Weiden PL, Grunbaum Z, Rasey JS, Kaplan HG, Graham MM, et al. Positron imaging feasibility studies. I: Characteristics of [3H]thymidine uptake in rodent and canine neoplasms: Concise communication. *J Nucl Med* 1981;22(10):869–874.
23. Shields AF, Larson SM, Grunbaum Z, Graham MM. Short-term thymidine uptake in normal and neoplastic tissues: Studies for PET. *J Nucl Med* 1984;25:759–764.
24. Christman D, Crawford EJ, Friedkin M, Wolf AP. Detection of DNA synthesis in intact organisms with positron-emitting (methyl-^{11}C)thymidine. *Proc Natl Acad Sci USA* 1972;69(4):988–992.
25. Sundoro-Wu BM, Schmall B, Conti PS, Dahl JR, Drumm P, Jacobsen JK. Selective alkylation of pyrimidyl-dianions: Synthesis and purification of ^{11}C labeled thymidine for tumor visualization using positron emission tomography. *Int J Appl Radiat Isotopes* 1984;35:705–708.
26. Vander Borght T, Labar D, Pauwels S, Lambotte L. Production of [2-^{11}C]Thymidine for quantification of cellular proliferation with PET. *Appl Radiat Isotopes* 1991;42:103–104.
27. Becherer A, Karanikas G, Szabo M, Zettinig G, Asenbaum S, Marosi C, et al. Brain tumour imaging with PET: A comparison between [18F]fluorodopa and [11C]methionine. *Eur J Nucl Med Mol Imaging* 2003;30(11):1561–1567.
28. Shields AF, Lim K, Grierson J, Link J, Krohn KA. Utilization of labeled thymidine in DNA synthesis: Studies for PET. *J Nucl Med* 1990;31(3):337–342.
29. Shields AF, Mankoff D, Graham MM, Zheng M, Kozawa SM, Link J, et al. Analysis of [2-^{11}C]thymidine blood metabolites for imaging with PET. *J Nucl Med* 1996;37:290–296.
30. Shields AF, Graham MM, Kozawa SM, Kozell LB, Link JM, Swenson ER, et al. Contribution of labeled carbon dioxide to PET imaging of carbon-11-labeled compounds. *J Nucl Med* 1992;33(4):581–584.
31. Mankoff DA, Shields AF, Graham MM, Link JM, Eary JF, Krohn KA. Kinetic analysis of 2-[carbon-11]thymidine PET imaging studies: Compartmental model and mathematical analysis. *J Nucl Med* 1998;39(6):1043–1055.
32. Mankoff DA, Shields AF, Graham MM, Link JM, Krohn KA. A graphical analysis method for estimating blood-to-tissue transfer constants for tracers with labeled metabolites. *J Nucl Med* 1996;37(12):2049–2057.
33. Wells P, Gunn RN, Alison M, Steel C, Golding M, Ranicar AS, et al. Assessment of proliferation in vivo using 2-[(11)C]thymidine positron emission tomography in advanced intra-abdominal malignancies. *Cancer Res* 2002;62(20):5698–5702.
34. Gunn RN, Yap JT, Wells P, Osman S, Price P, Jones T, et al. A general method to correct PET data for tissue metabolites using a dual-scan approach. *J Nucl Med* 2000;41(4):706–711.
35. Ritzel MW, Yao SY, Huang MY, Elliott JF, Cass CE, Young JD. Molecular cloning and functional expression of cDNAs encoding a human Na+-nucleoside cotransporter (hCNT1). *Am J Physiol* 1997;272(2 Pt 1):C707–C714.
36. Baldwin SA, Beal PR, Yao SY, King AE, Cass CE, Young JD. The equilibrative nucleoside transporter family, SLC29. *Pflugers Arch* 2004;447(5):735–743.
37. Sherley JL, Kelly TJ. Regulation of human thymidine kinase during the cell cycle. *J Biol Chem* 1988;263(17):8350–8358.
38. Shields AF, Coonrod DV, Quackenbush RC, Crowley JJ. Cellular sources of thymidine nucleotides: Studies for PET. *J Nucl Med* 1987;28:1435–1440.

39. Mankoff D, Shields A, Link J, Graham M, Muzi M, Peterson L, et al. Kinetic analysis of 2-[C-11]-thymidine PET imaging studies: Validation studies. *J Nucl Med* 1999;40(4):614–624.
40. Eary JF, Mankoff DA, Spence AM, Berger MS, Olshen A, Link JM, et al. 2-[C-11]Thymidine imaging of malignant brain tumors. *Cancer Res* 1999;59(3):615–621.
41. Martiat P, Ferrant A, Labar D, Cogneau M, Bol A, Michel C, et al. In vivo measurement of carbon-11 thymidine uptake in non-Hodgkin's lymphoma using positron emission tomography. *J Nucl Med* 1988;29:1633–1637.
42. van Eijkeren ME, De Schryver A, Goethals P, Poupeye E, Schelstraete K, Lemahieu I, et al. Measurement of short-term 11C-thymidine activity in human head and neck tumours using positron emission tomography (PET). *Acta Oncol* 1992;31(5):539–543.
43. Vander Borght T, Pauwels S, Lambotte L, Labar D, De Maeght S, Stroobandt G, et al. Brain tumor imaging with PET and 2-[carbon-11]thymidine. *J Nucl Med* 1994;35(6):974–982.
44. Wells P, Gunn RN, Steel C, Ranicar AS, Brady F, Osman S, et al. 2-[11C]Thymidine positron emission tomography reproducibility in humans. *Clin Cancer Res* 2005;11(12):4341–4347.
45. De Reuck J, Santens P, Goethals P, Strijckmans K, Lemahieu I, Boon P, et al. [Methyl-11C]thymidine positron emission tomography in tumoral and non- tumoral cerebral lesions. *Acta Neurol Belg* 1999;99(2):118–125.
46. Propper DJ, McDonald AC, Man A, Thavasu P, Balkwill F, Braybrooke JP, et al. Phase I and pharmacokinetic study of PKC412, an inhibitor of protein kinase C. *J Clin Oncol* 2001;19(5):1485–1492.
47. Wells P, West C, Jones T, Harris A, Price P. Measuring tumor pharmacodynamic response using PET proliferation probes: The case for 2-[(11)C]-thymidine. *Biochim Biophys Acta* 2004;1705(2):91–102.
48. Wells P, Aboagye E, Gunn RN, Osman S, Boddy AV, Taylor GA, et al. 2-[11C]Thymidine positron emission tomography as an indicator of thymidylate synthase inhibition in patients treated with AG337. *J Natl Cancer Inst* 2003;95(9):675–682.
49. Heidelberger C, Chaudhuri NK, Danneberg P, et al. Fluorinated pyrimidines, a new class of tumor-inhibitory compounds. *Nature* 1957;179:663.
50. Eidinoff ML, Cheong L, Gurpide EG, Benua RS, Ellison RR. Incorporation of 5-iodouracil labelled with iodine-131 into the deoxyribonucleic acid of human leukaemic leucocytes following in vivo administration of 5-iododeoxyuridine labelled with iodine-131. *Nature* 1959;183(4676):1686–1687.
51. Philip PA, Bagshawe KD, Searle F, Green AJ, Begent RH, Newlands ES, et al. In vivo uptake of 131I-5-iodo-2-deoxyuridine by malignant tumours in man. *Br J Cancer* 1991;63(1):134–135.
52. Tjuvajev JG, Macapinilac HA, Daghighian F, Scott AM, Ginos JZ, Finn RD, et al. Imaging of brain tumor proliferative activity with iodine-131-iododeoxyuridine. *J Nucl Med* 1994;35(9):1407–1417.
53. Kriss JP, Maruyama Y, Tung LA, Bond SB, Revesz L. The fate of 5-bromodeoxycytodine and 5-iododeoxyuridine in man. *Cancer Res* 1963;23:260–273.
54. Bergstrom M, Lu L, Fasth KJ, Wu F, Bergstrom-Pettermann E, Tolmachev V, et al. In vitro and animal validation of bromine-76-bromodeoxyuridine as a proliferation marker. *J Nucl Med* 1998;39(7):1273–1279.
55. Gudjonsson O, Bergstrom M, Kristjansson S, Wu F, Nyberg G, Fasth KJ, et al. Analysis of 76Br-BrdU in DNA of brain tumors after a PET study does not support its use as a proliferation marker. *Nucl Med Biol* 2001;28(1):59–65.
56. Fowler JS, Finn RD, Lambrecht RM, Wolf AP. The synthesis of ^{18}F-5-fluorouracil. VII. *J Nucl Med* 1973;14:63–64.
57. Dimitrakopoulou-Strauss A, Strauss LG, Schlag P, Hohenberger P, Mohler M, Oberdorfer F, et al. Fluorine-18-fluorouracil to predict therapy response in liver metastases from colorectal carcinoma. *J Nucl Med* 1998;39(7):1197–1202.
58. Abe Y, Fukuda H, Ishiwata K, Yoshioka S, Yamada K, Endo S, et al. Studies on ^{18}F-labeled pyrimidines. Tumor uptakes of ^{18}F-5-fluorouracil, ^{18}F-5-fluorouridine, and ^{18}F-5-fluoro-2′-deoxyuridine in animals. *Eur J Nucl Med* 1983;8:258–261.
59. Shani J, Wolf W, Schlesinger T, Atkins HL, Bradley-Moore PR, Casella V, et al. Distribution of 18F-5-fluorouracil in tumor-bearing mice and rats. *Int J Nucl Med Biol* 1978;5(1):19–28.
60. Crawford EJ, Friedkin M, Wolf AP, Fowler JS, Gallagher BM, Lambrecht RM, et al. ^{18}F-5-Fluorouridine, a new probe for measuring the proliferation of tissue in vivo. *Adv Enzyme Regul* 1982;20:3–22.

61. Seitz U, Wagner M, Vogg AT, Glatting G, Neumaier B, Greten FR, et al. In vivo evaluation of 5-[(18)F]fluoro-2'-deoxyuridine as tracer for positron emission tomography in a murine pancreatic cancer model. *Cancer Res* 2001;61(10):3853–3857.
62. Buchmann I, Vogg AT, Glatting G, Schultheiss S, Moller P, Leithauser F, et al. [18F]5-Fluoro-2-deoxyuridine-PET for imaging of malignant tumors and for measuring tissue proliferation. *Cancer Biother Radiopharm* 2003;18(3):327–337.
63. Conti P, Alauddin M, Fissekis J, Schmall B, Watanabe K. Synthesis of 2'-fluoro-5-[11C]-methyl-1-beta-D-arabinofuranosyluracil ([11C]-FMAU): A potential nucleoside analog for in vivo study of cellular proliferation with PET. *Nucl Med Biol* 1995;22(6):783–789.
64. Lu L, Bergstrom M, Fasth KJ, Langstrom B. Synthesis of [76Br]bromofluorodeoxyuridine and its validation with regard to uptake, DNA incorporation, and excretion modulation in rats. *J Nucl Med* 2000;41(10):1746–1752.
65. Nimmagadda S, Mangner TJ, Sun H, Klecker RW, Jr., Muzik O, Lawhorn-Crews JM, et al. Biodistribution and radiation dosimetry estimates of 1-(2'-deoxy-2'-(18)F-fluoro-1-beta-D-arabinofuranosyl)-5-bromouracil: PET imaging studies in dogs. *J Nucl Med* 2005;46(11):1916–1922.
66. Shields A, Grierson J, Dohmen B, Machulla H-J, Stayanoff J, Lawhorn-Crews J, et al. Imaging proliferation in vivo with [F-18]FLT and positron emission tomography. *Nature Med* 1998;4:1334–1336.
67. Shields AF, Grierson JR, Kozawa SM, Zheng M. Development of labeled thymidine analogs for imaging tumor proliferation. *Nuclear Med Biol* 1996;23(1):17–22.
68. Mangner T, Klecker R, Anderson L, Shields A. Synthesis of 2'-[18F]fluoro-2'-deoxy-β-D-arabinofuranosyl nucleotides, [18F]FAU, [18F]FMAU, [18F]FBAU and [18F]FIAU, as potential PET agents for imaging cellular proliferation. *Nucl Med Biol* 2003(30):215–224.
69. Langen P, Etzold G, Hintsche R. 3'-Deoxy-3'-fluorothymidine, a new selective inhibitor of DNA-synthesis. *Acta Biol Med Ger* 1969;23(6):759–766.
70. Matthes E, Lehmann C, Scholz D, Rosenthal HA, Langen P. Phosphorylation, anti-HIV activity and cytotoxicity of 3'-fluorothymidine. *Biochem Biophys Res Commun* 1988;153(2):825–831.
71. Lundgren B, Bottiger D, Ljungdahl-Stahle E, Norrby E, Stahle L, Wahren B, et al. Antiviral effects of 3'-fluorothymidine and 3'-azidothymidine in cynomolgus monkeys infected with simian immunodeficiency virus. *J Acquir Immune Defic Syndr* 1991;4(5):489–498.
72. Flexner C, van der Horst C, Jacobson MA, Powderly W, Duncanson F, Ganes D, et al. Relationship between plasma concentrations of 3'-deoxy-3'-fluorothymidine (alovudine) and antiretroviral activity in two concentration-controlled trials. *J Infect Dis* 1994;170(6):1394–1403.
73. Grierson J, Shields A. A strategy for the labeling of [F-18]-3'-deoxy-3'-fluorothymidine: [F-18]FLT. *J Labelled Comp Radiopharm* 1995;37:606–607.
74. Grierson JR, Shields AF. An improved synthesis of [18F]FLT. *J Labelled Comp Radiopharm* 1999;42(Suppl 1):S525–S526.
75. Grierson JR, Shields AF. Radiosynthesis of 3'-deoxy-3'-[(18)F]fluorothymidine: [(18)F]FLT for imaging of cellular proliferation in vivo. *Nucl Med Biol* 2000;27(2):143–156.
76. Machulla H-J, Blocher A, Kuntzsch M, Wei R, Grierson J. Simplified labeling approach for synthesizing 3'-deoxy-3'-[18F]fluorothymidine ([18F]FLT). *J Radioanalyt Nucl Chem* 2000;243:843–846.
77. Muzi M, Vesselle H, Grierson JR, Mankoff DA, Schmidt RA, Peterson L, et al. Kinetic analysis of 3'-deoxy-3'-fluorothymidine PET studies: Validation studies in patients with lung cancer. *J Nucl Med* 2005;46(2):274–282.
78. Shields AF, Briston DA, Chandupatla S, Douglas KA, Lawhorn-Crews J, Collins JM, et al. A simplified analysis of [18F]3'-deoxy-3'-fluorothymidine metabolism and retention. *Eur J Nucl Med Mol Imaging* 2005;32(11):1269–1275.
79. Wagner M, Seitz U, Buck A, Neumaier B, Schultheiss S, Bangerter M, et al. 3'-[18F]Fluoro-3'-deoxythymidine ([18F]-FLT) as positron emission tomography tracer for imaging proliferation in a murine B-cell lymphoma model and in the human disease. *Cancer Res* 2003;63(10):2681–2687.
80. Grierson JR, Schwartz JL, Muzi M, Jordan R, Krohn KA. Metabolism of 3'-deoxy-3'-[F-18]fluorothymidine in proliferating A549 cells: Validations for positron emission tomography. *Nucl Med Biol* 2004;31(7):829–837.
81. Seitz U, Wagner M, Neumaier B, Wawra E, Glatting G, Leder G, et al. Evaluation of pyrimidine metabolising enzymes and in vitro uptake of 3'-[(18)F]fluoro-3'-deoxythymidine ([(18)F]FLT) in pancreatic cancer cell lines. *Eur J Nucl Med Mol Imaging* 2002;29(9):1174–1181.

82. Munch-Petersen B, Cloos L, Tyrsted G, Eriksson S. Diverging substrate specificity of pure human thymidine kinases 1 and 2 against antiviral dideoxynucleosides. *J Biol Chem* 1991;266(14): 9032–9038.
83. Jansson O, Bohman C, Munch-Petersen B, Eriksson S. Mammalian thymidine kinase 2: Direct photoaffinity labeling with [^{32}P]dTTP of the enzyme from spleen, liver, heart and brain. *Eur J Biochem* 1992;206:485–490.
84. Shields A, Grierson JR, Muzik O, Stayanoff JC, Lawhorn-Crews J, Obradovich JE, et al. Kinetics of 3′-deoxy-3′-[F-18]fluorothymidine uptake and retention in dogs. *Mol Imaging Biol* 2002:83–89.
85. Visvikis D, Francis D, Mulligan R, Costa DC, Croasdale I, Luthra SK, et al. Comparison of methodologies for the in vivo assessment of 18FLT utilisation in colorectal cancer. *Eur J Nucl Med Mol Imaging* 2004;31(2):169–178.
86. Muzi M, Mankoff DA, Grierson JR, Wells JM, Vesselle H, Krohn KA. Kinetic modeling of 3′-deoxy-3′-fluorothymidine in somatic tumors: Mathematical studies. *J Nucl Med* 2005;46(2):371–380.
87. Kenny LM, Vigushin DM, Al-Nahhas A, Osman S, Luthra SK, Shousha S, et al. Quantification of cellular proliferation in tumor and normal tissues of patients with breast cancer by [18F]fluorothymidine-positron emission tomography imaging: Evaluation of analytical methods. *Cancer Res* 2005; 65(21):10104–10112.
88. Gjedde A. Calculation of cerebral glucose phosphorylation from brain uptake of glucose analogs in vivo: A re-examination. *Brain Res Rev* 1982;4:237–274.
89. Patlak CS, Blasberg RG, Fenstermacher JD. Graphical evaluation of blood-to-brain transfer constants from multiple-time uptake data. *J Cereb Blood Flow Metab* 1983;3:1–7.
90. Minn H, Zasadny KR, Quint LE, Wahl RL. Lung cancer: Reproducibility of quantitative measurements for evaluating 2-[F-18]-fluoro-2-deoxy-D-glucose uptake at PET. *Radiology* 1995;196(1): 167–173.
91. Weber WA, Ziegler SI, Thodtmann R, Hanauske AR, Schwaiger M. Reproducibility of metabolic measurements in malignant tumors using FDG PET. *J Nucl Med* 1999;40(11):1771–1777.
92. Shields A, Lawhorn-Crews J, Briston D, Douglas K, Mangner T, Muzik O. The Reproducibility of FLT PET in patients with untreated non-small cell lung cancer. *J Nucl Med* 2005;46:426P.
93. Tseng JR, Dandekar M, Subbarayan M, Cheng Z, Park JM, Louie S, et al. Reproducibility of 3′-deoxy-3′-(18)F-fluorothymidine microPET studies in tumor xenografts in mice. *J Nucl Med* 2005;46(11):1851–1857.
94. Mankoff DA, Shields AF, Krohn KA. PET imaging of cellular proliferation. *Radiol Clin North Am* 2005;43(1):153–167.
95. Buck AK, Halter G, Schirrmeister H, Kotzerke J, Wurziger I, Glatting G, et al. Imaging proliferation in lung tumors with PET: 18F-FLT versus 18F-FDG. *J Nucl Med* 2003;44(9):1426–1431.
96. Cobben DC, Elsinga PH, Suurmeijer AJ, Vaalburg W, Maas B, Jager PL, et al. Detection and grading of soft tissue sarcomas of the extremities with (18)F-3′-fluoro-3′-deoxy-L-thymidine. *Clin Cancer Res* 2004;10(5):1685–1690.
97. Francis DL, Freeman A, Visvikis D, Costa DC, Luthra SK, Novelli M, et al. In vivo imaging of cellular proliferation in colorectal cancer using positron emission tomography. *Gut* 2003;52(11): 1602–1606.
98. Vesselle H, Grierson J, Muzi M, Pugsley JM, Schmidt RA, Rabinowitz P, et al. In vivo validation of 3′deoxy-3′-[(18)F]fluorothymidine ([(18)F]FLT) as a proliferation imaging tracer in humans: Correlation of [(18)F]FLT uptake by positron emission tomography with Ki-67 immunohistochemistry and flow cytometry in human lung tumors. *Clin Cancer Res* 2002;8(11):3315–3323.
99. Smyczek-Gargya B, Fersis N, Dittmann H, Vogel U, Reischl G, Machulla HJ, et al. PET with [18F]fluorothymidine for imaging of primary breast cancer: A pilot study. *Eur J Nucl Med Mol Imaging* 2004;31(5):720–724.
100. van Westreenen HL, Cobben DC, Jager PL, van Dullemen HM, Wesseling J, Elsinga PH, et al. Comparison of 18F-FLT PET and 18F-FDG PET in esophageal cancer. *J Nucl Med* 2005;46(3): 400–404.
101. Dittmann H, Dohmen BM, Paulsen F, Eichhorn K, Eschmann SM, Horger M, et al. [18F]FLT PET for diagnosis and staging of thoracic tumours. *Eur J Nucl Med Mol Imaging* 2003;30(10): 1407–1412.
102. Francis DL, Visvikis D, Costa DC, Arulampalam TH, Townsend C, Luthra SK, et al. Potential impact of [18F]3′-deoxy-3′-fluorothymidine versus [18F]fluoro-2-deoxy-D-glucose in positron emission tomography for colorectal cancer. *Eur J Nucl Med Mol Imaging* 2003;30(7):988–994.

103. Chen W, Cloughesy T, Kamdar N, Satyamurthy N, Bergsneider M, Liau L, et al. Imaging proliferation in brain tumors with 18F-FLT PET: Comparison with 18F-FDG. *J Nucl Med* 2005;46(6): 945–952.
104. Choi SJ, Kim JS, Kim JH, Oh SJ, Lee JG, Kim CJ, et al. [18F]3'-Deoxy-3'-fluorothymidine PET for the diagnosis and grading of brain tumors. *Eur J Nucl Med Mol Imaging* 2005;32(6):653–659.
105. Sun H, Sloan A, Mangner TJ, Vaishampayan U, Muzik O, Collins JM, et al. Imaging DNA synthesis with [18F]FMAU and positron emission tomography in patients with cancer. *Eur J Nucl Med Mol Imaging* 2005;32(1):15–22.
106. Oyama N, Ponde DE, Dence C, Kim J, Tai YC, Welch MJ. Monitoring of therapy in androgen-dependent prostate tumor model by measuring tumor proliferation. *J Nucl Med* 2004;45(3): 519–525.
107. Leyton J, Latigo JR, Perumal M, Dhaliwal H, He Q, Aboagye EO. Early detection of tumor response to chemotherapy by 3'-deoxy-3'-[18F]fluorothymidine positron emission tomography: The effect of cisplatin on a fibrosarcoma tumor model in vivo. *Cancer Res* 2005;65(10):4202–4210.
108. Sugiyama M, Sakahara H, Sato K, Harada N, Fukumoto D, Kakiuchi T, et al. Evaluation of 3'-deoxy-3'-18F-fluorothymidine for monitoring tumor response to radiotherapy and photodynamic therapy in mice. *J Nucl Med* 2004;45(10):1754–1758.
109. Waldherr C, Mellinghoff IK, Tran C, Halpern BS, Rozengurt N, Safaei A, et al. Monitoring antiproliferative responses to kinase inhibitor therapy in mice with 3'-deoxy-3'-18F-fluorothymidine PET. *J Nucl Med* 2005;46(1):114–120.
110. Dittmann H, Dohmen BM, Kehlbach R, Bartusek G, Pritzkow M, Sarbia M, et al. Early changes in [(18)F]FLT uptake after chemotherapy: An experimental study. *Eur J Nucl Med Mol Imaging* 2002; 29(11):1462–1469.
111. Bading JR, Shahinian AH, Bathija P, Conti PS. Pharmacokinetics of the thymidine analog 2'-fluoro-5-[(14)C]-methyl-1-beta-D-arabinofuranosyluracil ([(14)C]FMAU) in rat prostate tumor cells. *Nucl Med Biol* 2000;27(4):361–368.
112. Sun H, Mangner TJ, Collins JM, Muzik O, Douglas K, Shields AF. Imaging DNA synthesis in vivo with 18F-FMAU and PET. *J Nucl Med* 2005;46(2):292–296.
113. Collins JM, Klecker RW, Katki AG. Suicide prodrugs activated by thymidylate synthase: Rationale for treatment and noninvasive imaging of tumors with deoxyuridine analogues. *Clin Cancer Res* 1999;5(8):1976–1981.

9 Estrogen-Receptor Imaging and Assessing Response to Hormonal Therapy of Breast Cancer

Farrokh Dehdashti, MD, and Barry A. Siegel, MD

CONTENTS

INTRODUCTION
TREATMENT OF BREAST CANCER
ESTROGEN-RECEPTOR IMAGING
PREDICTING RESPONSE OF BREAST CANCER TO
  HORMONAL THERAPY

1. INTRODUCTION

One of the most important applications of positron emission tomography (PET) in clinical oncology is monitoring and assessing tumor response to treatment (as discussed in Chapter 1). In contrast to conventional anatomic imaging, which is insensitive for early assessment of therapeutic response, molecular imaging by PET can provide unique information about the likelihood of tumor responsiveness to therapy before initiation of treatment or early during a course of treatment. Additionally, PET is more sensitive and specific than conventional imaging for defining a complete or near-complete response after a course of treatment has ended. One of the most challenging aspects of managing patients with breast cancer is determining the most appropriate therapeutic regimen for an individual patient, based on the tumor's biological features. Additionally, it is difficult to identify patients who are not responding to the selected therapy shortly after starting treatment, so that an alternative therapy can be initiated. The traditional criteria for assessing therapeutic response in breast cancer are based on changes in size of measurable disease or on decline of tumor markers. Unfortunately, these criteria are not particularly useful in distinguishing responders from nonresponders early after therapy is begun. Additionally, patients with predominantly or only osseous metastatic disease represent a particularly difficult problem for treating physicians, as their disease is not usually measurable or easily evaluable, and several months of

From: *Cancer Drug Discovery and Development
In Vivo Imaging of Cancer Therapy*
Edited by: A.F. Shields and P. Price © Humana Press Inc., Totowa, NJ

therapy are needed before radiographs or bone scintigraphy can be used to determine the effectiveness of therapy. The disease status of these patients can be monitored by changes in clinical symptoms, in particular pain, and in tumor markers. However, not all such patients are symptomatic nor do all have abnormal tumor marker levels to monitor. The major premise underlying the use of PET in assessment of therapeutic response is based on its ability to delineate alterations in cell biology associated with response. With appropriate radiolabeled molecular probes, PET can be used to interrogate a variety of targets, including a specific change in cellular physiology, tumor-specific antigen or receptor, or a specific gene. In patients with breast cancer, several factors, such as proliferative rate and receptor status, have been recognized to be predictive of response to therapy. In this review, we will discuss the importance of the estrogen receptor (ER) in breast cancer, as well as its relationship to selection of therapy, and in predicting and assessing response to hormonal therapy of this cancer.

2. TREATMENT OF BREAST CANCER

Breast cancer is the most common malignancy of women. It is estimated that in the year 2006 that there will be 214,640 new cases of breast cancer and 41,430 breast cancer-related deaths in the United States *(1)*. The selection of systemic treatment of breast cancer, whether neoadjuvant, adjuvant, or palliative, is guided by the tumor's ER and/or progesterone receptor (PRg) status. Thus, *in vitro* analysis of tumor tissue for ER and PRg is routinely performed and is considered standard of care. The majority of breast cancers are estrogen-receptor positive (ER^+) and/or progesterone-receptor positive (PRg^+). When compared with hormone-negative [estrogen-receptor-negative (ER^-) and/or progesterone-receptor-negative (PRg^-)] breast cancer, hormone-positive (ER^+ and/or PRg^+) breast cancers are more likely to have clinical response to hormonal manipulation *(2)* and are less aggressive *(3)*. In addition, the natural history of receptor-positive disease differs from that of receptor-negative disease in terms of time to recurrence, site of recurrence, and overall pace of the disease. Hormonal therapy, when effective, is associated with significant improvements in disease-free and overall survival; moreover, the morbidity of hormonal therapy is generally lower than that of chemotherapy. However, prediction of tumor response to hormonal therapy based on ER and PRg status assessed by *in vitro* assays is only moderately accurate. Only 55–60% of patients with hormone-positive tumors and about 10% of patients with hormone-negative tumors actually respond to hormonal therapy *(4, 5)*. This is likely due to the fact that *in vitro* assays, now most typically immunohistochemical methods, provide limited information about the functional status of the receptors *(6)*. In addition, *in vitro* assays are unable to address intrinsic heterogeneity of receptor expression within individual lesions or the concordance or discordance between the original primary tumor and metastatic or recurrent lesions, unless biopsies of all of lesions can be obtained.

Despite the advantages of hormonal therapy, many oncologists choose chemotherapy over hormonal therapy for several reasons including the uncertain response of receptor-positive tumors to hormonal therapy, the belief that response to hormonal therapy occurs more slowly than response to chemotherapy, and the limited ability of conventional methods (clinical and radiological) to predict response or to assess response early after institution of hormonal therapy. Thus, an improvement in the ability to predict the outcome to hormonal therapy would allow many patients to avoid unnecessary morbidity associated with chemotherapy. In addition, it could enhance the prognostic stratification of patients with receptor-positive disease.

In hormone-responsive ER^+ breast cancer, the ER is essential for tumor growth, although, it does not act alone to stimulate tumor growth. It serves as a transcription factor for estrogen-regulated genes as well as a coactivator for other nuclear transcription factors. It has been demonstrated that ER imposes its regulatory function through classical and nonclassical pathways *(7)*. In the classical pathway, ER functions as a major transcription factor; estrogen binds to ER and activates DNA binding to estrogen response elements in the promoter of target genes, which recruits coactivator proteins, which then activates signal transduction pathways that increase gene transcription important in controlling cell growth. In the nonclassical pathway, ER does not function as the major transcription factor; rather it acts as coactivator proteins by stabilizing the DNA binding of the transcription factor complex or by recruiting other coactivators to these complexes. This pathway is responsible for transcription of several genes important in growth factor signal transduction pathways of breast cancer *(7, 8)*. Therefore, the ER is targeted by various interventions for treatment of hormone-sensitive breast cancer, and hormonal therapy is designed to block ER function. At one time, therapy for breast cancer could include altering hormone production by techniques such as removal of the ovaries in premenopausal women and either adrenalectomy or high-dose estrogen therapy in postmenopausal women whose ovaries were nonfunctional. In premenopausal women with hormone-sensitive breast cancer, oophorectomy has been replaced by medical castration prior to antiestrogen therapy. Currently, as discussed below, various types of endocrine therapy are available for treatment of patients with hormone-sensitive breast cancer. For many years, tamoxifen has been the mainstay of hormonal therapy in patients with hormone-sensitive breast cancer. Tamoxifen exerts its therapeutic efficacy primarily from its antiproliferative action by binding competitively to the ERs, thereby blocking the mitogenic effect of biologically active estrogens *(9)*. However, tamoxifen can only partially block ER activity. Currently, a variety of hormonal agents are available for treatment of patients with hormone-sensitive breast cancer and these agents exert their antiestrogenic effects by several different mechanisms. These mechanisms include estrogen antagonism through enhancement of progesterone pathways (megesterol acetate), suppression of endogenous estrogen production (aromatase inhibitors, e.g., anastrazole, exemestane, and letrozole), and degradation of ERs (fulvestrant) *(10)*. In addition, ovarian ablation and luteinizing hormone-releasing hormone antagonists reduce circulating estrogen levels and thus inhibit ligand-induced activation of ER *(7)*.

3. ESTROGEN-RECEPTOR IMAGING

Because of the importance of ERs in breast cancer and the limitations of *in vitro* receptor assays, noninvasive assessment of ERs has been the subject of many investigations. The presence of ERs provides a mechanism for tumor imaging via selective uptake of radiolabeled hormones. Receptor-based imaging can provide information about the location of the tumor and assess the level and functional status of the receptor. Determination of the presence or absence of functional receptors can be important in directing therapy in breast cancer. Particularly in advanced disease, where within-site or site-to-site heterogeneity of receptor expression can occur, imaging methods to assess regional receptor expression can offer significant advantages over biopsy-based methods in directing therapy. Thus over the past several decades, there has been considerable effort to identify a radioligand with high affinity for the ER, high target-to-nontarget selectivity, high specific activity, appropriate *in vivo* metabolism and clearance, and physical properties suitable for imaging. Several radioligands for conventional single-photon gamma imaging and for imaging with PET have been developed *(11)*.

3.1 Estrogen-Receptor Imaging with Single-Photon Gamma Scintigraphy

The most promising single-photon gamma ER imaging agent is ^{123}I-labeled *cis*-11β-methoxy-17α-iodovinylestradiol (Z^{123}I-MIVE) *(11)*. This agent has been shown to have high sensitivity and specificity for the *in vivo* detection of ER$^+$ breast cancer. It has been shown to have high ER binding affinity in both rat and human mammary tumors *(12, 13)*.

3.2 Clinical Z^{123}I-MIVE Studies

In patients with primary and metastatic breast cancer, there is good agreement between Z^{123}I-MIVE uptake and *in vitro* immunohistochemical analysis of ER *(14)*. Rijks *et al.* have shown that the binding of Z^{123}I-MIVE to ER$^+$ breast cancer is a receptor-mediated process and there is a good correlation between of Z^{123}I-MIVE uptake and *in vitro* analysis of ER levels (agreement of 90% in primary and 82% in metastatic breast cancer). Bennink *et al.* studied 22 patients with palpable breast cancer and demonstrated that Z^{123}I-MIVE scintigraphy has a sensitivity of 100% with single-photon emission computed tomography (SPECT) and 94% with planar scintigraphy for determining tumor ER status *(15)*. In addition, there was a good correlation between immunohistological and planar scintigraphic scores of ER status ($r = 0.72$, $p < 0.01$). However in their series, there was an underestimation of ER positivity using planar scintigraphy. This could be related to the heterogeneous distribution of ER within the tumor as well as tissue attenuation of Z^{123}I-MIVE radioactivity, as attenuation correction was not applied. Although an uptake ratio of tumor-to-contralateral normal breast tissue was calculated on the planar images, the lack of correction for soft tissue attenuation limited the accuracy of these measurements. Since count density on SPECT images is subject to multiple factors, such as reconstruction filters and parameters, depth dependency, and nonuniform attenuation, SPECT uptake ratios were not calculated, although SPECT improved contrast and lesion detection.

Bennink *et al.* studied 23 patients who had metastatic breast cancer before and 4 weeks after treatment with tamoxifen with Z^{123}I-MIVE scintigraphy *(11)* in order to determine whether changes in tumor uptake of Z^{123}I-MIVE are predictive of subsequent response to tamoxifen therapy. After initiation of antiestrogen treatment, 17 of 21 patients with clear uptake on baseline scintigraphy showed complete blockade of ER activity on Z^{123}I-MIVE scintigraphy. The remaining four patients showed mixed or no ER blockade. All patients with faint baseline uptake or mixed or no ER blockade after tamoxifen showed progressive disease despite antiestrogen treatment. Patients with clear baseline uptake and complete ER blockade after tamoxifen had a significantly longer progression-free interval (mean ± SEM, 14.4 ± 1.6 versus 1.8 ± 0.8 months; $p < 0.01$).

3.3 Estrogen-Receptor Imaging with Positron Emission Tomography

The most promising and well-characterized radioligand for PET imaging is the estradiol analogue, 16α-[^{18}F]fluoro-17β-estradiol (FES), which also has been the most extensively studied ER-based radioligand in patients with breast cancer. It has been shown to have high specific activity, high selective ER binding *in vitro*, and high affinity for ER$^+$ target tissues in animal models *(16–18)*. Because of the favorable imaging characteristics of FES associated with the ^{18}F label, we and others have used this radioligand for *in vivo* detection and quantification of ER levels in patients with breast cancer.

3.4 Clinical 16α-[^{18}F]Fluoro-17β-estradiol-Positron Emission Tomography Studies

We and others have shown that tumor FES uptake reliably reflects the ER content of breast cancer; the FES uptake in the primary tumor, measured quantitatively on PET images, is significantly correlated with the ER concentration determined by quantitative ligand binding assays or immunohistochemical staining of tumor tissue obtained from women with untreated primary breast cancer ($r = 0.96$, $p < 0.001$) *(19, 20)*. In a subsequent study of women with ER$^+$ metastatic breast cancer, we demonstrated that FES PET has a sensitivity of 93% (53 of 57 lesions) for detecting hormone-sensitive metastatic foci *(21)*. In that study, we also demonstrated that tumor FES uptake decreased following institution of antiestrogen therapy, further supporting the hypothesis that tumor uptake of FES is a receptor-mediated process, and suggesting that FES PET could be used to evaluate the availability of functional ERs in breast cancer in order to predict the likelihood of response to antiestrogen therapy. Subsequently, in patients with untreated advanced (locally advanced, metastatic, and recurrent) breast cancer, we demonstrated an overall agreement rate of 88% between tumor uptake of FES and *in vitro* ER levels *(22)*. This level of agreement is similar to that observed with replicate *in vitro* assays, where disagreements have been explained by factors such as interlaboratory variability, interassay variability, and specimen integrity variability.

A number of parameters are known to affect ER expression and thus its bioavailability to interact with FES. Mankoff *et al.* demonstrated a significant association between FES uptake and menopausal status, serum estradiol level, serum sex steroid binding protein (SBP) level, and prior hormonal therapy in patients with primary and metastatic ER$^+$ breast cancer *(20)*. Higher average standardized uptake values (SUVs) for FES were noted in tumors of women who were postmenopausal, had lower serum estradiol and SBP levels, and had been previously treated with hormonal agents.

It is known that ER$^+$ tumors are generally less aggressive than ER$^-$ tumors. It also has been shown, in breast cancer and in several other tumors, that fluorodeoxyglucose (FDG) uptake is correlated with tumor aggressiveness of the tumor. Thus, it is possible that the ER status of breast cancer could be predicted by the FDG uptake as a surrogate measure of tumor aggressiveness. In a study of patients with untreated advanced breast cancer, we found no significant relationship between tumor FDG uptake and either tumor ER status or FES uptake, despite the expectation that ER$^+$ tumors should be less aggressive than ER$^-$ tumors, and thus should exhibit less FDG uptake *(22)*. The mean SUV for FDG in ER$^+$ tumors was 4.0 ± 2.1 and for ER$^-$ tumors was 4.5 ± 3.0 ($p < 0.65$). Also, we found no significant correlation between tumor FDG uptake and tumor FES uptake in 43 malignant lesions subjected to quantitative analysis ($r = 0.15$;

p = NS). Thus, FES PET provides unique information about the ER status of breast cancer that cannot be obtained indirectly with FDG PET. Survival of women with ER$^+$ disease is known to be better than that of women with ER$^-$ disease independent of the stage of disease. Similarly, Mortimer *et al.* found that the median survival of women with FES$^-$ disease was shorter than that of women with FES$^+$ breast cancer *(23)*.

In breast cancer, there is intrinsic heterogeneity of receptor expression within individual lesions, as well as discordance between the receptor status of the primary tumor and that of metastatic or recurrent lesions in 20–25% of patients *(24, 25)*. However, since it is generally not possible or practical to assess regional receptor expression using biopsy-based methods, treatment decisions are thus often based on an incomplete characterization of tumor biology. It has been shown that FES PET is a useful means for addressing this problem of heterogeneous receptor expression. In a group of patients with advanced ER$^+$ breast cancer, we used FES PET to study tumor heterogeneity and within-patient ER concordance between primary and metastatic foci *(23)*. Complete concordance among multiple lesions within a patient was observed in only 76% of patients. The level of concordance observed by FES PET is comparable to that found by *in vitro* ER assays when multiple sites have been biopsied. Mankoff *et al.* also showed that FES uptake within breast cancer is heterogeneous. In patients with multiple sites of disease, 10% had one or more sites with a complete absence of FES. The quantitative heterogeneity of FES uptake, measured by the coefficient of variation of SUV, was 30%. Moreover, the heterogeneity of FES uptake did not correlate with heterogeneity of FDG uptake within the same tumor *(20)*.

In addition, FES PET is associated with radiation risks that are within accepted limits. Based on the biodistribution of FES in patients with breast cancer, Mankoff *et al.* demonstrated that the organ and whole-body radiation doses associated with FES PET are comparable to those associated with other commonly used clinical nuclear medicine studies *(26)*. The effective dose equivalent is 0.022 mSv/MBq (80 mrem/mCi). The organ that receives the highest dose is the liver [0.13 mGy/MBq (470 mrad/mCi)], followed by the gallbladder [0.10 mGy/MBq (380 mrad/mCi)] and the urinary bladder [(0.05 mGy/MBq (190 mrad/mCi)]. The radiation dose with FES is well below the maximum individual study and annual total-body doses of 30 and 50 mGy, respectively, permitted for investigational radiopharmaceuticals by the FDA regulations at 21 CFR 361.1 *(26)*.

Thus, FES PET provides a reliable *in vivo* imaging technique that can provide information about the location of the tumor and assess the level and functional status of ER. Determination of the presence and the functional status of receptors in tumors is important in directing therapy, particularly in advanced disease, where within-site or site-to-site heterogeneity of receptor expression can occur. Imaging methods to assess regional receptor expression can offer significant advantages over biopsy-based methods in directing therapy.

4. PREDICTING RESPONSE OF BREAST CANCER TO HORMONAL THERAPY

Hormonal therapy of advanced breast cancer offers several advantages compared to chemotherapy, including lower morbidity, lower cost, and improved survival in patients with hormonally responsive tumors. Current clinical predictors of response to hormonal agents include a long disease-free interval, nonvisceral metastases, high tumor ER levels, the presence of PRgs, and the development of a clinical flare reaction. The so-called "clinical flare reaction" occurs in 5–20% of women with breast cancer who receive hormonal therapy. This phenomenon has been reported to occur after treatment with a variety of different hormonal agents, but most commonly after institution of tamoxifen. Within 7–10 day after starting tamoxifen, patients who have a flare reaction have subjective and objective findings suggesting disease progression. Soft tissue lesions may increase in size, pain from osseous metastases may become more severe, and hypercalcemia may develop (27, 28). It is postulated that this transient "progression" of disease is due to the initial agonist effects of the drug, which immediately precede the down-regulation of the hormone receptor and subsequent tumor regression (28, 29). Thus, the flare reaction is an indicator of functioning ERs and a predictor of therapeutic responsiveness; 80% of patients who have a flare reaction will exhibit disease response with continuation of the hormonal agent (28). However, clinically, it is often impossible to distinguish a flare reaction from disease progression and this, as well as the low frequency of clinical flare, makes it unreliable as a predictive index.

Since the clinical flare reaction is a good, albeit infrequent, predictor of response to tamoxifen, it is possible that a larger fraction of patients who ultimately respond to hormone treatment would experience a subclinical "metabolic flare" characterized by an increase in FDG uptake early during a course of tamoxifen treatment. An early estrogen-agonist effect of tamoxifen has been documented in studies of immature female rats (30). Similar to estrogen, tamoxifen causes prompt increases in FDG accumulation in the uteri of immature female rats; the increase with estrogen is approximately twice that observed with tamoxifen administration (30, 31). Presumably, both estrogen and tamoxifen initially stimulate cell proliferation and glucose metabolism and, thus, cause increased FDG uptake. These observations in animal studies suggested that augmentation of tumor FDG uptake ("metabolic flare") early during a course of tamoxifen treatment would be indicative of an agonist effect of the drug on *functional* ERs and, thus, predictive of a good response to therapy. In addition, functional ERs should be characterized by high tumor FES uptake before therapy. In a clinical study of patients with advanced ER$^+$ breast cancer, we have shown that the pattern of functional ERs identified by PET (high tumor uptake of FES prior to therapy and an increase in tumor uptake of FDG 7–10 days after initiation of tamoxifen therapy) was predictive of response (32, 33). We found that the positive- and negative-predictive values for response with an increase from baseline in tumor FDG uptake (measured by SUV) of ≥ 10% (which was arbitrarily selected as the cutoff criterion for defining metabolic flare) were 91% and 94%, respectively. The baseline FES was superior to ER and PR status determined *in vitro* in predicting response to hormonal therapy. The positive- and negative-predictive values for a baseline SUV for FES uptake >2.0 (which was arbitrarily selected as the cutoff SUV for defining functional ERs) were 79% and 88%, respectively (33) (Figs. 1 and 2).

Similarly in a recent study, Linden *et al.* also demonstrated that FES PET was superior to *in vitro* ER in predicting response to hormonal therapy (34). The investigators have studied 47 patients with ER$^+$ primary or recurrent breast cancer with FES PET before hormonal therapy. All patients received hormonal therapy for at least 6 months unless there was evidence of tumor progression. Eleven of the 47 patients (23%)

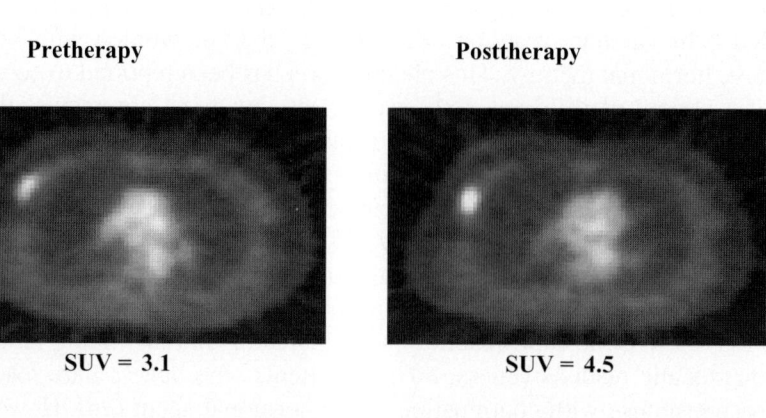

Fig. 1. Positron emission tomography assessment of ER function: responder. Selected transaxial FDG PET (upper row) and FES PET (lower row) images before (left) and after (right) tamoxifen therapy in a patient with locally advanced ER$^+$ breast cancer. On the pretreatment images, there is intense FDG and FES uptake in a primary right breast cancer. One week after therapy, there is an increase in tumor FDG uptake (reflected by an increase in the maximum SUV of the tumor) and a concomitant decrease in FES uptake.

had an objective response. Quantitative FES uptake and response were significantly associated; none of the 15 patients with an initial FES SUV < 1.5 responded to hormonal therapy while 11 of the 32 patients (34%) with SUV > 1.5 responded to therapy ($p <$ 0.01). While none of the patients with absent FES uptake responded to hormone therapy, the association between qualitative FES PET results and response was not significant ($p = 0.14$). In addition, these investigators demonstrated that in the subset of patients whose tumors did not overexpress HER2neu, 11 of 24 (46%) patients with SUV > 1.5 responded. Thus while FES uptake was highly predictive of response to hormonal therapy in patients without HER2 overexpression, it was considerably less predictive in patients whose tumors overexpressed HER2. It thus appears that overexpression of HER2 in breast cancer defines a subset of more aggressive tumors that are less sensitive to endocrine treatment (35).

Recently, several new hormonal therapeutic agents have been approved for treatment of hormone-sensitive breast cancer that unlike tamoxifen lack estrogenic effect. Based on the hormonal challenge test, an old concept in the management of breast cancer (36), we hypothesized that development of a "metabolic flare" in response to a challenge pulse of estradiol will be predictive of response to any type of therapy that either targets or is mediated via functional estrogen receptors. We are currently investigating whether the "metabolic flare" in response to a challenge pulse of estradiol can predict the likelihood of response to new hormonal agents such as aromatase inhibitors and fulvestrant, since these drugs are now more widely used than tamoxifen for treating advanced breast cancer *(37, 38)*.

In summary, ER is an important prognostic factor that also has a significant role in the growth of ER$^+$ breast cancer. Hormonal therapy is the most effective treatment for ER$^+$ breast cancer and is designed to block ER function. Assessment of response to hormonal therapy is difficult early after institution of therapy, because several months of therapy are needed before response can be assessed. The ER status of the tumor determined by *in vitro* assays is predictive of response in slightly more than half of the patients with ER$^+$ tumors. Thus, a more effective method is needed to predict response to hormonal therapy. We and others have shown that PET with FES predicts therapeutic response with moderate reliability. We also have shown that a metabolic flare resulting from interaction between functional ER and the initial estrogenic effect of tamoxifen can be detected by FDG. This appears to be an even more reliable method to identify which patients with hormone-sensitive breast cancer will respond to tamoxifen early during therapy. As noted, a similar approach involving FDG PET before and after a

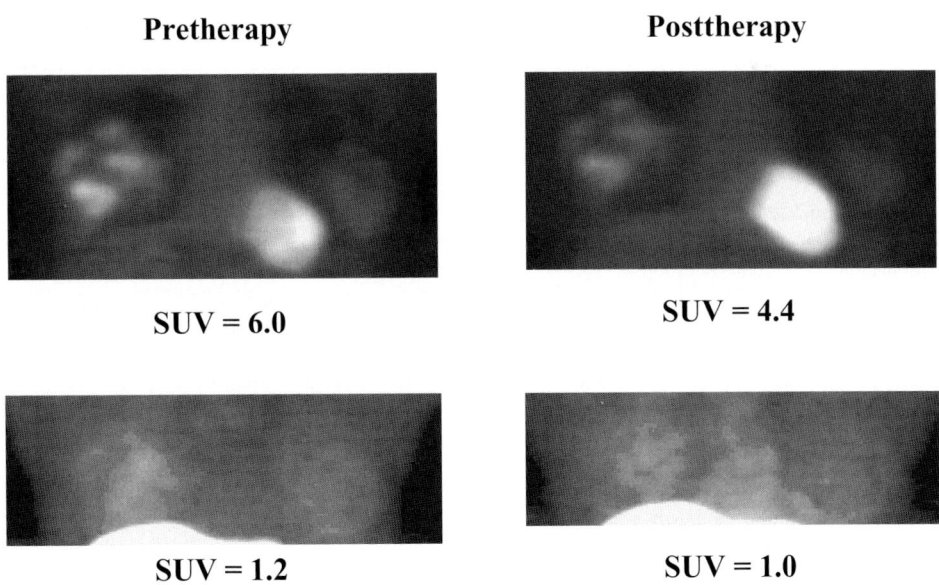

Fig. 2. Positron emission tomography assessment of ER function: nonresponder. Anterior maximum intensity reprojection FDG PET (upper row) and FES PET (lower row) images before (left) and after (right) tamoxifen therapy in a patient with locally advanced, multifocal ER$^+$ breast cancer. On the pretreatment images, there is intense FDG uptake and very low FES uptake in the primary tumors in the right breast. One week after beginning therapy, there is no evidence of metabolic flare on FDG PET images and no significant change in the low FES uptake within the right breast.

challenge pulse of estradiol may be able to predict the likelihood of response to newer types of hormonal therapy before therapy is initiated. We expect that the information provided by PET will allow tailoring of systemic therapy, thereby providing an improved therapeutic index in patients with advanced breast cancer.

REFERENCES

1. Jemal A, Siegel R, Ward E, Murray T, et al. Cancer Statistics, 2006. *CA Cancer J Clin* 2006; 56:106–130.
2. Early Breast Cancer Trialists' Collaborative Group. Tamoxifen for early breast cancer: An overview of the randomized trials. *Lancet* 1998;351:1451–1467.
3. Henderson IC, Patek AJ. The relationship between prognostic and predictive factors in the management of breast cancer. *Breast Cancer Res Treat* 1998;52:261–288.
4. Hellman S, Harris JR. Natural history of breast cancer. In: Harris JR, Lippman ME, Marrow M, Osborne CK, eds. Diseases of the Breast, 2nd ed. Philadelphia, PA: Lippincott Williams & Wilkins, 2000:471–488.
5. Osborne CK. Steroid hormone receptors in breast cancer management. *Breast Cancer Res Treat* 1998;51:227–238.
6. Sledge GL, McGuire W. Steroid hormone receptors in human breast cancer. *Adv Cancer Res* 1983; 38:61–75.
7. Osborne CK, Schiff R. Estrogen-receptor biology: Continuing progress and therapeutic implications. *J Clin Oncol* 2005;23:1616–1622.
8. Segars JH, Driggers PH. Estrogen action and cytoplasmic signaling cascades. Part I: Membrane-associated signaling complexes. *Trends Endocrinol Metab* 2002;13:349–354.
9. Jordan VC. A current view of tamoxifen for the treatment and prevention of breast cancer. *Br J Pharmacol* 1993;110:507–517.
10. Robertson JF. Selective oestrogen receptor modulators/new antioestrogens: A clinical perspective. *Cancer Treat Rev* 2004;30:695–706.
11. Bennink RJ, van Tienhoven G, Rijks LJ, et al. In vivo prediction of response to antiestrogen treatment in estrogen receptor-positive breast cancer. *J Nucl Med* 2004;45:1–7.
12. Rijks LJ, Boer GJ, Endert E, et al. The stereoisomers of 17α-[^{123}I]iodovinyloestradiol and its 11β-methoxy derivative evaluated for their oestrogen receptor binding in human MCF-7 cells and rat uterus, and their distribution in immature rats. *Eur J Nucl Med* 1996;23:295–307.
13. Rijks LJ, Boer GJ, Endert E, de Bruin K, Janssen AG, van Royen EA. The Z-isomer of 11β-methoxy-17α-[^{123}I]iodovinylestradiol is a promising radioligand for estrogen receptor imaging in human breast cancer. *Nucl Med Biol* 1997;24:65–75.
14. Rijks LJ, Bakker PJ, van Tienhoven G, et al. Imaging of estrogen receptors in primary and metastatic breast cancer patients with iodine-123-labeled Z-MIVE. *J Clin Oncol* 1997;15:2536–2545.
15. Bennink RJ, Rijks LJ, van Tienhoven G, Noorduyn LA, Janssen AG, Sloof GW. Estrogen receptor status in primary breast cancer: Iodine 123-labeled cis-11β-methoxy-17α-iodovinyl estradiol scintigraphy. *Radiology* 2001;220:774–779.
16. Katzenellenbogen JA. Designing steroid receptor-based radiotracers to image breast and prostate tumors. *J Nucl Med* (Suppl) 1995;36:8–13.
17. Kiesewetter DO, Kilbourn MR, Landvatter SW, Heiman DF, Katzenellenbogen JA, Welch MJ. Radiochemistry and radiopharmaceuticals. *J Nucl Med* 1984;25:1212–1221.
18. Mathias CJ, Welch MJ, Katzenellenbogen JA, et al. Characterization of the uptake of 16α-[^{18}F]fluoro-17β-estradiol in DMBA-induced mammary tumors. *Int J Rad Appl Instrum [B]* 1987;14:15–25.
19. Mintun MA, Welch MJ, Siegel BA, et al. Breast cancer. PET imaging of estrogen receptors. *Radiology* 1988;169:45–48.
20. Mankoff DA, Peterson, LM, Petra PH, et al. Factors affecting the level and heterogeneity of uptake of [^{18}F]fluoroestradiol (FES) in patients with estrogen-receptor (ER+) breast cancer. *J Nucl Med* 2002;43:286.
21. McGuire AH, Dehdashti F, Siegel BA, et al. Positron tomographic assessment of 16α-[^{18}F]fluoro-17β-estradiol uptake in metastatic breast carcinoma. *J Nucl Med* 1991;32:1526–1531.

22. Dehdashti F, Mortimer JE, Siegel BA, et al. Positron tomographic assessment of estrogen receptors in breast cancer. Comparison with FDG-PET and in vitro receptor assays. *J Nucl Med* 1995; 36:1766–1774.
23. Mortimer JE, Dehdashti F, Siegel BA, Katzenellenbogen JA, Fracasso P, Welch MJ. Positron emission tomography with 2-[^{18}F]fluoro-2-deoxy-D-glucose and 16α-[^{18}F]fluoro-17β-estradiol in breast cancer: Correlation with estrogen receptor status and response to systemic therapy. *Clin Cancer Res* 1996; 2:933–939.
24. Campbell FC, Blamey RW, Elston CW, et al. Quantitative oestradiol receptor values in primary breast cancer and response of metastases to endocrine therapy. *Lancet* 1981;2:1317–1319.
25. Butler JA, Trezona T, Vargas H, State D. Value of measuring hormone receptor levels of regional metastatic carcinoma of the breast. *Arch Surg* 1989;124:1131–1136.
26. Mankoff DA, Peterson LM, Tewson TJ, et al. [^{18}F]Fluoroestradiol radiation dosimetry in human PET studies. *J Nucl Med* 2001;42:679–684.
27. Plotkin D, Lechner J, Jung W, Rosen PJ. Tamoxifen flare in advanced breast cancer. *JAMA* 1978; 240:2644–2646.
28. Vogel CL, Schoenfelder J, Shemano I, Hayes DF, Gams RA. Worsening bone scan in the evaluation of antitumor response during hormonal therapy of breast cancer. *J Clin Oncol* 1995;13:1123–1128.
29. Legha SS. Tamoxifen in the treatment of breast cancer. *Ann Intern Med* 1988;109:219–228.
30. Welch MJ, Bonasera TA, Sherman EIC, Katzenellenbogen JA, Dehdashti F, Siegel BA. [F-18]Fluorodeoxyglucose (FDG) and 16α[F-18]fluoroestradiol-17β (FES) uptake in estrogen-receptor (ER)-rich tissues following tamoxifen treatment: A preclinical study. *J Nucl Med* 1995;36:39P.
31. Wahl RL, Cody R, Fisher S. FDG uptake before and after estrogen receptor stimulation: Feasibility studies for functional receptor imaging. *J Nucl Med* 1991;32:1011.
32. Dehdashti F, Flanagan FL, Mortimer JE, Katzenellenbogen JA, Welch MJ, Siegel BA. PET assessment of "metabolic flare" to predict response of metastatic breast cancer to antiestrogen therapy. *Eur J Nucl Med* 1999;26:51–56.
33. Mortimer JE, Dehdashti F, Siegel BA, Trinkaus K, Katzenellenbogen JA, Welch MJ. Metabolic flare: An indicator of hormone responsiveness in advanced breast cancer. *J Clin Oncol* 2001;19: 2797–2803.
34. Linden HM, Stekhova S, Link JM, et al. Quantitative fluoroestradiol (FES) PET imaging predicts response to endocrine treatment. *J Clin Oncol* 2006;24:566.
35. Ellis MJ, Coop A, Singh B, et al. Letrozole is more effective neoadjuvant endocrine therapy than tamoxifen for ErbB-1- and/or ErbB-2-positive, estrogen receptor-positive primary breast cancer: Evidence from a phase III randomized trial. *J Clin Oncol* 2001;19:3808–3816.
36. Nathanson IT, Kelley RM. Hormonal treatment of cancer. *N Engl J Med* 1952;246:135–145.
37. Bonneterre J, Thurlimann B, Robertson JFR, et al. Anastrozole versus tamoxifen as first-line therapy for advanced breast cancer in 668 postmenopausal women: Results of the Tamoxifen or Arimidex Randomized Group Efficacy and Tolerability study. *J Clin Oncol* 2000;18:3748–3757.
38. Nabholtz JM, Buzdar A, Pollak M, et al. Anastrozole is superior to tamoxifen as first-line therapy for advanced breast cancer in postmenopausal women: Results of a North American multicenter randomized trial. *J Clin Oncol* 2000;18:3758–3767.

10 Quantitative Approaches to Positron Emission Tomography

Adriaan A. Lammertsma, PhD

Contents

    Introduction
    Scope for Quantification
    2-[^{18}F]Fluoro-2-deoxy-d-glucose
    Analytical Methods
    T/N Ratio
    Standardized Uptake Value
    Nonlinear Regression
    Graphic (Patlak) Analysis
    Simplified Kinetic Method
    Quantification for Response Monitoring
    Standardization
    Future Directions
    Conclusions

1. INTRODUCTION

Over the past decade positron emission tomography (PET) has become the fastest growing medical imaging technology. This is primarily based on its performance as a diagnostic tool in oncology. In particular, its sensitivity for detecting metastases using whole body scans and 2-[^{18}F]fluoro-2-deoxy-D-glucose ([^{18}F]FDG) as a tracer is unrivaled, resulting in reimbursement for a steadily increasing number of indications. The development of PET/computed tomography (CT) scanners has further stimulated the use of PET, as investment in such a scanner is now also feasible for smaller hospitals.

It should be noted, however, that originally PET was developed as a technique for the noninvasive *in vivo* quantification of functional processes and molecular interactions *(1)*. In fact, many different physiological, biochemical, and pharmacokinetic parameters can be measured with high selectivity and sensitivity in the picomolar to nanomolar range *(2)*. Apart from glucose metabolism, processes that can be measured include blood flow, blood volume, oxygen utilization, presynaptic and postsynaptic

From: *Cancer Drug Discovery and Development
In Vivo Imaging of Cancer Therapy*
Edited by: A.F. Shields and P. Price © Humana Press Inc., Totowa, NJ

receptor density and affinity, neurotransmitter release, enzyme activity, drug delivery and uptake, and gene expression.

2. SCOPE FOR QUANTIFICATION

The detection of distant metastases using whole body [^{18}F]FDG PET does not rely on quantification. Due to the high glycolytic rate of most tumors *(3)* and the kinetic properties of [^{18}F]FDG, uptake of [^{18}F]FDG in malignant tissues is increased and, consequently, detection of positive lymph nodes and/or metastases involves identification of areas with increased uptake (i.e., hot spots) within a background (normal tissue) of lower uptake. Clearly, for this purpose, visual assessment of the whole body images will suffice.

Qualitative FDG images can even be useful for assessing response to chemotherapy. It is particularly useful if in repeat whole body scans new sites with increased uptake are detected, indicating progressive disease. In addition, if uptake in a tumor disappears during treatment, there is good reason to believe that the treatment is effective. On the other hand, if there is no change in uptake it can be assumed that there is no response. The difficulty arises in (the majority of) intermediate cases, where some reduction in uptake might be seen. Clearly, a quantitative method would potentially allow for the definition of objective cut-off values for response or, more likely, the definition of response probabilities associated with a certain reduction in [^{18}F]FDG uptake.

In essence, PET is a technique that allows for quantification of functional processes and molecular interactions. This makes it ideally suited as a tool for the objective assessment of therapeutic efficacy, both with respect to monitoring response to an existing treatment in an individual patient and to assessing the efficacy of new drugs *(4)*.

It should be noted that although presently most oncological studies are based on [^{18}F]FDG, PET is not restricted to [^{18}F]FDG. It is likely that in the future, response will be measured using more tumor-specific markers than [^{18}F]FDG. Also in those cases, quantification of the most appropriate tracer parameters will remain important, if response is to be measured objectively.

3. 2-[^{18}F]FLUORO-2-DEOXY-D-GLUCOSE

As mentioned above, most PET studies on cancer therapy are based on [^{18}F]FDG, an analogue of glucose, that is transported into the cell by the glucose transporter. There it is phosphorylated to [^{18}F]FDG-6-PO$_4$ by hexokinase. In contrast to phosphorylated natural glucose, [^{18}F]FDG-6-PO$_4$ is not a substrate for further metabolism. In addition, in most tissues including tumors, the rate of dephosphorylation is negligible. Due to this lack of tissue clearance, [^{18}F]FDG accumulates in proportion to glucose metabolism *(5, 6)*. Together with the long half-life of ^{18}F (~2 h) relative to study duration (1 h), this guarantees a high signal-to-noise ratio, which is ideal for quantitative studies. The main disadvantage of [^{18}F]FDG for monitoring response to therapy is the fact that it is an analogue of glucose with different affinities for the glucose transporter and hexokinase *(5)*. Therefore, irrespective of the method of analysis being used (i.e., even in case of visual inspection), it has to be assumed that the relative affinities of [^{18}F]FDG and glucose for glucose transporter and hexokinase do not change as a result of therapy, i.e., that the so-called lumped constant remains indeed constant.

4. ANALYTICAL METHODS

As a result of its widespread availability, a variety of methods for the analysis of [^{18}F]FDG data have been developed. These range from qualitative (visual) through semiquantitative (e.g., standardized uptake value) to fully quantitative (glucose metabolism) approaches. The main limitation of a qualitative method (i.e., visual inspection) has already been mentioned. In the next sections advantages and shortcomings of the semiquantitative and quantitative methods will be summarized. More detailed descriptions can be found elsewhere *(7)*.

5. T/N RATIO

A very simple method of "quantifying" [^{18}F]FDG uptake in a tumor (T) is by normalizing it to uptake in normal tissue (N), the T/N ratio. This semiquantitative method (Table 1) requires only a static emission scan and no (arterial) input function. As normal tissue serves as an internal standard, it is not even necessary to (cross)-calibrate the scanner against a well counter or dose calibrator. However, as unidirectional uptake of [^{18}F]FDG increases over time (with different rates in tumor and normal tissue!), the T/N ratio will be a (complex) function of time. Therefore, the emission scan should always be acquired at the same time after injection.

The major drawback of this method is that a representative region of normal tissue needs to be defined, which could be difficult for some tumor locations. In addition, in many cases, it is not easy to define exactly the same (normal) tissue in repeat scans. Moreover, during the course of systemic and toxic chemotherapy, this normal tissue will also have been exposed, yet it has to be assumed that it is not affected. Furthermore, as uptake in normal tissue is low in (fasting) cancer patients, the T/N ratio will be sensitive to noise, especially if there is nonhomogeneous uptake in the normal tissue.

6. STANDARDIZED UPTAKE VALUE

The most popular method is also a simple semiquantitative method, the so-called standardized uptake value (SUV). In older literature this has also been named differential uptake ratio (DUR) or differential absorption ratio (DAR). In contrast to T/N, in SUV calculations (Table 2), tumor uptake is not normalized to that in normal tissue, but to injected dose and a factor that takes into account the total distribution space of injected [^{18}F]FDG. Originally, this factor was body weight *(8)*, but based on the altered uptake in fatty tissues, both body surface area *(9)* and lean body mass *(10)* have been proposed as potentially more accurate factors. To account for possible changes in plasma glucose levels *(11)* during therapy, a correction for plasma glucose has also

Table 1
Properties of T/N Ratio

Single image–static scan
No arterial input function required
No (cross)-calibration required
Time dependent
Normal tissue is available
Normal tissue is "normal"

Table 2
Properties of Standardized Uptake Values

Single image–static scan
No arterial input function required
Plasma clearance is assumed to be "normal"
Time dependent
Correction for plasma glucose optional
Correction for either
  Body weight
  Body surface area
  Lean body mass

been proposed. Note that a combination of all these correction factors results in a total of six different SUV definitions, making it difficult to compare results from different institutes, even for SUV alone.

The main advantage over the T/N ratio method is that no normal tissue (with all its inherent limitations) needs to be defined. Otherwise the same advantages (single scan, no blood sampling) and disadvantages (time dependency) apply. A further disadvantage is that injected dose needs to be measured accurately and that PET scanner and dose calibrator are cross-calibrated. In addition, if therapy affects plasma clearance of [^{18}F]FDG (i.e., by changing uptake in other parts of the body), the relationship between uptake at a certain time and injected dose will be different for the posttherapy scan as compared with the pretherapy scan. In Fig. 1 an example (hypothetical) is shown to

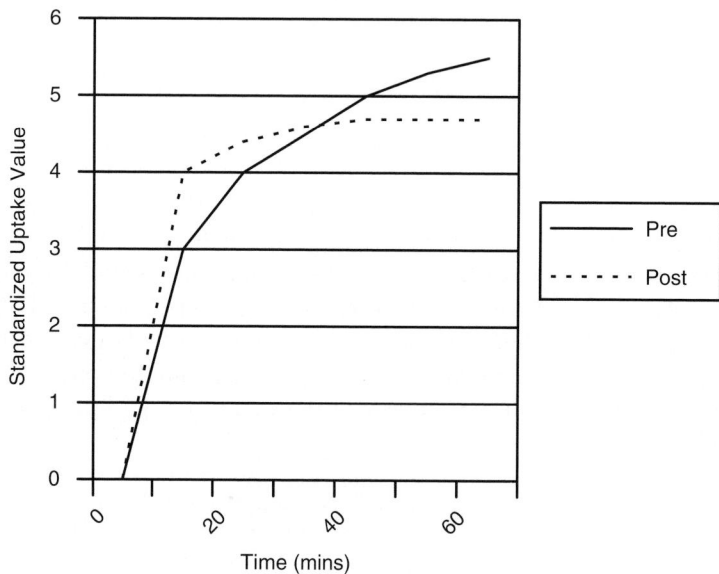

Fig. 1. The time dependency of SUV calculations. In this hypothetical case SUV values will be the same for only one specific time after injection. Earlier times will give an increase in posttherapy SUV, while later times will give a decrease. In practice, the exact curves are not known from a single scan, indicating that the relationship between SUV and glucose metabolism is assumed to be constant. This might not be the case if the body distribution of [^{18}F]FDG changes under the influence of therapy.

illustrate the danger of using a single scan (snapshot) to characterize a dynamic physiological process. As can be seen, interpretation of results (increase or decrease in uptake following therapy) could differ for different scanning times. Note that in this case it will not help to scan at a fixed time point as the kinetics for a certain patient are not known a priori.

7. NONLINEAR REGRESSION

The time dependency of SUV stems from the fact that tissue uptake is a continuing process that depends on a number of physiological entities. As uptake is irreversible, no equilibrium is reached and a single image represents only a snapshot in time. To describe the behavior of [^{18}F]FDG uptake over time, use has to be made of a kinetic model. The familiar compartmental model *(6)* for [^{18}F]FDG is shown in Fig. 2. The corresponding model equations are

$$dC_f(t)/dt = K_1 C_p(t) - (k_2 + k_3)C_f(t) + k_4 C_m(t) \tag{1}$$

$$dC_m(t)/dt = k_3 C_f(t) - k_4 C_m(t) \tag{2}$$

$$C_{tis}(t) = C_f(t) + C_m(t) \tag{3}$$

where C denotes concentration as a function of time t, the subscripts $p, f, m,$ and *tis* stand for [^{18}F]FDG in arterial plasma, free [^{18}F]FDG in tissue, phosphorylated (metabolized) [^{18}F]FDG in tissue, and total tissue, respectively, and the rate constants k express the rate of exchange between the various compartments.

It should be noted that it is not possible to measure the brain concentration C_{tis} *in vivo* as it is not possible to separate tissue from blood. Therefore, an intravascular component should be taken into account. The final operational equation is therefore

$$C_{PET}(t) = (1 - V_b)C_{tis}(t) + V_b C_{wb}(t) \tag{4}$$

where V_b represents the fractional blood volume in tissue and C_{wb} the concentration in whole blood (not plasma).

From this set of equations, it can be seen that tissue uptake depends on (the history of) the plasma concentration and on the four rate constants describing the rate of

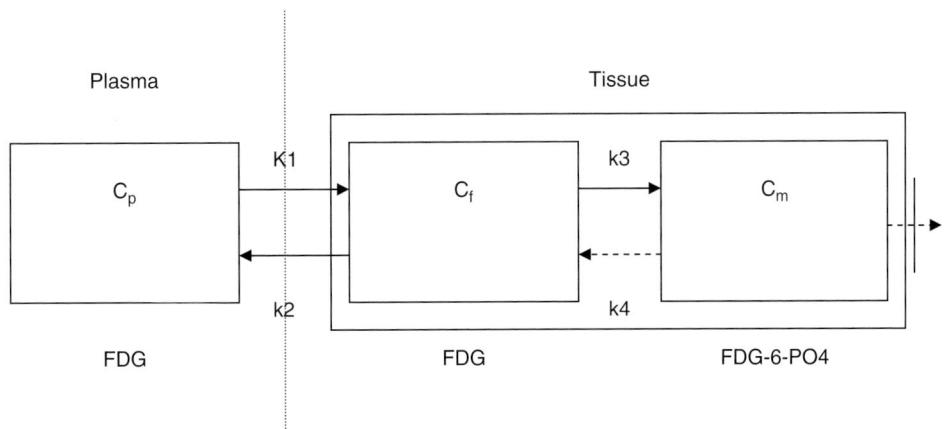

Fig. 2. Standard compartment model for describing [^{18}F]FDG uptake in tissue. The left side illustrates the plasma concentration. The right side shows the various compartments as seen by PET. This actually includes an intravascular component (not shown in the figure).

exchange between different compartments (plasma versus free [^{18}F]FDG in tissue: K_1 and k_2; free versus phophorylated [^{18}F]FDG in tissue: k_3 and k_4). In physiological terms, K_1 represents flow multiplied by extraction, thereby indicating its relationship with the expression of GLUT (glucose transporter). The rate of phosphorylation (i.e., hexokinase activity) is represented by k_3 and the rate of dephosphorylation by k_4. As the rate of dephosphorylation is negligible in most tissues, including tumors, k_4 can be set to zero in most applications, thereby simplifying the equations.

Even if $k_4 = 0$, the above equations contain a number of parameters that need to be estimated and it is clear that this cannot be achieved using a single scan. Instead, following injection, [^{18}F]FDG kinetics are measured using dynamic scanning. In addition, fast (preferably on-line) arterial blood sampling is required to measure the plasma input function. The various parameters (rate constants and vascular fraction) can then be estimated using standard nonlinear regression techniques and, from these parameters, glucose consumption can be calculated using

$$MR_{glu} = (C_{glu}/LC)(K_1 k_3)/(k_2 + k_3) \qquad (5)$$

where C_{glu} is the plasma concentration of (stable) glucose and LC is the so-called lumped constant relating [^{18}F]FDG kinetics to that of glucose *(5, 6)*.

A major advantage of nonlinear regression (Table 3) is that glucose metabolism is obtained, independent of time. The main assumption is that the lumped constant, describing differences in kinetics between [^{18}F]FDG and glucose, is known and constant between repeat scans. Note that although this is never mentioned, this assumption applies to all methods, even visual inspection, as it is a direct consequence of using [^{18}F]FDG rather than native glucose. Further advantages of nonlinear regression over all other methods are that changes in GLUT (K_1) and hexokinase (k_3) activity can be addressed separately, that possible dephosphorylation (k_4) can be taken into account, and that results are independent of the fate of glucose in the rest of the body [i.e., the method is independent of changes in plasma clearance; $C_p(t)$ is measured].

Apart from the complex scanning protocol, including arterial blood sampling, the major limitation of nonlinear regression is its sensitivity to noise, limiting the precision of derived parameters for smaller regions. This, for example, precludes its use for pixel-by-pixel calculations. Although the relatively complex calculation method (nonlinear regression) is often listed as a limitation, this is nonsense. Reconstructions are more complex calculations and these are never listed as a problem. Once implemented, calculations can be performed in an automatic manner and this also applies to nonlinear regression [provided regions of interest (ROI) has been defined]. The disadvantage of

Table 3
Properties of Nonlinear Regression

Provides glucose metabolism
Provides hexokinase activity
Provides GLUT activity
Accounts for dephosphorylation
Arterial input function required
Fast dynamic scanning required
Sensitive to noise

arterial sampling does not apply to studies of tumors in the thorax, where the input function can be derived from the vascular structures within the field of view *(12)*, particularly the ascending aorta (image-derived input function). A few venous samples at late times are recommended, however, for quality control of this image-derived input function *(13)*.

8. GRAPHIC (PATLAK) ANALYSIS

As mentioned above, the main limitation of nonlinear regression is its sensitivity to noise. Linear regression does not suffer from this shortcoming. Therefore, an interesting alternative to the nonlinear regression method is the so-called Patlak or Patlak/Gjedde analysis *(14)*, which is a linearization of the compartmental equation for irreversible tracers (i.e., $k_4 = 0$). It can be shown that plotting C_t/C_p against $\int C_p/C_p$ for $k_4 = 0$ will result in a straight line after an initial equilibration period (for [^{18}F]FDG typically some 10 min). Moreover, the slope of this straight line will be equal to the net rate of influx K_i, which corresponds to

$$K_i = K_1 k_3/(k_2 + k_3) \tag{6}$$

and glucose metabolism can be calculated using this slope according to

$$MR_{glu} = (C_{glu}/LC) \, K_i \tag{7}$$

where K_i is typically obtained over an interval of 10–60 min after injection.

Although dynamic scanning is still required (Table 4), fast frames over the initial phase are not required. Scanning can be started some 10 min after injection and only a few frames are required. In addition, fast arterial sampling during the first 10 min is not required as only the integral of the arterial input curve over that interval is needed. Arterial samples, however, are still required at later times, although arterialized venous or even venous samples might be a viable alternative at later times (due to the much smaller arteriovenous differences at later times after injection).

Disadvantages compared with nonlinear regression analysis are that separate assessment of GLUT and hexokinase activity is not possible and it is assumed that dephosphorylation is negligible. This latter assumption is valid for most tumors, but should be investigated before a Patlak analysis can be performed. A significant advantage, however, is the possibility of performing calculations at the pixel level, thereby generating functional images of glucose metabolism *(15)*. This can be a major advantage for tumors located close to vascular structures as the contrast between tumor and blood will be much higher for MR_{glu} than for "raw" [^{18}F]FDG images.

Table 4
Properties of Patlak

Provides glucose metabolism
"Slow" dynamic scanning required
Arterial input function required
    Possibly venous or arterialized venous blood sufficient
Insensitive to noise
Pixel by pixel calculations possible–functional glucose
    metabolism maps
Requires dephosphorylation to be negligible

9. SIMPLIFIED KINETIC METHOD

Patlak analysis still requires dynamic scanning and therefore it does not allow a survey of MR_{glu} over the entire body, i.e., it cannot be combined with a whole body scan. One possibility to combine accurate quantification with an overview of the body is to perform a dynamic scan over the primary tumor, followed by a whole body scan to identify and evaluate metastases. An alternative could be the simplified kinetic method (SKM) that combines a static scan with the calculation of MR_{glu} *(16)*. It does require at least one and preferably a few samples during the scan. These samples are used to scale a population-derived average plasma curve.

The key feature of SKM (Table 5) is that it does estimate MR_{glu} without the need for a dynamic scan and with a very reduced sampling protocol. The advantage over SUV is that it does, at least to some extent, take into account changes in plasma clearance. Therefore, it will be less sensitive than SUV to changes in plasma kinetics and possibly also to deviations in scanning start time (e.g., patient related delay). Disadvantages of SKM are that the correction for changes in plasma kinetics is only a first-order correction and that the method has not been used extensively, i.e., it has not been validated in a large patient population.

10. QUANTIFICATION FOR RESPONSE MONITORING

As mentioned previously, the level of quantification required for a study depends on the question being asked. If an [^{18}F]FDG PET study is performed for staging purposes, a qualitative whole body scan may suffice. If, however, the purpose of the study is to understand aspects of tumor physiology, the answer becomes less straightforward. Although, in theory, full kinetic analysis using nonlinear regression is the method of choice, and this is indeed the case if information is required about GLUT and hexokinase activity or if there is reason to believe that dephosphorylation is not negligible. On the other hand, if only glucose metabolism is required and it is known from previous studies that dephosphorylation is indeed negligible, Patlak analysis would be a better choice, not only because it is less sensitive to noise, but because it allows for the generation of functional images of glucose metabolism. These images would be extremely useful in assessing tumor heterogeneity.

For response monitoring purposes, the situation is even more complicated. Evidence is emerging that suggests that [^{18}F]FDG PET is a sensitive technique for predicting tumor response early during the course of therapy. It already starts to play an important role in drug development and eventually it is likely to enter routine clinical practice, where it could be used in optimizing treatment for individual patients (e.g., change of therapy when no response is apparent after one course of chemotherapy). It can,

Table 5
Properties of Simplified Kinetic Method

Single image–static scan
Few venous blood samples required
Provides glucose metabolism
First order correction for changes in plasma clearance

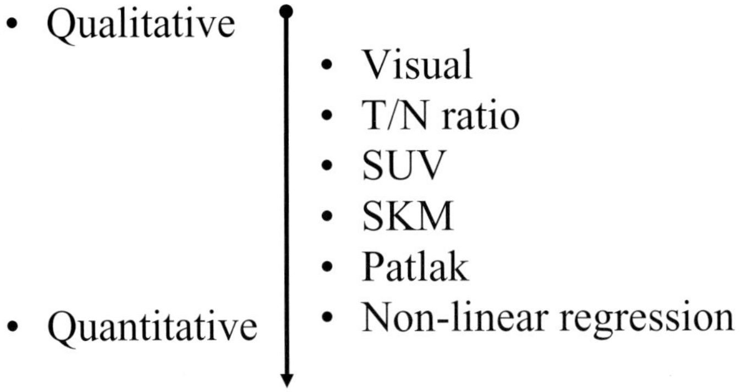

- Qualitative
  - Visual
  - T/N ratio
- Quantitative
  - SUV
  - SKM
  - Patlak
  - Non-linear regression

Fig. 3. Schematic diagram of the level of quantification achieved with the various methods presented in this chapter. Note that the level of quantification parallels the level of complexity of the scanning/analysis protocol.

however, be applied clinically only if its implementation is relatively straightforward. Nevertheless, accuracy should not be compromised by an inferior implementation, as it could lead to erroneous information about new drugs or wrong decisions in patient management. As a matter of fact, a full assessment of the value of [^{18}F]FDG PET for monitoring response has been seriously hampered by the existence of a multitude of analytical methods that have been used. Only a selection of the most common methods has been described in the previous sections. These are summarized again in Fig. 3, indicating the relative degree of quantification. Unfortunately, as discussed in the previous sections, there is a relationship between degree of quantification and degree of complexity. Clearly, the method of choice should be a trade-off between simplicity and accuracy. It should be noted that this optimal trade-off might be different for different tumors. A level of accuracy should be achieved that is sufficient to determine (with confidence) whether a change in uptake (or metabolism) represents a response.

11. STANDARDIZATION

Large-scale implementation of [^{18}F]FDG PET for monitoring tumor response to anticancer therapy requires worldwide standardization. The European Organisation for Research and Treatment of Cancer (EORTC) PET study group took the first initiative for standardization. Following two consensus meetings held in Brussels in 1998 and 1999, recommendations were published for the measurement of clinical and subclinical response using [^{18}F]FDG and PET *(17)*. These recommendations concerned all aspects of patient preparation, scanning protocols, methods of analysis, and definition of metabolic response criteria. The main aim was to create a framework that would enable the comparison (and pooling) of results from different centers, a prerequisite for multicenter trials. A set of guidelines from the National Cancer Institute (NCI) was published in 2006 *(18)*.

The complete EORTC guidelines are beyond the scope of the present chapter. Within the context of quantification, however, the EORTC guidelines on methods of analysis are of particular interest. The principle behind these specific guidelines was the definition of a minimum standard that could be adhered to by all clinical PET groups. This minimum standard was defined as SUV corrected for body surface area, but not for plasma glucose. The latter correction was considered to be small, as the scanning protocol prescribed that all patients were fasting for a minimum of 6 h. In addition, although measurement of plasma glucose (to check whether patients were fasting) was included in the guidelines, the EORTC PET study group was afraid that many clinical groups would use a very simple assay. As such an assay has a variability of 10–15%, they would reduce rather than improve the accuracy of SUV calculations. Interestingly, a number of studies that were performed after the guidelines were published *(19–21)* have shown that correcting SUV for plasma glucose (measured using the hexokinase method) significantly improved the correlation with nonlinear regression. It still needs to be determined whether this has clinical implications (i.e., with respect to determining response), otherwise this finding needs to be incorporated in a revision of the guidelines.

The EORTC PET study group also recommended that at least one center should perform a formal comparison of the above SUV results with those obtained from the more quantitative Patlak analysis. Such a comparison would be needed for each type of tumor until sufficient data are available about the relationship between SUV and Patlak analyses. If this is constant, then the Patlak analysis could be omitted in future studies. In a series of three studies on lung, breast, and gastroesophageal cancer *(19–21)*, Patlak and nonlinear regression produced nearly identical results. Moreover, there was a constant relationship between SUV and Patlak and between SKM and Patlak, suggesting that both simplified methods could be used for monitoring response to cancer therapy. In a recent study (unpublished results) with a new drug, however, the relationship between SUV and Patlak changed significantly, resulting in a lower SUV after therapy than would be expected on the basis of the Patlak (or nonlinear regression) analysis. In this case, using SUV would overestimate the efficacy of the drug. SKM performed better, but still an underestimation compared with Patlak was observed. This example makes it clear that when evaluating a new drug, the relationship between SUV (or SKM) and Patlak after therapy should always be investigated to avoid incorrect interpretation of the results of these simplified methods.

The EORTC did not provide very specific recommendations about ROI definition and analysis. The main recommendation was that the same ROI volumes should be sampled on subsequent scans and that they should be positioned as close to the original tumor volume as possible. In subsequent studies *(22, 23)* the impact of ROI definition on [^{18}F]FDG quantification was assessed. It was shown that consistency in defining ROI was extremely important for reliable quantitative results. The actual type of ROI (maximum, mean, manual) was less important for response studies as long as the same type was used on prescans and postscans. Only a fixed size ROI gave poor results. For absolute quantification, the type of ROI was more important and a threshold technique (e.g., all pixels within a 50% threshold between maximum pixel count and background) performed best.

12. FUTURE DIRECTIONS

The role of [^{18}F]FDG PET for assessing cancer therapy is still under investigation. The issue is no longer whether an early assessment of [^{18}F]FDG uptake during therapy (e.g., after one course) has prognostic value with respect to outcome. To date, the main issues are whether it can be used as a reliable tool for evaluating new drugs and whether it can be used to optimize therapy for individual patients. This implies that there is still a need for identifying the optimal method of quantification, which might be different for different tumors and drugs. Quantitative analysis becomes even more important if outcome is related not only to the rate of change of [^{18}F]FDG uptake, but also to the residual absolute uptake after one course of chemotherapy, as suggested recently *(24)*.

Assessment of glucose metabolism using [^{18}F]FDG is only one of many processes that can be studied with PET. There are several other, even more tumor specific, processes (e.g., protein synthesis, hypoxia, gene therapy) that would be good candidates for response monitoring, given the availability of suitable tracers. Assessment of response using such a tracer always requires full quantification based on a tracer kinetic model that describes its fate in the tumor. This is needed, because the relationship between uptake and underlying biological process is almost always more complex than that between [^{18}F]FDG and glucose consumption. That also implies that a simple SUV analysis is unsuitable for most tracers.

A well-known example is the measurement of blood flow using [^{15}O]H$_2$O *(25)*. Uptake of [^{15}O]H$_2$O is proportional to blood flow (first pass extraction is close to 100%) but, as [^{15}O]H$_2$O is freely diffusible, it is immediately cleared, again proportional to flow, to finally result in a tissue distribution that is governed by the partition coefficient of water. It is not possible to define an interval in which uptake reflects only blood flow (by definition, this interval itself would be flow dependent) and, therefore, it will be no surprise that there is also no relationship between SUV and blood flow for any interval *(26)*. If the purpose of a study is to assess the effects of antiangiogenic therapy by measuring blood flow, SUV analysis of a static [^{15}O]H$_2$O scan will not suffice.

A final example is the use of [^{18}F]FLT as a tracer of proliferation *(27)*. Although the tracer kinetic model is almost identical to that of [^{18}F]FDG, it remains to be seen whether a simple SUV analysis would be useful. In contrast to [^{18}F]FDG where glucose metabolism or K_i is the parameter of interest, this is not the case for [^{18}F]FLT. In theory, for [^{18}F]FLT, TK1 activity or k_3 is the parameter of interest and its relationship with "raw" uptake is more complex.

13. CONCLUSIONS

The possibility of evaluating response to cancer therapy at a very early stage during treatment is an exciting application of PET with implications for both developing new drugs and assessing efficacy of therapy in individual patients. At present [^{18}F]FDG is the tracer of choice, based on the increased glycolytic activity of most tumors. For objective assessment of response some form of quantification is required. In this respect, the development of [^{18}F]FDG has been hampered by the many different (semi)quantitative methods that have been used. Based on several studies it now seems that for many tumors and therapies an SUV analysis seems sufficient. For increased accuracy, normalization to plasma glucose levels is recommended. At the cost of only a few late venous samples, the SKM analysis provides better protection against potential therapy-induced changes in plasma clearance. For new drugs it is strongly recommended that the relationship with the quantitative Patlak analysis be evaluated first, as examples are emerging in which the relationship between SUV and Patlak (and, although to a lesser degree, also the relationship between SKM and Patlak) is greatly affected by the therapy itself, potentially leading to significant overestimation of response when using SUV. For all other tracers, including [^{18}F]FLT, full kinetic analysis is required. To avoid unnecessary delay, as previously seen with [^{18}F]FDG, any new simplification needs to be fully evaluated before it is used in large-scale studies.

REFERENCES

1. Phelps ME, Mazziotta, Schelbert HR. Positron Emission Tomography and Autoradiography. New York: Raven Press, 1986.
2. Jones T. The role of positron emission tomography within the spectrum of medical imaging. *Eur J Nucl Med* 1996;23:207–211.
3. Warburg O. On the origin of cancer cells. *Science* 1956;123:306–314.
4. Comar D. PET for Drug Development and Evaluation. Dordrecht: Kluwer Academic Publishers, 1995.
5. Sokoloff L, Reivich M, Kennedy C, Des Rosiers MH, Patlak CS, Pettigrew KD, Sakurada O, Shinohara M. The [14C]deoxyglucose method for the measurement of local cerebral glucose utilization: Theory, procedure, and normal values in the conscious and anesthetized albino rat. *J Neurochem* 1977;28:897–916.
6. Phelps ME, Huang SC, Hoffman EJ, Selin C, Sokoloff L, Kuhl DE. Tomographic measurement of local cerebral glucose metabolic rate in humans with (F-18)2-fluoro-2-deoxy-D-glucose: Validation of method. *Ann Neurol* 1979;6:371–388.
7. Hoekstra CJ, Paglianiti I, Hoekstra OS, Smit EF, Postmus PE, Teule GJJ, Lammertsma AA. Monitoring response to therapy in cancer using [^{18}F]-2-fluoro-2-deoxy-D-glucose and positron emission tomography: An overview of different analytical methods. *Eur J Nucl Med* 2000;27:731–743.
8. Wahl RL, Cody RL, Hutchins GD, Mudgett EE. Primary and metastatic breast carcinoma: Initial clinical evaluation with PET with the radiolabeled glucose analogue 2-[F-18]-fluoro-2-deoxy-D-glucose. *Radiology* 1991;179:765–770.
9. Kim CK, Gupta NC, Chandramouli B, Alavi A. Standardized uptake values of FDG: Body surface area correction is preferable to body weight correction. *J Nucl Med* 1994;35:164–167.
10. Zasadny KR, Wahl RL. Standardized uptake values of normal tissues at PET with 2-[fluorine-18]-fluoro-2-deoxy-D-glucose: Variations with body weight and a method for correction. *Radiology* 1993;189:847–850.
11. Lindholm P, Minn H, Leskinen-Kallio S, Bergman J, Ruotsalainen U, Joensuu H. Influence of the blood glucose concentration on FDG uptake in cancer–a PET study. *J Nucl Med* 1993;34:1–6.
12. Van der Weerdt AP, Klein LJ, Boellaard R, Visser CA, Visser FC, Lammertsma AA. Image-derived input functions for determination of MRGlu in cardiac (18)F-FDG PET scans. *J Nucl Med* 2001; 42:1622–1629.
13. Hoekstra CJ, Hoekstra OS, Lammertsma AA. On the use of image-derived input functions in oncological fluorine-18 fluorodeoxyglucose positron emission tomography studies. *Eur J Nucl Med* 1999;26: 1489–1492.
14. Patlak CS, Blasberg RG, Fenstermacher JD. Graphical evaluation of blood-to-brain transfer constants from multiple-time uptake data. *J Cereb Blood Flow Metab* 1983;3:1–7.
15. Messa C, Choi Y, Hoh CK, Jacobs EL, Glaspy JA, Rege S, Nitzsche E, Huang SC, Phelps ME, Hawkins RA. Quantification of glucose utilization in liver metastases: Parametric imaging of FDG uptake with PET. *J Comput Assist Tomogr* 1992;16:684–689.
16. Hunter GJ, Hamberg LM, Alpert NM, Choi NC, Fischman AJ. Simplified measurement of deoxyglucose utilization rate. *J Nucl Med* 1996;37:950–955.
17. Young H, Baum R, Cremerius U, Herholz K, Hoekstra O, Lammertsma AA, Pruim J, Price P on behalf of the European Organization for Research and Treatment of Cancer (EORTC) PET Study Group. Measurement of clinical and subclinical tumor response using [^{18}F]-fluorodeoxyglucose and positron emission tomography: Review and 1999 EORTC recommendations. *Eur J Cancer* 1999;35: 1773–1782.

18. Shankar LK, Hoffman JM, Bacharach S, Graham MM, Karp J, Lammertsma AA, Larson S, Mankoff DA, Siegel BA, van den Abbeele A, Yap J, Sullivan D. Consensus recommendations for the use of ^{18}F-FDG as an indicator of therapeutic response in patients in national cancer institute trials. *J Nucl Med* 2006;47:1059–1066.
19. Hoekstra CJ, Hoekstra OS, Stroobants SG, Vansteenkiste J, Nuyts J, Smit EF, Boers M, Twisk JWR, Lammertsma AA. Methods to monitor response to chemotherapy in non-small cell lung cancer with ^{18}F-FDG PET. *J Nucl Med* 2002;43:1304–1309.
20. Krak NC, van der Hoeven JJ, Hoekstra OS, Twisk JWR, van der Wall E, Lammertsma AA. Measuring [^{18}F]FDG uptake in breast cancer during chemotherapy: Comparison of analytical methods. *Eur J Nucl Med Mol Imaging* 2003;30:674–681.
21. Kroep JR, Van Groeningen CJ, Cuesta MA, Craanen ME, Hoekstra OS, Comans EFI, Bloemena E, Hoekstra CJ, Golding RP, Twisk JWR, Peters GJ, Pinedo HM, Lammertsma AA. Positron emission tomography using 2-deoxy-2-[^{18}F]-fluoro-D-glucose for response monitoring in locally advanced gastroesophageal cancer; a comparison of different analytical methods. *Mol Imaging Biol* 2003;5:337–346.
22. Boellaard R, Krak NC, Hoekstra OS, Lammertsma AA. Effects of noise, image resolution and ROI definition on the accuracy of standard uptake values: A simulation study. *J Nucl Med* 2004;45:1519–1527.
23. Krak NC, Boellaard R, Hoekstra OS, Twisk JWR, Hoekstra CJ, Lammertsma AA. Effects of ROI definition and reconstruction method on quantitative outcome and applicability in a response monitoring trial. *Eur J Nucl Med Mol Imaging* 2005;32:294–301.
24. Hoekstra CJ, Stroobants SG, Smit EF, Vansteenkiste J, van Tinteren H, Postmus PE, Golding R, Biesma B, Schramel FJHM, van Zandwijk N, Lammertsma AA, Hoekstra OS. Prognostic relevance of response evaluation using [^{18}F]-2-fluoro-2-deoxy-D-glucose positron emission tomography in patients with locally advanced non-small-cell lung cancer. *J Clin Oncol* 2005;23:8362–8370.
25. Lammertsma AA, Mazoyer BM. EEC concerted action on cellular degeneration and regeneration studied with PET: Modelling expert meeting blood flow measurement with PET. *Eur J Nucl Med* 1990;16:807–812.
26. Hoekstra CJ, Stroobants SG, Hoekstra OS, Smit EF, Vansteenkiste J, Lammertsma AA. Measurement of perfusion in stage IIIA-N2 non-small cell lung cancer using $H_2^{15}O$ and positron emission tomography. *Clin Cancer Res* 2002;8:2109–2115.
27. Shields AF, Grierson JR, Dohmen BM, Machulla HJ, Stayanoff JC, Lawhorn-Crews JM, Obradovich JE, Muzik O, Mangner TJ. Imaging proliferation in vivo with [F-18]FLT and positron emission tomography. *Nat Med* 1998;4:1334–1336.

11 Positron Emission Tomography Measurement of Drug Kinetics

Azeem Saleem, PhD, and P. Price, MD

CONTENTS

    INTRODUCTION
    PHARMACOKINETIC PROCESSES
    PLASMA PHARMACOKINETIC PARAMETERS
    PLASMA PHARMACOKINETIC MODELING
    PHARMACOKINETIC–PHARMACODYNAMIC OPTIMIZATION
    WHY DO WE NEED TISSUE PHARMACOKINETICS?
    HOW CAN POSITRON EMISSION TOMOGRAPHY AID DRUG DEVELOPMENT?
    POSITRON EMISSION TOMOGRAPHY TRACER KINETICS
    LINEAR AND NONLINEAR KINETICS
    POSITRON EMISSION TOMOGRAPHY PHARMACOKINETIC STUDIES
    POSITRON EMISSION TOMOGRAPHY PHARMACOKINETIC PARAMETERS
    DRUG METABOLISM
    POSITRON EMISSION TOMOGRAPHY MODELING TECHNIQUES
    POSITRON EMISSION TOMOGRAPHY KINETIC STUDIES WITH ANTICANCER AGENTS
    N-[2-(DIMETHYLAMINO)ETHYL]ACRIDINE-4-CARBOXAMIDE
    5-FLUOROURACIL
    TEMOZOLOMIDE
    SUMMARY

Positron emission tomography (PET) is a highly sensitive noninvasive functional imaging modality that can provide quantitative *in vivo* tissue data with high temporal resolution. Such information can be exploited to assess the behavior of a drug within the body (pharmacokinetics) and its effects on the biosystem (pharmacodynamics). Knowledge of *in vivo* drug pharmacology is especially invaluable in the assessment

From: *Cancer Drug Discovery and Development*
In Vivo Imaging of Cancer Therapy
Edited by: A.F. Shields and P. Price © Humana Press Inc., Totowa, NJ

and development of anticancer agents and is likely to play a significant role in the development of novel targeted therapies. Specifically, PET pharmacokinetic studies can provide information on drug access, kinetics, and drug concentration in tumors and normal tissues, all of which have a bearing on drug activity, tissue toxicity, and drug scheduling. In addition, such studies can provide proof of principle of the *in vivo* mechanism of drug action and *in vivo* targeting of molecular therapeutic targets. In this review, basic principles of PET drug kinetic measurement techniques are discussed, followed by examples of PET kinetic studies performed at various stages of the drug developmental process and their utility and contribution to anticancer drug development are highlighted.

1. INTRODUCTION

Pharmacokinetics is the study of the time course (kinetics) of different processes (absorption, distribution, metabolism, and excretion) that govern the fate of a drug in the body. Pharmacodynamics is the study of the intensity, duration, and type of action (therapeutic and/or adverse effects) of a drug. Pharmacokinetics reflects what the body does to the drug and pharmacodynamics what the drug does to the body.

Since the term pharmacokinetics was coined by Teorell in 1937, after his pioneering work on the kinetics of distribution of substances administered in the body *(1, 2)*, pharmacokinetics has found increasing acceptance in the evaluation of new therapeutic agents. The availability of new, sensitive, and specific analytical techniques, such as high-performance liquid chromatography (HPLC) and gas and liquid mass spectrometry, and the advent of powerful computers have also immensely contributed to the development of plasma pharmacokinetics in recent years.

Conventionally, repeated plasma samples are obtained usually up to a few days after drug administration to obtain the temporal plasma concentrations of the parent drug (and metabolites). From this, drug behavior within the body is summarized by derivation of pharmacokinetic parameters by application of kinetic modeling methods or methods independent of modeling. In the following sections, we shall initially discuss conventional pharmacokinetic methods followed by PET drug kinetic measurement techniques and finally illustrate the utility and contribution of PET kinetic studies in anticancer drug development.

2. PHARMACOKINETIC PROCESSES

The four processes that reflect the behavior of the drug in the body are absorption, distribution, metabolism, and excretion (ADME). The intravenous route is the most commonly used method of drug administration with anticancer agents. However, some important drugs such as tamoxifen, cyclophosphamide, and, more recently, capecitabine are administered orally. In addition to time delay, some drugs may undergo a significant amount of first-pass metabolism before reaching the systemic circulation when administered extravascularly *(3)*.

After absorption, drugs circulate in plasma, either bound to plasma proteins or in an unbound state, with an equilibrium existing, in most cases, between protein-bound and unbound drug. Bound drugs are restricted in their passage across capillaries and only the unbound drug is distributed to tissues. Drugs with low molecular weight diffuse readily into tissues from the vascular system as do lipophilic compounds. Finally, drug distribution is influenced by the ionization status of the drug, with uncharged drugs diffusing well across lipid membranes, compared to charged molecules. The ionization status of drug is dependent on the dissociation constant (pK_a) of the drug and the pH of the surrounding environment. Generally, at a pH 2 units higher or lower than the drug pK_a, the drugs may be either 99% ionized or nonionized *(4)*. Multidrug resistance proteins (p-glycoprotein and multidrug resistance-associated proteins) located in epithelial and endothelial cells are being increasingly recognized as critical determinants for the movement of a large number of commonly prescribed drugs across cellular barriers *(5)*. Within the tissues, drugs may be either free or bound specifically to sites of action such as receptors resulting in pharmacological or toxic effects or to a nonspecific binding site, which causes no effect.

Competing with the forces of distribution of the drug are those of elimination, namely metabolism and excretion. Certain organs such as liver, lung, and blood possess enzymes that metabolize drugs. For most drugs, metabolism occurs in the liver *(6)*. Although metabolism generally results in detoxification, some drugs may have cytotoxic circulating metabolites. Knowledge of the metabolic pathway of the drug is useful, as drug action could be modified either by inhibiting or inducing metabolism for maximal therapeutic gain. An area of rapidly increasing importance is genetically determined variability in drug metabolizing enzymes (pharmacogenetics) *(7)*. Such genetic variability can result in enhanced toxicity due to impaired detoxification *(8)*, enhanced activation, or lack of desired effect due to impaired activation *(9)*. Furthermore, genetically determined variability may also be a risk factor in carcinogenesis *(10)*.

Drug excretion takes place by renal or hepatobiliary routes for most drugs. Both are complex processes involving a chain of events, any of which can be modulated by disease processes or other medications *(11, 12)*. Cancer patients frequently have organ dysfunction following metastatic dissemination. Knowledge of a drug's elimination profile is therefore essential in providing optimal benefit and minimal risk.

3. PLASMA PHARMACOKINETIC PARAMETERS

Plasma pharmacokinetic parameters that summarize drug behavior in the body include drug half-life, clearance, area under the concentration–time curve (AUC), and maximal drug concentrations.

3.1 Plasma Concentration and Half-Life

Maximal drug concentrations in plasma (C_{max}) and the time to reach maximal concentrations (t_{max}) are derived from inspection of serial plasma data. The half-life is defined as the time required for drug concentrations to decrease by 50%. When a drug has more than one half-life, the terminal or elimination half-life is usually taken as the parameter of interest. Half-life is important because it determines the time required to reach steady state (C_{ss}) and the dosage interval. When the rate of drug infusion is equal to the elimination rate, steady-state plasma levels are reached.

3.2 Clearance

Clearance (CL) of a drug by an organ is the volume of blood cleared of the drug per unit time *(13)*. Physiologically, clearance is determined by the blood flow to the organ, which eliminates the drug, and the efficiency of the organ in extracting the drug. When organs have a high intrinsic clearance (i.e., enzymes have a large capacity to metabolize the drug), the drug clearance of the organ is equal to the blood flow to the organ. On the other hand, when the intrinsic clearance of an organ is low, the clearance of the drug from the organ is dependent on the product of unbound drug in the plasma and the intrinsic ability of the drug to clear unbound drug from the blood. Clearances in the various organs are additive to give the total clearance of the drug. Clearance can be calculated in one of two ways: either by measurement (or estimation) after a single dose or by determination of the steady-state concentration (C_{ss}) during continuous infusion *(14)*.

$$\text{Clearance} = \text{Dose}/\text{AUC} \qquad (1)$$

$$\text{Clearance} = \text{Dose rate}/C_{ss} \qquad (2)$$

3.4 Volume of Distribution

The systemic volume of distribution (V_d) can be defined as the volume the drug would need to occupy to account for the total drug within the body, which gives an indication of the distributive characteristics of the drug *(15)*. However, as the body is not a homogeneous organ, the size of the volume can provide clues only about the distribution of the drug in the body. If the drug is highly bound to plasma proteins, the volume will be close to plasma volume. On the contrary, if the drug is rapidly sequestrated by tissues, V_d will be large (e.g. >100 liters).

3.5 Area Under the Concentration–Time Curve

The area under the plasma concentration–time curve (AUC), also referred to as exposure, is probably the most important pharmacokinetic parameter in cancer chemotherapy. It is commonly used as a surrogate of tumor and normal tissue exposure and can be calculated as the ratio of dose and clearance (AUC = Dose/CL) in model-dependent techniques.

4. PLASMA PHARMACOKINETIC MODELING

4.1 Compartmental Modeling

Traditionally plasma pharmacokinetic modeling is performed by using either compartmental or noncompartmental methods. In compartmental analyses, the body is thought to consist of one (monocompartmental model) or several (multicompartmental model) compartments. These compartments are not necessarily physical compartments representing physiological disposition, but are a simplification of biological complexities whose elements represent key dynamics. The transfer of the drug into and out of the compartments is described by constants known as rate constants (e.g., k_{21} and k_{12}). Pharmacokinetic parameters are obtained by fitting a model to the plasma concentration–time curve. The fitted curve can consist of one or more exponentials, depending on the model, with each exponential describing the kinetics of the drug in the body. Dedicated software *(16, 17)* is widely available to model the pharmacokinetic data and obtain the various parameters.

4.2 Noncompartmental Modeling

Noncompartmental modeling is based on the theory of statistical moments and follows from the recognition that drug elimination is a stochastic process *(18, 19)*. In this approach, the movement of individual drug molecules through a body compartment is governed by probability. Thus, the residence time of the drug in the body can be viewed as a frequency distribution with a mean and variance around the mean. The AUC corresponds to the zero-order moment and is calculated using the trapezoidal method *(20)*. The first moment is defined as the AUC of the product of time (t) and plasma concentration (C), from time 0 to infinity. This area is defined as the area under the first moment curve (AUMC). Mean residence time (MRT), which is the time required to eliminate 63.2% of the drug, is given by the ratio of AUMC to AUC *(19)*:

$$\text{MRT} = \text{AUMC/AUC} \tag{3}$$

5. PHARMACOKINETIC–PHARMACODYNAMIC OPTIMIZATION

One way of optimization of therapy would be to relate the pharmacokinetic parameters with the therapeutic effects, such as tumor response and normal tissue toxicity (pharmacodynamic effect). If such a relationship was established, this would lead to the utilization of pharmacokinetic parameters for therapeutic monitoring and in selecting optimal dose and schedule *(21)*. To establish such a relationship, pharmacokinetic parameters would have to be identified that correlate with the pharmacodynamic outcome. Methotrexate *(22, 23)* and carboplatin *(24, 25)* are two antineoplastic agents for which pharmacokinetic parameters are used in the optimization of therapy.

A number of *in vitro* models have been proposed that relate dose (usually the survival fraction) *(26–28)*. These dose–response curves can take a variety of forms *(27)*, but the effect is usually exponential. In contrast to *in vitro* modeling, *in vivo* models are much more complex, and it is necessary to account for pharmacokinetic, biochemical, and cell kinetic parameters simultaneously in both normal and tumor tissue. Furthermore, there is a time lag between measured plasma concentrations and effect, with the pharmacological effect not being apparent while the drug is still detectable.

Most clinical pharmacodynamic studies to date have focused on modeling the extent of hematological toxicity, as myelosuppression is easily quantified, occurs at predictable times, and is usually reversible. Modeling of nonhematological toxicities is more difficult as these are often poorly quantified and based on subjective data. However, when nonhematological toxicity such as nephrotoxicity can be measured, models of toxicity can be constructed in a manner analogous to myelosuppression *(29)*. The greatest challenge is to model tumor response, as factors such as biochemical drug response and drug delivery may prevent response even at high drug concentrations. Some examples of pharmacokinetic–toxicity/tumor response relationships are given in Table 1 *(30–46)*.

6. WHY DO WE NEED TISSUE PHARMACOKINETICS?

Although pharmacokinetic parameters derived from plasma sampling have been used as a good surrogate of tissue and tumor pharmacokinetics (Table 1), an in-depth understanding of normal tissue and tumor pharmacokinetics is essential for rational anticancer drug development. This will enable exploitation of variations in drug kinetics between normal tissue and tumor so that the therapeutic index is maximized. Moreover, drug development is currently undergoing enormous changes, due to an increase in our understanding of the processes that induce and drive malignant transformation. This understanding has resulted in a shift in paradigm from the development of predominantly cytotoxic agents to compounds that target the specific alterations that drive malignant transformation. New targets include genes, antigens, and pathways involved in angiogenesis, cell cycle, signal transduction, cell death, drug resistance, invasion, and metastasis. Due to these new targeted therapies, the need to revise the way we test new drugs has become apparent. Consequently, in addition to plasma pharmacokinetics, tumor and normal tissue pharmacokinetic information is likely to be required at an early stage in drug development to ensure that adequate exposure to drug or active metabolites is being achieved. Furthermore, it is envisaged that hypothesis-testing clinical trial designs would be incorporated into phase I studies to provide early proof of principle of mechanism of action. Noninvasive technologies such as PET will play a key role in providing such information to support drug development.

Table 1
Relationship between Pharmacokinetic Parameters and Toxicity[a]

Drug	Pharmacokinetic parameter	Tumor response and toxicity
Busulfan	AUC	Hepatotoxicity (30)
Carboplatin	AUC	Leukopenia
	AUC	Thrombocytopenia (31, 32)
	AUC	Ovarian cancer (33)
Cisplatin	C_{max}, AUC	Nephrotoxicity (29)
Doxorubicin	C_{ss}	Leukopenia (34)
Docetaxel	AUC	Neutropenia (35)
Etoposide	$C_{ss} > 1.2\,\mu g/ml$	Non-small-cell lung cancer (36)
5-Fluorouracil	AUC	Myelosuppression, GI toxicity (37)
	C_{max}	Myelosuppression, GI toxicity (38)
	C_{ss}, AUC	GI toxicity (39)
	AUC	Head and neck cancer (38)
		Colorectal cancer (40)
Irinotecan	AUC	Neutropenia (41)
	Biliary index	Diarrhea (42)
Methotrexate	$C_{48h} > 0.9\,\mu M$	Myelosuppression (22)
	$C_{ss} > 16\,\mu M$	Acute lymphocytic leukemia (43)
Paclitaxel	Time $> 0.05\,\mu M$	Neutropenia (44)
Vinblastine	C_{ss}	Leukopenia (45)
Vincristine	AUC	Neurotoxicity (46)

[a] AUC, area under the curve; GI, gastrointestinal.

7. HOW CAN POSITRON EMISSION TOMOGRAPHY AID DRUG DEVELOPMENT?

As PET is a quantitative and highly sensitive dynamic imaging modality, it can provide tissue and tumor data with high temporal resolution, not available by other means. In general, PET can provide information on tumor and normal tissue distribution of drugs, as well as drug clearance. Mathematical modeling of tissue and plasma pharmacokinetic data enables important kinetic parameters relating to the uptake, distribution, and washout to be derived. Positron emission tomography can also provide information on target modulation and predict response based on assessment of the molecular/biochemical defect (pharmacodynamics). In addition to its value in the evaluation of the pharmacology of anticancer agents, PET can play an important role in the elucidation of pathophysiological processes that may in turn aid rational drug discovery. Data derived from plasma radioactive metabolite profiling during PET scanning can be important on its own, providing evidence of specific metabolic processes in humans or animals. In addition, as biological therapies in which the determination of optimal therapeutic dose will be the primary aim (MTD may be irrelevant) during early stages of clinical drug development, it is anticipated that PET will play an important role in the drug development process by helping determine optimal biological doses.

8. POSITRON EMISSION TOMOGRAPHY TRACER KINETICS

In physiology, a tracer is an analog of a biochemical species of interest that behaves identically *in vivo* to its counterpart without perturbing the physiological system under observation. When this molecule of interest is radiolabeled and utilized in PET and other nuclear imaging studies, it is called a radiotracer. External detection of the emitted activity from the very small amounts of administered radiotracer is made possible by the ability of radiochemists to produce molecules of high specific activity (activity/mole). In addition to studying physiological phenomena, radiotracers can be used to study the *in vivo* pharmacokinetics of drugs including anticancer agents *(47)*. For this, the radiolabeled drug should be identical in chemical and biological properties to the stable drug. This is achieved by replacing the stable nuclides with their positron-emitting counterparts. Positron emitters are available for commonly occurring elements such as carbon, nitrogen, and oxygen. Fluorine-18, a commonly used radionuclide, is used to replace fluorine present in compounds of interest such as 5-fluorouracil (5-FU). However, it can also be used to replace hydrogen atoms, of which it is isoteric, or hydroxyl groups, of which it is isoelectronic. Although these analogs are not guaranteed to retain the pharmacokinetic properties of the native drug, the substitutions are highly conservative and have yielded useful probes in many situations such as in fluorinated antiestrogens *(48)*.

9. LINEAR AND NONLINEAR KINETICS

Most drugs follow linear pharmacokinetics, which means that the serum concentrations change proportionally with drug dose. Some drugs do not show such a proportional change in drug concentrations with a change in dose. They are then said to follow nonlinear kinetics. A more than expected change in AUC, C_{ss}, or drug concentration

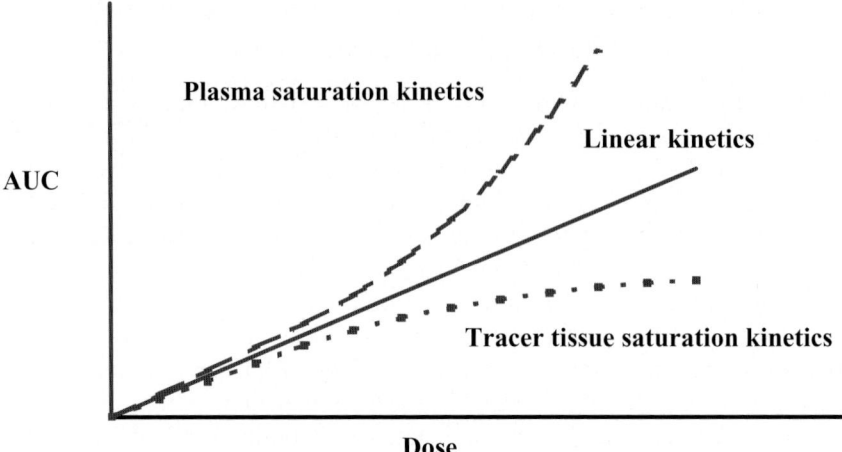

Fig. 1. Relationship between dose and AUC under linear and nonlinear conditions. An increase in dose administered results in a proportional increase in AUC when drugs follow linear kinetics. A more or less than proportional increase is seen in plasma and tissues when drugs follow nonlinear kinetics.

occurs due to saturation of elimination processes such as enzymatic biotransformation, biliary excretion, and renal tubular reassertion. This occurs when the maximum rate of metabolism (V_{max}) for the drug is approached. The kinetics of a saturable biosystem can be expressed by the following equation:

$$V = \frac{V_{max} C}{K_m + C} \qquad (4)$$

where V is the rate of metabolism and C is the serum concentration. The serum concentration at which the rate of metabolism equals $V_{max}/2$ is K_m. Practically speaking, K_m is the serum concentration at which nonproportional changes in AUC and C_{ss} start to occur when the dose is increased. Such a nonproportional and supralinear change in plasma drug concentrations or AUC with a change in dose is called Michaelis–Menten kinetics *(49)* (Fig. 1, top curve). Most drugs metabolized by hepatic enzymes still appear to follow linear kinetics at therapeutic concentration ranges. The reason for this disparity is that the therapeutic range for most drugs is well below the K_m of the enzyme systems that metabolize the drug. In a saturable biosystem, an increase in plasma drug concentrations above the K_m results in saturation of drug kinetics in specific tissues. Therefore, in PET tissue kinetic studies, a decrease in radiotracer uptake or exposure with increasing drug doses would demonstrate saturation of tissue uptake, metabolism, or excretion of the drug in that tissue (Fig. 1, bottom curve).

10. POSITRON EMISSION TOMOGRAPHY PHARMACOKINETIC STUDIES

PET studies could be employed at three main levels during the process of taking a cytotoxic drug from concept to licensure including (1) preclinical development level, (2) prephase I level (prior to conventional phase I studies), and (3) phase I/II/III level. *In vivo* tissue pharmacokinetics of the radiolabeled drug can be studied after administration of the radiotracer either alone (high specific activity), admixed with increasing or therapeutic quantities of unlabeled drug (low specific activity), or during a continuous infusion of the unlabeled stable drug. In the first instance, when the radiotracer is usually administered to evaluate pharmacokinetics at tracer doses, it is essential that the system is naive to the drug or is administered after a period, ensuring washout of previously administrated drug from the system (i.e., $C_0 = 0$). This will help prevent misinterpretation of results due to the presence of unlabeled drug in the body. The total amount of drug in such instances is minimal and doses as low as 1/1000 of the starting phase I dose of the drug can be administered. For most drugs, concentrations achieved at these doses are much lower than the K_m for saturable metabolic processes. Hence, the pharmacokinetics at these doses predict the drug pharmacokinetics only for the range of drug concentrations until the K_m is reached (i.e., within the range of drug concentrations in which the drug exhibits linear pharmacokinetics).

In contrast to conventional pharmacokinetic analyses, where plasma data are usually collected for at least 48 h after drug administration (depending on the $t_{1/2}$), the short half-lives of the commonly used positron emitters and patient comfort make tissue data collection in PET studies beyond a few hours almost impossible.

11. POSITRON EMISSION TOMOGRAPHY PHARMACOKINETIC PARAMETERS

Given the characteristic physical decay of the positron, PET tissue pharmacokinetic parameters are calculated after correction of tissue activity for radioactive decay. In addition, tissue data is normalized for other study variables such as the injected radioactivity and the body surface area of the patient. From this, tissue parameters are obtained.

11.1 Radioactive Decay

Although the amount of radioactive material that remains decreases with time, the rate of radioactive decay for the substance remains the same. The rate of decay that is exponential depends on the amount of the material and is given as

$$N = N_0 e^{-\lambda t} \tag{5}$$

where N_0 and N are, respectively, the number of radioactive nuclei present initially or after a time t. λ is the disassociation rate constant, which is characteristic of the isotope and is the probability that an atom will decay in a second. In PET pharmacokinetic studies, by correcting for radioactive decay, the biological half-life of the radiolabeled compound can be directly obtained from tissue data.

11.2 Tissue Radioactivity and Area Under the Curve

Tissue pharmacokinetic parameters such as maximal radioactivity (also referred to as C_{max}) and time to reach C_{max} (t_{max}) are calculated by simple visual inspection. As tissue radioactivity (MBq.mL^{-1}) is normalized for the injected dose per body surface area, it is consequently expressed as m^2.mL^{-1}. When the drug is not metabolized, drug concentration in tissue (mg.mL^{-1}) can also be calculated from the measured tissue radioactivity (tissue activity/specific activity).

The area under the radioactivity–time curve (also referred to as AUC) can be calculated relatively easily for the duration of the scan. This is done by integrating the activity in all time frames for the full duration of the dynamic scan. Radiotracer AUC is expressed as $m^2.mL^{-1}.sec$, after correction for radioactive decay and normalization for body surface area.

11.3 Half-Life, Clearance

After correcting for radioactive decay, it is possible to derive the drug $t_{1/2}$ and clearance by fitting an exponential equation to the time–activity curve (TAC) as in plasma kinetic modeling. It is important to remember that this may result in incorrect values when scan duration (dictated largely by radionuclide half-life) is less than at least twice the half-life of the drug. Hence, extrapolation of tissue AUC and clearance to infinity are not usually performed.

11.4 Uptake

The standardized uptake value (SUV) is defined as the tissue concentration of tracer as measured by a PET scanner divided by the activity injected divided by body weight *(50)*. Normalization to body surface instead of body weight has been shown to result in decreasing the variability of SUV *(51)*. SUV normalized to body surface area can be defined as

$$\text{SUV}_{bsa}(m^2.mL^{-1}) = \frac{\text{Tissue activity}(MBq.mL^{-1})}{\text{Injected activity}(MBq)/\text{Body suface area}(m^2)} \quad (6)$$

11.5 Partition Coefficient and Volume of Distribution

Partition coefficient is the concentration of substance in the tissue (C_t) over that in the plasma (C_p), provided the tracer has access to the whole tissue space *(52)*. It can also be defined more generally as the ratio between tissue and arterial blood concentration in equilibrium. The parameter volume of distribution (V_d) has a different meaning in PET pharmacokinetics, although the concept has been borrowed from clinical pharmacokinetics. V_d is defined as the ratio of volumes (or "spaces") making the tissue concentration equal to that in the plasma. The space then taken by the substance compared to the total volume is the V_d. Both V_d and partition coefficient are numerically identical and are unitless, although V_d is sometimes given the units of $mL.g^{-1}$ when density corrections are made. V_d is derived from the rate constants obtained by PET pharmacokinetic modeling.

12. DRUG METABOLISM

The kinetics of a drug can be quantified easily with PET if the drug is not metabolized during the scan duration, as the entire tissue activity would be due to the radiolabeled drug. However, when the drug is metabolized, it is difficult to differentiate between the chemical species carrying the radiolabel, as PET lacks *in vivo* chemical information. Knowledge of chemical composition may be important as tumor radioactivity is usually composed of parent drug and metabolites that may be active, inactive, or toxic to normal tissues.

When metabolism occurs, a number of strategies can be used to deal with the contamination arising from labeled metabolites. These include (1) mathematical modelling, (2) obtaining a correction for metabolites by performing an additional study after administration of the radiolabeled metabolite *(53)*, (3) washout strategies for radiotracers with a long physical half-life, in which nonspecific binding and metabolites are allowed to be eliminated leaving specifically bound species, which are imaged at a later time point *(54)*, and (4) inhibition of metabolism in one arm of a paired study to enable the contribution of metabolism to be assessed *(55)*.

13. POSITRON EMISSION TOMOGRAPHY MODELING TECHNIQUES

As in plasma kinetic modeling, PET modeling can also be divided broadly into two categories: (1) compartmental-based or model-led techniques and (2) multivariate based or data-led techniques. The data-led techniques such as principal component analysis *(56)*, cluster analysis *(57)*, and factor analysis *(58)* make no *a priori* assumptions of the model structure and dictate what can be identified from the data. However, they often fail to fully characterize the parameters of interest and are extensively used as first-pass analysis with new tracers when little is known about the tracer's behavior. Compartmental techniques themselves form a broad spectrum from rigidly model-led methods requiring *a priori* assumptions of the data (fluorodeoxyglucose model) to techniques such as spectral analysis *(59)*, which require few *a priori* assumptions and lie between the strictly data-led and highly structured methods.

Single-input/single-output systems typically characterize PET studies. In general, the system input is the plasma TAC and the system output is the tissue TAC, and a model is fitted that best explains their relationship. The plasma TAC for the parent drug is therefore also known as input function. This is derived from the continuous on-line monitoring (typically every second) of blood radioactivity, discrete (typically 5–10) sampling of blood, blood/plasma partitioning of radioactivity, and plasma metabolite profile throughout the scan duration. The input function has high temporal resolution (3600 time points for a 60-min scan). Similarly, temporal resolution of the tissue TAC or output function is high and is determined by the frame durations of the dynamic scans, which are usually short (usually 5 sec) at early time points to resolve the kinetics better. This gives rise to temporally and spatially rich data, allowing model determination for each of the tissues analyzed by the PET scanner. The relationship between input and output responses is modeled by a process known as convolution, a mathematical function distinct and different from the multiplicative function.

As examples, two modeling methods that have been utilized to describe drug kinetics are briefly discussed.

13.1 Graphic Analysis

Graphic or Patlak approaches were first used by Rutland *(60)* and developed in a more theoretical framework by Gjedde *(61)* and Patlak *(62)*. This method is used to measure the irreversible radiotracer uptake into the tissues and was originally developed to calculate blood to brain influx constant. In this method it is assumed that relatively rapid, free, and reversible exchange of the tracer occurs between the only source of the tracer, i.e., the plasma and tissue region made up of n compartments. It is also assumed that there is another tissue distribution region, called the "bound or irreversible" region, that may consist of one or more parts that can be mathematically lumped together into a single irreversible compartment. The tracer may enter, but not leave this compartment, and if the tracer is metabolized, this occurs only in the irreversible region and the metabolite is trapped there and is measurable.

Positron emission tomography data are transformed and the rate of the unidirectional flux of the tracer into the irreversible compartment (K_I) is determined. After transformation the Patlak model equation is defined as

$$C_t(t)/C_p(t) = K_I \int_0^t C_p(\tau)d\tau/C_p(t) + (V_p + V_o) \tag{7}$$

where V_o is the steady-state space of the exchangeable region, V_p is the plasma volume within the tissue, and $C_t(t)$ and $C_p(t)$ are tissue and plasma time courses of the tracer, respectively. K_I is the net clearance from plasma into tissues and is referred to as the net unidirectional influx constant or the net irreversible uptake rate constant.

The transformed data are plotted with $C_t(t)/C_p(t)$ on the y-axis (ordinate) and $\int_0^t C_p(\tau)d\tau/C_p(t)$ on the x-axis (abscissa). The transformation of the data on the abscissa results in transforming the bolus input function into an infusion function of the arterial plasma activity. For each measured time point, the integral of the plasma signal up to that time point is divided by the actual plasma concentration of that point in time. In other words, for each point in the abscissa a new time is calculated, namely the time that would have been needed to reach the actual plasma integral with the actual plasma activity at that time. The tissue concentration measured by PET is simply normalized to the actual plasma concentration in the Patlak plot. The abscissa of the Patlak plot is also called "stretched" time or "funny" time.

As a consequence of the transformation, the abscissa, which has the dimension of time, will, for larger time points, always reach infinity because as the numerator increases the denominator approaches 0. In addition, if the tissue levels follow the plasma level, because nothing is being trapped, then the tissue over plasma curve bends and becomes horizontal. If the signal is trapped into the tissue, the curve will always show a positive slope. Graphic analysis has also been applied to assess the uptake and retention of [^{18}F]fluorodeoxyglucose, whose metabolite [^{18}F]fluorodeoxyglucose-6-phosphate is trapped in pathological states.

13.2 Spectral Analysis

Spectral analysis *(59)* is a further development of an approach used by Tobler and Engel *(63)*, who used a set of hyperbolic basis functions to investigate *in vitro* binding data. This kinetic modeling technique lies between the strictly data-led and highly structured techniques and allows for the distinction between transient, reversible, and irreversible tracer kinetic components. When the biological half-life of the tracer is much longer compared to the physical/radioactive half-life, the effective half-life approaches the physical half-life of the radionuclide. This principle is utilized in spectral analysis, where nondecay-corrected TACs are used for modeling. In this method, the behavior of the radiotracer *in vivo* is defined by a number of kinetic components (β), which may be transient to irreversible. The data, uncorrected for decay, serve as a useful constraint in defining these components, with values approaching λ being associated with retention of the drug/metabolites in tissue.

Spectral analysis is based on the *a priori* definition that the tissue impulse response function (IRF) can be constructed from a sum of nonnegative exponential terms.

This model is defined as

$$\text{Tissue}(t) = IRF(t) \otimes \text{Plasma}(t) \qquad (8)$$

where $IRF = \sum_{i=1}^{i=k} \alpha_i \exp(-\beta_i t)$ and k is the number of identifiable kinetic components, β.

The discrete spectrum of exponentials (β) is prechosen and fixed to cover an appropriate spectral range. For *in vivo* studies involving short-lived positron-emitting isotopes, this range needs to extend from the slowest possible loss of radioactivity from the tissue (i.e., that associated with radioactive half-life of the isotope) up to a value appropriate for a transient phenomena (e.g., the passage of activity through the tissue vasculature). Positron emission tomography data that are not decay corrected thus provide a useful constraint on the range of values for β. For example, with studies involving ^{18}F [decay constant (λ) 0.000105 sec^{-1}], a suitable range is from 10^{-4} sec^{-1} to 1 sec^{-1}. Thus a β value of 1 sec^{-1} is associated with the fastest component and is usually due to transient blood volume effects. On the other hand, a β value of λ is associated with retention of activity in the tissue and is likely to be associated with tissue response. Kinetic components may range between 0 and λ with components tending toward irreversibility as they approach values of λ *(59)*.

The relative contribution of the components is indicated by α, the intensity of each of the components. Values for α may be obtained from a fit of the model to the measured time–activity data of the tissue using a constrained nonnegative least squares algorithm. It is convenient for display purposes to divide the range of spectral components logarithmically to give the maximum ($n = 100$) possible values for β, between 1 and λ. Although the model allows for such a relatively large set of basis functions to be used in the fitting of the PET data, the fit consists of only a small subset of these. Spectral analysis is especially useful in assessing drug pharmacokinetics where no *a priori* model assumptions can be made. This is especially useful in the assessment of anticancer agents *(64)*. In addition, the relationship between plasma and tissue activity given by the IRF can be used to correct for tissue metabolites.

14. POSITRON EMISSION TOMOGRAPHY KINETIC STUDIES WITH ANTICANCER AGENTS

A number of anticancer agents have been radiolabeled for PET kinetic studies such as cisplatin *(65)*, 1,3-bis-(2-chlorethyl)-1-nitrosourea (BCNU) *(66)*, tamoxifen *(67)*, *N*-[2-(dimethylamino)ethyl]acridine-4-carboxamide (DACA), 5-FU, and temozolomide. In this review, some of the PET kinetic studies performed with radiolabeled DACA, 5-FU, and temozolomide will be described.

15. *N*-[2-(DIMETHYLAMINO)ETHYL]ACRIDINE-4-CARBOXAMIDE

N-[2-(Dimethylamino)ethyl]acridine-4-carboxamide (Xenova: XR5000) (Fig. 2) is a third generation agent derived from the antileukemic agent amsacrine, [4-(9-acridinylamino)methanesulfon-*m*-anisidide]. It was a product of the synthesis and testing program for antitumor tricyclic carboxamide-based intercalating agents at the University of Auckland in New Zealand *(68)*. *N*-[2-(Dimethylamino)ethyl]acridine-4-carbox-

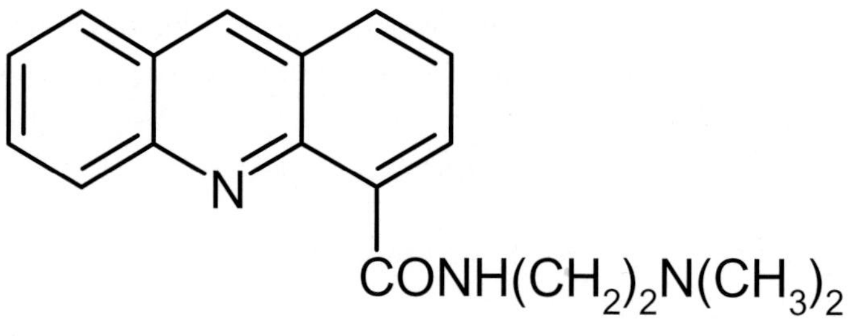

Fig. 2. Chemical structure of DACA.

amide stimulates DNA breakage via formation of cleavable complexes between DNA and topoisomerase I and II *(68, 69)*. Its high activity against experimental solid tumors is thought to stem from this dual interaction with both topoisomerase I and II, as well as its ability to overcome P-glycoprotein and "atypical" (topoisomerase II-mediated) multidrug resistance *(69–72)*. The lipophilicity of DACA together with suppression of ionization of the acridine nitrogen at physiological pH *(68)* were considered attractive distributive properties in regard to the ability to cross the blood–brain barrier to reach brain tumors. Animal studies demonstrated that the pharmacokinetics of DACA were linear up to the maximum tolerated dose in both mice *(73)* and rats *(74)*. Dose-limiting neurotoxicity was observed in mice following intravenous administration of DACA *(73)*, which was thought to be due to the high uptake and retention of DACA and/or DACA metabolites into normal brain *(75, 76)*.

15.1 Positron Emission Tomography Studies in Early Drug Development

On the basis of its novel mechanism of action and promising antitumor activity in preclinical models, DACA was selected for clinical trial under the auspices of the Cancer Research UK Phase I/II trials committee. As part of the drug development process, PET studies were performed preclinically *(76, 77)* and prior to phase I and in conjunction with phase I/II clinical studies in humans, aimed at providing intratumoral and normal tissue distribution data to aid drug development *(78, 79)*. Tumor and normal tissue pharmacokinetics of [^{11}C]DACA were evaluated at tracer concentrations prior to conventional phase I trials (prephase I) in 24 patients and compared with [^{11}C]DACA tracer studies in 5 patients receiving a 3-h infusion of DACA as part of a phase I clinical trial *(78)*. In the prephase I PET studies, a mean [^{11}C]DACA dose of 7.83 µg.m^{-2} was administered corresponding to less than 1/1000 of the phase I starting dose (9 mg. m^{-2}). Paired [^{11}C]DACA PET studies were also performed at tracer doses given alone and on the fourth day in three patients receiving the maximum tolerated phase I dose of DACA (3010 mg.m^{-2}) as a 120-h infusion *(79)*. Tissue perfusion parameters were also calculated after [^{15}O]H$_2$O PET scanning.

15.2 Preclinical Studies with [^{11}C]N-[2-(Dimethylamino)ethyl]acridine-4-carboxamide

The biodistribution and metabolism of [^{11}C]DACA were investigated in rats by plasma sampling, sacrifice experiments with tissue analyses, and imaging using PET scanning *(76)*. Rapid clearance of ^{11}C radioactivity from rat blood, plasma, and major organs was observed. The half-life of ^{11}C radioactivity clearance in rat blood between

15 and 90 min was calculated to be 3.2 h; the levels of [^{11}C]DACA in rat plasma decreased from 69 ± 3% (SD) at 2 min to 29 ± 1.5% at 25 min. A number of radioactive metabolites in rat plasma were observed and one metabolite was identified as the [^{11}C]DACA-N-oxide. Analysis of rat tissues showed rapid and extensive metabolism in tissues, particularly in liver and kidney; however, [^{11}C]DACA (i.e., the parent compound) was the major radioactive component in the lung, heart, and brain over 40 min. PET scanning using [^{11}C]DACA in the rat showed little retention of ^{11}C radioactivity in major organs with rapid excretion via gut and kidney. The rat data were consistent with animal (mouse and rat) preclinical data obtained with preexisting techniques with longer-lived isotopes *(73, 74)*. Most importantly, there were no unexpected interspecies differences in metabolism of DACA that would have indicated that changes should be made in the planned phase I study *(76)*.

15.3 Prephase I and Early Phase I Studies

Prephase I and phase I studies with a 3-h infusion schedule demonstrated that [^{11}C]DACA underwent rapid and extensive metabolism with a greater proportion of unmetabolized [^{11}C]DACA being present in phase I studies. Seven radioactive metabolites were observed in both prephase I and phase I studies as in animal studies *(76, 77)*. Inspection of cumulative PET images showed that the radiotracer was taken up by a number of tumor types (Fig. 3). Together with complementary rodent data that suggest that [^{11}C]DACA is the highest contributor of tumor radioactivity at 5 min and decreased rapidly compared to metabolites *(80)*, it can be inferred that [^{11}C]DACA is taken up

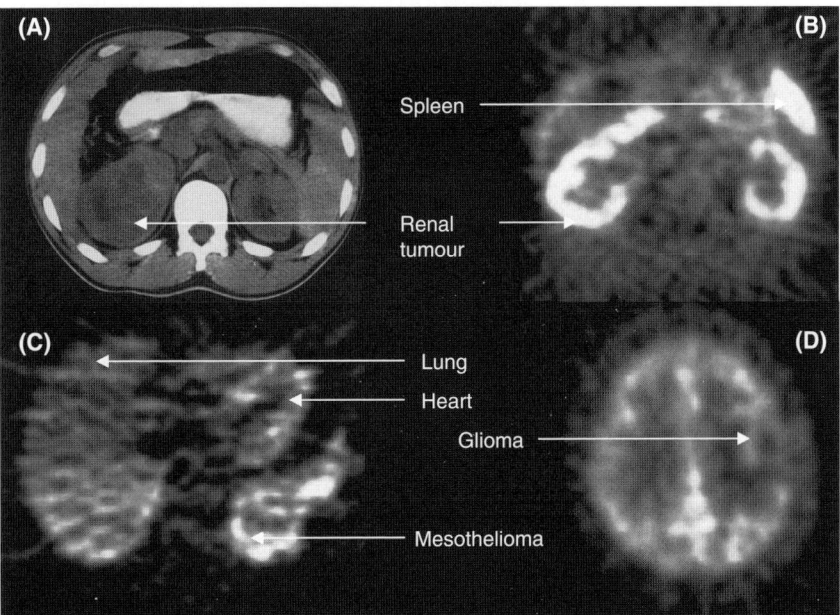

Fig. 3. Typical transabdominal CT scan (A) corresponding to a PET [^{11}C]DACA image (B) demonstrating uptake of the radiotracer in kidneys, spleen, and by the renal tumor. Uptake of the radiotracer is also seen in the heart, myocardium, and another tumor type, mesothelioma, in (C) and into the brain and a glial tumor (D). (*See* color plate.) [Reproduced with permission from *J Clin Oncol* 2001; 19(5):1424, Fig. 2.]

into the tumor. In keeping with the high lipophilicity of DACA and the fact that it is not a substrate for P-glycoprotein, brain uptake was observed (Fig. 3).

Overall, tissue exposure, comprising [^{11}C]DACA and [^{11}C]DACA metabolites, varied between and within tissues. Variability within sampled tissue was much lower compared to variability between patients. Examination of the TACs showed that pharmacokinetics of [^{11}C]DACA and metabolites in normal tissues showed a rapid peak and slower washout with the exception of the liver (Fig. 4). The characteristic profile of liver pharmacokinetics, together with the longer T_{max} and high SUV at 55 min, is indicative of high hepatic turnover and is consistent with its role as the primary tissue respon-

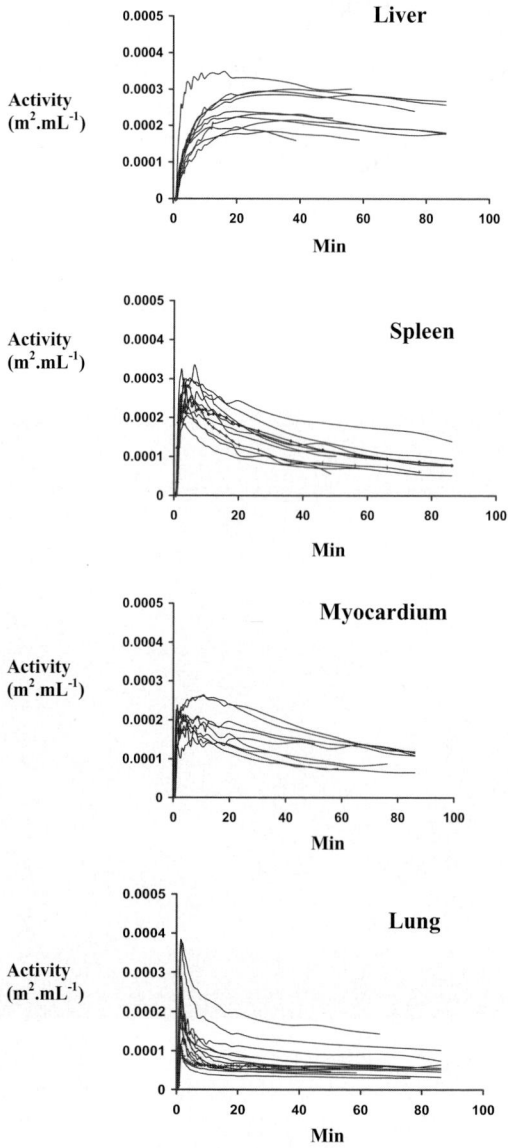

Fig. 4. [^{11}C]*N*-[2-(Dimethylamino)ethyl]acridine-4-carboxamide TACs for liver, spleen, myocardium, and lung in the prephase study group.

Table 2
Area Under the Curve (AUC) and Standardized Uptake Value (SUV) for Normal Tissues and Tumor with [^{11}C]N-[2-(Dimethylamino)ethyl]acridine-4-carboxamide

Tissue	$AUC_{0-60min}$ $(m^2.mL^{-1}.sec)^a$			SUV_{55min} $(\times 10^{-5} m^2.mL^{-1})^a$		
	Prephase I	Phase I	p value	Prephase I	Phase I	p value
Myocardium	0.490 (0.05)^a	0.316 (0.01)	0.04	5.642 (0.55)	2.971 (0.16)	0.004
Lung	0.309 (0.05)	0.219 (0.05)	0.43	4.016 (0.56)	2.376 (0.71)	0.15
Spleen	0.527 (0.05)	0.379 (0.04)	0.06	5.672 (0.60)	3.699 (0.36)	0.01
Liver	0.846 (0.07)	0.688 (0.12)	0.17	13.447 (0.89)	10.100 (1.71)	0.09
Brain	0.152 (0.01)	NC	NC^b	1.746 (0.43)	NC	NC
Vertebra	0.149 (0.01)	0.154 (0.03)	0.91	2.597 (0.38)	2.257 (0.38)	0.91
Kidney	0.275 (0.02)	NC	NC	3.393 (0.51)	NC	NC
Tumor	0.173 (0.02)	0.317 (0.03)	0.02	2.219 (0.23)	3.663 (0.37)	0.02

^{a} Mean (SE).
^{b} NC, not calculated.

sible for the metabolism of DACA *(81)*. Tumor TACs were highly variable in contrast to normal tissue TACs.

Comparison of prephase I and phase I tissue pharmacokinetic parameters demonstrated an overall decrease in C_{max}, AUC, and SUV for all normal tissues analyzed (Table 2). Of these, the decrease was statistically significant *($p < 0.05$)* for spleen (SUV) and myocardium (AUC and SUV) only (Table 2 and Fig. 5). This nonlinearity in splenic and myocardial pharmacokinetics with increasing dose could be due to saturable process

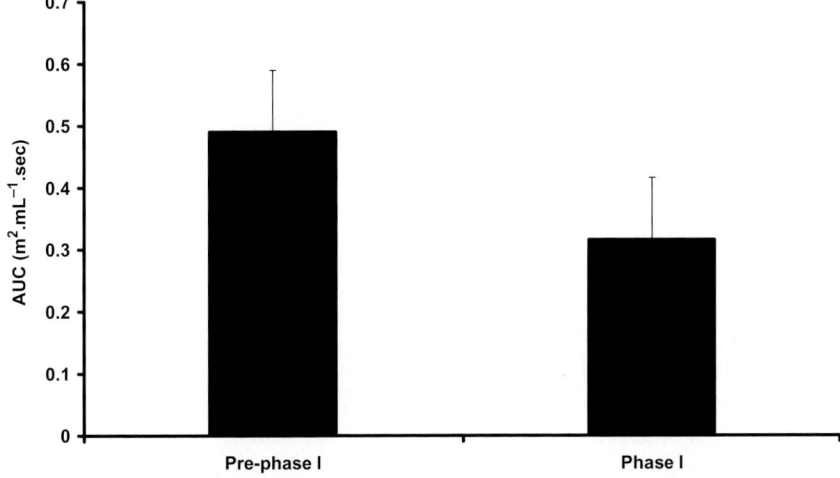

Fig. 5. Saturable myocardial kinetics. A significant decrease in myocardial [^{11}C]DACA AUC was observed when [^{11}C]DACA was administered during a phase I (3h) infusion of DACA.

in drug uptake, tissue binding, or metabolism. In addition, an unusually high uptake of radiotracer observed in the myocardium would alert us to possible cardiovascular side-effects. Dose-limiting pain in the infusion arm and one instance of myocardial ischemia observed in the phase I trial could be a manifestation of the cardiovascular toxicity of DACA, although the mechanism for these effects is unclear *(82, 83)* and a possible relationship would need to be established between tissue concentration and toxicity

The lower uptake of radiotracer in human brain compared to most of the other tissues studied (Table 2) may explain the low incidence of neurological side-effects with DACA *(82, 83)* as lethal neurotoxicity in rodents was attributed to high DACA C_{max} *(84)*. Similarly, the lower AUC and C_{max} observed in the vertebral body compared to other normal tissues analyzed suggested that myelotoxicity was unlikely to be dose limiting, as has been confirmed by further clinical studies *(82, 83)*.

In contrast to what is seen in normal tissues, tumor pharmacokinetic parameters (C_{max}, AUC, SUV) for [^{11}C]DACA and metabolites increased significantly, a finding that could be due in part to the decrease in exposure to normal tissues. *N*-[2-(Dimethyl amino)ethyl]acridine-4-carboxamide did not alter blood flow to normal tissues and tumors. In tumors, moderate but significant correlations were observed for blood flow versus tumor AUC ($r = 0.76$; $p = 0.02$) and blood flow versus SUV ($r = 0.79$; $p = 0.01$) in prephase I studies, emphasizing the importance of drug delivery in uptake and retention in tumors even with lipophilic drugs such as DACA.

15.4 Late Phase I/Phase II Studies

Paired [^{11}C]DACA PET studies performed at tracer doses given alone and during a 120-h infusion at the MTD *(79)* demonstrated an increase in tumor radiotracer exposure (AUC; mean ± SD in $m^2.mL^{-1}.sec$) from 0.209 ± 0.04 when [^{11}C]DACA was given alone compared to 0.242 ± 0.04 ($p < 0.05$) in the combination studies. This increase in tumor exposure would suggest maximal tumor drug levels were not attained at the MTD. It was concluded on the basis of PET findings that although an MTD was reached based on toxicity data, the absence of saturable kinetics in tumor could suggest that it was still possible to reach higher drug concentrations in the tumor, which may be of therapeutic benefit to the patients. However, this may not be practically possible with the current drug regimens, although other dosage regimens need to be explored. In regard to normal tissue toxicity, the TAC profile, C_{max}, and AUC for vertebral body were in the lower range, compared to other normal tissues, predictive of a low incidence of myelotoxicity with the 120-h infusion regimen of DACA, as has been confirmed by the clinical data *(79)*.

These studies with DACA have demonstrated the utility of using PET in early drug development and the invaluable information PET can provide in such situations.

16. 5-FLUOROURACIL

5-Fluorouracil (5-FU) is an antimetabolite widely used in the management of carcinoma of the colon, rectum, breast, stomach, pancreas, and other malignancies. It is currently the most commonly used cytotoxic drug for gastrointestinal malignancies *(85)*. As a single agent given intravenously, 5-FU has limited efficacy in the treatment of advanced colorectal cancer, with response rates less than 14% *(86)*. Attempts to increase the efficacy of 5-FU by biochemical modulation using leucovorin and methotrexate, or by schedule modification by giving it as a continuous infusion, have shown a doubling of tumor response, without a major impact on survival duration *(86–88)*. More recently, combining 5-FU and leucovorin with irinotecan *(89, 90)* or oxaliplatin *(91, 92)* leads to an increase in response rates with a modest improvement in survival in metastatic colorectal cancer compared with 5-FU and leucovorin.

The cytotoxic effects of 5-FU are the result of interference with both RNA and DNA. 5-Fluorouracil is converted intracellularly to 5-fluorouridine triphosphate (FUTP), 5-fluoro-2′-deoxyuridine monophosphate (FdUMP), and 5-fluoro-2′-deoxyuridine triphosphate (FdUTP). Incorporation of FUTP into RNA and FdUMP into DNA as fraudulent bases causes errors in RNA processing and DNA replication, respectively, while FdUMP binds to thymidylate synthetase (TS) with greater affinity than the natural substrate and inhibits production of thymidine monophosphate and, thus, DNA synthesis *(85)*. Up to 80% of administered 5-FU is primarily degraded in the liver by dihydropyrimidine dehydrogenase (DPD) into inactive catabolites, with α-fluoro-β-alanine (FBAL) being the ultimate catabolite.

16.1 Positron Emission Tomography Pharmacokinetic Studies

The ease in the chemical synthesis of 5-[^{18}F]FU *(93, 94)*, and the favorable half-life of fluorine ($t_{1/2}$ 110 min), has made it the most often monitored anticancer drug using PET. Shani and Wolf in 1977 first studied 5-[^{18}F]FU biodistribution in mice, where a direct relationship was found between response and tumor levels of 5-[^{18}F]FU *(95)*. Studies to establish the pharmacokinetics of 5-[^{18}F]FU soon followed in humans initially on a rectilinear scanner *(96)* and later with PET *(97–101)*. Work done by Harte et al. has indicated good reproducibility of PET imaging in 5-[^{18}F]FU kinetic studies and confirmed the utility of PET as a tool to monitor *in vivo* tissue and tumor pharmacokinetics of 5-[^{18}F]FU *(99)*.

Dimitrakopoulou et al. evaluated 50 patients with hepatic metastases from colorectal tumors using PET following intravenous infusion of 5-[^{18}F]FU. They found the highest uptake of radiotracer in liver, with low and highly variable uptake in liver metastases. They also demonstrated a relationship between perfusion, early uptake of 5-[^{18}F]FU at 8 min, and retention at 120 min in a subgroup of metastases *(102)*. A six-compartment model to describe the behavior of 5-[^{18}F]FU based on PET pharmacokinetic studies was soon proposed *(103)*. The same group also assessed the effect of drug delivery by intraarterial and intravenous infusion in 1998 in a similar group of patients. Although they found that intraarterial infusion led to increased 5-[^{18}F]FU influx, the major limiting factor for the low therapeutic effect was the high elimination rate of 5-[^{18}F]FU from the tumor cells *(98)*.

A pharmacodynamic relationship between the tumor uptake of 5-FU and response, first seen in mice (104) and later in humans with MRS studies *(105, 106)*, has also been demonstrated in humans by PET methods *(97, 101)*. These studies have demonstrated that colorectal liver metastases with a higher uptake of 5-[^{18}F]FU at 2 h (trapping), as measured by a greater SUV, responded better with a negative growth rate and increased survival *(97, 101)*.

16.2 Biomodulatory Studies

The biomodulation of tumor and normal tissue 5-[^{18}F]FU pharmacokinetics by *N*-phosphonacetyl-L-aspartate (PALA), folinic acid, and α-interferon has been assessed

(100). Blood flow to the tumor was found to be an important determinant of tumor exposure to total ^{18}F radioactivity (consisting of fluorine-18 radiolabeled 5-FU, anabolites, and catabolites). The importance of drug delivery in the initial uptake and retention of radioactivity uptake was supported by a significant correlation between tumor blood flow and tissue exposure to ^{18}F radioactivity at 8 and 60 min. Blood flow to the tumor, and hence tumor exposure to ^{18}F activity, decreased significantly ($p < 0.05$) after modulation with PALA and a nonsignificant increase in tumor blood flow and AUC was seen with α-interferon. On the other hand, no changes in tumor pharmacokinetics were seen with folinic acid biomodulation *(100)*.

16.3 Proof of Principle Studies

It was felt that the degradation of 5-FU, resulting in the loss of up to 80% of systemically administered drug, could be one reason for the poor response rates observed with 5-FU. Hence, strategies for enhancing the systemic exposure of 5-FU have focused on the catabolic pathway of 5-FU and specifically on modulation of the proximal and rate-limiting catabolic enzyme, dihydropyrimidine dehydrogenase (DPD). Eniluracil completely inhibits DPD catalytic activity in tumors and peripheral blood mononuclear cells *(107)* resulting in an increase in plasma 5-FU half-life and complete oral bioavailability *(108)*. Against this background, an important question for the clinical development of eniluracil was whether DPD inactivation modulated *in vivo* 5-FU pharmacokinetics in tumor and normal tissue in patients. To provide direct evidence of DPD inactivation by eniluracil in tissues, the pharmacokinetics of 5-[^{18}F]FU were compared in six patients who had not received eniluracil and after they had received two schedules of eniluracil including a 4-day course of oral eniluracil and a 28-day combination therapy of oral 5-FU and eniluracil *(109)*.

This study provided several key observations that provided proof of principle for the inactivation of DPD in tissues by eniluracil. First, a significant decrease in image intensity and in AUC of ^{18}F-labeled radioactivity in liver (Fig. 6 and Table 3), the organ with the highest levels of DPD *(110, 111)*, was observed following eniluracil administration. This decrease in uptake in the liver can be attributed to the lack of formation and retention of α-[^{18}F]fluoro-β-alanine *(103, 112)* in the liver with eniluracil. Second, there was a decrease in exposure of ^{18}F-labeled radioactivity in kidneys, which are the route of excretion of FBAL *(113, 114)*, after eniluracil administration, consistent with a lower uptake of [^{18}F]FBAL into kidney parenchymal cells and its elimination. This was supported by very low urinary FBAL levels observed after eniluracil administration in the study. Third, no radiotracer localization was observed in the gallbladder after eniluracil administration, probably due to the lack of [^{18}F]FBAL formation and elimination. The radiotracer localization in the gallbladder without eniluracil treatment is consistent with its role in the elimination of 5-[^{18}F]FU (Fig. 7). Indirect evidence for inactivation of DPD was also provided by the absence of ^{18}F-labeled catabolites in plasma, greatly decreased amounts of total α-fluoro-β-alanine in urine, and an increase in the plasma half-life and plasma AUC of 5-FU after eniluracil also observed in this study *(109)*.

In this study, the value of predicting normal tissue toxicity and tumor response was also investigated. Hematological toxic effects are more common with a 5-FU bolus than with 5-FU continuous infusion *(115)*. Fraile and colleagues *(116)* found that the maximum concentrations of 5-FU in the bone marrow after bolus doses were much higher than that following a continuous infusion and postulated a direct relationship

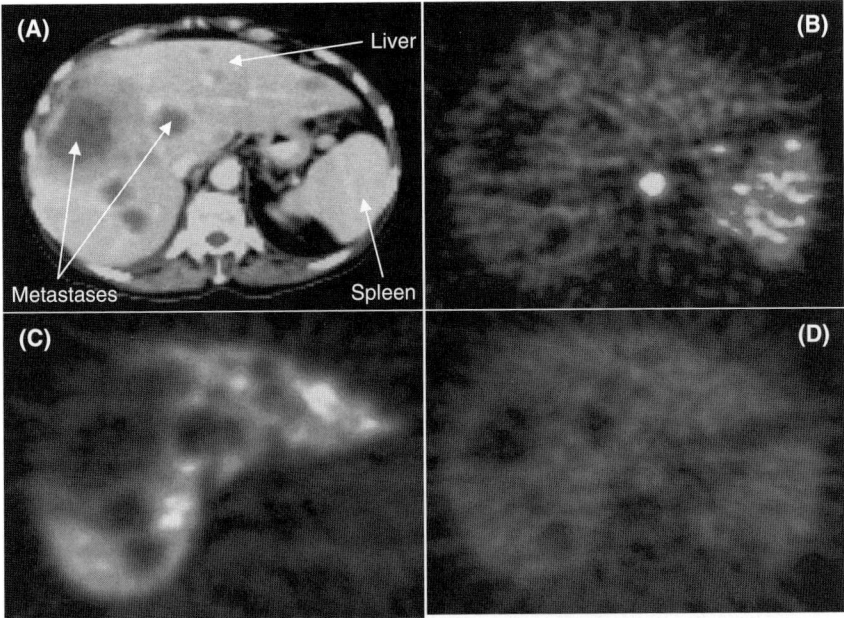

Fig. 6. Typical transabdominal computed tomograph (A) and corresponding PET blood flow (B) and PET 5-[^{18}F]FU images without eniluracil (C) and after eniluracil (D), showing liver, spleen, and multiple hepatic metastases. (*See* color plate.) [Reprinted with permission from Elsevier (*Lancet* 2000;355:2128, Fig. 2.).]

between maximum concentration in bone marrow and myelotoxicity. Maximal 5-FU (equivalent) concentrations achieved after 5-FU/eniluracil treatment in vertebral body (to indicate marrow concentrations) in this study were mean 0.65 µmol.L^{-1} 5-FU equivalent and similar to those previously reported by Fraile and colleagues for continuous infusion 5-FU treatment (of 1000–1100 mg/m^2/day). This finding may explain the low frequency of such effects in other studies with the 28-day dosing schedule *(117, 118)*.

Eniluracil inactivation of DPD did not change blood perfusion in tumors, suggesting that changes in tumor pharmacokinetics of 5-[^{18}F]FU after eniluracil administration

Table 3
Area Under the Curve up to 4 h in Normal Tissues and Tumor after 5-[^{18}F]Fluorouracil[a]

	Mean (SE) AUC_{0-4h} ($m^2.mL^{-1}.sec$)		
	Period 1	*Period 2*	*Period 3*
Liver	1.857 (0.169)	0.927 (0.086)	0.961 (0.137)
Kidney	4.981 (0.926)	1.071 (0.037)	1.096 (0.054)
Spleen	0.345 (0.030)	0.508 (0.042)	0.554 (0.044)
Vertebra	0.230 (0.021)	0.678 (0.258)	0.446 (0.055)
Tumor	0.431 (0.078)	0.543 (0.053)	0.550 (0.030)

[a] Period 1 was in eniluracil-naive patients. In periods 2 and 3, studies were performed after 3 and 27 days of eniluracil.

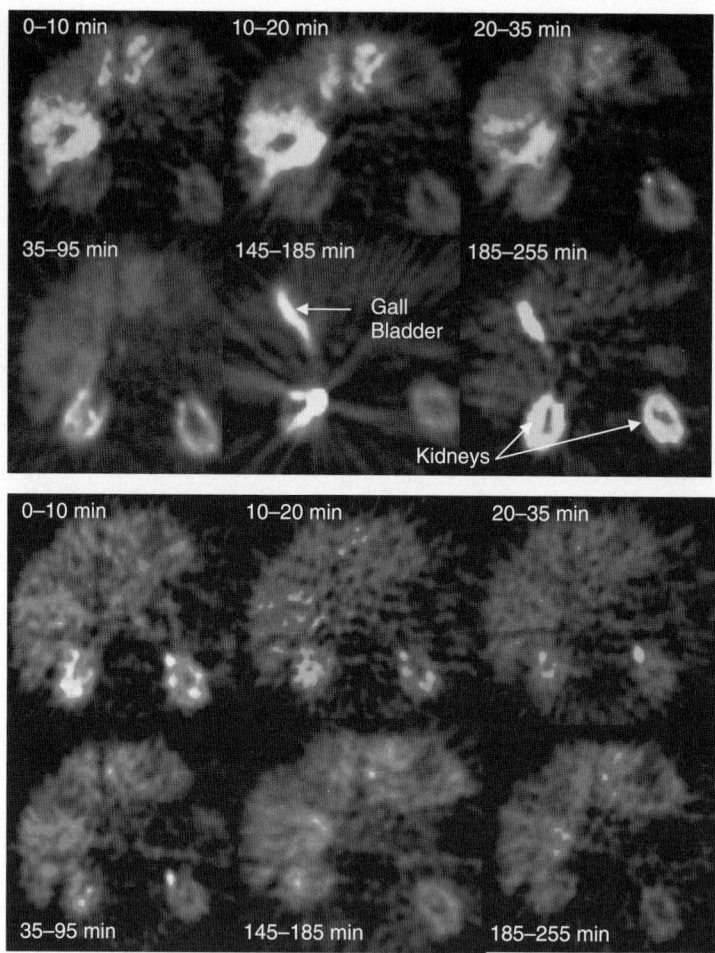

Fig. 7. Temporal representation of drug localization in a selected transabdominal plane passing through the base of the liver. Time frames have been added to provide a composite image between the periods indicated at the bottom of the figures. Upper panel is a dynamic sequence of ^{18}F-labeled tracer obtained when 5-[^{18}F]FU was given without eniluracil. Lower panel is a dynamic sequence of ^{18}F-labeled tracer obtained when 5-[^{18}F]FU was injected with eniluracil. (*See* color plate.) [Reprinted with permission from Elsevier (*Lancet* 2000;355:2128, Fig. 2.).]

were not due to changes in delivery of drug to the tumor. However, tumor perfusion was at least 3- to 4-fold lower in tumors compared to splenic perfusion and the mean fractional volume of distribution (V_d), defined as the fraction of tissue volume into which the [^{15}O]H$_2$O diffuses, was also lower in tumors (0.5) compared to spleen (0.8) and kidney (0.7). This could partly account for the low fluorine-18 radioactivity seen in tumors. It was also found that whereas liver and kidneys showed a decrease in AUC following eniluracil administration, there was no change in tumor AUC. Given the absence of radiolabeled catabolites after eniluracil administration, the data suggest increased tumor exposure to 5-[^{18}F]FU, its anabolites, or both.

In addition to demonstrating the *in vivo* mechanism of action of an enzyme inactivator aimed at enhancing systemic exposure of an anticancer drug in humans, this study

16.4 5-Fluorouracil Tissue Pharmacokinetic Modeling

Although pharmacokinetic data predicted a favorable response to treatment with 5-FU/eniluracil, clinical results using this regimen have been disappointing *(118)*. One reason for the absence of therapeutic benefit could be the poor tumor perfusion observed in the PET study that may result in decreased drug delivery to the tumors. In addition, other tissue factors that may contribute to the efficacy (or lack of efficacy) of 5-FU can be assessed using pharmacokinetic modeling methods. However, the presence of radiolabeled catabolites in tissues and the inability of PET to distinguish between labeled chemical forms of a compound limit the pharmacokinetic information derived from PET studies *(100, 102)*. Attempts to evaluate the contribution of the various chemical forms using compartmental methods have been made, although these are associated with a number of assumptions *(103)*.

The ability to obtain a "pure" 5-FU (plus anabolite) tissue PET signal by blocking catabolism of 5-FU by eniluracil, as described in the previous section, enabled the application of tissue modeling approaches, which have less inherent assumptions *(59, 62)*. This allowed the derivation of a relationship between tissue and plasma 5-FU, from which the tissue contribution of catabolites in the absence of eniluracil and the rate constants for net clearance of 5-FU from plasma into tumor and liver could be calculated.

The contribution of catabolites to tissue data involved derivation of the relationship between plasma 5-[^{18}F]FU levels and tissue response (5-[^{18}F]FU plus ^{18}F-labeled anabolites), referred to as the 5-[^{18}F]FU unit impulse response function (IRF_{FU}). Given that eniluracil completely inhibits 5-[^{18}F]FU catabolism *(107, 109)*, spectral analysis can be used to obtain the following when 5-[^{18}F]FU is injected after eniluracil treatment:

$$[\text{Total tissue}_a](t) = [\text{Plasma 5-FU}](t) \otimes IRF_{FU}(t) \qquad (9)$$

where [Total tissue$_a$] (t) and [Plasma 5-FU] (t) denote the concentration of total radiolabel in tissue and 5-[^{18}F]FU in plasma, respectively, as a function of time, and $\otimes$ is the convolution operator. Total tissue in the presence of eniluracil is 5-[^{18}F]FU plus ^{18}F-labeled anabolites. In the absence of eniluracil, Total tissue also includes ^{18}F-labeled catabolites.

It was assumed that (1) other than catabolism, 5-[^{18}F]FU behaves similarly before and after eniluracil and (2) the amount of catabolites that reaches tumors from circulation is much higher than any catabolites produced by tumor. These assumptions are supported by previous studies *(103, 119, 120)* and from the fact that tumor catabolite profiles follow that of plasma *(109)*. The following equation then holds for the concentration of tissue 5-[^{18}F]FU plus ^{18}F-labeled anabolites ([Tissue 5-FU]):

$$[\text{Tissue 5-FU}](t) = [\text{Plasma 5-FU}](t) \otimes IRF_{FU}(t) \qquad (10)$$

The contribution of tissue catabolites (predominantly [^{18}F]FBAL) can then be derived as follows:

$$[\text{Tissue catabolites}](t) = [\text{Total tissue}_b](t) - [\text{Tissue 5-FU}] \qquad (11)$$

where [Tissue catabolites] (t) and [Total tissue$_b$] (t) denote the tissue concentration of catabolites and total radiolabel in eniluracil-naive patients, respectively, as a function of time.

Deconvolution of tissue data (Figs. 8 and 9) was achieved by a spectral analysis algorithm as previously described *(59)*. Figure 8A and B shows representative plasma input function and corresponding TACs for liver metastases in a patient. This relationship between plasma input function and corresponding tissue output activity (IRF$_{FU}$) was calculated from these curves using Eq. (8) and is illustrated as a spectrum of kinetic components in Fig. 8C and as a curve in Fig. 8D. The spectra in Fig. 8C consist of a number of components, with different frequencies. Kinetic components with high frequency that lie close to or coincident with the upper level of the predefined range [$\beta = 1$ sec^{-1}, log (β) = 0] are due either to rapid transit times of the tracer in the vasculature or to the dispersion of blood counts measured online. The intermediate and low-frequency components of the spectrum reflect the extravascular behavior of the tracer such as tissue retention and subsequent release of tracer. If the lowest frequency component is coincident with or close to the limit set by the decay constant for the isotope [for ^{18}F, $\beta = 0.0001053$ sec^{-1}, log (β) = -4], then irreversible or near irreversible trapping of tracer is indicated. The sums of these spectral components (ignoring the high frequency component when present) in Fig. 8C, after correction for radioactive decay of the isotope (^{18}F), are plotted as a unit impulse response function of the metastases to tracer in the plasma in Fig. 8D. Figure 9 illustrates the result of deconvolution and the individual TACs for total radioactivity, radiolabeled parent and anabolites, and radiolabeled catabolites are plotted.

In contrast to metabolite uncorrected data *(109)*, the AUC$_{0-95\,min}$ was significantly different between eniluracil-treated and eniluracil-naive patients not only for liver but also for tumor ($p<0.05$). This confirmed a higher tumor exposure to 5-[^{18}F]FU/anabolites after inactivation of DPD by eniluracil. After DPD inactivation by eniluracil a 7-fold increase in tumor exposure to 5-[^{18}F]FU/anabolites was observed. Mean (SE) AUC$_{0-95\,min}$ (m^2.mL^{-1}.sec) values for tumor prior to and after eniluracil were 0.034 (0.004) and 0.247 (0.019), respectively *(55)*. The percentage of catabolites in liver and tumor up to 95 min in eniluracil-naive patients was 95% and 83%, respectively *(55)*. In Fig. 9C, the tissue levels of ^{18}F-labeled catabolites appear to follow that of the plasma input function supporting the assertion that tumor catabolites are derived predominantly from circulating catabolites. Tumor AUC was calculated between 0 and 95 min only, since continuous arterial sampling was not performed beyond 95 min, and hence it was possible to derive an input function between 0 and 95 min only for modeling purposes.

The tissue 5-[^{18}F]FU signal after eniluracil administration (which contains no catabolites) was used to calculate the net unidirectional extraction of 5-[^{18}F]FU into tumors using Patlak analysis *(62)*. Although the presence of a linear phase of the curve (Fig. 10A and B) indicated that unidirectional uptake of 5-[^{18}F]FU occurred in tumors, the magnitude of uptake was low. The mean K_I (mL plasma.mL tissue^{-1}.min^{-1}) for 5-[^{18}F]FU extraction by tumors (0.0036) was 8-fold less than that for fluorodeoxyglucose (0.0295) in a tumor with a standardized uptake value of 12 (Fig. 10C). For comparison, the initial (up to 10 min) extraction and trapping of 5-[^{18}F]FU through catabolism by the liver in eniluracil-naive patients (Fig. 10D) was 205-fold higher with a mean K_I of 0.738 mL plasma.mL tissue^{-1}.min^{-1}. These data provide very strong evidence to suggest

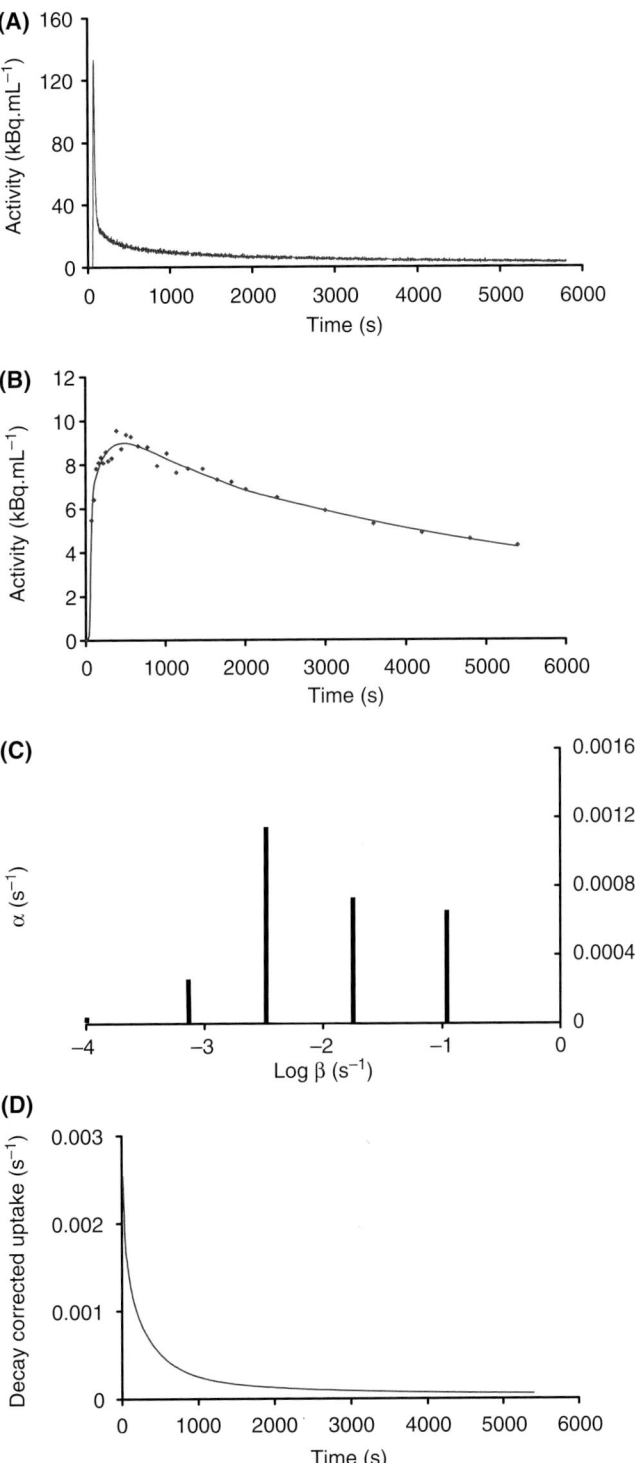

Fig. 8. Spectral analysis of tumor data for a patient. (A) Arterial plasma input function after intravenous injection of 5-[^{18}F]FU. (B) Corresponding time–activity curve for a liver metastasis showing line of best fit. (C) Tumor unit impulse response function displayed as a spectrum of kinetic components. (D) Tumor unit impulse response function displayed as a curve. [Reproduced with permission from *Cancer Research* 2001;61:4939, Fig. 3.]

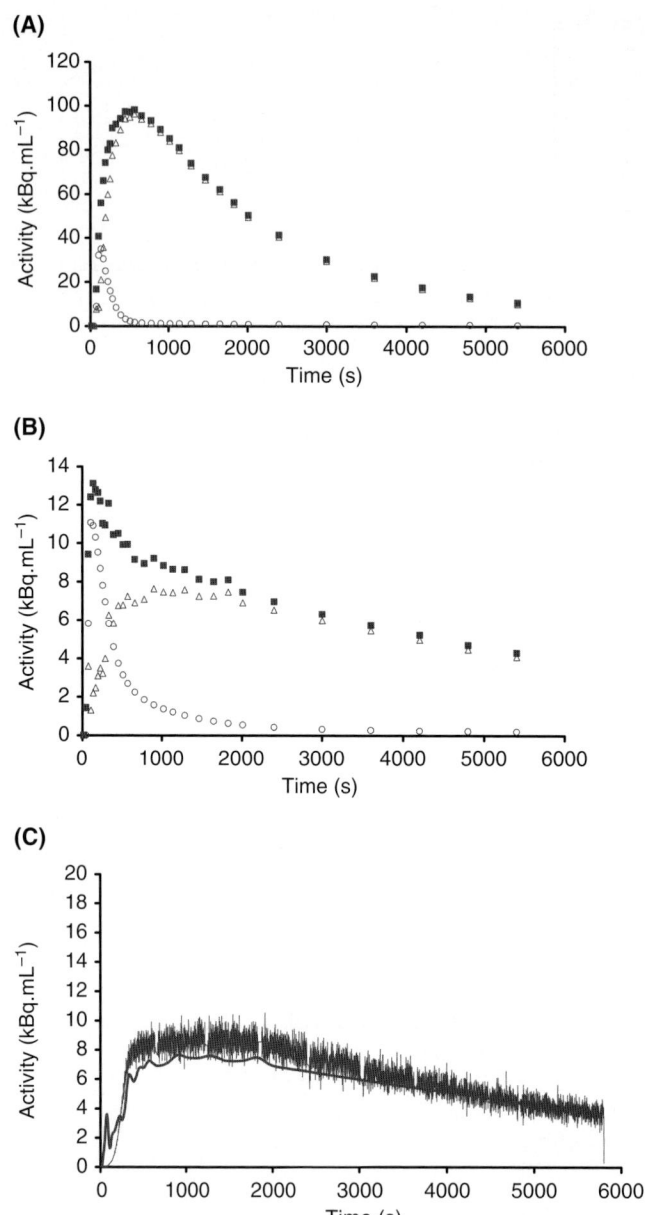

Fig. 9. Deconvolution of total tissue radioactivity data (■) into catabolites (Δ) and parent plus anabolites (○) components for (A) tumor and (B) liver of a patient. (C) Comparison of activity–time curves for catabolites in plasma (wavy line) and tumor (solid line). Tumor catabolite levels followed plasma levels. [Reproduced with permission from *Cancer Research* 2001;61:4939, Fig. 4.]

that the low efficacy of 5-FU could be attributable, in part, to the low net clearance of 5-FU by tumors (K_I = 0.0036 ± 0.0005 mL plasma.mL tissue^{-1}.min^{-1}) *(55)*.

In conclusion, the blocking of 5-FU catabolism by eniluracil allowed the magnitude of 5-[^{18}F]FU catabolism to be determined and allowed unidirectional extraction of 5-[^{18}F]FU by tumor and liver in patients. These have confirmed the extensive presence

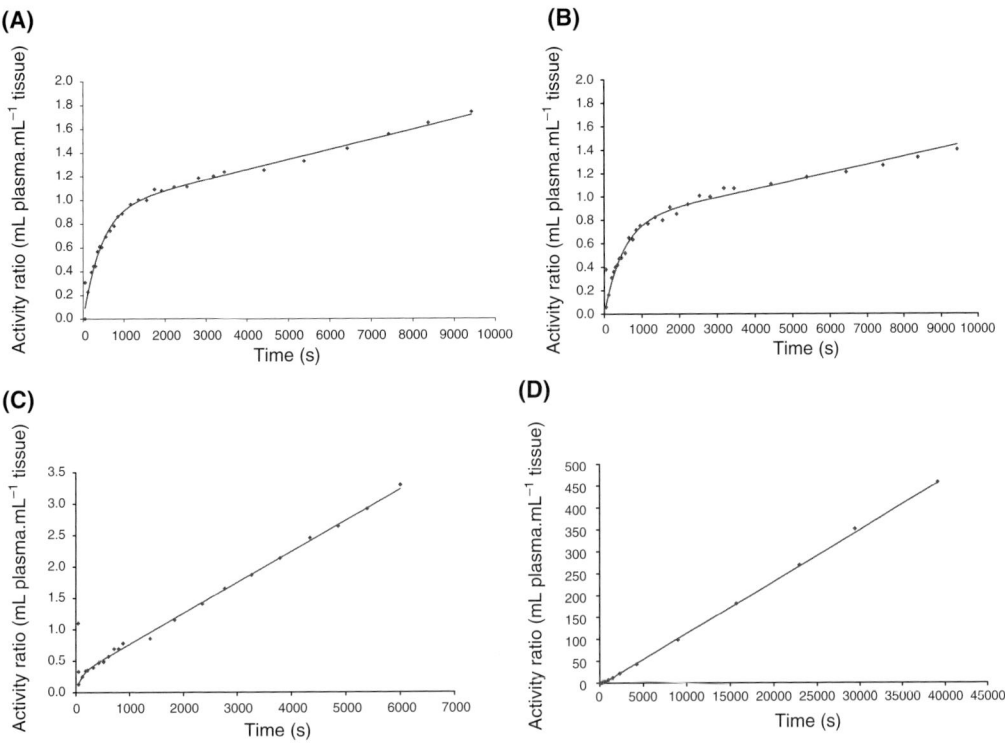

Fig. 10. Results of Patlak analysis showing unidirectional uptake. (A and B) Data from two metastatic regions within the liver of a patient in whom catabolism of 5-FU was inhibited by eniluracil and line of best fit. The presence of a linear phase of the curve indicates unidirectional uptake. (C) For comparison, Patlak fluorodeoxyglucose data from another patient with a cerebral tumor and a standardized uptake value of 12 and (D) initial (up to 10 min) uptake by liver of catabolites in a patient whose catabolism was not inhibited and line of best fit for the same patient. Parent 5-[^{18}F]FU and ^{18}F-labeled anabolite radioactivity were removed from the total liver radioactivity data.

of noncytotoxic 5-FU catabolites in the tumor and limited extraction of 5-[^{18}F]FU by tumors. The low uptake of 5-FU by tumors as well as the low systemic availability due to hepatic catabolism may compromise the cytotoxicity of 5-FU. It is therefore likely that biomodulators that may influence these properties in addition to agents that are likely to improve tumor drug delivery may add to the efficacy of 5-FU.

17. TEMOZOLOMIDE

Temozolomide is an alkylating agent of the imidazo[5,1-*d*]-1,2,3,5-tetrazine series *(121)* and is structurally related to the antimelanoma drug dacarbazine; both agents require conversion to 5-(3-methyltriazen-1-yl)imidazole-4-carboxamide (MTIC) for their clinical activity. It has good oral bioavailability *(122)* and unlike 5-(3,3-dimethyltriazen-1-yl)imidazole-4-carboximide (DTIC), which requires metabolic activation to MTIC in the liver, the conversion of temozolomide to MTIC is postulated to be spontaneous and pH dependent *(123)*. Temozolomide has demonstrated significant activity against gliomas *(124, 125)*, malignant melanomas *(126)*, and pediatric solid tumors *(127)*. The most commonly employed dosage regimen is 200 mg.m^{-2} daily for 5 days, once every 28 days. The main adverse effect is myelosuppression, which does not appear to be cumulative in nature. Other schedules such as the extended continuous oral schedule have also been evaluated *(128)*.

17.1 [¹¹C]Temozolomide Positron Emission Tomography Studies

Positron emission tomography studies have been conducted with a tracer dose of temozolomide labeled in the *3-N-methyl* positions. It has been found that tumor exposure to carbon-11-labeled temozolomide was significantly higher ($p < 0.001$) compared to normal brain *(129)*. A pharmacodynamic relationship was also established, with response to temozolomide in recurrent high-grade gliomas being related to tumor drug concentration *(130)*.

It has been proposed that temozolomide undergoes decarboxylation and ring opening to form MTIC, which is further fragmented to produce the highly reactive methyldiazonium ion that alkylates DNA (Fig. 11). Temozolomide is robustly stable under acid conditions, but the rate of degradation increases rapidly on passing through neutral to basic pH *(131)*. This pH-dependent activation of temozolomide may provide an important basis of targeted therapy directed toward tumors (such as gliomas) that are known to have a higher pH compared to surrounding brain tissue *(132)*.

The *in vivo* mechanism of action of temozolomide was investigated using PET by using a dual labeling strategy. Paired PET studies were performed after injection of [¹¹C]temozolomide radiolabeled in two different positions: at the *4-carbonyl* and *3-N-methyl* positions of the molecule. It was hypothesized that if the proposed mechanism of action was true, then ring opening of [¹¹C]temozolomide at the 3–4 position would

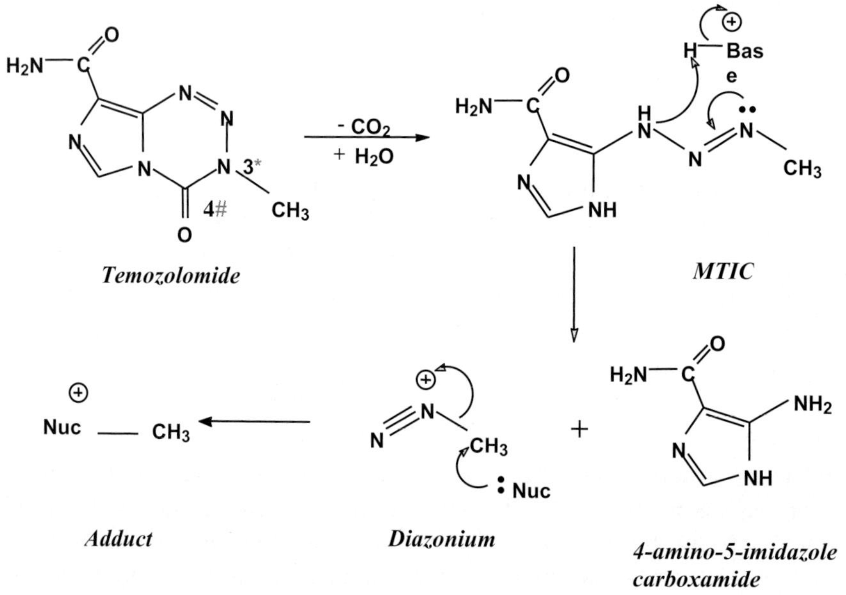

Fig. 11. Mechanism of action of temozolomide. It was postulated that radiolabel in the *3-N-methyl* (*) position of temozolomide would be retained ultimately by the alkylating species after ring opening of temozolomide. On the other hand, the radiolabel in the *4-carbonyl* (#) position will become converted to [¹¹C]carbon dioxide, which can be detected in the exhaled air and plasma.

lead to the formation of $[^{11}C]CO_2$ with $[4-^{11}C\text{-}carbonyl]$temozolomide, whereas with $[3\text{-}N\text{-}^{11}C\text{-}methyl]$temozolomide the label will ultimately be incorporated into DNA (Fig. 11). Spectral analysis was used to elucidate the contribution of $[^{11}C]CO_2$ to the tissue image. This required an additional PET study after the injection of carbon-11-radiolabeled bicarbonate (which rapidly equilibrates with $[^{11}C]CO_2$ in blood aided by carbonic anhydrase in red blood cells) to derive a relationship between plasma and tissue $[^{11}C]CO_2$. It was therefore possible to deduce tissue pharmacokinetics of $[^{11}C]$temozolomide with both $[3\text{-}N\text{-}^{11}C\text{-}methyl]$temozolomide and $[4\text{-}^{11}C\text{-}carbonyl]$temozolomide.

In addition, to ascertain if temozolomide possessed tumor specificity, any differential in the chemical conversion of temozolomide in tumor compared to plasma and normal tissue was evaluated. It was postulated that if the hypothetical mechanism of chemical breakdown of temozolomide was true, then the generation of $[^{11}C]CO_2$ after administration of $[4\text{-}^{11}C\text{-}carbonyl]$temozolomide would be indicative of the ring opening of $[^{11}C]$temozolomide and the amount of $[^{11}C]CO_2$ generated would enable quantification of the total ring opening in the body for the scan duration (90 min).

Ring opening over 90 min was therefore derived after administration of $[4\text{-}^{11}C\text{-}carbonyl]$temozolomide from the ratio of total $[^{11}C]$temozolomide activity to the total ^{11}C-labeled tracer activity [Eq. (12)] and expressed as the percentage of ring opening ($\times 100\ \%$):

$$\text{Ring opening over 90 min} = 1 - \frac{\text{AUC}_{0-90}\,[^{11}C]\text{temozolomide}}{\text{AUC}_{0-90}\,[^{11}C]\text{total tracer}} \qquad (12)$$

Thus if there were no ring opening, then all the activity over 90 min in the $[4\text{-}^{11}C\text{-}carbonyl]$ temozolomide scan would be from $[^{11}C]$temozolomide. Using this method, ring opening over 90 min was calculated in plasma, normal tissue, and tumor. This method assumes that breakdown of temozolomide occurs only by ring opening at the 3–4 position, with decarboxylation resulting in the generation of $[^{11}C]CO_2$ from the radiolabeled carbon atom in the C-4 position. The methodology used to determine ring opening in tissues has a potential drawback in that it reflects both tissue-specific decarboxylation and influx of $[^{11}C]$temozolomide and $[^{11}C]CO_2$ from the bloodstream. Further, the calculation of the tissue metabolite correction is dependent on the method of analysis, which in the past has proven to be robust *(53)*.

A number of PET tissue data confirmed the postulated mechanism of action of temozolomide. First, a 5-fold higher amount of exhaled $[^{11}C]CO_2$ was sampled with $[4\text{-}^{11}C\text{-}carbonyl]$temozolomide administration. Second, a significant concentration of plasma $[^{11}C]CO_2$ was detected with $[4\text{-}^{11}C\text{-}carbonyl]$emozolomide in contrast to small quantities of $[^{11}C]CO_2$ detected in plasma with $[3\text{-}N\text{-}^{11}C\text{-}methyl]$temozolomide. Third, a decrease in tissue exposure ($\text{AUC}_{0-90\,\text{min}}$) to $[^{11}C]$temozolomide was observed with $[4\text{-}^{11}C\text{-}carbonyl]$temozolomide compared to $[3\text{-}N\text{-}^{11}C\text{-}methyl]$temozolomide, indicating the loss of radiolabel as $[^{11}C]CO_2$. Of potential therapeutic value in the clinical efficacy of temozolomide was the higher tumor exposure ($\text{AUC}_{0-90\,\text{min}}$) seen with temozolomide and total radiotracer compared to surrounding normal tissue *(133)*. The higher $\text{AUC}_{0-90\,\text{min}}$ observed for $[^{11}C]$temozolomide in tumors compared to white and gray matter may provide a beneficial therapeutic index that may account for the clinical efficacy of temozolomide seen in gliomas *(124)*. It is worth noting that the higher $\text{AUC}_{0-90\,\text{min}}$ seen

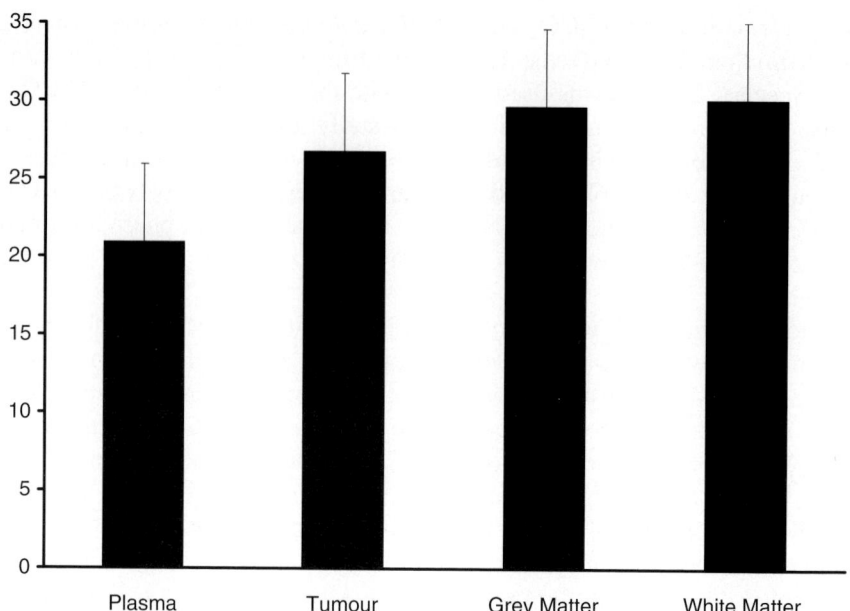

Fig. 12. Percentage ring opening of temozolomide. The ring opening in tissue was greater than in plasma ($p < 0.05$), but there was no difference in ring opening between tumor and normal brain.

in brain tumors compared to normal brain may be related to a compromised blood–brain barrier and hence higher delivery, rather than to retention of temozolomide.

Having confirmed the mechanism of breakdown of temozolomide, it was then necessary to determine if there was a differential in ring opening between plasma, normal tissue, and tumor that may represent a targeted method of drug action in the tumor. If such a differential existed this would lend some support to the original hypothesis on temozolomide metabolism in which it was proposed that metabolic conversion occurred in DNA *(131)*. In this study, the percentage ring opening in plasma over 90 min (20.89%) was less ($p < 0.05$) than that observed in tumor (26.78%), gray matter (29.70%), and white matter (30.13%) (Fig. 12). There were, however, no differences in the amount of observed ring opening between tumor and normal tissues ($p > 0.05$) *(133)*. The absence of a difference in ring opening between tumors and normal tissue suggested that the ring opening of temozolomide was tissue specific but not tumor specific.

In summary, PET pharmacokinetic studies confirm the *in vivo* mechanism of action of temozolomide. In addition, they confirm a higher exposure to temozolomide in tumors compared to normal brain. However, it does not confirm that the ring opening of temozolomide occurs preferentially in tumors compared to normal tissue *(133)*.

18. SUMMARY

Knowledge of drug pharmacokinetics is invaluable in the assessment and development of anticancer agents. In addition to plasma pharmacokinetic parameters, *in vivo* normal tissue and tumor information can be provided by PET. Specifically, PET pharmacokinetic studies can provide information on drug access, kinetics, and drug concentration in tumors and normal tissues, all of which have a bearing on drug activity, tissue toxicity, and drug scheduling. In addition, such studies can provide proof of principle of the *in vivo* mechanism of drug action and *in vivo* targeting of molecular therapeutic targets.

REFERENCES

1. Teorell T. Kinetics of distribution of substances administered to the body. I: The extravascular modes of administration. *Arch Int Pharmacodynam* 1937;57:205–225.
2. Teorell T. Kinetics of distribution of substances administered to the body. II: The intravascular modes of administration. *Arch Int Pharmacodynam* 1937;57:226–240.
3. Pond SM, Tozer TN. First-pass elimination. Basic concepts and clinical consequences. 1984; 9(1):1–25.
4. Laurence DR, Bennett PN, Brown MJ. General pharmacology. In: Clinical Pharmacology, 8th ed. Edinburgh: Churchill Livingstone, 1997.
5. Ayrton A, Morgan P. Role of transport proteins in drug absorption, distribution and excretion. *Xenobiotica* 2001;31(8–9):469–497.
6. Sitar DS. Human drug metabolism in vivo. *Pharmacol Ther* 1989;43(3):363–375.
7. Meyer UA, Zanger UM, Skoda RC, Grant D, Blum M. Genetic polymorphisms of drug metabolism. *Prog Liver Dis* 1990;9:307–323.
8. Diasio RB, Beavers TL, Carpenter JT. Familial deficiency of dihydropyrimidine dehydrogenase. Biochemical basis for familial pyrimidinemia and severe 5-fluorouracil-induced toxicity. *J Clin Invest* 1988;81(1):47–51.
9. Desmeules J, Gascon MP, Dayer P, Magistris M. Impact of environmental and genetic factors on codeine analgesia. *Eur J Clin Pharmacol* 1991;41(1):23–26.
10. Idle JR, Armstrong M, Boddy AV, *et al.* The pharmacogenetics of chemical carcinogenesis. *Pharmacogenetics* 1992;2(6):246–258.
11. Kintzel PE, Dorr RT. Anticancer drug renal toxicity and elimination: Dosing guidelines for altered renal function. *Cancer Treat Rev* 1995;21(1):33–64.
12. LeBlanc GA. Hepatic vectorial transport of xenobiotics. *Chem Biol Interact* 1994;90(2):101–120.
13. Gibaldi M, Koup JR. Pharmacokinetic concepts—drug binding, apparent volume of distribution and clearance. *Eur J Clin Pharmacol* 1981;20(4):299–305.
14. Ratain MJ. Pharmacology of cancer chemotherapy. In: DeVita VT, Hellman S, Rosenberg SA, eds. Cancer: Principles and Practice of Oncology, 5th ed. Philadelphia: Lippincott-Raven, 1997: 375–385.
15. Riegelman S, Loo J, Rowland M. Concept of a volume of distribution and possible errors in evaluation of this parameter. *J Pharm Sci* 1968;57(1):128–133.
16. D'Argenio DZ, Schumitzky A. A program package for simulation and parameter estimation in pharmacokinetic systems. *Comput Programs Biomed* 1979;9(2):115–134.
17. Weiner DL. NONLIN84/PCNONLIN: Software for the statistical analysis of nonlinear models. *Methods Find Exp Clin Pharmacol* 1986;8(10):625–628.
18. Yamaoka K, Nakagawa T, Uno T. Statistical moments in pharmacokinetics. *J Pharmacokinet Biopharm* 1978;6(6):547–558.
19. Cutler DJ. Theory of the mean absorption time, an adjunct to conventional bioavailability studies. *J Pharm Pharmacol* 1978;30(8):476–478.
20. Yeh KC, Kwan KC. A comparison of numerical integrating algorithms by trapezoidal, Lagrange, and spline approximation. *J Pharmacokinet Biopharm* 1978;6(1):79–98.
21. Kobayashi K, Jodrell DI, Ratain MJ. Pharmacodynamic-pharmacokinetic relationships and therapeutic drug monitoring. *Cancer Surv* 1993;17:51–78.
22. Stoller RG, Hande KR, Jacobs SA, Rosenberg SA, Chabner BA. Use of plasma pharmacokinetics to predict and prevent methotrexate toxicity. *N Engl J Med* 1977;297(12):630–634.
23. Monjanel S, Rigault JP, Cano JP, Carcassonne Y, Favre R. High-dose methotrexate: Preliminary evaluation of a pharmacokinetic approach. *Cancer Chemother Pharmacol* 1979;3(3):189–196.
24. Calvert AH, Newell DR, Gumbrell LA, *et al.* Carboplatin dosage: Prospective evaluation of a simple formula based on renal function. *J Clin Oncol* 1989;7(11):1748–1756.

25. Newell DR, Siddik ZH, Gumbrell LA, et al. Plasma free platinum pharmacokinetics in patients treated with high dose carboplatin. *Eur J Cancer Clin Oncol* 1987;23(9):1399–1405.
26. Chou TC. Derivation and properties of Michaelis-Menten type and Hill type equations for reference ligands. *J Theor Biol* 1976;59(2):253–276.
27. Drewinko B, Roper PR, Barlogie B. Patterns of cell survival following treatment with antitumor agents in vitro. *Eur J Cancer* 1979;15(1):93–99.
28. Wagner JG. Kinetics of pharmacologic response. I. Proposed relationships between response and drug concentration in the intact animal and man. *J Theor Biol* 1968;20(2):173–201.
29. Reece PA, Stafford I, Russell J, Khan M, Gill PG. Creatinine clearance as a predictor of ultrafilterable platinum disposition in cancer patients treated with cisplatin: Relationship between peak ultrafilterable platinum plasma levels and nephrotoxicity. *J Clin Oncol* 1987;5(2):304–309.
30. Grochow LB, Jones RJ, Brundrett RB, et al. Pharmacokinetics of busulfan: Correlation with venoocclusive disease in patients undergoing bone marrow transplantation. *Cancer Chemother Pharmacol* 1989;25(1):55–61.
31. Egorin MJ, Van Echo DA, Tipping SJ, et al. Pharmacokinetics and dosage reduction of cis-diamine(1,1-cyclobutanedicarboxylato)platinum in patients with impaired renal function. *Cancer Res* 1984; 44(11):5432–5438.
32. Newell DR, Pearson AD, Balmanno K, et al. Carboplatin pharmacokinetics in children: The development of a pediatric dosing formula. The United Kingdom Children's Cancer Study Group. *J Clin Oncol* 1993;11(12):2314–2323.
33. Jodrell DI, Egorin MJ, Canetta RM, et al. Relationships between carboplatin exposure and tumor response and toxicity in patients with ovarian cancer. *J Clin Oncol* 1992;10(4):520–528.
34. Ackland SP, Ratain MJ, Vogelzang NJ, Choi KE, Ruane M, Sinkule JA. Pharmacokinetics and pharmacodynamics of long-term continuous-infusion doxorubicin. *Clin Pharmacol Ther* 1989; 45(4):340–347.
35. Extra JM, Rousseau F, Bruno R, Clavel M, Le Bail N, Marty M. Phase I and pharmacokinetic study of Taxotere (RP 56976; NSC 628503) given as a short intravenous infusion. *Cancer Res* 1993;53(5):1037–1042.
36. Kunitoh H, Watanabe K. Phase I/II and pharmacologic study of long-term continuous infusion etoposide combined with cisplatin in patients with advanced non-small-cell lung cancer. *J Clin Oncol* 1994;12(1):83–89.
37. Santini J, Milano G, Thyss A, et al. 5-FU therapeutic monitoring with dose adjustment leads to an improved therapeutic index in head and neck cancer. *Br J Cancer* 1989;59(2):287–290.
38. Vokes EE, Mick R, Kies MS, et al. Pharmacodynamics of fluorouracil-based induction chemotherapy in advanced head and neck cancer. *J Clin Oncol* 1996;14(5):1663–1671.
39. Thyss A, Milano G, Renee N, Vallicioni J, Schneider M, Demard F. Clinical pharmacokinetic study of 5-FU in continuous 5-day infusions for head and neck cancer. *Cancer Chemother Pharmacol* 1986;16(1):64–66.
40. Milano G, Etienne MC, Renee N, et al. Relationship between fluorouracil systemic exposure and tumor response and patient survival. *J Clin Oncol* 1994;12(6):1291–1295.
41. Canal P, Gay C, Dezeuze A, et al. Pharmacokinetics and pharmacodynamics of irinotecan during a phase II clinical trial in colorectal cancer. Pharmacology and Molecular Mechanisms Group of the European Organization for Research and Treatment of Cancer. *J Clin Oncol* 1996; 14(10):2688–2695.
42. Mick R, Gupta E, Vokes EE, Ratain MJ. Limited-sampling models for irinotecan pharmacokinetics-pharmacodynamics: Prediction of biliary index and intestinal toxicity. *J Clin Oncol* 1996; 14(7):2012–2019.
43. Evans WE, Crom WR, Abromowitch M, et al. Clinical pharmacodynamics of high-dose methotrexate in acute lymphocytic leukemia. Identification of a relation between concentration and effect. *N Engl J Med* 1986;314(8):471–477.
44. Gianni L, Kearns CM, Giani A, et al. Nonlinear pharmacokinetics and metabolism of paclitaxel and its pharmacokinetic/pharmacodynamic relationships in humans. *J Clin Oncol* 1995;13(1):180–190.
45. Ratain MJ, Vogelzang NJ. Phase I and pharmacological study of vinblastine by prolonged continuous infusion. *Cancer Res* 1986;46(9):4827–4830.
46. Desai ZR, Van den Berg HW, Bridges JM, Shanks RG. Can severe vincristine neurotoxicity be prevented? *Cancer Chemother Pharmacol* 1982;8(2):211–214.

47. Saleem A, Aboagye EO, Price PM. In vivo monitoring of drugs using radiotracer techniques. *Adv Drug Deliv Rev* 2000;41(1):21–39.
48. Mintun MA, Welch MJ, Siegel BA, *et al.* Breast cancer: PET imaging of estrogen receptors. *Radiology* 1988;169(1):45–48.
49. Metzler CM, Tong DD. Computational problems of compartment models with Michaelis-Menten-type elimination. *J Pharm Sci* 1981;70(7):733–737.
50. Zasadny KR, Wahl RL. Standardized uptake values of normal tissues at PET with 2-[fluorine-18]-fluoro-2-deoxy-D-glucose: Variations with body weight and a method for correction. *Radiology* 1993;189(3):847–850.
51. Kim CK, Gupta NC, Chandramouli B, Alavi A. Standardized uptake values of FDG: Body surface area correction is preferable to body weight correction. *J Nucl Med* 1994;35(1):164–167.
52. Kety SS, Schmidt CF. The nitrous oxide method for quantitative determination of cerebral blood flow in man; theory, procedure and normal values. *J Clin Invest* 1948;27:476–483.
53. Gunn RN, Yap JT, Wells P, *et al.* A general method to correct PET data for tissue metabolites using a dual-scan approach. *J Nucl Med* 2000;41(4):706–711.
54. Blasberg RG, Roelcke U, Weinreich R, *et al.* Imaging brain tumor proliferative activity with [124I]iododeoxyuridine. *Cancer Res* 2000;60(3):624–635.
55. Aboagye EO, Saleem A, Cunningham VJ, Osman S, Price PM. Extraction of 5-fluorouracil by tumor and liver: A noninvasive positron emission tomography study of patients with gastrointestinal cancer. *Cancer Res* 2001;61(13):4937–4941.
56. Pedersen F, Bergstrom M, Bengtsson E, Langstrom B. Principal component analysis of dynamic positron emission tomography images. *Eur J Nucl Med* 1994;21(12):1285–1292.
57. O'Sullivan F, Muzi M, Graham MM, Spence A. Parametric imaging by mixture analysis in 3D validation for dual-tracer glucose studies. In: Myers R, Cunningham VJ, Bailey DL, Jones T, eds. Quantification of Brain Function Using PET. San Diego: Academic Press, 1996:297–300.
58. Yap JT, Cooper M, Chen CT, Cunningham VJ. Generation of parametric images using factor analysis. In: Myers R, Cunningham VJ, Bailey DL, Jones T, eds. Quantification of Brain Function Using PET. San Diego: Academic Press, 1996:292–296.
59. Cunningham VJ, Jones T. Spectral analysis of dynamic PET studies. *J Cereb Blood Flow Metab* 1993;13(1):15–23.
60. Rutland MD. A single injection technique for subtraction of blood background in 131I-hippuran renograms. *Br J Radiol* 1979;52(614):134–137.
61. Gjedde A. Calculation of cerebral glucose phosphorylation from brain uptake of glucose analogs in vivo: A re-examination. *Brain Res* 1982;257(2):237–74.
62. Patlak CS, Blasberg RG, Fenstermacher JD. Graphical evaluation of blood-to-brain transfer constants from multiple-time uptake data. *J Cereb Blood Flow Metab* 1983;3(1):1–7.
63. Tobler HJ, Engel G. Affinity spectra: A novel way for the evaluation of equilibrium binding experiments. *Naunyn Schmiedebergs Arch Pharmacol* 1983;322(3):183–192.
64. Meikle SR, Matthews JC, Brock CS, *et al.* Pharmacokinetic assessment of novel anti-cancer drugs using spectral analysis and positron emission tomography: A feasibility study. *Cancer Chemother Pharmacol* 1998;42(3):183–193.
65. Ginos JZ, Cooper AJ, Dhawan V, *et al.* [13N]cisplatin PET to assess pharmacokinetics of intra-arterial versus intravenous chemotherapy for malignant brain tumors. *J Nucl Med* 1987;28(12):1844–1852.
66. Tyler JL, Yamamoto YL, Diksic M, *et al.* Pharmacokinetics of superselective intra-arterial and intravenous [11C]BCNU evaluated by PET. *J Nucl Med* 1986;27(6):775–780.
67. Inoue T, Kim EE, Wallace S, *et al.* Preliminary study of cardiac accumulation of F-18 fluorotamoxifen in patients with breast cancer. *Clin Imaging* 1997;21(5):332–336.
68. Atwell GJ, Rewcastle GW, Baguley BC, Denny WA. Potential antitumor agents. 50. In vivo solid-tumor activity of derivatives of N-[2-(dimethylamino)ethyl]acridine-4-carboxamide. *J Med Chem* 1987;30(4):664–669.
69. Finlay GJ, Marshall E, Matthews JH, Paull KD, Baguley BC. In vitro assessment of N-[2-(dimethyl amino)ethyl]acridine-4- carboxamide, a DNA-intercalating antitumour drug with reduced sensitivity to multidrug resistance. *Cancer Chemother Pharmacol* 1993;31(5):401–406.
70. Finlay GJ, Baguley BC. Selectivity of N-[2-(dimethylamino)ethyl]acridine-4-carboxamide towards Lewis lung carcinoma and human tumour cell lines in vitro. *Eur J Cancer Clin Oncol* 1989;25(2):271–277.

71. Baguley BC, Holdaway KM, Fray LM. Design of DNA intercalators to overcome topoisomerase II-mediated multidrug resistance. *J Natl Cancer Inst* 1990;82(5):398–402.
72. Baguley BC, Zhuang L, Marshall E. Experimental solid tumour activity of N-[2-(dimethylamino)ethyl]-acridine-4-carboxamide. *Cancer Chemother Pharmacol* 1995;36(3):244–248.
73. Paxton JW, Young D, Evans SM, Kestell P, Robertson IG, Cornford EM. Pharmacokinetics and toxicity of the antitumour agent N-[2- (dimethylamino)ethyl]acridine-4-carboxamide after i.v. administration in the mouse. *Cancer Chemother Pharmacol* 1992;29(5):379–384.
74. Paxton JW, Young D, Robertson IG. Pharmacokinetics of acridine-4-carboxamide in the rat, with extrapolation to humans. *Cancer Chemother Pharmacol* 1993;32(4):323–325.
75. Cornford EM, Young D, Paxton JW. Comparison of the blood–brain barrier and liver penetration of acridine antitumor drugs. *Cancer Chemother Pharmacol* 1992;29(6):439–444.
76. Osman S, Luthra SK, Brady F, et al. Studies on the metabolism of the novel antitumor agent [N-methyl-11C]N- [2-(dimethylamino)ethyl]acridine-4-carboxamide in rats and humans prior to phase I clinical trials. *Cancer Res* 1997;57(11):2172–2180.
77. Brady F, Luthra SK, Brown G, et al. Carbon-11 labelling of the antitumour agent N-[2- (dimethylamino)ethyl]acridine-4-carboxamide (DACA) and determination of plasma metabolites in man. *Appl Radiat Isot* 1997;48(4):487–492.
78. Saleem A, Harte RJ, Matthews JC, et al. Pharmacokinetic evaluation of N-[2-(dimethylamino)ethyl]acridine-4-carboxamide in patients by positron emission tomography. *J Clin Oncol* 2001;19(5):1421–1429.
79. Propper DJ, de Bono J, Saleem A, et al. Use of positron emission tomography in pharmacokinetic studies to investigate therapeutic advantage in a phase I study of 120-hour intravenous infusion XR5000. *J Clin Oncol* 2003;21(2):203–210.
80. Osman S, Rowlinson-Busza G, Luthra SK, et al. Comparative biodistribution and metabolism of carbon-11-labeled N-[2-(dimethylamino)ethyl]acridine-4-carboxamide and DNA-intercalating analogues. *Cancer Res* 2001;61(7):2935–2944.
81. Schofield PC, Robertson IG, Paxton JW, et al. Metabolism of N-[2-(Dimethylamino)ethyl]acridine-4-carboxamide in cancer patients undergoing a phase I clinical trial. *Cancer Chemother Pharmacol* 1999;44(1):51–58.
82. Twelves CJ, Gardner C, Flavin A, et al. Phase I and pharmacokinetic study of DACA (XR5000): A novel inhibitor of topoisomerase I and II. CRC Phase I/II Committee. *Br J Cancer* 1999;80(11):1786–1791.
83. McCrystal MR, Evans BD, Harvey VJ, Thompson PI, Porter DJ, Baguley BC. Phase I study of the cytotoxic agent N-[2-(dimethylamino)ethyl]acridine- 4-carboxamide. *Cancer Chemother Pharmacol* 1999;44(1):39–44.
84. Evans SM, Young D, Robertson IG, Paxton JW. Intraperitoneal administration of the antitumour agent N-[2- (dimethylamino)ethyl]acridine-4-carboxamide in the mouse: Bioavailability, pharmacokinetics and toxicity after a single dose. *Cancer Chemother Pharmacol* 1992;31(1):32–36.
85. Pinedo HM, Peters GF. Fluorouracil: Biochemistry and pharmacology. *J Clin Oncol* 1988;6(10):1653–1664.
86. Modulation of fluorouracil by leucovorin in patients with advanced colorectal cancer: Evidence in terms of response rate. Advanced Colorectal Cancer Meta-Analysis Project [see comments]. *J Clin Oncol* 1992;10(6):896–903.
87. Meta-analysis of randomized trials testing the biochemical modulation of fluorouracil by methotrexate in metastatic colorectal cancer. Advanced Colorectal Cancer Meta-Analysis Project. *J Clin Oncol* 1994;12(5):960–969.
88. Efficacy of intravenous continuous infusion of fluorouracil compared with bolus administration in advanced colorectal cancer. Meta-analysis Group In Cancer. *J Clin Oncol* 1998;16(1):301–308.
89. Saltz LB, Cox JV, Blanke C, et al. Irinotecan plus fluorouracil and leucovorin for metastatic colorectal cancer. Irinotecan Study Group. *N Engl J Med* 2000;343(13):905–914.
90. Douillard JY, Cunningham D, Roth AD, et al. Irinotecan combined with fluorouracil compared with fluorouracil alone as first-line treatment for metastatic colorectal cancer: A multicentre randomised trial. *Lancet* 2000;355(9209):1041–1047.
91. Chau I, Webb A, Cunningham D, et al. Oxaliplatin and protracted venous infusion of 5-fluorouracil in patients with advanced or relapsed 5-fluorouracil pretreated colorectal cancer. *Br J Cancer* 2001;85(9):1258–1264.

92. de Gramont A, Figer A, Seymour M, *et al.* Leucovorin and fluorouracil with or without oxaliplatin as first-line treatment in advanced colorectal cancer. *J Clin Oncol* 2000;18(16):2938–2947.
93. Brown GD, Khan SR, Steel CJ, *et al.* A practical synthesis of 5-[18F]fluorouracil using HPLC and a study of its metabolic profile in rats. *J Label Compd Radiopharm* 1993;32:521–522.
94. Vine EN, Young D, Vine WH, Wolf W. An improved synthesis of 18F-5-fluorouracil. *Int J Appl Radiat Isot* 1979;30(7):401–405.
95. Shani J, Young D, Schlesinger T, *et al.* Dosimetry and preliminary human studies of 18F-5-fluorouracil. *Int J Nucl Med Biol* 1982;9(1):25–35.
96. Young D, Vine E, Ghanbarpour A, Shani J, Siemsen JK, Wolf W. Metabolic and distribution studies with radiolabeled 5-fluorouracil. *Nuklearmedizin* 1982;21(1):1–7.
97. Dimitrakopoulou-Strauss A, Strauss LG, Schlag P, *et al.* Fluorine-18-fluorouracil to predict therapy response in liver metastases from colorectal carcinoma. *J Nucl Med* 1998;39(7):1197–1202.
98. Dimitrakopoulou-Strauss A, Strauss LG, Schlag P, *et al.* Intravenous and intra-arterial oxygen-15-labeled water and fluorine-18-labeled fluorouracil in patients with liver metastases from colorectal carcinoma. *J Nucl Med* 1998;39(3):465–473.
99. Harte RJ, Matthews JC, O'Reilly SM, Price PM. Sources of error in tissue and tumor measurements of 5-[18F]fluorouracil. *J Nucl Med* 1998;39(8):1370–1376.
100. Harte RJ, Matthews JC, O'Reilly SM, *et al.* Tumor, normal tissue, and plasma pharmacokinetic studies of fluorouracil biomodulation with N-phosphonacetyl-L-aspartate, folinic acid, and interferon alfa. *J Clin Oncol* 1999;17(5):1580–158.
101. Moehler M, Dimitrakopoulou-Strauss A, Gutzler F, Raeth U, Strauss LG, Stremmel W. 18F-labeled fluorouracil positron emission tomography and the prognoses of colorectal carcinoma patients with metastases to the liver treated with 5-fluorouracil. *Cancer* 1998;83(2):245–253.
102. Dimitrakopoulou A, Strauss LG, Clorius JH, *et al.* Studies with positron emission tomography after systemic administration of fluorine-18-uracil in patients with liver metastases from colorectal carcinoma. *J Nucl Med* 1993;34(7):1075–1081.
103. Kissel J, Brix G, Bellemann ME, *et al.* Pharmacokinetic analysis of 5-[18F]fluorouracil tissue concentrations measured with positron emission tomography in patients with liver metastases from colorectal adenocarcinoma. *Cancer Res* 1997;57(16):3415–3423.
104. Shani J, Wolf W, Schlesinger T, *et al.* Distribution of 18F-5-fluorouracil in tumor-bearing mice and rats. *Int J Nucl Med Biol* 1978;5(1):19–28.
105. Presant CA, Wolf W, Albright MJ, *et al.* Human tumor fluorouracil trapping: Clinical correlations of in vivo 19F nuclear magnetic resonance spectroscopy pharmacokinetics. *J Clin Oncol* 1990; 8(11):1868–1873.
106. Presant CA, Wolf W, Waluch V, *et al.* Association of intratumoral pharmacokinetics of fluorouracil with clinical response. *Lancet* 1994;343(8907):1184–1187.
107. Ahmed FY, Johnston SJ, Cassidy J, *et al.* Eniluracil treatment completely inactivates dihydropyrimidine dehydrogenase in colorectal tumours. *J Clin Oncol* 1999;17(8):2439–2445.
108. Baker SD, Khor SP, Adjei AA, *et al.* Pharmacokinetic, oral bioavailability, and safety study of fluorouracil in patients treated with 776C85, an inactivator of dihydropyrimidine dehydrogenase. *J Clin Oncol* 1996;14(12):3085–3096.
109. Saleem A, Yap J, Osman S, *et al.* Modulation of fluorouracil tissue pharmacokinetics by eniluracil: In-vivo imaging of drug action. *Lancet* 2000;355(9221):2125–2131.
110. Lu Z, Zhang R, Diasio RB. Population characteristics of hepatic dihydropyrimidine dehydrogenase activity, a key metabolic enzyme in 5-fluorouracil chemotherapy. *Clin Pharmacol Ther* 1995; 58(5):512–522.
111. Naguib FN, el Kouni MH, Cha S. Enzymes of uracil catabolism in normal and neoplastic human tissues. *Cancer Res* 1985;45(11 Pt 1):5405–5412.
112. Brix G, Bellemann ME, Gerlach L, Haberkorn U. Intra- and extracellular fluorouracil uptake: Assessment with contrast-enhanced metabolic F-19 MR imaging. *Radiology* 1998;209(1):259–267.
113. Heggie GD, Sommadossi JP, Cross DS, Huster WJ, Diasio RB. Clinical pharmacokinetics of 5-fluorouracil and its metabolites in plasma, urine, and bile. *Cancer Res* 1987;47(8):2203–2206.
114. Zhang RW, Soong SJ, Liu TP, Barnes S, Diasio SB. Pharmacokinetics and tissue distribution of 2-fluoro-beta-alanine in rats. Potential relevance to toxicity pattern of 5-fluorouracil. *Drug Metab Dispos* 1992;20(1):113–119.
115. Toxicity of fluorouracil in patients with advanced colorectal cancer: Effect of administration schedule and prognostic factors. Meta-Analysis Group In Cancer. *J Clin Oncol* 1998;16(11):3537–3541.

116. Fraile RJ, Baker LH, Buroker TR, Horwitz J, Vaitkevicius VK. Pharmacokinetics of 5-fluorouracil administered orally, by rapid intravenous and by slow infusion. *Cancer Res* 1980;40(7): 2223–2228.
117. Baker SD, Diasio RB, O'Reilly S, *et al.* Phase I and pharmacologic study of oral fluorouracil on a chronic daily schedule in combination with the dihydropyrimidine dehydrogenase inactivator eniluracil. *J Clin Oncol* 2000;18(4):915–926.
118. Schilsky RL, Levin J, West WH, *et al.* Randomized, open-label, phase III study of a 28-day oral regimen of eniluracil plus fluorouracil versus intravenous fluorouracil plus leucovorin as first-line therapy in patients with metastatic/advanced colorectal cancer. *J Clin Oncol* 2002; 20(6):1519–1526.
119. Brix G, Bellemann ME, Haberkorn U, Gerlach L, Lorenz WJ. Assessment of the biodistribution and metabolism of 5-fluorouracil as monitored by 18F PET and 19F MRI: A comparative animal study. *Nucl Med Biol* 1996;23(7):897–906.
120. Ikenaka K, Shirasaka T, Kitano S, Fujii S. Effect of uracil on metabolism of 5-fluorouracil in vitro. *Gann* 1979;70(3):353–359.
121. Stevens MF, Hickman JA, Stone R, *et al.* Antitumor imidazotetrazines. 1. Synthesis and chemistry of 8-carbamoyl-3-(2-chloroethyl)imidazo[5,1-d]-1,2,3,5-tetrazin-4(3 H)-one, a novel broad-spectrum antitumor agent. *J Med Chem* 1984;27(2):196–201.
122. Baker SD, Wirth M, Statkevich P, *et al.* Absorption, metabolism, and excretion of 14C-temozolomide following oral administration to patients with advanced cancer. *Clin Cancer Res* 1999;5(2): 309–317.
123. Clark AS, Deans B, Stevens MF, *et al.* Antitumor imidazotetrazines. 32. Synthesis of novel imidazotetrazinones and related bicyclic heterocycles to probe the mode of action of the antitumor drug temozolomide. *J Med Chem* 1995;38(9):1493–1504.
124. Newlands ES, O'Reilly SM, Glaser MG, *et al.* The Charing Cross Hospital experience with temozolomide in patients with gliomas. *Eur J Cancer* 1996;32A(13):2236–2241.
125. Brada M, Hoang-Xuan K, Rampling R, *et al.* Multicenter phase II trial of temozolomide in patients with glioblastoma multiforme at first relapse. *Ann Oncol* 2001;12(2):259–266.
126. Bleehen NM, Newlands ES, Lee SM, *et al.* Cancer Research Campaign phase II trial of temozolomide in metastatic melanoma. *J Clin Oncol* 1995;13(4):910–913.
127. Estlin EJ, Lashford L, Ablett S, *et al.* Phase I study of temozolomide in paediatric patients with advanced cancer. United Kingdom Children's Cancer Study Group. *Br J Cancer* 1998; 78(5):652–661.
128. Brock CS, Newlands ES, Wedge SR, *et al.* Phase I trial of temozolomide using an extended continuous oral schedule. *Cancer Res* 1998;58(19):4363–4367.
129. Brock CS, Matthews JC, Brown G, *et al.* The kinetic behavior of temozolomide in man (Meeting abstract). In: Annual Meeting of the American Society of Clinical Oncology, 1996.
130. Brock CS, Matthews JC, Brown G, *et al.* Response to temozolomide (TEM) in recurrent high grade gliomas (HGG) is related to tumour drug concentration. (Meeting abstract). *Ann Oncol* 1998;9(Suppl 1):174.
131. Denny BJ, Wheelhouse RT, Stevens MF, Tsang LL, Slack JA. NMR and molecular modeling investigation of the mechanism of activation of the antitumor drug temozolomide and its interaction with DNA. *Biochemistry* 1994;33(31):9045–9051.
132. Vaupel P, Kallinowski F, Okunieff P. Blood flow, oxygen and nutrient supply, and metabolic microenvironment of human tumors: A review. *Cancer Res* 1989;49(23):6449–6465.
133. Saleem A, Brown GD, Brady F, *et al.* Metabolic activation of temozolomide measured in vivo using positron emission tomography. *Cancer Res* 2003;63(10):2409–2415.

12 Imaging Genes for Viral and Adoptive Therapies

Inna Serganova, PhD, Vladimir Ponomarev, MD, PhD, Phillipp Mayer-Kuckuk, PhD, Ekaterina Doubrovina, MD, PhD, Michael Doubrovin, MD, PhD, and Ronald G. Blasberg, MD

CONTENTS

    INTRODUCTION AND BACKGROUND
    THERAPEUTIC GENES THAT CAN BE IMAGING GENES
    RECEPTOR IMAGING GENES
    OPTICAL IMAGING GENES
    ARRANGEMENT OF THERAPEUTIC AND IMAGING GENES IN A VECTOR DELIVERY SYSTEM
    IMAGING ADOPTIVE IMMUNE CELL THERAPIES
    IMAGING STEM CELLS
    ISSUES FOR THE FUTURE

1. INTRODUCTION AND BACKGROUND

    The concept of using gene therapy for cancer treatment was initially met with enthusiasm. The possibility of replacing or altering damaged genes, the introduction of suicide genes into cancer cells, and the alteration of cell function as a consequence of exogenous gene expression were advocated. Therapeutic genes can be transferred to patients through a variety of vehicles. These include retroviruses, herpes viruses, adenoviruses, adeno-associated viruses, lentiviruses, baculoviruses, liposomes, bacterial hosts, naked DNA, DNA precipitates, and protein–DNA conjugates (Table 1) *(1, 2)*. However, the practical application of gene therapy to treat cancer has been somewhat disappointing so far. Major obstacles remain, including the inability to target appropriate tissues and deliver therapeutic genes to a sufficient number of target cells, the inability to monitor the level of expression of the therapeutic gene, the loss of

Table 1
Characteristics of Most Commonly Used Vectors

Type	Insert size	Genome	Cell division required	Duration of expression	Advantages	Disadvantages
Retrovirus	5–7 kb	RNA	Yes	Long-term	Potential to integrate into genome of target cells	Insertional mutagenesis
Lentivirus	10–12 kb	RNA, part retrovirus family	No	Long-term	Integrate into genome of nondividing target cells	Nonspecific integration
Adeno-associated virus	2–4 kb	DNA	No	Long-term	High transduction efficiency into muscle and brain	Insertional mutagenesis; difficulties with production; do not work in all organs
Adenovirus	7–35 kb	DNA	No	Transient	Relative high transduction efficiency into normal and tumor cells; easy production and at high titers; tropism can be modified	Local tissue inflammation and immune response
Herpes simplex virus	Up to 30 kb	DNA	Yes	Transient	High transduction efficiency	Difficult to obtain long-term gene expression; the cytopathic nature; difficult to target
Nonviral vectors	No limitation	RNA or DNA	No	Transient	Repetitive and safe administration feasible	Low efficiency gene transfer

therapeutic gene expression over time, and the inability to correlate the level and duration of gene expression with therapeutic outcome.

One improvement in the implementation of gene therapy protocols would be to monitor the expression of the therapeutic gene noninvasively. Under ideal conditions, the therapeutic gene would also be an imaging gene, as is the case with herpes simplex virus thymidine kinase (HSV1-TK). Alternatively, it is possible to include a therapeutic gene with a second, imaging gene in the same cDNA expression cassette. In this case, both therapeutic and imaging genes are expressed together. The location and the level of therapeutic gene expression will be reflected by the expression of the imaging gene. Before discussing specific issues related to imaging genes, it would be helpful to briefly outline three currently used strategies for noninvasive monitoring and quantification of molecular events. These strategies are broadly defined as "direct," "indirect," and "biomarker" imaging. They have been discussed in detail in several recent reviews *(3–10)* and in other perspectives on molecular imaging *(11–17)*.

Direct molecular imaging strategies are usually described in terms of a specific target and a target-specific probe. The imaging of specific antigens on the cell surface with radiolabeled antibodies and genetically engineered antibody fragments (minibodies) is an example of direct molecular imaging that has evolved over the past 30 years. In addition, *in vivo* imaging of receptor density/occupancy using small radiolabeled ligands has also been widely used, particularly in neuroscience research over the past two decades. These two examples represent some of the first molecular imaging applications used in clinical nuclear medicine. More recent research has focused on the preparation of paramagnetic nanoparticles and small radiolabeled or fluorescent molecules that target specific receptors (e.g., the estrogen or androgen receptors) *(18, 19)* or are activated by endogenous proteases *(20)*. However, the use of direct imaging strategies is limited by the need to develop and validate a specific probe for each molecular target. Each probe requires detailed characterization including sensitivity, specificity, and safety. The time and cost for new probe development can be substantial. For example, the development, validation, and regulatory approval for [^{18}F]fluorodeoxyglucose positron emission tomography [^{18}F]FDG PET imaging of glucose utilization in tumors have taken over 20 years. Nevertheless, once a new imaging probe has been "approved," it may have wide clinical application, as is the case with [^{18}F]FDG.

Indirect imaging strategies are more complex. One example of indirect imaging that is now being widely used is reporter gene imaging. It requires "pretargeting" (delivery) of the reporter gene to the target tissue by transfection or transduction, and it usually includes transcriptional control components that can function as "molecular-genetic sensors" that can regulate and initiate reporter gene expression. This strategy has been widely applied in optical-based *(21–23)* and radionuclide-based imaging *(24–28)*, and to a lesser degree in magnetic resonance imaging (MRI) *(29, 30)*. The first reporter imaging approaches used the bacterial chloramphenicol acetyltransferase (CAT) gene *(31)* and the lacZ gene *(32)*. However, postmortem tissue sampling and processing (e.g., β-galactosidase assay) were required. More recent studies have focused on noninvasive imaging techniques involving live animals and humans *(33)*.

A general paradigm for noninvasive reporter gene imaging using radiolabeled probes was initially described in 1995 *(24)* and three examples are shown in Fig. 1. This paradigm requires the appropriate combination of a reporter/marker transgene and a reporter/marker probe. The reporter transgene usually encodes for an enzyme, receptor, or

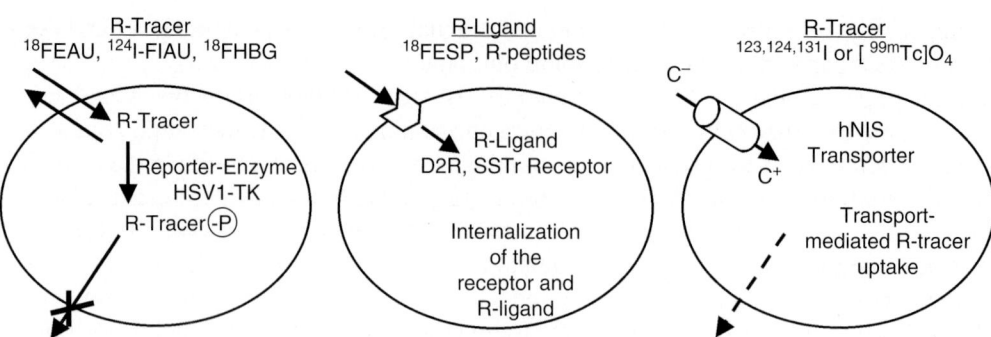

Fig. 1. Different radionuclide-based reporter systems. The reporter gene is transfected into target cells by a delivery system (e.g., a virus). The reporter gene product can be a cytoplasmic or nuclear enzyme. The imaging probe, a radioactive tracer, must cross the cell membrane and be metabolized within cytoplasm or nucleus to a product that is "trapped" within the cell (the most commonly used enzymatic reaction is phosphorylation). As a result, the phosphorylated tracer becomes incapable of exiting by recrossing the plasma membrane and is trapped within the cell (A). A receptor at the cell surface can be the product of reporter gene expression and the imaging ligand binds to this receptor, resulting in the accumulation of the detectible ligand in the transduced tissue (B). A transporter incorporated into the cell membrane can also be the product of reporter gene expression, and the imaging probe concentrates in the cells expressing the reporter gene (C). The level of probe concentration is usually proportional to the level of reporter gene product and can reflect several processes, including the level of transcription, the modulation and regulation of translation, protein–protein interactions, and posttranslational regulation of protein conformation and degradation.

transporter that selectively interacts with a radiolabeled probe and results in accumulation of radioactivity in the transduced cell. In addition, reporter systems based on the expression of fluorescence proteins (broadly used in cell culture and embryogenesis studies) *(34)* are becoming more widely applied in small animal imaging *(35)*.

Biomarker imaging or surrogate marker imaging can be used to assess downstream effects of one or more endogenous molecular genetic processes. This approach is particularly attractive for potential translation into clinical studies in the near term, because existing radiopharmaceuticals and imaging paradigms may be useful for monitoring downstream effects of alterations in specific cellular pathways that occur in diseases such as cancer.

The biomarker approach is very likely to be less specific and more limited with respect to the number of molecular genetic processes that can be imaged. Nevertheless, it benefits from the use of radiolabeled probes that have already been developed and studied in human subjects. Thus, the translation of biomarker imaging paradigms into clinical applications will be far easier than either the direct imaging paradigms outlined above or the reporter transgene imaging paradigms outlined below. However, it remains to be shown whether there is a sufficiently high correlation between biomarker imaging and direct molecular assays that reflects the activity of a particular molecular/genetic pathway of interest.

In this chapter, we will emphasize the development of reporter genes for noninvasive, quantitative imaging in small animals and the potential for translation to comparable studies in patients. One focus includes animal models of cancer and the potential for novel studies in patients with cancer, although the opportunity for reporter gene studies in other genetically based human diseases certainly exists. This chapter begins with a description of the PET-based imaging genes and the probes that we think will be the first candidates in clinical trials. Then we will describe other imaging genes, mostly for optical imaging, that have been developed by investigators working with a variety of cancer models in mice. The optical reporters are unlikely to enter the clinic, at least not in the near term. The last part of the chapter is dedicated to the possible arrangements of imaging genes in various delivery systems and their application in gene and adoptive therapies.

2. THERAPEUTIC GENES THAT CAN BE IMAGING GENES

2.1 Genes Encoding Enzymes

2.1.1 HERPES SIMPLEX VIRUS I THYMIDINE KINASE AS A THERAPEUTIC AND A REPORTER GENE

The herpes simplex virus type 1 thymidine kinase gene has gained considerable importance in clinical medicine and as a research tool. The HSV1-TK enzyme, like mammalian TKs, phosphorylates thymidine (TdR). Unlike mammalian TKs, viral TKs can also phosphorylate acycloguanosines (e.g., acyclovir, ACV; ganciclovir, GCV; penciclovir, PCV) as well as TdR analogs that are not (or minimally) phosphorylated by eukaryotic enzymes *(36)*. Viral enzymes convert acycloguanosine monophosphates to diphosphates and triphosphates, which facilitates their incorporation into elongating DNA by cellular DNA polymerase and results in chain termination and cell death. This property of acycloguanosine analogs, such as ACV and GCV, has been used for the treatment of viral infections. For this reason HSV1-TK has been studied extensively as a therapeutic gene. HSV1-TK has also been used in gene therapy clinical trials performed in the United States and Europe. These trials have been performed primarily to assess drug sensitivity following retroviral transfer of the HSV1-TK gene into tumor cells followed by systemic treatment with the GCV *(37)*. These suicide gene therapy protocols depend on the expression of HSV1-TK in target tissue. Several important issues have been raised during these trials, including whether the viral transduction of the target tissue has been successful, what level of transgene expression is achieved in the target tissue, and what is the optimal time for beginning GCV treatment. Another important clinical issue is monitoring for potential toxicity. Imaging the distribution and expression level of the therapeutic gene in nontarget normal tissues provides a level of safety in individual patients undergoing gene therapy.

In the mid-1990s, a number of potential marker/reporter probes for imaging HSV1-TK gene expression were studied in our laboratory. They include 2′-deoxy-2′-fluoro-5-iodo-1-[β]-D-arabinofuranosyluracil (FIAU), 5-iodo-2′-deoxyuridine (IUdR), and GCV (Fig. 2A). Of these, FIAU had been previously radiolabeled for imaging viral infections *(38)*. After *in vitro* determinations of HSV1-TK sensitivity and selectivity for FIAU, this compound was found to have good imaging potential. In addition, a variety of radionuclides (^{11}C, ^{124}I, ^{18}F ^{131}I, ^{123}I) can be used for FIAU labeling. FIAU contains a 2′-fluoro substitution in the sugar that impedes cleavage of the *N*-glycosidic bond by nucleoside phosphorylases. This results in a significant prolongation of the nucleoside in plasma and an increase in delivery of nondegraded radiolabeled tracer to the target tissues. The first series of imaging experiments involving HSV1-TK transduced tissue and FIAU were performed in rats bearing intracerebral RG2 tumors using

A

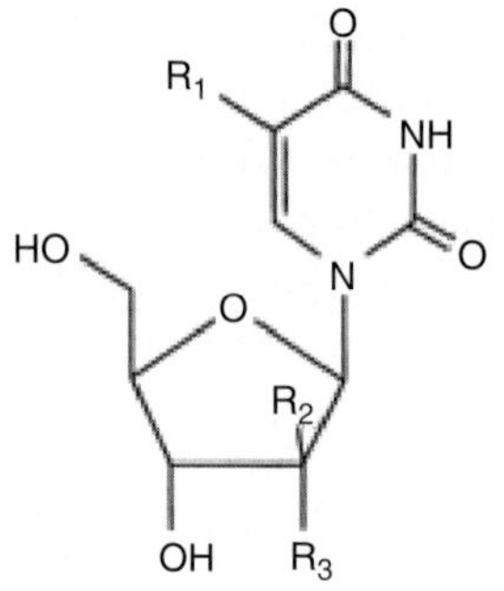

Probe	R1	R2	R3
FIAU	I	F	H
FIRU	I	H	F
FMAU	CH$_3$	F	H
IVFRU	CH$_2$=CH$_2$-I	H	F
IUdR	I	H	H
BrUdR	Br	H	H

B

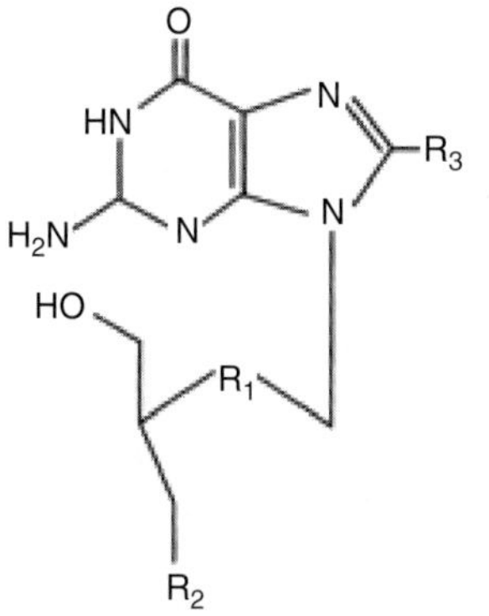

Probe	R1	R2	R3
GCV	O	OH	H
PCV	CH$_2$	OH	H
FGCV	O	OH	F
FPCV	CH$_2$	OH	F
FHPG	O	F	H
FHBG	CH$_2$	F	H

Fig. 2. Chemical structures of pyrimidine (A) and acycloguanosine (B) nucleoside probes.

quantitative autoradiography (QAR) techniques *(23)* (Fig. 3). This was subsequently followed by gamma camera, single-photon emission computed tomography (SPECT), and PET imaging studies *(24, 25)*.

Investigators from the University of California, Los Angeles (UCLA) have used other radiolabeled compounds for PET imaging of HSV1-TK expression. Their choice of acycloguanosine derivatives (Fig. 2B) as reporter probes was based on the ability of these nucleosides to be radiolabeled with short-lived fluorine-18 ($t_{1/2}$ = 110 min) and no affinity to the mammalian TK-1. A goal of these researchers was to develop methods for repetitive imaging (every 6–8 h) of the reporter protein. A list of ^{18}F-labeled acycloguanosine analogs is shown in Fig. 2B and the appropriate references are given *(10, 26, 27)*. After several years of comparative studies, a new radiolabeled acycloguanine, 9-(4-[^{18}F]fluoro-3-hydroxymethylbutyl)guanine or [^{18}F]FHBG *(39)*, was developed at the University of Southern California (USC). In parallel, the UCLA investigators evaluated a mutant HSV1-TK enzyme (HSV1-sr39TK) with increased ACV and GCV suicidal efficacy. They showed higher affinity and uptake of [^{18}F]FHBG in HSV1-sr39TK transduced cells *(40)*. The mutant, HSV1-sr39TK, enhances [^{18}F]FHBG uptake by 2-fold compared to wild-type HSV1-TK, thus improving the imaging capabilities of the enzyme *(41)*. Recently, [^{18}F]FHBG has been studied in normal human volunteers and the biodistribution, biosafety, and dosimetry have been determined; it was found to be safe and potentially useful for human applications *(42)*. The preliminary findings in a phase I/II clinical trial of gene therapy for recurrent glioblastoma showed that FIAU PET imaging of HSV-1-TK expression in patients is feasible and that vector-mediated gene expression may predict the therapeutic effect *(43)*.

Noninvasive monitoring of the distribution of transgene expression over time is highly desirable and will have a critical impact on the development of standardized

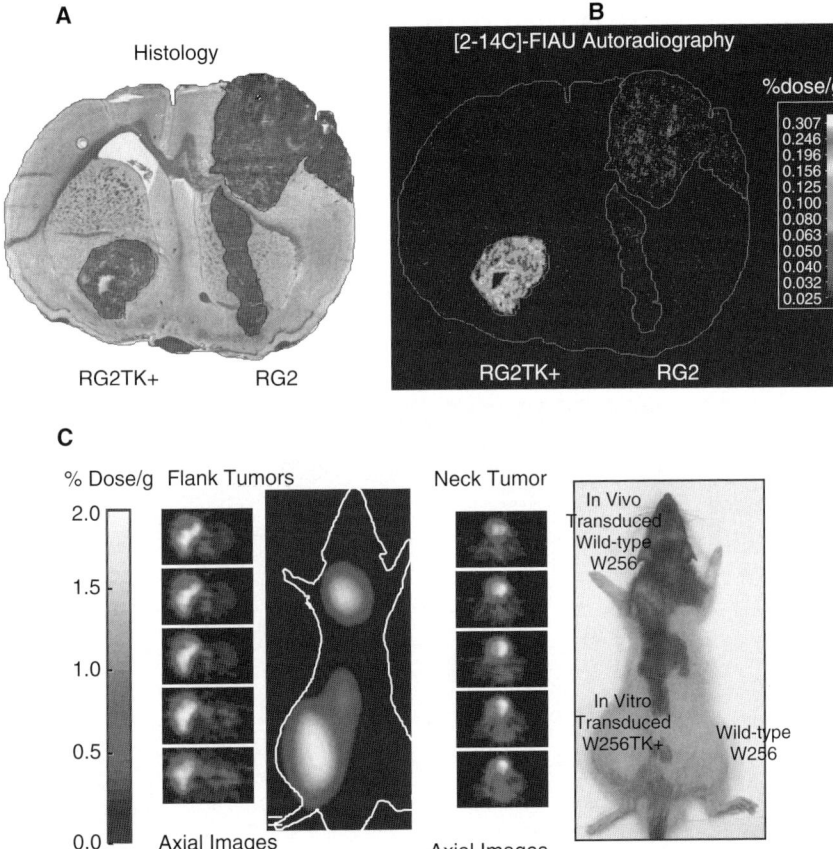

Fig. 3. Autoradiographic imaging of HSV1-TK expression (A). A rat brain with a stably transduced RG2TK⁺ brain tumor in the left hemisphere and a wild-type (nontransduced) RG2 tumor in the right hemisphere is shown. The histology and autoradiographic images were generated from the same tissue section (A and B). Both tumors are clearly seen in the toluidine blue-stained histological section (A). Twenty-four hours after intravenous administration of [^{14}C]FIAU, the RG2TK⁺ tumor is clearly visualized in the autoradiographic image (B), whereas the RG2 tumor is barely detectable; the surrounding brain is at background levels. [Adapted from Tjuvajev *et al. (24)*.] PET imaging HSV1-TK expression (C). Three tumors were produced in rnu rats. A W256TK⁺ (positive control) tumor was produced from stably transduced W256TK⁺ cells and is located in the left flank, and two wild-type W256 tumors were produced in the dorsum of the neck (test) and in the right flank (negative control). The neck tumor was inoculated with 10^6 gp-STK-A2 vector-producer cells (retroviral titer: 10^6–10^7 cfu/ml) to induce HSV1-TK transduction of the wild-type tumor *in vivo*. Fourteen days after gp-STK-A2 cell inoculation, no carrier added [^{124}I]FIAU (25 µCi) was injected intravenously and PET imaging was performed 30 h later. Localization of radioactivity is clearly seen in the left flank tumor (positive control) and in the *in vivo*-transduced neck tumor (test), but only low background levels of radioactivity were observed in the wild-type right flank tumor (negative control). (*See* color plate.) [Adapted from Tjuvajev *et al. (26)*.]

gene therapy protocols and on efficient and safe vector applications in human beings (Fig. 4). It is most likely that [^{124}I]FIAU and [^{18}F]FHBG will be the first radiolabeled probes that will be introduced into the clinic for the imaging of HSV1-TK gene expression.

Other applications of HSV1-TK as a reporter gene are imaging endogenous biological processes. Imaging the transcriptional regulation of endogenous genes in living animals using noninvasive imaging techniques can provide a better understanding of normal and cancer-related biological processes. Recent papers from our group have shown that p53 and hypoxia inducible factor-1 (HIF-1)-dependent gene expression can be imaged *in vivo* with PET and by *in situ* fluorescence *(44, 45)*. Retroviral vectors were generated by placing the herpes simplex virus type 1 thymidine kinase (TK) and enhanced green fluorescent protein fusion gene (*HSV1-TK/eGFP*, a dual-reporter gene) under control of a specific response element for p53, as well as HIF-1. Upregulation of these transcriptional factors was demonstrated and correlated with the expression of dependent downstream genes [p21, vascular endothelial growth factor (VEGF), corre-

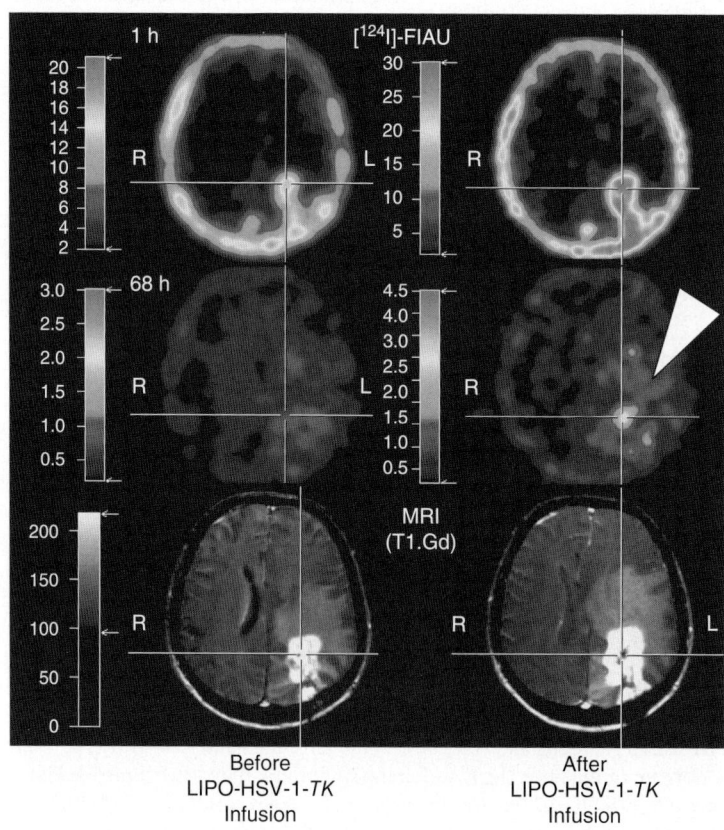

Fig. 4. HSV1-TK reporter gene imaging in patients. Coregistration of FIAU-PET and MRI before (left column) and after (right column) vector application. A region of specific [^{124}I]FIAU retention (at 68 h) within the tumor after liposome–HSV-1-TK complex transduction is visualized (white arrow). This tumor region showed signs of necrosis (cross-hairs, right column) after ganciclovir treatment. (*See* color plate.) [Adapted from Jacobs *et al. (43)*.]

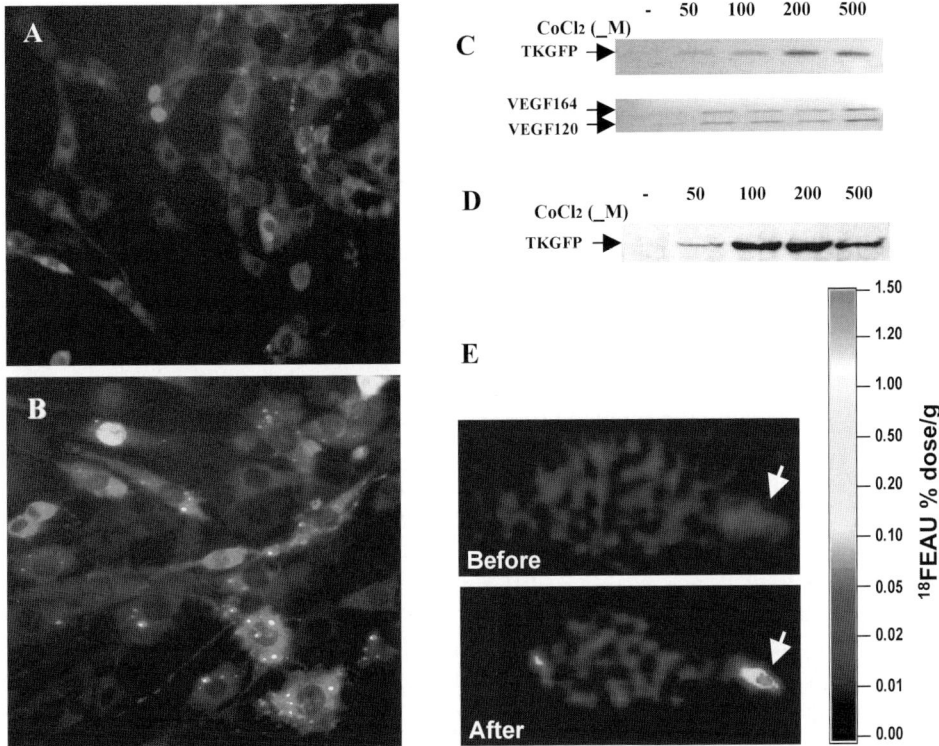

Fig. 5. Characterization of a hypoxia-sensitive specific reporter system *in vitro* and *in vivo*. Fluorescence microscopy of #4C6 reporter cells under baseline conditions (A) and following exposure to 200 μM $CoCl_2$ for 24 h (B). Expression of VEGF and a herpes simplex virus 1 thymidine kinase–green fluorescence protein (HSV1-TK/GFP) in response to hypoxic conditions. Agarose gel electrophoresis of the RT-PCR products (C) was performed to validate a new hypoxia-dependent reporter system. Western blotting (D) of the expression level of TKGFP confirms the integrity of the reporter system. Assays were performed 24 h after exposure to different concentrations of $CoCl_2$. *In vivo* microPET imaging of ischemia-reperfusion injury-induced HIF-1 transcriptional activity. (E) Axial PET images of HIF-1-mediated TKGFP expression in subcutaneous #4C6 xenografts growing in both anterior limbs of the same mouse before and after tourniquet application to the left anterior limb proximal to the tumor. The subcutaneous #4C6 tumor xenograft growing in the right limb was not affected and served as a control *(45)*. (*See* color plate.)

spondently] (Fig. 5). Positron emission tomography imaging of p53 and HIF-1 transcriptional activity in tumors using *cis*-reporter systems was developed and validated *(44, 45)*. These could be used to assess the effects of new drugs or other novel therapeutic paradigms that are mediated through these pathways. Imaging endogenous gene expression may be hampered when weak promoters, in their usual *cis* configuration, are used to activate the transcription of the reporter gene. This results in weak transcriptional activity of the reporter gene.

To address this limitation, a "two-step transcriptional amplification" (TSTA) approach can be used to enhance transcriptional activity. This was used to image activation of the androgen-responsive prostate-specific antigen (PSA) promoter with firefly luciferase and mutant herpes simplex virus type 1 thymidine kinase (HSV1-sr39TK) reporter genes in a prostate cancer cell line (LNCaP) *(46)*. Further improvements of the androgen-responsive TSTA system for reporter gene expression were made using a "chimeric" TSTA system that uses duplicated variants of the PSA gene enhancer to express GAL4 derivatives fused to one, two, or four VP16 activation domains. A very encouraging result was the demonstration that the TSTA system was androgen concentration sensitive, suggesting a continuous rather than binary reporter response. Another study *(47)* validated methods to enhance the transcriptional activity of the carcinoembryonic antigen (CEA) promoter using a *trans* system (similar to the TSTA described above). To increase promoter strength while maintaining tissue specificity, a recombinant adenovirus was constructed that contained a TSTA system with a tumor-specific CEA promoter driving a transcription transactivator, which then activates a minimal promoter to drive expression of the HSV1-TK suicide/reporter gene. This ADV/CEA-binary-tk system resulted in equal or greater cell killing of transduced cells by ganciclovir in a CEA-specific manner, compared with ganciclovir killing of all cells transduced with a CEA-independent vector containing a constitutive viral promoter driving HSV1-TK expression (ADV/RSV-TK). However, as observed with the PSE-TSTA reporter system above, the *in vivo* imaging comparison of the TSTA and *cis* reporter systems showed substantially less dramatic differences than those obtained by the *in vitro* analyses *(46, 47)*.

Gene expression levels are also regulated by posttranscriptional modulation, including the translation of mRNA. A recent study demonstrated that imaging posttranscriptional regulation of gene expression is feasible. This was shown by exposing cells to antifolates and inducing a rapid increase in the levels of the enzyme dihydrofolate reductase (DHFR). Several studies indicated that the DHFR binds to its own mRNA in the coding region, and that inhibition of DHFR by methotrexate (MTX) releases the DHFR enzyme from the mRNA. Consequently, this release results in an increase in translation of DHFR protein. In addition to the described translational regulation of DHFR in *Cancer Cell*s exposed to MTX, increased levels of DHFR also result through DHFR gene amplification, a common mechanism of acquired resistance to this drug. In contrast to rapid translational modulation of DHFR, gene amplification occurs in response to chronic exposure to antifolates, and elevated cellular levels of DHFR result from transcription of multiple DHFR gene copies. Recently, Mayer-Kuckuk *et al.* showed that this adaptive cellular response mechanism could be used to determine whether posttranscriptional regulation of gene expression could be monitored by reporter PET imaging *(48)*. The results of this study indicated that the increase in reporter protein and enzyme (DHFR-HSV1-TK) activity was occurring at a translational level, rather than at a transcriptional level. This effect could be visualized by [^{124}I]FIAU and PET imaging studies that were performed on nude rats bearing DHFR-HSV1-TK-transduced HCT-8 xenografts.

2.2 Genes Encoding Transporters

2.2.1 hNIS as a Therapeutic and Reporter Gene

Radioactive iodide (^{131}I) therapy is one approach in the treatment of human thyroid cancer. Thyrocytes are physiologically capable of accumulating iodine because of the presence of the sodium iodide symporter (NIS) in their plasma membranes *(49)*; NIS is also expressed, although at lower levels, in many other organs including the salivary and lacrimal glands, stomach, kidney epithelial cells, and placenta *(50, 51)*. It is an intrinsic membrane glycoprotein with 13 putative transmembrane domains. Detailed studies of cells expressing NIS show that the symporter transports two sodium ions with one iodide ion across the cell membrane *(52)*. Thus NIS can transport many other anions coupled with sodium, such as ClO_3^-, SCN^-, NO_3^-, Br^-, TcO_4^-, and RhO_4^- *(53)*. Since cloning of the NIS gene in 1996, interest has developed in the use of NIS as an imaging reporter gene. First, NIS is not a foreign gene; thus, it is nonimmunogenic. Second, the tissue expression distribution of endogenous NIS protein is limited; as a result, imaging of exogenous NIS function can be performed in a variety of tissues due to limited background expression (stomach and thyroid are major exceptions). Third, NIS mediates the uptake of simple radiopharmaceuticals; therefore, complicated syntheses and labeling of substrate molecules are not required for imaging. Fourth, most of the radiotracers are specific only to NIS-expressing cells; therefore the background signal is significantly reduced. Fifth, both NIS-mediated radiotracer uptake and background radioactivity clear rapidly, making them ideally suited for noninvasive imaging.

The human NIS (hNIS) gene has been used in various vectors to produce stable transduced cell lines. High iodide uptake levels have been achieved in such transduced cells and transduced xenografts *(54–58)*. A feature of the bidirectional NIS transporter is the rapid washout of iodide from most cells, except thyrocytes bearing thyroperoxidase. In normal thyroid tissue, this enzyme iodinates thyroglobulin tyrosine residues. Incorporating iodine atoms into thyroid hormone results in the retention of accumulated radioactivity in these cells. In an attempt to overcome the rapid excretion of radioiodide from NIS-transfected tumors, the thyroperoxidase (TPO) gene was cotransduced into tumor cells *(59)*. The transfection with both human NIS and TPO genes resulted in some increase in radioiodide uptake and retention, and an enhanced rate of tumor cell apoptosis, but this has not been consistently achieved. Other therapeutic studies have used more energetic β emitters (e.g., ^{188}Re) or α emitters (e.g., ^{211}At), in place of ^{131}I, in conjunction with the NIS transporter *(60, 61)*.

The sodium iodide symporter can serve as both a therapeutic and a reporter gene. Noninvasive imaging of therapeutic transgenes provides the opportunity to modify therapy directed at transfected cells or tumors. For example, quantification of NIS expression is currently used to plan subsequent radioiodine therapy. Experimental ^{131}I therapy of NIS-transfected myeloma in SCID mice *(62)* was successful because transgene expression was high (up to 18-fold) in transduced myeloma cells, with negligible expression in other cells. Myeloma xenografts containing wild-type and hNIS-expressing cells could be imaged with a gamma camera. They were completely eradicated with a single therapeutic dose of [^{131}I]iodide, without recurrence for up to 5 months after therapy. The treatment was successful even though hNIS was not transduced into every myeloma cell *(63)*. The likely explanation of this response is that nontransduced cells were killed by radioactivity emitted by [^{131}I]iodide from neighboring cells, the "bystander" effect *(63)*.

Progress in the molecular and functional characterization of NIS during the past few years has clearly created new opportunities for the development of diagnostic and therapeutic applications for NIS *(64–66)*. These applications are especially relevant in the field of nuclear medicine, and for the prospect of using administered radioisotopes in a highly targeted fashion to effectively destroy a wide variety of cancer cells by internal, rather than external, radiation.

Control of hNIS gene expression by endogenous transcription factors and transcription factor complexes is actively being investigated and has led to the development of novel strategies to image signaling pathway activity in cancer cells. A number of promoter elements have been used to control or regulate hNIS expression. The first transfer of the hNIS gene into tumors for targeted radiotherapy was performed with a recombinant adenovirus, AdNIS, where expression of the rat NIS gene was under the control of the constitutive cytomegalovirus (CMV) promoter *(54)*. Later, the NIS reporter gene was used for imaging retinoic acid receptor activity using an artificial *cis*-acting retinoic acid responsive element *(67)*. Recently, the same group has shown that p53 expression can be monitored both *in vitro* and *in vivo* using the NIS reporter gene in a *cis*-p53RE-hNIS construct *(65)*.

Recently we developed a self-inactivating retroviral vector containing a dual-reporter gene cassette (hNIS-IRES-eGFP) with the hNIS and eGFP genes, separated by an internal ribosome entry site (IRES) element, and driven by a constitutive CMV promoter. A stably transduced rat glioma (RG2) cell line was generated with this construct and used for *in vitro* and *in vivo* imaging studies of [^{131}I]iodide and ^{99m}TcO$_4$-pertechnetate accumulation, as well as eGFP fluorescence. The experiments clearly showed a correlation between the expression of hNIS and eGFP. Gamma camera imaging studies performed on RG2-hNIS-IRES-GFP tumor-bearing mice demonstrated that the IRES-linked dual reporter gene is functional and stable. Optical and nuclear imaging of tumors produced from the cell lines carrying the hNIS-IRES-GFP cassette (Fig. 6) will provide the opportunity to monitor tumor growth and response to therapy *(68)*.

2.3 Receptors

2.3.1 SOMATOSTATIN RECEPTOR AS A THERAPEUTIC AND REPORTER GENE

A peptide, somatostatin, inhibits the release of growth hormone and was originally detected in the hypothalamus of rats. It was subsequently shown to be a cyclic peptide consisting of 14 amino acids *(69, 70)*. Somatostatin belongs to a phylogenetically ancient, multigene family of peptides with two important bioactive products: somatostatin-14 and somatostatin-28. Somatostatin modulates neurotransmission in the central nervous system (as a neurotransmitter) and regulates the release of growth hormone and thyrotropin (as a neurohormone). It also has a regulatory role in the gastrointestinal tract, as well as in the exocrine and endocrine pancreas. When synthesized and released into the gastrointestinal tract and pancreas, somatostatin acts in an autocrine and paracrine manner to inhibit glandular secretion. It is also a regulator of neurotransmission, smooth-muscle contractility, and absorption of nutrients *(71)*. The various actions of somatostatin are mediated through specific membrane receptors (SSTRs), which have been demonstrated in various regions of the brain, anterior pituitary and leptomeninges, the endocrine and exocrine pancreas, and the mucosa of the gastrointestinal tract, as well as in cells of the immune system *(72)*. There are six SSTRs (types 1, 2A and 2B, 3, 4, and 5) and they all belong to a 7-transmembrane domain family of receptors associated with G-proteins. Expression of the type 2 somatostatin receptor (SSTr2) occurs primarily in the pituitary gland and this somatostatin receptor has high affinity for octreotide. Octreotide is an 8-amino acid peptide; it was the first synthetic somatostatin analog introduced for clinical use. It inhibits the release of

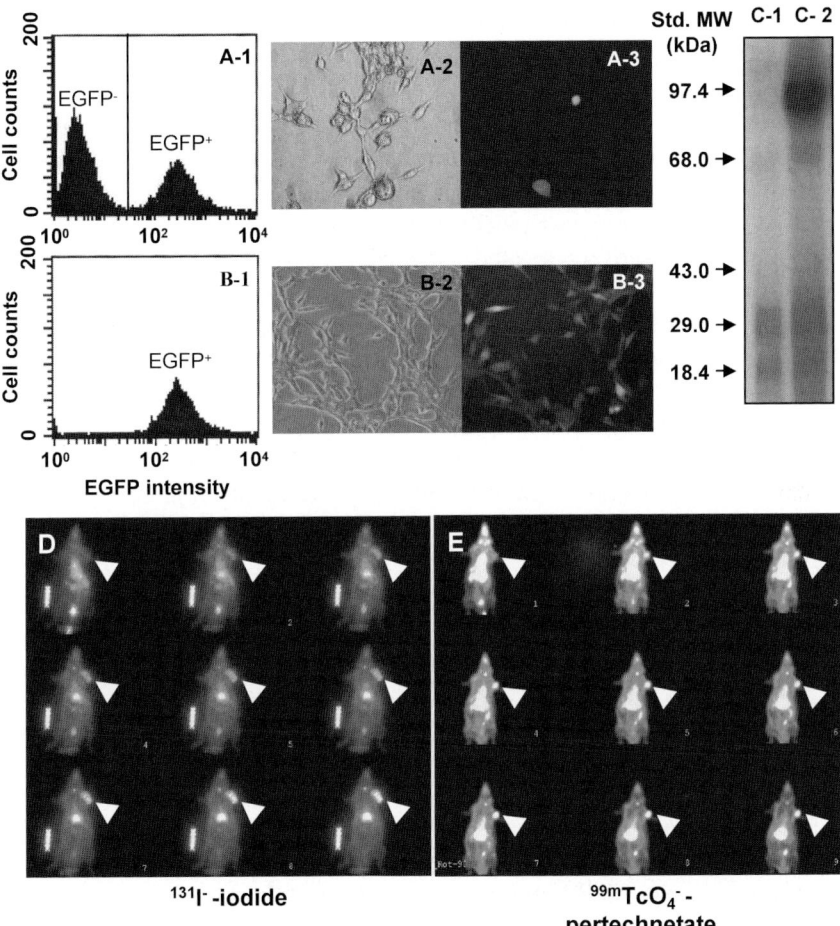

Fig. 6. *In vitro* and *in vivo* characterization of the hNIS-IRES-eGFP reporter in RG2 cells. (A-1) FACS analysis of RG2 transduced cells (bulk culture). (A-2) Phase-contrast microscopy of the same cells in A-1 before FACS sorting. (A-3) Fluorescence microscopy in the same region of A-2. (B-1) FACS profile of RG2-pQCNIG cells after sorting. (B-2) Phase-contrast microscopy of FCS-sorted GFP-positive cells. (B-3) Fluorescence microscopy shows the eGFP$^+$ cells in the same region of B-2. (C) Western blot analysis of hNIS protein in the membranes of wild-type RG2 (lane 1) and RG2-pQCNIG cells (lane 2). Dynamic gamma camera images of [^{131}I]iodide and ^{99m}TcO$_4$-pertechnetate accumulation in RG2-pQCNIG and RG2 wild-type xenografts in SCID mice (D and E, respectively). Arrows identify the RG2-pQCNIG xenograft in each image (the wild-type RG2 xenograft is located in the opposite, left shoulder). (*See* color plate.) [Adapted from J. Che *et al.* *(68)*.]

growth hormone, glucagon, and insulin more effectively than somatostatin-14 *(73)*. Octreotide is more stable and resistant to *in vivo* degradation compared to the endogenous 14-amino acid somatostatin peptide. It has been labeled with ^{111}In and ^{99m}Tc and successfully used for gamma camera imaging of endogenous SSTr2 expression in tumors *(74)*. The ^{99m}Tc-labeled P829, a somatostatin-avid peptide, and its ^{188}Re-labeled analog have also been used to image exogenous SSTr2 expression in mice following transfection of tumors with an adenovirus vector expressing human SSTR2 *(75, 76)*.

The ^{188}Re-labeled analog, which is not FDA approved, may also be useful for therapy because it decays with high-energy β-emission that is known to induce a "bystander effect."

The human SSTr2 gene, incorporated into a replication-incompetent adenoviral vector (Ad5-CMVhSSTr2), has also been used as a radionuclide-based reporter gene for noninvasive imaging. The transduction of A-427 cells by AdSSTr2 to induce somatostatin receptor expression was performed to demonstrate that ^{111}In-DTPA-D-Phe^1-octreotide could be used to located AdSSTr2-transfected A-427 tumors and to demonstrate therapeutic efficacy with ^{90}Y-DOTA-D-Phe^1-Tyr3-octreotide (^{90}Y-SMT 487). ^{90}Y-DOTA-D-Phe^1-Tyr3-octreotide also had a significant antigrowth effect on A-427 lung cancer xenografts *(77)*.

Several somatostatin analogs labeled with ^{111}In, ^{90}Y, ^{64}Cu, ^{177}Lu, and ^{188}Re have been used for therapeutic applications in preclinical models *(78–81)* and in clinical trials. Complete and partial responses were obtained in 25% of patients, and 55% showed stable disease lasting at least 3 month following administration of ^{90}Y-1,4,7,10-tetraazacyclododecane-N,N',N'',N'''-tetraacetic acid (DOTA)-D-Phe^1-Tyr^3-octreotide (SMT 487) in a phase I trial *(81, 82)*.

3. RECEPTOR IMAGING GENES

3.1 Dopamine D2 Receptor as a Reporter Gene

Dopamine (DA) is the predominant catecholamine neurotransmitter in the mammalian brain, where it controls a variety of functions including locomotor activity, cognition, emotion, positive reinforcement, food intake, and endocrine regulation. The five subtypes of dopamine receptors, D1 to D5, are members of a seven-transmembrane-spanning heterotrimeric GTP-binding protein (G-protein)-coupled receptor (GPCR) family. They can be further subdivided into D1-like (D1 and D5) and D2-like (D2, D3, and D4) receptors based on DNA sequence similarity *(83)*. The D2 receptor is a 415 amino acid protein that is expressed at highest levels in striatum and pituitary *(84, 85)*. This receptor interacts with 3-(2′-[^{18}F]fluoroethyl)spiperone (FESP), a radiolabeled probe that was developed to image dopaminergic neurons *(86)*. FESP, which can be synthesized at high specific activity, is currently used for SPECT and PET imaging of the D2 receptor in human neurodegenerative diseases such as Parkinson's disease *(87)*. The dopamine D2 receptor can also be used as a reporter gene in nonneural tissue that has little or no D2R expression (Fig. 7) *(88)*. However, expression of ligand-binding receptors could alter the signaling pathways of target cells and lead to a reduction in the level of cyclic-AMP. This problem was resolved with replacement of amino acid 80 from Asp to Ala in the D2 receptor (D2R80A) *(89)*. The mutant protein lacks the ability to be regulated by cyclic-AMP, but retains the affinity for FESP. This was elegantly demonstrated in a correlation study using a bicistronic adenoviral vector carrying both the mutated receptor and HSV1-sr39TK genes *(90)*. A potential problem associated with the strong expression of membrane proteins as reporter gene products is proper protein folding, intracellular trafficking, and insertion of these proteins into the plasma membrane so they retain their function. Despite these concerns, it is clear that quantitative determination of the D2 receptor expression can be performed *in vivo* with FESP.

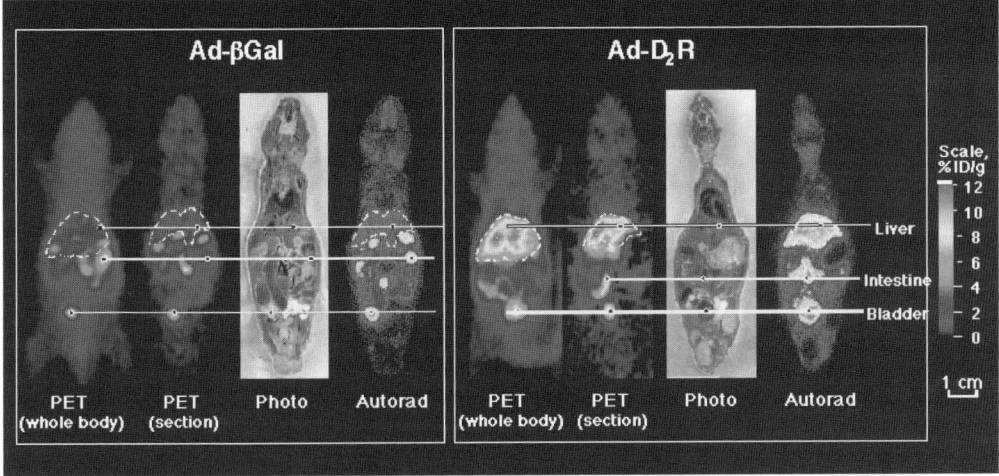

Fig. 7. Positron emission tomography and autoradiographic images of fluoroethylspiperone (FESP) following Ad-D2R and Ad-Bgal virus administration. Nude mice were injected via the tail vein with (A) 9×10^9 pfu of Ad-Bgal virus or (B) 9×10^9 pfu Ad2R virus. Two days after virus administration both mice were injected via the tail vein with [^{18}F]FESP (200 µCi, 200 µl). Three hours after the FESP injection the animals were imaged with microPET. A whole body coronal projection image of the ^{18}F activity distribution is displayed on the left. The liver outline is shown in white. The second images are coronal microPET sections, approximately 2 mm thick. After their PET scans, the mice were killed, frozen, sectioned, and photographed (third image from the left); the images on the right are autoradiographs of the tissue sections. The color scale represents the percent injected dose per gram of tissue (%ID/g). Images are displayed on the same quantitative color scale to allow signal intensity comparisons among the panels. (*See* color plate.) [Figure provided by S. Gambhir *(89)*.]

4. OPTICAL IMAGING GENES

Optical-based (bioluminescence and fluorescence) reporter systems are receiving increased attention because of their efficiency for sequential imaging, operational simplicity, and substantial cost benefits.

4.1 Bioluminescence Imaging

Bioluminescence reporter genes are being widely used in many laboratories for whole body imaging of small animals (Fig. 8). The most commonly used bioluminescence reporter systems include the firefly (FLuc) or *Renilla* (RLuc) luciferase genes *(91–93)*. As with nuclear and magnetic resonance reporter systems, bioluminescence imaging depends on the delivery of a specific substrate to the cells expressing the reporter gene. Furthermore, the light-emitting bioluminescence reaction, catalyzed by luciferases, depends on the presence of oxygen *(94)*. In the case of FLuc, an additional cofactor, ATP, is required. The firefly and *Renilla* luciferase reporter systems, in combination with their corresponding luminescent substrates (luciferin and coelenterazine), have several advantages for imaging small living animals. Autobioluminescence in most cases is essentially nonexistent and results in very low background light emission. This contributes to the very high sensitivity and specificity of this optical imaging technique *(95)*. Semiquantitative accuracy and reproducibility require that luciferin,

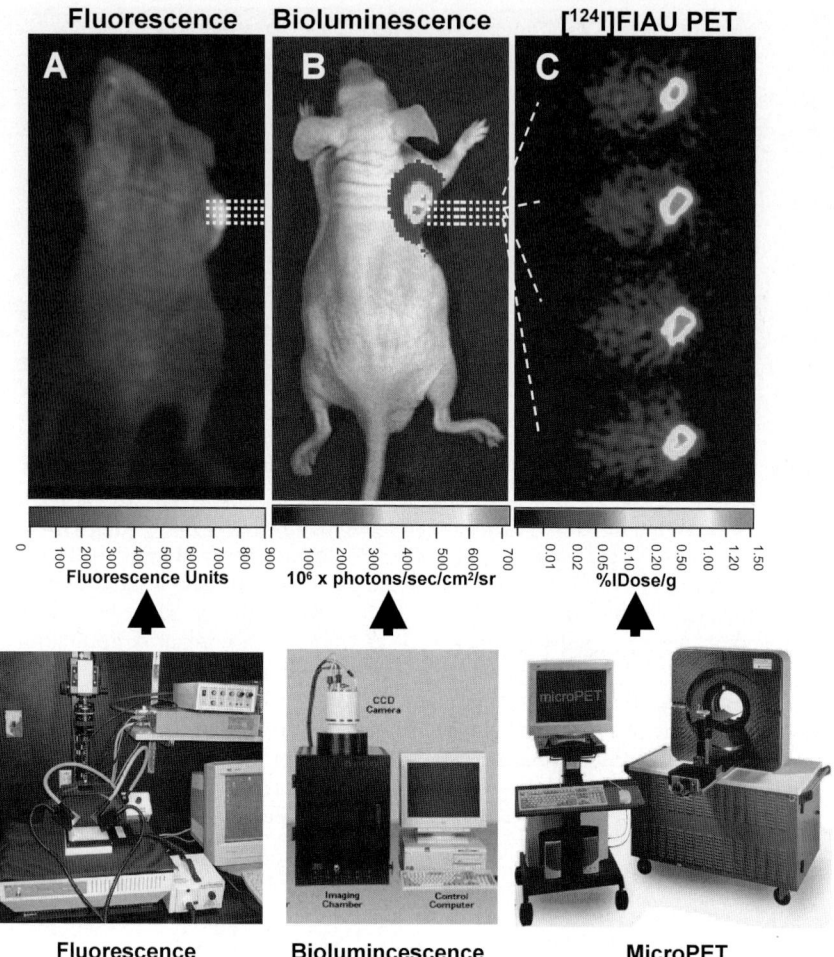

Fig. 8. Noninvasive *in vivo* multimodality imaging in mice bearing subcutaneous xenografts produced from U87-NES-HSV1-TK/GFP-cmvFluc and wild-type U87 cells. (A) Whole body fluorescence imaging; (B) whole body bioluminescence imaging; (C) axial PET images of [^{124}I]FIAU accumulation obtained at the levels indicated by the dotted white lines. (*See* color plate.) [Adapted from Ponomorev *et al.* *(98)*.]

ATP, and oxygen levels are not the rate-determining factors, but rather are present in excess at near saturation levels. Under these conditions, the photon emission flux (light intensity) is directly correlated with reporter gene expression and with the level of reporter gene product, namely, luciferase.

Another potential concern is the fact that the substrate for *Renilla* luciferase, coelenterazine, is a substrate for the MDR1 transporter. It has recently been shown that coelenterazine is rapidly exported from cell lines that express MDR1, and this could impact the photon emission flux from the coelenterazine–*Renilla* luciferase reporter system in these cells *(96)*. *In vivo* bioluminescence imaging has been successfully applied to many novel reporter systems and is rapidly expanding in the molecular and cell biology communities.

4.2 Fluorescence Imaging

In the past 10 years, GFP has evolved from a little known protein to a common widely used tool in molecular biology and cell biology. It is particularly useful because of its stability and the fact that its chromophore is formed by autocatalytic cyclization that does not require a cofactor. Furthermore, it appears that fusion of GFP to other proteins does not significantly alter its fluorescent properties or the intracellular location of the fusion protein *(97, 98)*. Fluorescent protein-based reporter gene systems started with different spectral shifted variants of *Aequorea victoria* GFP, including an eGFP *(99–106)*. A number of red fluorescent proteins, including *Discosoma* species (dsRed1 and dsRed2) *(107)* and *Heteractis crispa* (HcRed) *(108)*, have also been described. Fluorescence imaging has been shown to be useful for *in vitro* applications such as tracking the translocation of proteins within cells, identifying and selecting transduced cells using FACS, and cost-effective *in vitro* assays to validate the function and sensitivity of specific inducible reporter systems. The development of whole body transcutaneous fluorescence imaging technology provides for (1) imaging reporter gene expression in small living animals (Fig. 8), and (2) localizing transduced cells and/or the expression of inducible reporter systems (e.g., expression of HIF-1, Fig. 5) in tissue sections at the microscopic level by *in situ* fluorescence imaging. Limitations of fluorescence reporter imaging include (1) the requirement of an external source of light for activation of the chromophore, (2) tissue attenuation and scatter of both transmitted and emitted light, which limit the resolution and depth of imaging, and (3) endogenous autofluorescence of tissues, which frequently results in a substantial background emission that limits the sensitivity and specificity of fluorescence imaging. However, the use of selective filters or the application of spectral analysis can significantly reduce the contribution of autofluorescence to the acquired images. In addition, new classes of red fluorescent proteins and near-infrared dyes provide better deep tissue imaging characteristics *(107–109)* and are a focus of current research development.

Nevertheless, *in vivo* bioluminescence reporter imaging currently remains more sensitive than *in vivo* fluorescence reporter imaging due to the absence of autobioluminescence and low background activity. Luciferase is well suited to monitor transcription due to its relatively fast induction *(110)* and to the considerable short biological half-life of both luciferin and luciferase *(111)*. However, this advantage over the longer-lived eGFP has been recently mitigated by the development of short-lived, rapidly degradable variants of eGFP. These short-lived variants have been used for higher temporal resolution imaging of eGFP chimeric proteins within cells. Combining these reporter genes into a single fusion gene could provide additional tools for the analysis of cancer cells both *in vivo* and *ex vivo*. Such a dual-function reporter gene was created and the single encoded protein was shown to be both fluorescent and bioluminescent *(112)*.

5. ARRANGEMENT OF THERAPEUTIC AND IMAGING GENES IN A VECTOR DELIVERY SYSTEM

5.1 Fusion Gene Constructs for Therapy and Imaging

The product of a fusion gene is a single chimeric protein consisting of several domains, one of which could be the product of a therapeutic gene and another could be the product of an imaging gene (Fig. 9a and b). However, it would be problematic

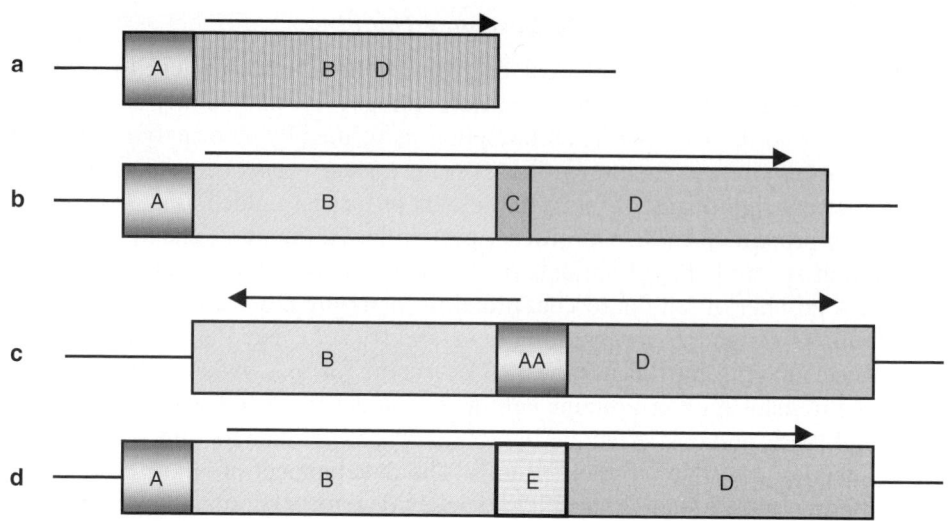

Fig. 9. Arrangement of therapeutic and imaging genes in a delivery system. (A) indicates the promoter element, which can be constitutive or inducible; (B) indicates the therapeutic gene; (D) indicates an imaging gene; (C) indicates a linker sequence between fusion genes; and (E) is an internal ribosomal entry site (IRES). The arrows indicate mRNA transcripts. (a) The therapeutic gene and the imaging gene are the same and result in a single protein. (b) The therapeutic gene and the imaging gene are fused to produce a chimeric protein. (c) The therapeutic gene and the reporter gene are driven from a bidirectional promoter. (d) The therapeutic gene and the reporter gene are expressed on a common message through an IRES element.

to develop fusion genes for all possible therapeutic modalities, where each part of the fusion protein retains its native conformation and has an equal level of function. In addition, many therapeutic genes and noninvasive imaging reporter genes are not suitable for such molecular manipulations because of the complexity of the tertiary protein structure. The HSV1-TK/GFP fusion gene was one of the first developed constructs with HSV1-TK for radiotracer-based noninvasive imaging that could be combined with *ex vivo* GFP fluorescence imaging *(113, 114)*. To optimize the sensitivity of imaging HSV1-TK/GFP reporter gene expression, a series of HSV1-TK/GFP mutants was developed with altered nuclear localization and better cellular enzymatic activity, compared to that of the native HSV1-TK/GFP fusion protein (HSV1-TK/GFP). These modifications of the HSV1-TK/GFP reporter gene included targeted inactivating mutations in the nuclear localization signal (NLS), the addition of a nuclear export signal (NES), a combination of both mutation types, and a truncation of the first 135 bp of the native *hsv1-TK* coding sequence containing a "cryptic" testicular promoter and the NLS *(97)*. A fusion gene containing HSV1-TK, FLuc, and the neomycin resistance gene has also been developed *(115)*. Two triple fusion genes have also been developed recently. We were able to construct a fusion gene containing HSV1-TK, GFP, and FLuc components, which have been used for fluorescence, bioluminescence, and nuclear imaging *(98)*. The HSV1-TK domain within these fusion constructs retains its therapeutic potential (our unpublished data). A triple fusion reporter vector harboring a bioluminescence synthetic *Renilla* luciferase (hRLuc) reporter gene, a reporter gene encoding the monomeric red fluorescence protein (mRFP), and a mutant herpes simplex virus type 1 sr39 thymidine kinase [HSV1-truncated sr39TK (tTK); a PET reporter gene] was also found to retain the activity of each protein component *(116)*.

The attempt to construct fusion genes that allow both imaging and therapeutic action is a worthwhile endeavor, since it would simplify the monitoring of therapeutic gene expression by noninvasive imaging and provide for relating gene expression to therapeutic efficacy. However, there is no guarantee that the fusion construct will result in a functional gene product. This could be due to a change in the conformational structure of the native protein or result in an alteration in the subcellular localization of the fusion protein, and result in a loss of activity in one of its components. Modulation of the fusion mRNA or a change in the clearance (breakdown) of the fusion protein may also be sufficiently different compared to each of the native proteins (gene products of the two native genes). Such differences could have a significant impact on the level of the fusion gene product, and, thereby, on the level of its biological activity. Fusion proteins are larger than each of the corresponding native proteins and are more likely to generate an immunological response and to result in a more rapid degradation of the fusion protein and reduction in the therapeutic benefit of the gene therapy. Thus, fusion gene technology cannot be generalized and may not be widely applicable in clinical imaging of therapeutic gene expression. However, when a fusion gene product is functional and nonimmunogenic, it may be a very useful construct for monitoring therapeutic gene expression.

5.2 Bidirectional Promoters for Therapeutic Gene and a Reporter Expression Gene

Bidirectional promoters can drive gene expression in both the 5′ and 3′ direction. They can be constitutive promoters or inducible promoters, and can be regulated by endogenous or pharmacological means (Fig. 9c). Gossen *et al. (117)* described an inducible promoter system that is regulated by the administration of inexpensive and readily available drugs (tetracycline and tetracycline analogs). These drugs freely diffuse throughout the body and can be used to control the expression of any single target gene in a dose-dependent manner. Many laboratories have used the tetracycline inducible system to control gene expression in both cell culture and in animals. Baron *et al. (118)* recently enhanced the tetracycline-inducible system by constructing a new vector in which a single bidirectional tetracycline inducible promoter can be used to control the expression of any pair of genes in a correlated, dose-dependent manner. A stable transduced HeLa cell line was created in which the D2R and HSV1-sr39TK PET reporter genes were driven by this bidirectional promoter *(119)*, and these cells were used to produce tumors in mice. When these tumor-bearing mice were exposed to tetracycline in their drinking water, both reporter genes were coexpressed. The level of reporter gene induction was imaged by sequential microPET imaging and analysis of FESP and FHBG retention. Following removal of the tetracycline, a repeat microPET analysis of FESP and FHBG retention in these tumors demonstrated that both D2R and HSV1-sr39TK expression returned to preinduction levels. These results demonstrated that bidirectional vectors can be used to monitor the coexpression of a therapeutic gene and an imaging gene, and that modulation of vector-introduced genes by a tetracycline-inducible promoter can be used to develop a novel experimental–clinical protocol.

5.3 Vectors Expressing an Internal Ribosomal Entry Site-Linked Therapeutic Gene and a Reporter Gene

Many viruses express several proteins from polycistronic messages. This distinguishes gene expression in viruses from that in mammalian cells, where "one transcript means one protein." In internal ribosomal entry site (IRES)-linked constructs, the most proximal cistron is translated by conventional cap-dependent initiation. The more distal cistron(s) are initiated from a cap-independent IRES *(120)*. Molecular biologists have used a large variety of artificial bicistronic messages to express two separate proteins from a common transcript (Fig. 9d). Utilization of bicistronic vectors to study the coordinated expression of therapeutic and imaging genes in gene therapy models has been used by a number of laboratories. In one of the first reports using a retroviral construct, it was shown that imaging of HSV1-TK can provide quantitative as well as topographical information related to the expression of a second, IRES-linked transgene *(121)*. In this case, HSV1-TK and β-galactosidase expression was shown to be stable over a wide range of values in the transduced xenografts. Both reporters are encoded in a single bicistronic message driven by the same retroviral promoter. Subsequently, microPET imaging was used to analyze the ability of reporter genes to measure and correlate the expression of two proteins from a bicistronic message delivered in an adenoviral vector. A replication-deficient adenovirus that expressed the D2R and HSV1-sr39TK PET reporter genes from a bicistronic message driven by the CMV promoter was repeatedly monitored by microPET with [^{18}F]FESP and [^{18}F]FHBG (tracers for D2R and HSV1-sr39TK, respectively). They demonstrated hepatic localization and a strong correlation ($r^2 = 0.89$) between HSV-sr39TK and D2R PET reporter gene expression over a 3-month period, in which absolute expression from the bicistronic message varied over a 10-fold range *(89)*. Recently the self-inactivated bicistronic retroviral vector bearing hNIS and GFP was developed in our group as we discussed above *(68)*. A major drawback associated with any IRES-based bicistronic vector is that the downstream transgene expression is often attenuated and expression levels may vary in different cell types. For future application of the bicistronic vector, it will be ideal to place the therapeutic gene upstream of IRES if maximal therapeutic effect is desired or the reporter gene upstream if supreme imaging sensitivity is needed. Alternatively, a "super-IRES" element can be engineered from short segments of cellular mRNA and cloned into the bicistronic vector to enhance downstream transgene expression by as much as 63-fold over the EMCV IRES element *(90)*.

6. IMAGING ADOPTIVE IMMUNE CELL THERAPIES

The invasive nature of classical pathology precludes the possibility of repetitive monitoring of cellular trafficking in the same subject over time. A noninvasive and repetitive evaluation of adoptively administered cells is necessary to study trafficking, homing, tumor targeting, activation, proliferation, and persistence of adoptively transferred cells. Such studies would significantly aid in the development and clinical implementation of new therapeutic approaches based on adoptive transfer of immune cells.

6.1 Ex Vivo *Radiolabeling and Nuclear Imaging*

Noninvasive imaging of lymphocyte trafficking dates back to the early 1970s, when the first experiments were performed with extracorporeal labeling of lymphocytes

(122, 123). These methods were applied to different immune cells using various metallic radioisotopes and chelation attachments for labeling (e.g., ^{111}In, ^{67}Co, ^{64}Cu, ^{51}Cr, ^{99m}Tc) *(122–127)*. ^{111}In in particular has been widely used in oncology as an imaging agent for monitoring studies with tumor-infiltrating lymphocytes *(127, 128)*. A major limitation of *ex vivo* labeling of lymphocytes is the relatively low level of radioactivity per cell that can be attained by labeling cells with radiotracers such as the [^{111}In]oxime and [^{64}Cu]PTSM. The exposure of cells to higher doses of radioactivity during labeling is also limited by radiotoxicity. Another shortcoming of the *ex vivo* radiolabeling approach is the short period for cell monitoring, which is limited by radioactivity decay and biological clearance.

6.2 Labeling with Supermagnetic Agents and Magnetic Resonance Imaging

Recent developments in MR imaging have enabled *in vivo* imaging at near microscopic resolution *(129, 130)*. This approach permits visualization and tracking of magnetically tagged cells using MRI. Conventional cell labeling techniques rely on the surface attachment of magnetic beads ranging in size from several hundred nanometers to micrometers. Although these methods are efficient for *in vitro* cell separation, cell surface labeling is generally not suitable for *in vivo* use due to rapid reticuloendothelial recognition and clearance of the labeled cells. Alternatively, lymphocytes and other cells have been labeled with small monocrystalline nanoparticles ranging in size from 10 to 40 nm *(131–135)* using fluid-phase or receptor-mediated endocytosis to achieve internalization of the nanoparticles. Unfortunately, this technique provides a low labeling efficiency, particularly in differentiated and nondividing cells. Several alternative methods have been developed for labeling cells at higher efficiencies using superparamagnetic iron-oxide nanoparticles or ^{111}I cross-linked to the HIV-1 TAT peptide, which facilitates transport across the cell membrane. For example, Dodd *et al. (136)* demonstrated that murine T cells loaded with superparamagnetic iron oxide nanoparticles preferentially migrated to the spleen. Although a clear reduction in signal intensity in the spleen was observed, the duration of the latter study did not exceed a 24-h period. A similar study by Kirscher *et al.* was reported, where OVA-specific T cells were labeled with highly cross-linked iron oxide nanoparticles (CLIO-HD). These OVA-specific T cells were shown to accumulate in the melanoma tumor over a period of 5 days *(137)*. These labeling techniques improved imaging the initial migration (within several days) of adoptively transferred lymphoid cells to sites providing supportive microenvironments. However, *ex vivo* labeling of T cells with MR contrast does not provide an opportunity to monitor their functional status, such as activation upon antigen recognition, cytokine secretion, proliferation, and cytolytic functions.

6.3 Genetic Labeling of Cells for Adoptive Therapy

Stable genetic labeling of adoptively transferred cells, such as lymphocytes, with various reporter genes has been used to circumvent the temporal limitations of *in vitro* radiolabeling or magnetic labeling of cells. The effectiveness of T cell-mediated gene therapy largely depends on efficient gene delivery to T-lymphocyte populations and targeted transgene expression in an appropriate progeny of transduced T cells. Retroviral-mediated transduction has proven to be one of the most effective means to deliver transgenes into T cells and results in high levels of sustained transgene expression *(138, 139)*. For example, long-term circulation of the Epstein–Barr virus (EBV)-specific cytotoxic donor-derived T cells has been shown to occur in patients treated for post-bone marrow transplantation EBV-induced lymphoproliferative diseases. Retroviral transduced T cells with the neomycin resistance or low-affinity nerve growth factor receptor (LNGFR) and HSV1-TK genes were detectable in peripheral blood samples from patients by polymerase chain reaction (PCR) or fluorescent-activated cell sorting (FACS) analysis *(140–142)*.

Genetic labeling of lymphocytes with the luciferase (FLuc) reporter gene and non-invasive bioluminescence imaging (BLI) of mice have been reported *(143, 144)*. Costa *et al.* showed the migration of myelin basic protein-specific, Luc-transduced $CD4^+$ T cells in the central nervous system *(145)*. The distribution of cytotoxic T-lymphocytes (CTL) can also be followed throughout the organism and monitored over time using BLI of Luc-expressing CTLs. However, BLI is a semiquantitative assay at best, because signal intensity depends largely on distance from the surface and on the variable optical characteristics of different tissues due to differences in attenuation and scatter of the emitted photons. Nevertheless, BLI of Luc expression has great potential in preclinical mouse-model studies, where high sensitivity, low cost, and technical simplicity are important for rapid screening.

The long-term trafficking and localization of T-lymphocytes are important components of the immune response, and in the elimination of abnormal cells and infectious agents from the body. Passive (*ex vivo*) labeling of T cells with radioactive isotopes can be unstable and does not account for proliferation of activated T cells in the body. Our group demonstrated the feasibility of long-term *in vivo* monitoring of adoptively transferred antigen-specific T cells that were transduced to express a radionuclide-based reporter gene for *in vivo* radiolabeling and PET imaging *(146)*. Epstein–Barr virus-specific T cells (CTLs) were obtained and stably transduced with a constitutively expressed dual reporter gene (HSV1TK/GFP fusion gene). SCID mice bearing four tumors [(1) autologous $HLA-A0201^+$ EBV-transformed B cells (EBV BLCL); (2) allogeneic EBV BLCL expressing the HLA-A0201 allele; (3) allogeneic HLA mismatched EBV BLCL; and (4) EBV-negative $HLA-A0201^+$ B cell acute lymphoblastic leukemia (B-ALL)] were treated with HSV1-TK/GFP transduced EBV-specific CTLs. Specific accumulation and localization of radioactivity were observed only in the autologous and allogeneic $HLA-A0201^+$ EBV-BLCL; no T cell infiltration was seen in the allogeneic HLA-A0201-matched, EBV-negative B-ALL or HLA-mismatched EBV BLCL xenografts (Fig. 10). Sequential imaging over 15 days after T cell injection permitted long-term monitoring of the HSV1-TK/GFP transduced cells and demonstrated tumor-specific migration and targeting of the CTLs. Infusion of EBV-specific CTLs led to the elimination of subcutaneous autologous EBV-BLCL tumor and $HLA-A0201^+$ allogeneic EBV-BLCL xenografts. This tumor rejection was abolished by administration of GCV, which eliminated the HSV1-TK-transduced T cells (our unpublished data). These studies demonstrate the feasibility of long-term *in vivo* monitoring of targeting and migration of antigen-specific CTLs that are transduced to constitutively express a radionuclide-based reporter gene. This paradigm provides the opportunity for repeated visualization of transferred T cells within the same animal over time using noninvasive reporter gene PET imaging and it is potentially transferable to clinical studies in patients with EBV^+ cancer.

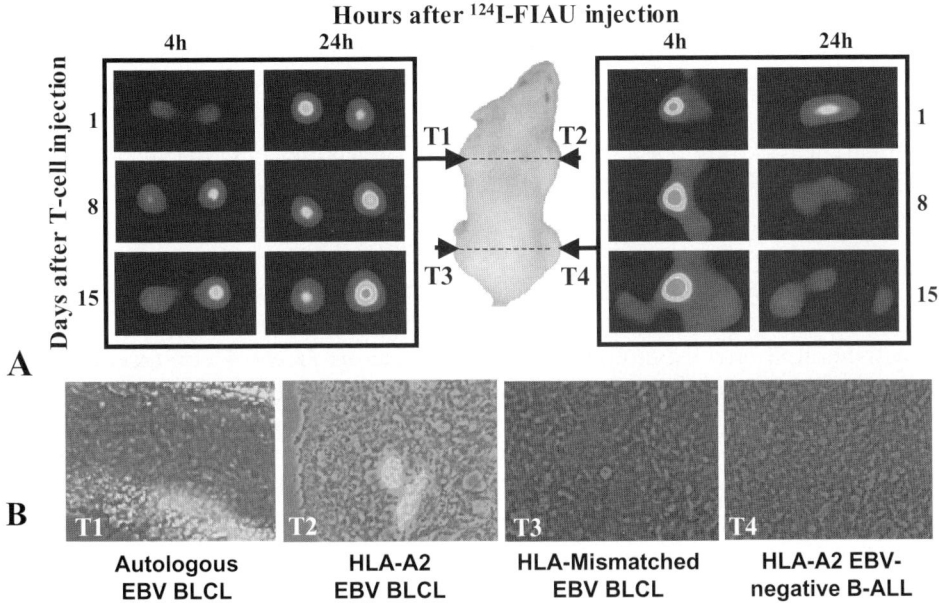

Fig. 10. MicroPET imaging of T cell migration and targeting. (A) Sequential axial cross-sectional images through the shoulders (left panel) and thighs (right panel) of mice bearing autologous EBV-BLCL (T1), *HLA-A0201*-matched EBV-BLCL (T2), HLA-mismatched EBV-BLCL (T3), and *HLA-A0201*[+] EBV[−] B-ALL (T4) tumors in the left and right shoulders and the left and right thighs, respectively, 4 and 24 h after each intravenous injection of [^{124}I]FIAU is administered are shown (vertical columns). Sequential microPET imaging is shown 1, 8, and 15 days after T cell infusion (horizontal rows). All images are from a single representative mouse. Axial images at the shoulder level demonstrate selective uptake of [^{124}I]FIAU in the autologous (T1) and *HLA-A0201*[+] allogeneic EBV[+] (T2) xenografts. No activity is detected in the lungs, reflecting clearance of T cells from the lung by 24 h after transfer. Axial cross-sectional images at the thigh demonstrate [^{124}I]FIAU in the bladder (Bl) at 4 h. Radioactivity in the bladder and abdominal organs is very low by 24 h after [^{124}I]FIAU infusion. No accumulation of [^{124}I]FIAU was detected in the EBV[+] *HLA-A0201* (T3) or EBV[−] *HLA-A0201*[+] B-ALL (T4) xenografts. (B) Fluorescence microscopy of corresponding tissue cryosections. CTL-TKGFP fluorescence was seen in the autologous EBV-BLCL (T1) and *HLA-A0201*-matched allogeneic EBV-BLCL (T2) xenografts. No CTL-TKGFP fluorescence was observed in the HLA-mismatched EBV-BLCL (T3) and *HLA-A0201*[+] EBV[−] B-ALL (T4) xenografts. Images were obtained from 20-mm tissue sections with ×400 magnification. (*See* color plate.) [(Adapted from Koehne *et al.* *(146)*.]

In another study we have shown tumor-specific trafficking and tumoricidal activity of Wilms tumor protein (WT1)-specific T cells that were transduced with HSV1-TK/GFP fusion reporter gene and administered to animals bearing WT1-positive tumors *(147)*. Similar studies were conducted by the UCLA group showing a specific targeting of murine sarcoma virus antigen-positive tumor by antigen-specific T cells that were transduced with PET and BLI reporter genes *(148)*. In these studies, a bicistronic retroviral vector for T cell labeling with HSV1-TK and GFP was used *(148)*, and a lentivirus encoding a triple modality reporter gene was used in a follow-up study *(149)*.

The potential of PET imaging for quantifying cell signals in regions of anatomic interest exists. However, little is known about the constraints and parameters for using PET signal detection to establish cell numbers in different regions of interest. Su *et al.*

determined the correlation of PET signal to cell number, and characterized the cellular limit of detection for PET imaging. These studies using human T cells transduced with HSV1-TK reporter gene revealed a cell number-dependent signal, with a limit of detection calculated as 10^6 cells in a region of interest of 0.1 ml volume. Quantitatively similar parameters were observed with stably transduced N2a glioma cells and primary T lymphocytes *(150)*.

6.4 T Cell Activation

An essential component of the immune response in many normal and disease states is T cell activation. Our group has monitored and assessed T cell receptor (TCR)-dependent activation *in vivo* using noninvasive PET imaging *(151)*. T cell receptor interactions with MHC-peptide complexes expressed on antigen-presenting cells initiate T cell activation, resulting in transcription that is mediated by several factors. Several of these factors, including interleukin-2 (IL-2) and other cytokines, contribute to the regulation of a number of target genes through several activating pathways and involve several transcription factors such as nuclear factor of activated T cells (NFAT) *(152)*. Furthermore, this activation can be arrested clinically by the use calcineurin inhibitors such as cyclosporin A and FK506 *(153)*. When combined with imaging of NFAT-mediated activation of T cells, noninvasive PET imaging should allow monitoring of the trafficking, proliferation, and antigen-specific activation of T cells in antitumor vaccination trials.

7. IMAGING STEM CELLS

Scientists and the general public alike have been intrigued by the existence of stem cells, and this fascination is rooted in their unique biological properties. Stem cells have the capacity for indefinite reproduction, together with the ability to produce differentiated progeny. Evidence shows that stem cells can form single or multiple tissues and hence it is believed that these cells can generate and maintain human organs without becoming exhausted. Scientists have attempted to capitalize on the exceptional regenerative capacity of stem cells in the development of novel treatments for a wide variety of human diseases, such as Parkinson's and Alzheimer's diseases, stroke, burns, heart disease, and osteoarthritis.

Beyond their regenerative capacity, intrinsic properties such as the cancer tropism of certain types of stem and progenitor cells have been documented. Two prominent examples that motivated the imaging studies discussed in this section are the recruitment of endothelial precursor cells (EPCs) into the tumor vasculature and tumor targeting of marrow stromal cells (MSCs). We will also discuss *in vivo* imaging of transplanted hematopoietic stem cells.

7.1 Endothelial Precursor Cells

Angiogenesis of neoplasms is of great interest to cancer biologists as tumor development is critically dependent on new blood vessel formation. Endothelial precursor cells have the ability to mature into the cells that line the lumen of blood vessels and they have been implicated in both reendothelialization and neovascularization. Hence, imaging of EPCs and neoangiogenesis may offer powerful tools for cancer diagnostics and treatment. A portfolio of advanced methods has been developed for functional imaging of various aspects of tumor angiogenesis, including the number and geometry of blood vessels, as well as blood flow and vascular permeability *(154)*. The origin of cells that contribute to new tumor blood vessel formation is not well understood, but in an important contribution Lyden *et al.* demonstrated that tumor recruitment of bone marrow-derived EPCs is necessary for neoangiogenesis *(155, 156)*. This finding prompted a recent study aimed at imaging EPCs *in vivo*.

Anderson and colleagues investigated the neovasculature of murine gliomas in immunodeficient mice *(157)*. Prior to transplantation, an Sca^+ bone marrow cell population that contains endothelial precursor cells was labeled with MRI "visible" iron oxide. Paramagnetic iron oxide produces large susceptibility artifacts enabling its detection as hypointense areas by MRI *(158)* and these particles can be used to label cells *ex vivo*. By utilizing iron oxide-labeled EPCs and *in vivo* MRI, systemically transplanted cells in the vicinity of the tumor were detected as early as 9 days after infusion *(158)*. The study provides proof of principle that imaging of EPCs plus an appropriate mouse model can be combined for the noninvasive assessment of EPC tumor migration. Although the applied imaging modality requires sophisticated MRI, the iron oxide labeling method is fast, passive, and nontoxic. In future studies, this technique may be useful for labeling highly purified EPC populations without any genetic alterations. Taken together, imaging of tumor migration of EPCs complements the previous progress in functional imaging of tumor angiogenesis.

7.2 Marrow Stromal Cells

Tumor targeting of MSCs for drug delivery was described by Studeny *et al.* in 2002 *(159)* and was confirmed by the same group in 2004 *(160)*. Human MSCs were genetically modified to produce interferon-β and subsequently were transplanted systemically into immunodeficient mice that develop cancer metastatic to the lungs. Preferential tumor targeting of the administered cells was detected by histology and could be related to a therapeutic effect in terms of increased overall survival *(158, 159)*.

These encouraging findings followed an imaging study by Zhang *et al.* who explored brain tumor targeting of MSCs after intravenous administration *(161)*. By using iron oxide cell labeling in combination with MRI, they demonstrated tumor tropism of the transplanted MSCs *(161)*. The observations were confirmed by histology and supported the findings made earlier by Studeny and colleagues.

7.3 Hematopoietic Stem Cells

The driving force for exploring the transplantation biology of hematopoietic stem cells (HSCs) in regard to cancer treatment is the use of bone marrow transplantation in the management of certain, mainly hematological cancers, such as leukemia, lymphoma, and myeloma. Moreover, it has been demonstrated that HSCs are valuable targets for the transfer of genes that confer resistance to anticancer drugs *(162)*. Such a myeloprotective strategy aims to increase cancer cell kill by dose escalation of the drug. Generally, there is a synergy between gene therapy approaches and imaging because, as outlined earlier in this chapter, many imaging strategies rely on the use of reporter genes. Hence, in an established strategy requiring gene transfer the therapeutic gene can be combined with or substituted for a suitable imaging reporter.

The application of molecular imaging for *in vivo* assessment of HSCs has lagged somewhat behind the technical developments of current imaging techniques. This has been partly due to the successful and convenient use of antibody-based FACS analysis of peripheral blood containing cells derived from transplanted HSCs. Nevertheless, imaging provides striking advantages. For example, the ability to monitor HSCs trafficking spatially in the whole body prompted Wang et al. *(163)* to explore luciferase reporter gene-based bioluminescence imaging of HSCs. Partially purified human HSCs were transduced to express the luciferase reporter gene and then transplanted into immunodeficient mice. The transduced HSCs were subsequently monitored for body distribution. The study demonstrated proof of principle that BLI can monitor the fate of HSCs in a mouse model. A more elegant, in-depth analysis has been presented by Contag's laboratory *(164)*. The investigators derived purified, luciferase-marked HSCs from transgenic donor animals. These transgenic reporter HSCs, together with inert support cells, were systemically transplanted into irradiated recipients. The use of BLI revealed the dynamics of hematopoietic reconstitution over time. Of interest is the attempt to monitor reconstitution from single HSC transplants. The data support the concept that HSCs preferentially home to the spleen and vertebrae, despite the fact that homing sites tend to be variable and are not distinct in all animals. Although very informative, BLI for the dissection of HSC transplantation biology may be limited by the achievable detection sensitivity, particularly in deeper organs of the mouse. Also, current BLI methods provide only two-dimensional images; hence there is still a need for *ex vivo* histological correlation to validate interpretation of the *in vivo* bioluminescence images.

8. ISSUES FOR THE FUTURE

Noninvasive reporter gene imaging is a very exciting indirect imaging strategy that can be fully exploited in experimental and transgenic animals. However, reporter gene imaging applications will be more limited in patients due to the necessity of transducing target tissue with specific reporter constructs. Ideal vectors for targeting specific organs or tissue (tumors) in patients do not exist at this time, although vector development is a very active area of human gene therapy research. At least *two* different reporter constructs will be required in most cases for optimal reporter imaging studies: one will be a "constitutive" reporter that will be used to identify the site, extent, and duration of vector delivery and efficiency of tissue transduction (the normalizing or denominator term), and one will be an "inducible" reporter that is sensitive to the functional status of the transduced cells as described above.

The initial application of such double-reporter systems in patients will most likely be performed as part of a gene therapy protocol *(43)* or an adoptive therapy protocol where the patient's own cells are harvested (e.g., lymphocytes, T cells, or blood- or marrow-derived progenitor/stem cells). These cells can be transduced and expanded *ex vivo*, and then adoptively readministered to the patient. This scenario couples reporter gene imaging with existing adoptive therapies and allows for *ex vivo* transduction and expansion of harvested cells.

Each new vector (and imaging probe) requires extensive validation and time-consuming safety testing prior to government approval for human administration. However, once a reporter-gene and reporter-probe combination has been validated and approved for human studies, this reporter system can potentially be used in many different reporter systems and vectors. That is not the case with direct imaging probes, where the number of probes is closely related to the number of potential direct imaging targets. Although highly specific images can sometimes be obtained with direct imaging probes, the development and validation of new probes are similar to the development, testing, and validation of new drugs. In contrast, the development and validation of different reporter gene constructs are far simpler than that for new imaging probes. The wider application and more rapid development of inducible reporter-imaging systems (to image endogenous transcriptional regulation, posttranscriptional modulation, protein–protein interactions, protein degradation, pathway-specific signaling activity, etc.) are likely to result in the translation of reporter gene imaging into patient studies sooner than the application of corresponding direct imaging probes. Nevertheless, direct imaging probes do have certain advantages and they will continue to be developed and make significant contributions to molecular imaging. A major advantage of direct imaging probes is that once developed and validated, they do not require the transduction of target tissue by a reporter gene-bearing vector.

The development of versatile and sensitive assays that do *not* require tissue samples will be of considerable value for monitoring molecular–genetic and cellular processes in animal models of human disease, as well as for studies in human subjects in the future. Noninvasive imaging will compliment established *ex vivo* molecular–biological assays that require tissue sampling, and imaging will provide a spatial as well as a temporal dimension to our understanding of various diseases. The benefits of noninvasive monitoring (imaging) of transgene expression in gene therapy protocols are substantial; it will provide a practical and clinically useful way to identify successful gene transduction and expression in target (and nontarget) tissue over time. This is particularly true for adoptive therapy protocols where constitutively expressed reporter genes can be used to monitor the distribution, targeting, and persistence of administered cells; similarly, it may also be important to monitor the activation and functional status of these cells using inducible promoters to initiate expression of different reporter genes. In all cases, an objective and quantitative measure of the level and duration of therapeutic gene expression or adoptive cell targeting and persistence can be related to therapeutic outcome.

Government approval will be required for all new vectors and all new direct imaging probes prior to their human administration. The translation of molecular imaging research into patient studies and clinical application must proceed stepwise and must be carefully monitored to ensure safe and effective use.

ACKNOWLEDGMENTS

A special acknowledgment is given to our friend and colleague Juri Gelovani-Tjuvajev, who joined our group in 1991 and has recently accepted a well-deserved appointment as Chairman of the Department of Experimental Diagnostic Imaging at the MD Anderson Cancer Center in Houston. He has been a leading investigator and initiated many of the projects in our laboratory.

REFERENCES

1. Buchsbaum DJ, Curiel DT. Gene therapy for the treatment of cancer. *Cancer Biother Radiopharm* 2001;16(4):275–288.
2. Somia N, Verma IM. Gene therapy: Trials and tribulations. *Nature Rev* 2000;1:91–99.

3. Blasberg R, Tjuvajev J. In vivo monitoring of gene therapy by radiotracer imaging. In: Ernst Shering Research Foundation Workshop 22: Impact of Molecular Biology and New Technical Developments on Diagnostic Imaging. Berlin-Heidelberg: Springer-Verlag, 1997.
4. Gambhir SS, Herschman HR, Cherry SR, Barrio JR, Satyamurthy N, Toyokuni T, Phelps ME, Larson SM, Balatoni J, Finn R, Sadelain M, Tjuvajev J, Blasberg R. Imaging transgene expression with radionuclide imaging technologies. *Neoplasia* 2000;2:118–138.
5. Tavitian B. In vivo antisense imaging. *Quart J Nucl Med* 2000;3:236–255.
6. Ray P, Bauer E, Iyer M, Barrio JR, Satyamurthy N, Phelps ME, Herschman HR, Gambhir SS. Monitoring gene therapy with reporter gene imaging. *Semin Nuclear Med* 2001;312–320.
7. Blasberg RG, Gelovani J. Molecular-genetic imaging: A nuclear medicine-based perspective. *Mol Imaging* 2002;3:280–300.
8. Luker GD, Sharma V, Piwnica Worms D. Visualizing protein-protein interactions in living animals. *Methods* 2003;1:110–122.
9. Weissleder R, Ntziachristos V. Shedding light onto live molecular targets. *Nature Med* 2003;1:123–128.
10. Gelovani Tjuvajev J, Blasberg RG. In vivo imaging of molecular-genetic targets for cancer therapy. *Cancer Cell* 2003;4:327–332.
11. Berger F, Gambhir SS. Recent advances in imaging endogenous or transferred gene expression utilizing radionuclide technologies in living subjects: Applications to breast cancer. *Breast Cancer Res* 2001;1:28–35.
12. Contag CH, Ross BD. It's not just about anatomy: In vivo bioluminescence imaging as an eyepiece into biology. *J Magn Reson Imaging* 2002;16:378–387.
13. Gambhir SS. Molecular imaging of cancer with positron emission tomography. *Nat Rev Cancer* 2002;2:683–693.
14. Blasberg RG, Tjuvajev JG. Molecular-genetic imaging: Current and future perspectives. *J Clin Invest* 2003;11:1620–1629.
15. Weissleder R, Ntziachristos V. Shedding light onto live molecular targets. *Nature Med* 2003;9:123–128.
16. Min JJ, Gambhir SS. Gene therapy progress and prospects: Noninvasive imaging of gene therapy in living subjects. *Gene Ther* 2004;2:115–125.
17. Shah K, Jacobs A, Breakefield XO, Weissleder R. Molecular imaging of gene therapy for cancer. *Gene Ther* 2004;11:1175–1187.
18. Dehdashti F, Mortimer JE, Siegel BA, Griffeth LK, Bonasera TJ, Fusselman MJ, Detert DD, Cutler PD, Katzenellenbogen JA, Welch MJ. Positron tomographic assessment of estrogen receptors in breast cancer: Comparison with FDG-PET and in vitro receptor assays. *J Nucl Med* 1995;10:1766–1774.
19. Larson SM, Morris M, Gunther I, Beattie B, Humm JL, Akhurst TA, Finn RD, Erdi Y, Pentlow K, Dyke J, Squire O, Bornmann W, McCarthy T, Welch M, Scher H. Tumor localization of 16beta-18F-fluoro-5alpha-dihydrotestosterone versus 18F-FDG in patients with progressive, metastatic prostate cancer. *J Nucl Med* 2004;3:366–373.
20. Jaffer FA, Tung CH, Gerszten RE, Weissleder, R. In vivo imaging of thrombin activity in experimental thrombi with thrombin-sensitive near-infrared molecular probe. *Arterioscler Thromb Vasc Biol* 2002;22:1929–1935.
21. Contag CH, Spilman SD, Contag PR, Oshiro M, Eames B, Dennery P, Stevenson DK, Benaron DA. Visualizing gene expression in living mammals using a bioluminescent reporter. *Photochem Photobiol* 1997;4:523–531.
22. Contag PR, Olomu IN, Stevenson DK, Contag CH. Bioluminescent indicators in living mammals. *Nature Med* 1998;2:245–247.
23. Rehemtulla A, Stegman LD, Cardozo SJ, Gupta S, Hall DE, Contag CH, Ross BD. Rapid and quantitative assessment of cancer treatment response using in vivo bioluminescence imaging. *Neoplasia* 2000;6:491–495.
24. Tjuvajev JG, Stockhammer G, Desai R, Uehara H, Watanabe H, Gansbacher B, Blasberg RG. Imaging the expression of transfected genes in vivo. *Cancer Res* 1995;55:6126–6132.
25. Tjuvajev JG, Finn R, Watanabe K, Joshi R, Oku T, Kennedy J, Beattie B, Koutcher J, Larson S, Blasberg RG. Noninvasive imaging of herpes virus thymidine kinase gene transfer and expression: A potential method for monitoring clinical gene therapy. *Cancer Res* 1996;56:4087–4095.

26. Tjuvajev JG, Avril N, Oku T, Sasajima T, Miyagawa T, Joshi R, Safer M, Beattie B, DiResta G, Daghighian F, Augensen F, Koutcher J, Zweit J, Humm J, Larson SM, Finn R, Blasberg R. Imaging herpes virus thymidine kinase gene transfer and expression by positron emission tomography. *Cancer Res* 1998;58:4333–4341.
27. Gambhir SS, Barrio JR, Wu L, Iyer M, Namavari M, Satyamurthy N, Bauer E, Parrish C, MacLaren DC, Borghei AR, Green LA, Sharfstein S, Berk AJ, Cherry SR, Phelps ME, Herschman HR. Imaging of adenoviral-directed herpes simplex virus type 1 thymidine kinase reporter gene expression in mice with radiolabeled ganciclovir. *J Nucl Med* 1998;11: 2003–2011.
28. Gambhir SS, Barrio JR, Phelps ME, Iyer M, Namavari M, Satyamurthy N, Wu L, Green LA, Bauer E, MacLaren DC, Nguyen K, Berk AJ, Cherry SR, Herschman HR. Imaging adenoviral-directed reporter gene expression in living animals with positron emission tomography. *Proc Natl Acad Sci USA* 1999;5:2333–2338.
29. Weissleder R, Simonova M, Bogdanova A, Bredow S, Enochs WS, Bogdanov A. MR imaging and scintigraphy of gene expression through melanin induction. *Radiology* 1997;2:425–429.
30. Louie AY, Huber MM, Ahrens ET, Rothbacher U, Moats R, Jacobs RE, Fraser SE, Meade TJ. In vivo visualization of gene expression using magnetic resonance imaging. *Nature Biotechnol* 2000; 3:321–325.
31. Overbeek PA, Chepelinsky AB, Khillan JS, Piatigorsky J, Westphal H. Lens-specific expression and developmental regulation of the bacterial chloramphenicol acetyltransferase gene driven by the murine alpha A-crystallin promoter in transgenic mice. *Proc Natl Acad Sci USA* 1985;82: 7815–7819.
32. Forss-Petter S, Danielson PE, Catsicas S, Battenberg E, Price J, Nerenberg M, Sutcliffe JG. Transgenic mice expressing beta-galactosidase in mature neurons under neuron-specific enolase promoter control. *Neuron* 1990;5:187–197.
33. Balaban RS, Hampshire VA. Challenges in small animal noninvasive imaging. Review. *ILAR J* 2001;42:248–262.
34. March JC, Rao G, Bentley WE. Biotechnological applications of green fluorescent protein. *Appl Microbiol Biotechnol* 2003;62:303–315.
35. Hoffman RM. In vivo imaging with fluorescent proteins: The new cell biology. *Acta Histochem* 2004;106:77–87.
36. Fyfe JA, Keller PM, Furman PA, Miller RL, Elion GB. Thymidine kinase from herpes simplex virus phosphorylates the new antiviral compound, 9-(2-hydroxyethoxymethyl)guanine. *J Biol Chem* 1978; 253:8721–8727.
37. Oldfield EH, Ram Z, Culver KW, Blaese RM, DeVroom HL, Anderson WF. Gene therapy for the treatment of brain tumors using intra-tumoral transduction with the thymidine kinase gene and intravenous ganciclovir. *Hum Gene Ther* 1993;4:39–69.
38. Saito Y, Price RW, Rottenberg DA, Fox JJ, Su TL, Watanabe KA, Philips FS. Quantitative autoradiographic mapping of herpes simplex virus encephalitis with a radiolabeled antiviral drug. *Science* 1982;217:1151–1153.
39. Iyer M, Barrio JR, Namavari M, Bauer E, Satyamurthy N, Nguyen K, Toyokuni T, Phelps ME, Herschman HR, Gambhir SS. 8-[18F]Fluoropenciclovir: An improved reporter probe for imaging HSV1-tk reporter gene expression in vivo using PET. *J Nucl Med* 2001;42:96–105.
40. Gambhir SS, Bauer E, Black ME, Liang Q, Kokoris MS, Barrio JR, Iyer M, Namavari M, Phelps ME, Herschman HR. A mutant herpes simplex virus type 1 thymidine kinase reporter gene shows improved sensitivity for imaging reporter gene expression with positron emission tomography. *Proc Natl Acad Sci USA* 2000;97:2785–2790.
41. Alauddin MM, Conti PS. Synthesis and preliminary evaluation of 9-(4-[18F]-fluoro-3-hydroxymethylbutyl)guanine ([18F]FHBG): A new potential imaging agent for viral infection and gene therapy using PET. *Nucl Med Biol* 1998;25:175–180.
42. Yaghoubi SS, Barrio JR, Namavari M, Satyamurthy N, Phelps ME, Herschman HR, Gambhir SS. Imaging progress of herpes simplex virus type 1 thymidine kinase suicide gene therapy in living subjects with positron emission tomography. *Cancer Gene Ther* 2005;12:329–339.
43. Jacobs A, Voges J, Reszka R, Lercher M, Gossmann A, Kracht L, Kaestle C, Wagner R, Wienhard K, Heiss WD. Positron-emission tomography of vector-mediated gene expression in gene therapy for gliomas. *Lancet* 2001;358:727–729.

44. Doubrovin M, Ponomarev V, Beresten T, Balatoni J, Bornmann W, Finn R, Humm J, Larson S, Sadelain M, Blasberg R, Gelovani Tjuvajev J. Imaging transcriptional regulation of p53-dependent genes with positron emission tomography *in vivo*. *Proc Natl Acad Sci USA* 2001; 98:9300–9305.
45. Serganova I, Doubrovin M, Vider J, Ponomarev V, Soghomonyan S, Beresten T, Ageyeva L, Serganov A, Cai S, Balatoni J, Blasberg R, Gelovani J. Molecular imaging of temporal dynamics and spatial heterogeneity of hypoxia-inducible factor-1 signal transduction activity in tumors in living mice. *Cancer Res* 2004;64:6101–6108.
46. Zhang L, Adams JY, Billick E, Ilagan R, Iyer M, Le K, Smallwood A, Gambhir SS, Carey M, Wu L. Molecular engineering of a two-step transcription amplification (TSTA) system for transgene delivery in prostate cancer. *Mol Ther* 2002;5:223–232.
47. Qiao J, Doubrovin M, Sauter BV, Huang Y, Guo ZS, Balatoni J, Akhurst T, Blasberg RG, Tjuvajev JG, Chen SH, Woo SL. Tumor-specific transcriptional targeting of suicide gene therapy. *Gene Ther* 2002;9:168–175.
48. Mayer-Kuckuk P, Banerjee D, Malhotra S, Doubrovin M, Iwamoto M, Akhurst T, Balatoni J, Bornmann W, Finn R, Larson S, Fong Y, Gelovani Tjuvajev J, Blasberg R, Bertino JR. Cells exposed to antifolates show increased cellular levels of proteins fused to dihydrofolate reductase: A method to modulate gene expression. *Proc Natl Acad Sci USA* 2002;99:3400–3405.
49. Dai G, Levy O, Carrasco N. Cloning and characterization of the thyroid iodide transporter. *Nature* 1996;379:458–460.
50. Selmi-Ruby S, Watrin C, Trouttet-Masson S, *et al.* The porcine sodium/iodide symporter gene exhibits an uncommon expression pattern related to the use of alternative splice sites not present in the human or murine species. *Endocrinology* 2003;144:1074–1085.
51. Tazebay UH, Wapnir IL, Levy O, Dohan O, Zuckier LS, Zhao QH, Deng HF, Amenta PS, Fineberg S, Pestell RG, Carrasco N. The mammary gland iodide transporter is expressed during lactation and in breast cancer. *Nat Med* 2000;6:871–878.
52. Eskandari S, Loo DDF, Day G, Levy O, Wright EW, Carrasco N. Thyroid Na^+/I^- symporter: Mechanism, stoichiometry, and specificity. *J Biol Chem* 1997;272:27230–27238.
53. Van Sande J, Massart C, Beauwens R, Schoutens A, Costagliol S, Dumon JE, Wolff J. Anion selectivity by the sodium iodide symporter. *Endocrinology* 2003;144:247–252.
54. Boland A, Ricard M, Opolon P, Bidart JM, Yeh P, Filetti S, Schlumberger M, Perricaudet M. Adenovirus-mediated transfer of the thyroid sodium/iodide symporter gene into tumors for a targeted radiotherapy. *Cancer Res* 2000;60:3484–3492.
55. Kakinuma H, Bergert ER, Spitzweg C, Cheville JC, Lieber MM, Morris JC. Probasin promoter (ARR(2)PB)-driven, prostate-specific expression of the human sodium iodide symporter (h-NIS) for targeted radioiodine therapy of prostate cancer. *Cancer Res* 2003;63:7840–7844.
56. Schipper ML, Weber A, Behe M, Goke R, Joba W, Schmidt H, Bert T, Simon B, Arnold R, Heufelder AE, Behr TM. Radioiodide treatment after sodium iodide symporter gene transfer is a highly effective therapy in neuroendocrine tumor cells. *Cancer Res* 2003;63:1333–1338.
57. Dingli D, Peng KW, Harvey ME, Greipp PR, O'Connor MK, Cattaneo R, Morris JC, Russell SJ. Image-guided radiovirotherapy for multiple myeloma using a recombinant measles virus expressing the thyroidal sodium iodide symporter. *Blood* 2004;103:1641–1646.
58. Spitzweg C, O'Connor MK, Bergert ER, Tindall DJ, Young CY, Morris JC. Treatment of prostate cancer by radioiodine therapy after tissue-specific expression of the sodium iodide symporter. *Cancer Res* 2000;60:6526–6530.
59. Huang M, Batra RK, Kogai T, Lin YQ, Hershman JM, Lichtenstein A, Sharma S, Zhu LX, Brent GA, Dubinett SM. Ectopic expression of the thyroperoxidase gene augments radioiodide uptake and retention mediated by the sodium iodide symporter in non-small cell lung cancer. *Cancer Gene Ther* 2001;8:612–618.
60. Moon DH, Lee SJ, Park KY, Park KK, Ahn SH, Pai MS, Chang H, Lee HK, Ahn IM. Correlation between 99mTc-pertechnetate uptakes and expressions of human sodium iodide symporter gene in breast tumor tissues. *Nucl Med Biol* 2001;28:829–834.
61. Groot-Wassink T, Aboagye EO, Glaser M, Lemoine NR, Vassaux G. Adenovirus biodistribution and noninvasive imaging of gene expression in vivo by positron emission tomography using human sodium/iodide symporter as reporter gene. *Hum Gene Ther* 2002;13:1723–1735.
62. Dingli D, Diaz RM, Bergert ER, O'Connor MK, Morris JC, Russell SJ. Genetically targeted radiotherapy for multiple myeloma. *Blood* 2003;102:489–496.

63. Buchsbaum DJ, Chaudhuri TR, Zinn KR. Radiotargeted gene therapy. *J Nucl Med* 2005; 46:179S–186S.
64. Miyagawa M, Beyer M, Wagner B, Anton M, Spitzweg C, Gansbacher B, Schwaiger M, Bengel FM. Cardiac reporter gene imaging using the human sodium/iodide symporter gene. *Cardiovasc Res* 2005;65:195–202.
65. Kim KI, Chung JK, Kang JH, Lee YJ, Shin JH, Oh HJ, Jeong JM, Lee DS, Lee MC. Visualization of endogenous p53-mediated transcription in vivo using sodium iodide symporter. *Clin Cancer Res* 2005;11:123–128.
66. Faivre J, Clerc J, Gerolami R, Herve J, Longuet M, Liu B, Roux J, Moal F, Perricaudet M, Brechot C. Long-term radioiodine retention and regression of liver cancer after sodium iodide symporter gene transfer in wistar rats. *Cancer Res* 2004;64:8045–8051.
67. So MK, Kang JH, Chung JK, Lee YJ, Shin JH, Kim KI, Jeong JM, Lee DS, Lee MC. In vivo imaging of retinoic acid receptor activity using a sodium/iodide symporter and luciferase dual imaging reporter gene. *Mol Imaging* 2004;3:163–171.
68. Che J, Doubrovin M, Serganova I, Ageyeva L, Zanzonico P, Blasberg R. hNIS-IRES-eGFP dual reporter gene imaging. *Mol Imaging* 2005;4:128–136.
69. Krulich L, Dhariwal AP, McCann SM. Stimulatory and inhibitory effects of purified hypothalamic extracts on growth hormone release from rat pituitary in vitro. *Endocrinology* 1968;83:783–790.
70. Brazeau P, Vale W, Burgus R, Ling N, Butcher M, Rivier J, Guillemin R. Hypothalamic polypeptide that inhibits the secretion of immunoreactive pituitary growth hormone. *Science* 1973;179:77–79.
71. Reichlin S. Somatostatin. *N Engl J Med* 1983;309:1495–1501.
72. Reubi JC, Kvols L, Krenning E, Lamberts SW. Distribution of somatostatin receptors in normal and tumor tissue. *Metabolism* 1990;39:78–81.
73. Bauer W, Briner U, Doepfner W, Haller R, Huguenin R, Marbach P, Petcher TJ, Pless. SMS 201–995: A very potent and selective octapeptide analogue of somatostatin with prolonged action. *Life Sci* 1981;31:1133–1140.
74. Forssell-Aronsson EB, Nilsson O, Bejegard SA, Kolby L, Bernhardt P, Molne J, Hashemi SH, Wangberg B, Tisell LE, Ahlman H. 111In-DTPA-D-Phe1-octreotide binding and somatostatin receptor subtypes in thyroid tumors. *J Nucl Med* 2000;41:636–642.
75. Zinn KR, Buchsbaum DJ, Chaudhuri TR, Mountz JM, Grizzle WE, Rogers BE. Noninvasive monitoring of gene transfer using a reporter receptor imaged with a high-affinity peptide radiolabeled with ^{99m}Tc or ^{188}Re. *J Nucl Med* 2000;41:887–895.
76. Kundra V, Mannting F, Jones AG, Kassis AI. Noninvasive monitoring of somatostatin receptor type 2 chimeric gene transfer. *J Nucl Med* 2002;43:406–412.
77. Rogers BE, Zinn KR, Lin CY, Chaudhuri TR, Buchsbaum DJ. Targeted radiotherapy with [(90)Y]-SMT 487 in mice bearing human nonsmall cell lung tumor xenografts induced to express human somatostatin receptor subtype 2 with an adenoviral vector. *Cancer* 2002;94:1298–1305.
78. Lewis JS, Lewis MR, Cutler PD, et al. Radiotherapy and dosimetry of ^{64}Cu-TETA-Tyr^3-octreotate in a somatostatin receptor-positive, tumor-bearing rat model. *Clin Cancer Res* 1999;5:3608–3616.
79. de Jong M, Breeman WA, Bernard BF, Bakker WH, Schaar M, van Gameren A, Bugaj JE, Erion J, Schmidt M, Srinivasan A, Krenning EP. [^{177}Lu-DOTA^0,Tyr^3] octreotate for somatostatin receptor-targeted radionuclide therapy. *Int J Cancer* 2001;92:628–633.
80. Paganelli G, Zoboli S, Cremonesi M, Macke HR, Chinol M. Receptor-mediated radionuclide therapy with ^{90}Y-DOTA-D-Phe^1-Tyr^3-octreotide: Preliminary report in cancer patients. *Cancer Biother Radiopharm* 1999;14:477–483.
81. Kwekkeboom DJ, Bakker WH, Kooij PP, Konijnenberg MW, Srinivasan A, Erion JL, Schmidt MA, Bugaj JL, de Jong M, Krenning EP. [^{177}Lu-DOTA^0,Tyr^3]octreotate: Comparison with [^{111}In-DTPA^0]octreotide in patients. *Eur J Nucl Med* 2001;28:1319–1325.
82. de Jong M, Kwekkeboom D, Valkema R, Krenning EP. Radiolabelled peptides for tumour therapy: Current status and future directions—plenary lecture at the EANM 2002. *Eur J Nucl Med Mol Imaging* 2003;30:463–469.
83. Sibley DR, Monsma FJ Jr. Molecular biology of dopamine receptors. *Trends Pharmacol Sci* 1992; 13:61–69.
84. Bunzow JR, Van Tol HH, Grandy DK, Albert P, Salon J, Christie M, Machida CA, Neve KA, Civelli O. Cloning and expression of a rat D$_2$ dopamine receptor cDNA. *Nature* 1988;367:783–787.
85. Missale C, Nash SR, Robinson SW, Jaber M, Caron MG. Dopamine receptors: From structure to function. *Physiol Rev* 1998;78:189–225.

86. Satyamurthy N, Barrio JR, Bida GT, Huang SC, Mazziotta JC, Phelps ME. 3-(2'-[18F]Fluoroethyl)s piperone, a potent dopamine antagonist: Synthesis, structural analysis and in-vivo utilization in humans. *Int J Rad Appl Instrum [A]* 1990;41:113–129.
87. Barrio JR, Satyamurthy N, Huang SC, Keen RE, Nissenson CH, Hoffman JM, Ackermann RF, Bahn MM, Mazziotta JC, Phelps ME. 3-(2'-[18F]Fluoroethyl)spiperone: In vivo biochemical and kinetic characterization in rodents, nonhuman primates, and humans. *J Cereb Blood Flow Metab* 1989; 9:830–839.
88. MacLaren DC, Gambhir SS, Satyamurthy N, Barrio JR, Sharfstein S, Toyokuni T, Wu L, Berk AJ, Cherry SR, Phelps ME, Herschman HR. Repetitive, non-invasive imaging of the dopamine D2 receptor as a reporter gene in living animals. *Gene Ther* 1999;6:785–791.
89. Liang Q, Satyamurthy N, Barrio JR, Toyokuni T, Phelps MP, Gambhir SS, Herschman HR. Noninvasive, quantitative imaging in living animals of a mutant dopamine D2 receptor reporter gene in which ligand binding is uncoupled from signal transduction. *Gene Ther* 2001;8:1490–1498.
90. Chen IY, Wu JC, Min JJ, Sundaresan G, Lewis X, Liang Q, Herschman HR, Gambhir SS. Micro-positron emission tomography imaging of cardiac gene expression in rats using bicistronic adenoviral vector-mediated gene delivery. *Circulation* 2004;109:1415–1420.
91. Gross S, Piwnica-Worms D. Spying on cancer; molecular imaging in vivo with genetically encoded reporters. *Cancer Cell* 2005;7:5–15.
92. Yu YA, Timiryasova T, Zhang Q, Beltz R, Szalay AA. Optical imaging: Bacteria, viruses, and mammalian cells encoding light-emitting proteins reveal the locations of primary tumors and metastases in animals. *Anal Bioanal Chem* 2003;377:964–972.
93. Wilson T, Hastings JW. Bioluminescence. *Annu Rev Cell Dev Biol* 1998;14:197–230.
94. Contag CH, Spilman SD, Contag PR, Oshiro M, Eames B, Dennery P, Stevenson DK, Benaron DA. Visualizing gene expression in living mammals using a bioluminescent reporter. *Photochem Photobiol* 1997;4:523–531.
95. Bhaumik S, Gambhir S. Optical imaging of Renilla luciferase reporter gene expression in living mice. *Proc Natl Acad Sci USA* 2002;99:377–382.
96. Pichler A, Prior JL, Piwnica-Worms D. Imaging reversal of multidrug resistance in living mice with bioluminescence: MDR1 P-glycoprotein transports coelenterazine. *Proc Natl Acad Sci USA* 2004; 6;1702–1707.
97. Ponomarev V, Doubrovin M, Serganova I, Beresten T, Vider J, Shavrin A, Ageyeva L, Balatoni J, Blasberg R, Tjuvajev JG. Cytoplasmically retargeted HSV1-tk/GFP reporter gene mutants for optimization of noninvasive molecular-genetic imaging. *Neoplasia* 2003;5:245–254.
98. Ponomarev V, Doubrovin M, Serganova I, Vider J, Shavrin A, Beresten T, Ivanova A, Ageyeva L, Tourkova V, Balatoni J, Bornmann W, Blasberg R, Gelovani Tjuvajev J. A novel triple modality reporter gene for whole body fluorescent, bioluminescent and nuclear noninvasive imaging. *Eur J Nucl Med* 2004;5:740–751.
99. Levy JP, Muldoon RR, Zolotukhin S, Link CJ Jr. Retroviral transfer and expression of a humanized, red-shifted green fluorescent protein gene into human tumor cells. *Nat Biotechnol* 1996;14: 610–614.
100. Lalwani AK, Han JJ, Walsh BJ, Zolotukhin S, Muzyczka N, Mhatre AN. Green fluorescent protein as a reporter for gene transfer studies in the cochlea. *Hear Res* 1997;114:139–147.
101. Ellenberg J, Lippincott Schwartz J, Presley JF. Dual-colour imaging with GFP variants. *Trends Cell Biol* 1999;9:52–56.
102. Matz M, Matz MV, Fradkov AF, Labas YA, Savitsky AP, Zaraisky AG, Markelov ML, Lukyanov SA. Fluorescent proteins from nonbioluminescent Anthozoa species. *Nat Biotechnol* 1999; 17:969–973.
103. Falk MM, Lauf U. High resolution, fluorescence deconvolution microscopy and tagging with the autofluorescent tracers CFP, GFP, and YFP to study the structural composition of gap junctions in living cells. *Microsc Res Technol* 2001;52:251–262.
104. Hadjantonakis AK, Nagy A. The color of mice: In the light of GFP-variant reporters. *Histochem Cell Biol* 2001;115:49–58.
105. Labas YA, Gurskaya NG, Yanushevich YG, Fradkov AF, Lukyanov KA, Lukyanov SA, Matz MV. Diversity and evolution of the green fluorescent protein family. *Proc Natl Acad Sci USA* 2002; 99:4256–4261.
106. Campbell RE, Tour O, Palmer AE, Steinbach PA, Baird GS, Zacharias DA, Tsien RY. A monomeric red fluorescent protein. *Proc Natl Acad Sci USA* 2002;99:7877–7882.

107. Mathieu S, El-Battari A. Monitoring E-selectin-mediated adhesion using green and red fluorescent proteins. *J Immunol Methods* 2003;272:81–92.
108. Gurskaya NG, Fradkov AF, Terskikh A, Matz MV, Labas YA, Martynov VI, Yanushevich YG, Lukyanov KA, Lukyanov SA. GFP-like chromoproteins as a source of far-red fluorescent proteins. *FEBS Lett* 2001;507:16–20.
109. Yang M, Baranov E, Jiang P, Sun F, Li XM, Li LN, Hasegawa S, Bouvet M, Al Tuwaijri M, Chishima T, Shimada H, Moossa AR, Penman S, Hoffman RM. Whole-body optical imaging of green fluorescent protein expressing tumors and metastases. *Proc Natl Acad Sci USA* 2000;97:1206–1211.
110. Kolb VA, Makeyev EV, Spirin AS. Co-translational folding of an eukaryotic multidomain protein in a prokaryotic translation system. *J Biol Chem* 2000;275;16597–16601.
111. Thompson JF, Hayes LS, Lloyd DB. Modulation of firefly luciferase stability and impact on studies of gene regulation. *Gene* 1991;103:171–177.
112. Day RN, Kawecki M, Berry D. Dual function reporter protein for analysis of gene expression in living cells. *Biotechnology* 1998;25:852–854.
113. Loimas S, Wahlfors J, Janne J. Herpes simplex virus thymidine kinase-green fluorescent protein fusion gene: New tool for gene transfer studies and gene therapy. *Biotechniques* 1998;24:614–618.
114. Jacobs A, Dubrovin M, Hewett J, Sena-Esteves M, Tan CW, Slack M, Sadelain M, Breakefield XO, Tjuvajev JG. Functional coexpression of HSV-1 thymidine kinase and green fluorescent protein: Implications for noninvasive imaging of transgene expression. *Neoplasia* 1999;1:154–161.
115. Strathdee CA, McLeod MR, Underhill TM. Dominant positive and negative selection using luciferase, green fluorescent protein and beta-galactosidase reporter gene fusions. *Biotechniques* 2000; 28:210–214.
116. Ray P, De A, Min JJ, Tsien RY, Gambhir SS. Imaging tri-fusion multimodality reporter gene expression in living subjects. *Cancer Res* 2004;64(4):1323–1330.
117. Gossen M, Bujard H. Tight control of gene expression in mammalian cells by tetracycline-responsive promoters. *Proc Natl Acad Sci USA* 1992;89:5547–5551.
118. Baron U, Gossen M, Bujard H. Tetracycline-controlled transcription in eukaryotes: Novel transactivators with graded transactivation potential. *Nucleic Acids Res* 1997;25:2723–2729.
119. Sun X, Annala AJ, Yaghoubi SS, Barrio JR, Nguyen KN, Toyokuni T, Satyamurthy N, Namavari M, Phelps ME, Herschman HR, Gambhir SS. Quantitative imaging of gene induction in living animals. *Gene Ther* 2001;8:1572–1579.
120. Martinez-Salas E. Internal ribosome entry site biology and its use in expression vectors. *Curr Opin Biotechnol* 1999;10:458–464.
121. Tjuvajev JG, Joshi A, Callegari J, Lindsley L, Joshi R, Balatoni J, Finn R, Larson SM, Sadelain M, Blasberg RG. A general approach to the non-invasive imaging of transgenes using cis-linked herpes simplex virus thymidine kinase. *Neoplasia* 1999;1:315–320.
122. Gobuty AHRR, Barth RF. Organ distribution of 99mTc- and 51Cr-labeled autologous peripheral blood lymphocytes in rabbits. *J Nucl Med* 1977;18:141–146.
123. Papierniak CKBR, Kretschmer RR, Gotoff SP, Colombetti LG. Technetium-99m labeling of human monocytes for chemotactic studies. *J Nucl Med* 1976;17:988–992.
124. Korf JV-DL, Brinkman-Medema R, Niemarkt A, de Leij LF. Divalent cobalt as a label to study lymphocyte distribution using PET and SPECT. *J Nucl Med* 1998;39:836–841.
125. Rannie GH TM, Ford WL. An experimental comparison of radioactive labels with potential application to lymphocyte migration studies in patients. *Clin Exp Immunol* 1977;29:509–514.
126. Adonai N NK, Walsh J, Iyer M, Toyokuni T, Phelps ME, McCarthy T, McCarthy DW, Gambhir SS. Ex vivo cell labeling with 64Cu-pyruvaldehyde-bis(N4-methylthiosemicarbazone) for imaging cell trafficking in mice with positron-emission tomography. *Proc Natl Acad Sci USA* 2002;99: 3030–3035.
127. Kasi LP LL, Saranti S, Podoloff DA, Freedman RS. Indium-111 labeled leukocytes in evaluation of active specific immunotherapy responses. *Int J Gynecol Cancer* 1995;5:226–232.
128. Dillman ROHS, Schiltz PM, Barth NM, Beutel LD, Nayak SK, O'Connor AA. Tumor localization by tumor infiltrating lymphocytes labeled with indium-111 in patients with metastatic renal cell carcinoma, melanoma, and colorectal cancer. *Cancer Biother Radiopharm* 1997;12:65–71.
129. Jacobs REAE, Meade TJ, Fraser SE. Looking deeper into vertebrate development. *Trends Cell Biol* 1999;9:73–76.
130. Johnson GABH, Black RD, Hedlund LW, Maronpot RR, Smith BR. Histology by magnetic resonance microscopy. *Magn Reson Q* 1993;9:1–30.

131. Weissleder RCH, Bogdanova A, Bogdanov A Jr. Magnetically labeled cells can be detected by MR imaging. *J Magn Reson Imaging* 1997;7:258–263.
132. Schoepf UME, Melder RJ, Jain RK, Weissleder R. Intracellular magnetic labeling of lymphocytes for in vivo trafficking studies. *Biotechniques* 1998;24:642–646.
133. Dodd SJWM, Suhan JP, Williams DS, Koretsky AP, Ho C. Detection of single mammalian cells by high-resolution magnetic resonance imaging. *Biophys J* 1999;76:103–109.
134. Hawrylak NGP, Broadus J, Schlueter C, Greenough WT, Lauterbur PC. Nuclear magnetic resonance (NMR) imaging of iron oxide-labeled neural transplants. *Exp Neurol* 1993;121:181–192.
135. Weissleder RMA, Mahmood U, Bhorade R, Benveniste H, Chiocca EA, Basilion JP. In vivo magnetic resonance imaging of transgene expression. *Nat Med* 2000;6:351–355.
136. Dodd CH, Chu WJ, Yang P, Zhang HG, Mountz JD Jr, Zinn K, Forder J, Josephson L, Weissleder R, Mountz JM, Mountz JD. Normal T-cell response and in vivo magnetic resonance imaging of T cells loaded with HIV transactivator-peptide-derived superparamagnetic nanoparticles. *J Immunol Methods* 2001;256:89–105.
137. Kircher MFAJ, Graves EE, Love V, Josephson L, Lichtman AH, Weissleder R. In vivo high resolution three-dimensional imaging of antigen-specific cytotoxic T-lymphocyte trafficking to tumors. *Cancer Res* 2003;63:6838–6846.
138. Hagani ABRI, Tan C, Krause A, Sadelain M. Activation conditions determine susceptibility of murine primary T-lymphocytes to retroviral infection. *J Gene Med* 1999;1:341–351.
139. Gallardo HF, Tan C, Ory D, Sadelain M. Recombinant retroviruses pseudotyped with the vesicular stomatitis virus G glycoprotein mediate both stable gene transfer and pseudotransduction in human peripheral blood lymphocytes. *Blood* 1997;90:952–957.
140. Rooney CM, Ng CY, Loftin S, Li C, Krance RA, Brenner MK, Heslop HE. Use of gene-modified virus-specific T lymphocytes to control Epstein-Barr-virus-related lymphoproliferation. *Lancet* 1995;345:9–13.
141. Verzeletti SBC, Marktel S, Nobili N, Ciceri F, Traversari C, Bordignon C. Herpes simplex virus thymidine kinase gene transfer for controlled graft-versus-host disease and graft-versus-leukemia: Clinical follow-up and improved new vectors. *Hum Gene Ther* 1998;9:2243–2251.
142. Bonini CFG, Verzeletti S, Servida P, Zappone E, Ruggieri L, Ponzoni M, Rossini S, Mavilio F, Traversari C, Bordignon C. HSV-TK gene transfer into donor lymphocytes for control of allogeneic graft-versus-leukemia. *Science* 1997;276:1719–1724.
143. Hardy JEM, Bachmann MH, Negrin RS, Fathman CG, Contag CH. Bioluminescence imaging of lymphocyte trafficking in vivo. *Exp Hematol* 2001;29:1353–1360.
144. Zhang W FJ, Harris SE, Contag PR, Stevenson DK, Contag CH. Rapid in vivo functional analysis of transgenes in mice using whole body imaging of luciferase expression. *Transgenic Res* 2001;10:423–434.
145. Costa GLSM, Nakajima A, Nguyen EV, Taylor-Edwards C, Slavin AJ, Contag CH, Fathman CG, Benson JM. Adoptive immunotherapy of experimental autoimmune encephalomyelitis via T cell delivery of the IL-12 p40 subunit. *J Immunol* 2001;167:2379–2387.
146. Koehne G, Doubrovin M, Doubrovina E, Zanzonico P, Gallardo HF, Ivanova A, Balatoni J, Teruya-Feldstein J, Heller G, May C, Ponomarev V, Ruan S, Finn R, Blasberg RG, Bornmann W, Riviere I, Sadelain M, O'Reilly RJ, Larson SM, Gelovani Tjuvajev JG. Serial in vivo imaging of the targeted migration of human HSV-TK-transduced antigen-specific lymphocytes. *Nat Biotechnol* 2003;21:405–413.
147. Doubrovina ES, Doubrovin M, Lee S, Shieh JH, Heller G, Pamer E, O'Reilly RJ. In vitro stimulation with WT1 peptide-loaded Epstein-Barr virus-positive B cells elicits high frequencies of WT1 peptide-specific T cells with in vitro and in vivo tumoricidal activity. *Clin Cancer Res* 2004;10:7207–7219.
148. Dubey SH, Adonai N, Du S, Rosato A, Braun J, Gambhir SS, Witte ON. Quantitative imaging of the T cell antitumor response by positron-emission tomography. *Proc Natl Acad Sci USA* 2003;100:1232–1237.
149. Kim YJDP, Ray P, Gambhir SS, Witte ON. Multimodality imaging of lymphocytic migration using lentiviral-based transduction of a tri-fusion reporter gene. *Mol Imaging Biol* 2004;6:331–340.
150. Su H, Gambhir SS, Braun J. Quantitation of cell number by a positron emission tomography reporter gene strategy. *Mol Imaging Biol* 2004;6:139–148.
151. Ponomarev V, Doubrovin M, Lyddane C, Beresten T, Balatoni J, Bornman W, Finn R, Akhurst T, Larson S, Blasberg R, Sadelain M, Tjuvajev JG. Imaging TCR-dependent NFAT-mediated T-cell activation with positron emission tomography in vivo. *Neoplasia* 2001;3:480–488.

152. Li W HR. Regulation of the nuclear factor of activated T cells in stably transfected Jurkat cell clones. *Biochem Biophys Res Commun* 1996;219:96–99.
153. Kiani ARA, Aramburu J. Manipulating immune responses with immunosuppressive agents that target NFAT. *Immunity* 2000;12:359–372.
154. McDonald DM, Choyke PL. Imaging of angiogenesis: From microscope to clinic. *Nat Med* 2003; 9:713–725.
155. Lyden D, Hattori K, Dias S, Costa C, Blaikie P, Butros L, Chadburn A, Heissig B, Marks W, Witte L, Wu Y, Hicklin D, Zhu Z, Hackett NR, Crystal RG, Moore MA, Hajjar KA, Manova K, Benezra R, Rafii S. Impaired recruitment of bone-marrow-derived endothelial and hematopoietic precursor cells blocks tumor angiogenesis and growth. *Nat Med* 2001;7:1194–1201.
156. Lyden D, Hattori K, Dias S, Costa C, Blaikie P, Butros L, Chadburn A, Heissig B, Marks W, Witte L, Wu Y, Hicklin D, Zhu Z, Hackett NR, Crystal RG, Moore MA, Hajjar KA, Manova K, Benezra R, Rafii S. Noninvasive MR imaging of magnetically labeled stem cells to directly identify neovasculature in a glioma model. *Blood* 2005;105:420–425.
157. Anderson SA, Glod J, Arbab AS, Noel M, Ashari P, Fine HA, Frank JA. Noninvasive MR imaging of magnetically labeled stem cells to directly identify neovasculature in a glioma model. *Blood* 2005;105:420–425.
158. Bulte JW, Arbab AS, Douglas T, Frank JA. Preparation of magnetically labeled cells for cell tracking by magnetic resonance imaging. *Methods Enzymol* 2004;386:275–299.
159. Studeny M, Marini FC, Champlin RE, Zompetta C, Fidler IJ, Andreeff M. Bone marrow-derived mesenchymal stem cells as vehicles for interferon-beta delivery into tumors. *Cancer Res* 2002; 62:3603–3608.
160. Studeny M, Marini FC, Dembinski JL, Zompetta C, Cabreira-Hansen M, Bekele BN, Champlin RE, Andreeff M. Mesenchymal stem cells: Potential precursors for tumor stroma and targeted-delivery vehicles for anticancer agents. *J Natl Cancer Inst* 2004;96:1593–1603.
161. Zhang Z, Jiang Q, Jiang F, Ding G, Zhang R, Wang L, Zhang L, Robin AM, Katakowski M, Chopp M. In vivo magnetic resonance imaging tracks adult neural progenitor cell targeting of brain tumor. *Neuroimage* 2004;23:281–287.
162. Banerjee D, Bertino JR. Myeloprotection with drug-resistance genes. *Lancet Oncol* 2002;3: 154–158.
163. Wang X, Rosol M, Ge S, Peterson D, McNamara G, Pollack H, Kohn DB, Nelson MD, Crooks GM. Dynamic tracking of human hematopoietic stem cell engraftment using in vivo bioluminescence imaging. *Blood* 2003;102:3478–3482.
164. Cao YA, Wagers AJ, Beilhack A, Dusich J, Bachmann MH, Negrin RS, Weissman IL, Contag CH. Shifting foci of hematopoiesis during reconstitution from single stem cells. *Proc Natl Acad Sci USA* 2004;101:221–226.

13 *In Vivo* Magnetic Resonance Spectroscopy in Clinical Oncology

Arend Heerschap, PhD

CONTENTS

INTRODUCTION
^{1}H MAGNETIC RESONANCE SPECTROSCOPY DATA ACQUISITION PROTOCOLS
ASSESSMENT OF BRAIN TUMORS BY *IN VIVO* ^{1}H MAGNETIC RESONANCE SPECTROSCOPY
ASSESSMENT OF PROSTATE CANCER BY *IN VIVO* ^{1}H MAGNETIC RESONANCE SPECTROSCOPY
ASSESSMENT OF BREAST CANCER BY *IN VIVO* ^{1}H MAGNETIC RESONANCE SPECTROSCOPY
CONCLUSIONS

1. INTRODUCTION

Imaging is an essential step in the diagnostic pathway for patients with clinical signs pointing to the presence of a tumor. Anatomical imaging is routinely applied to uncover the presence of a suspicious lesion. Then a biopsy specimen, taken of this lesion, is analyzed by histopathology, which is the gold standard for the confirmation of the presence of cancer and its further identification. Imaging methods have become an important complementary element in the differentiation between malignant and benign lesions and in the determination of the local or metastatic extent of the tumor. Moreover, if cancer tissue is present, newer (bio)imaging methods may help to establish the type, grade, and stage of the tumor. All this information is crucial in the further management of disease, such as treatment planning, prediction of progression, and response to treatment. Magnetic resonance (MR) is often the major modality in the imaging of cancer patients. In routine clinical practice MR is commonly used to obtain anatomical information, but this technique is very versatile and offers many possibilities to acquire more functional information, in particular, information of a

From: *Cancer Drug Discovery and Development*
In Vivo Imaging of Cancer Therapy
Edited by: A.F. Shields and P. Price © Humana Press Inc., Totowa, NJ

physiological and metabolic nature. To increase the specificity and sensitivity of common magnetic resonance imaging (MRI), more functional approaches are increasingly being included in clinical examinations of patients with tumors. For instance, these may include perfusion weighted imaging (PWI) to assess vascular functionality, diffusion weighted imaging (DWI) to assess tissue characteristics associated with water movement, and MR spectroscopy (MRS) to assess tissue metabolism and physiology.

Methods such as PWI and DWI are based on the measurement of the signal of ^{1}H nuclei in water. A much broader range of (bio)molecules can be viewed by MRS, either by employing the signals of ^{1}H nuclei or the signals of other nuclei such as ^{31}P, ^{13}C, or ^{19}F in these molecules. The specific property of MRS that makes this possible is the so-called chemical shift, which causes unique resonance frequencies for nuclei of different molecular groups. Specific spectral profiles, which can be observed in an MR spectrum, obtained from a location in the body, reflect the identity of (bio)chemicals present at that location. Additionally, the physiological state and environment of biomolecules may also affect their spectral profiles. The intensity of the spectral signals is related to the tissue levels of these compounds. As the tissue levels of biomolecules are orders lower than that of water in the body, they give much lower signal intensities. In practice the detection of molecules is restricted to those present at tissue levels of more than 0.1–1 mM (mostly metabolites). Also, for this reason, MRS is commonly not used for anatomical imaging, but to assess metabolism or physiology at a cruder spatial scale in single or multiple selected locations (spatial mapping of metabolism). It thus offers a direct view on the (dynamic) levels of some metabolites and compounds and their physiological state and environment in body tissues.

One of the first applications of MRS to a patient with a tumor was the detection of an abnormal ^{31}P MR spectrum of a rhabdosarcoma as compared to that of muscle tissue *(1)*. A typical tumor feature, already evident in this spectrum, was the relatively high level of the so-called phosphomonoester peak, which contains resonances from phosphorylated choline and ethanolamine *(2)*. Later, when ^{1}H MRS was applied to patients with brain tumors, a relatively high signal was observed for a peak at about 3.2 ppm on the MRS chemical shift scale *(3)*. From *in vitro* nuclear magnetic resonance (NMR) studies of biopsy extracts this peak turned out to be mainly composed of the resonances originating from protons in methyl groups of "choline compounds" such as choline, phosphocholine, and glycerophosphocholine, of which the ^{1}H chemical shift dispersion is too small to be resolved in the *in vivo* spectrum. Further MRS studies of other human tumors also revealed the presence of relatively high levels of choline compounds, indicating that this was a general neoplastic phenomenon; this attracted much attention as it could serve as a potential biomarker in cancer diagnosis (detection, grading, and staging) and treatment response *(2, 4)*. The choline compounds are involved in the biosynthesis and degradation of phospholipids such as phosphatidylcholine, which is required for the build-up and maintenance of cell membranes (Fig. 1). Choline compounds are differentially increased in tumors depending on the type and grade of the tumor. The exact reason behind this increase is still a matter of research, but it may be caused by increased choline transport into tumor cells, increased choline kinase activity, and increased phospholipase expression and activity in tumors *(4–7)*. The composite peak at about 3.2 ppm in the ^{1}H MRS spectrum is commonly referred to as the total

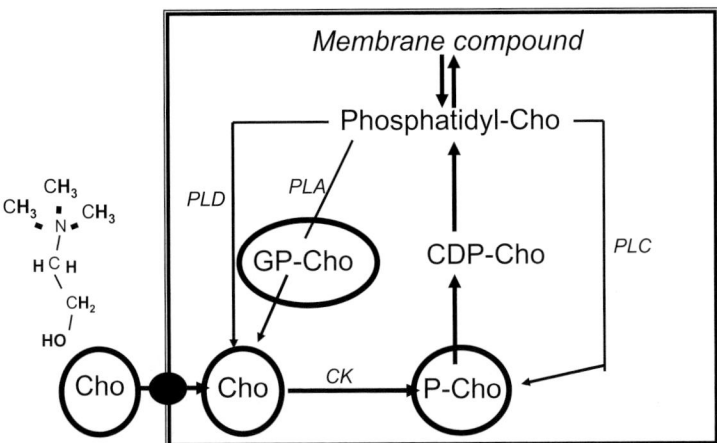

Fig. 1. Schematic view of the metabolic pathways involving (phospho)choline compounds. At the left is the chemical structure of choline (Cho). The methyl protons of choline and of the other encircled choline compounds (P-Cho, phosphocholine; GP-Cho, glycerophosphocholine) contribute to the dominating peak of these compounds at about 3.2 ppm in the *in vivo* ^{1}H MR spectrum. Biosynthetic enzymatic pathways are indicated by thick lines and catabolic reactions by thin lines. CK, choline kinase; PLA, PLC, PLD, phospholipase A, C, and D.

choline peak (tCho), although it may also contain (smaller) contributions from other compounds (e.g., taurine or myoinositol). Increases in the tCho peak have also been associated with increased cell density *(8)* and tumor hypoxia *(9)*.

In addition to the characteristic (relatively) increased tissue content in tCho, MRS of human tumors has uncovered abnormal tissue levels of other metabolites, reflecting changes in metabolism, morphology, or physiology due to neoplastic growth. Several of these metabolites are specific for the tissue from which the tumor originates, but abnormal levels of the individual compounds are generally not specific for tumor growth only and may occur in other pathologies. However, a typical composition of several metabolite resonances together, in a metabolic profile, may be characteristic of a particular tumor growth.

In clinical applications of MRS the ^{1}H nucleus has played a dominant role, mainly because this nucleus is present in most body metabolites and can be detected with high sensitivity. In addition, protons can be employed relatively easily on common clinical MRI machines, which are dedicated to the detection of protons in water and fat. However, other MR-sensitive nuclei such as ^{13}C, ^{31}P, ^{19}F, and ^{23}Na may provide highly relevant and unique information on tumor metabolism and physiology, but their application in a clinical setting has been limited until now. As higher field MR systems are being introduced in the clinic, it may become more attractive to make use of these nuclei in clinical examinations of tumors. Although interesting clinical results have been obtained in human tumor studies using other nuclei, e.g., ^{19}F *(10)* and ^{31}P *(11)*, this chapter is restricted to the main clinical applications of MRS to oncological problems using the ^{1}H nucleus, i.e., in the brain, prostate, and breast. Rather than giving a complete overview of all literature on clinical MRS of these three tumor types this chapter aims to provide the reader with a brief summary of some advances in key clinical applications.

2. ^{1}H MAGNETIC RESONANCE SPECTROSCOPY DATA ACQUISITION PROTOCOLS

Robust acquisition methods to obtain localized ^{1}H MR spectra from single and multiple volumes have been available since the 1990s for clinical applications at 1.5 T in the brain. But only recently have such methods become available for prostate and breast. ^{1}H MRS of a single voxel (SVS) is the easiest and quickest way to obtain metabolic information on tumor tissue. Commonly, localized MR spectra are obtained by so-called STEAM or PRESS pulse sequences at long echo time (about 270 msec), intermediate echo time (about 135 msec), or short echo time (about 30 msec or less). At increasing echo times signals of different compounds are differentially attenuated by T2* relaxation and J-modulation. In practice this means that at long echo times less metabolite signals are visible, but as the resonances are also less cluttered data processing becomes easier.

To measure viable tumor tissue by SVS the voxel (typically with a volume between about 1 and 8 ml) is positioned by MRI guidance using T1- and T2-weighted images. As these images are rather nonspecific for the presence of tumor tissue, a T1-weighted MRI is often obtained after intravenous application of a contrast agent containing gadolinium (Gd) to detect areas with abnormal vascularity in the tumor. For instance, in the brain the blood–brain barrier (BBB) may be disrupted by tumor growth, thus causing signal enhancement in T1-weighted MRI as Gd can spread in the interstitial space after its intravenous application. Assuming that these enhancing areas contain the viable part of the tumor, the placement of voxels for SVS is then guided by hyperintense areas on Gd-enhanced MR images. In principle, the presence of Gd may interfere with the tCho signal in MRS measurements if this is performed shortly after contrast MRI *(12–14)*, but at short echo times the effects on spectral signals are usually acceptable. A more serious drawback of this approach is that Gd enhancement may not occur despite the presence of a tumor, for instance, because of coopting growth of tumors *(15)*, or the signal enhancement in MRI may be rather nonspecific, requiring detailed analysis of time-dependent uptake of the contrast agent to identify tumor presence, such as done in the prostate *(16, 17)*. Moreover, during treatment a tumor vascularity may "normalize" *(18, 19)*, and treatment assessment with Gd-enhanced MRI may give the false impression that the tumor has disappeared. A way to circumvent ambiguities in volume selection is to use a multivoxel or spectroscopic imaging approach (MRSI), by which a large volume is usually selected that also covers nontumor tissue, which is divided up in smaller voxels (typically ~0.5 cm^3 or more) by so-called phase-encoding methods. For each metabolite a 2D or 3D spatial metabolic map can be reconstructed from signals in spectra of each voxel. In this way the heterogeneous nature of tumors (necrosis, viable tumor tissue, etc.) can also be assessed. A typical example of localized data acquisition in ^{1}H MRS of a brain tumor is shown in Fig. 2. A thorough description of the technical details of acquisition methods is beyond the scope of this chapter, but some particular aspects will be addressed below.

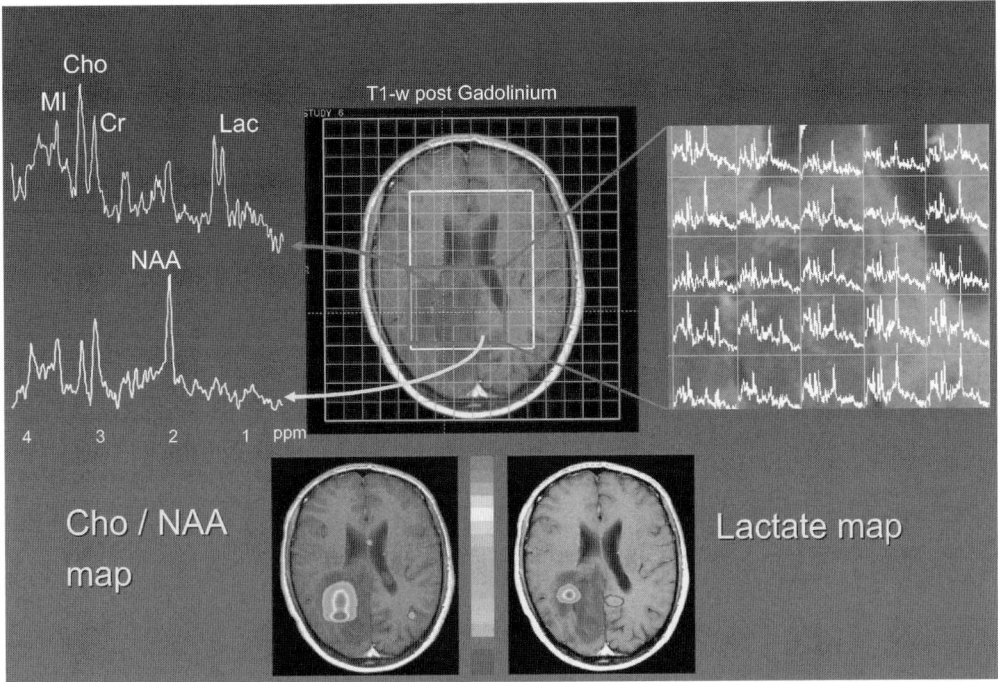

Fig. 2. A 2D MRSI of a patient with a low-grade oligodendroglioma. Spectral data were obtained from a 15-mm-thick slice by a STEAM sequence using a repetition time of 2500 msec and echo time of 20 msec. The FOV was 200 mm and the matrix size was 16 × 16. In the middle is a T1-weighted MR image obtained after Gd contrast application. A low intensity lesion is visible, but without clear contrast enhancement, indicating a still intact blood–brain barrier. As an overlay, the preselected volume and the spectroscopic imaging grid are indicated. At the right a blow-up is shown of the indicated box with voxels and spectra. At the left two MR spectra are shown. At the bottom left a normal appearing MR spectrum is shown outside the T1 lesion. At the top left an abnormal MR spectrum is shown from the center of the T1 lesion. The peak for N-acetylaspartate (NAA) at 2 ppm is strongly reduced and the peak for choline compounds (Cho) at 3.2 ppm is increased. An additional peak is observed at 1.3 ppm originating from methyl protons of lactate. At the bottom two metabolite maps are shown: at the bottom left a map of the Cho/NAA ratio and at the bottom right a lactate map. (*See* color plate.)

3. ASSESSMENT OF BRAIN TUMORS BY *IN VIVO* ^{1}H MAGNETIC RESONANCE SPECTROSCOPY

In the radiological examination of a patient suspected of having a brain tumor, the first step is to search for a space-occupying lesion that is characteristic of a tumor or a metastasis in the brain. For this, CT and conventional T2- and T1-weighted MRI, with the application of Gd as a contrast agent to detect an enhancing lesion, are often diagnostic. However, as outlined above, tumor areas may not always become visible with Gd, especially lower grade tumors. The differential diagnosis between neoplastic and nonneoplastic lesions may still remain problematic in some cases. The histopathological examination of biopsy material is the decisive step in the diagnosis of a brain tumor to establish type and grade, which in turn determine which additional treatment procedures are to be followed. Although biopsy material is commonly available, there are multiple cases in which an adequate noninvasive assessment would be desirable to avoid a biopsy, e.g., in cases with difficulties in differential diagnoses with nonneoplastic diseases or with high risks of morbidity or mortality. In addition, due to imaging uncertainties about the exact location of viable tumor tissue, biopsies may be obtained from the wrong area and better biopsy guidance is needed.

In treatment planning and monitoring and prediction of tumor progression multiple areas require improved noninvasive assessment. For instance, in surgery, but in particular in focused radiotherapy such as intensity modulated radiotherapy (IMRT), it is important to know the margins of the tumor and the most aggressive parts, which may be difficult to determine in some tumors such as gliomas. Also in the assessment of treatments by surgery or radiotherapy and chemotherapy, more functional mapping of the tumor presence is important. For instance, sometimes it is difficult to discriminate between radiation necrosis and tumor recurrence.

As has been demonstrated in numerous studies, ^{1}H MRS can contribute significantly to MR examinations in the management of brain tumors, i.e., to address the clinical problems described above. It provides unique metabolic information that can be diagnostic for tumor presence, tumor type, and grade, and may serve as a tool in the planning and evaluation of treatments and in the prediction of tumor progression and treatment response.

The main metabolites visible in a ^{1}H MR spectrum of the human brain obtained at long, intermediate, and short echo times are *N*-acetylaspartate (NAA) and total creatine (tCr) and choline (tCho) compounds (see Fig. 2). Most characteristic for tumor tissue in the brain is an increase in the tCho level as compared to unaffected tissue. The tCr content is decreased in some brain tumors. As creatine is an important compound in energy metabolism, this points to differences in energy metabolism or creatine uptake in the tumor cells. A reduction in NAA is a general observation in adult brain tumors. This reflects the replacement of healthy neuronal tissue, from which NAA predominantly originates, by tumor tissue, which is mostly not of neuronal origin. A reduction in NAA is a rather nonspecific observation as it also occurs in other brain pathologies with neuronal damage. In MR spectra of tumor tissue a doublet signal for lactate may often be observed. This observation initially raised much interest, as lactate is an end product of aerobic glycolysis, which is an important trait of more aggressive tumors. However, a lactate signal may also be seen due to the presence of regional hypoxia or because it is not cleared from tumor tissue due to an accumulation in necrotic or cystic regions, which is not necessarily associated with increased glycolysis *(20, 21)*. At shorter echo times additional signals are visible in MR spectra of brain tissue, such as glutamate, glutamine, and myoinositol, which may also have diagnostic potential.

In the differential diagnosis between neoplastic and nonneoplastic tissue MRI is of considerable value. However, standard imaging is not always able to discriminate between a lesion of a tumor in the brain and a lesion of another origin, such as that of a stroke. In these situations other MRI modalities, like MRS, may be considered as helpful additional tools. Characteristic spectral tumor features such as increased tCho and decreased NAA can be used for this purpose. In general, this has to be done with some caution as some pathologies such as reactive gliosis or sclerosis may show tumor-like MR spectra characteristic of low-grade tumors *(22, 23)*. More advanced data acquisition and processing may improve the specificity of MRS to allow it to differentiate tumor from nontumor cases *(24)*. Certain brain pathologies can be easily differentiated as they show MR spectra that are very different from those typical for tumors, for instance, those of abscesses *(25–27)*. The complementary use of other MRI methods such as PWI to determine relative cerebral tumor volume or DWI may be helpful in the differential diagnosis between neoplastic and nonneoplastic disease.

To identify the type and grade of tumors in the brain MRS may be particular helpful, next to the gold standard, i.e., histopathology of biopsy material. Among the primary brain tumors astrocytomas, glioblastomas, and meningiomas are most common, but in addition to these there are a large number of other rarer tumor types occurring in less than 5–10% of all brain tumor cases. Typical MR spectra have been identified for the three major primary brain tumors, e.g., glioblastomas have high lipid signals and an increased alanine signal is observed for meningiomas *(28, 29)*. Next to characteristic changes in NAA, creatine, and tCho levels, the particular levels of compounds observable at short echo times such as myoinositol, glutathione, glutamate, and glutamine may also help to differentiate low and high grade gliomas *(30, 31)*, gliomatosis ceribri from low grade gliomas *(32, 33)*, astrocytomas, schwannomas, and hemangiopericytomas from meningiomas *(29, 34–36)*, and oligodendrogliomas from astrocytomas *(37)*. The latter is of interest as oligodendrogliomas may better respond to chemotherapy. The tCho level appears to be correlated with the malignancy of the tumors as expressed in proliferation activity, grade, or cellular density *(8, 21, 38–40)*, but in most studies overlap in the data precludes individual assignments based on the level of this peak only. The use of MRSI for spatial mapping and the analysis of resonances of multiple compounds may be helpful in the grading of astrocytomas *(41)*. Lipid and macromolecular signals are of special interest in the grading of brain tumors as the high intensity of these signals is very characteristic of high-grade tumors *(39, 42)*, which may be related to membrane breakdown and (micro)necrosis *(43)* or intracellular triglyceride droplets *(44)*. The specific profile of lipids may help to differentiate glioblastomas from metastases, which otherwise have comparable spectra *(45)*. As glioblastomas show infiltrative growth they can also be discriminated from metastasis by multivoxel MRS *(46)*. In attempts to characterize the rarer brain tumor cases by MRS as much as possible, multisite projects have been initiated, such as the EU project INTERPRET *(47, 48)*.

The heterogeneous nature of brain tumors is an important aspect to be taken into account for biopsy guidance and for the planning, monitoring, and evaluation of treatments, such as surgery, radiotherapy, and chemotherapy. These procedures are commonly based on information from T2-weighted and Gd-enhanced T1-weighted MRI. Therefore, it is of particular importance that MRS can show gross abnormalities in addition to Gd-enhancing and T2 lesions, due to infiltrative tumor growth, as commonly occurs in gliomas *(49–51)*. In stereotactic procedures MRS can help to obtain biopsies from the proper tumor locations, i.e., the most malignant parts *(52–54)*, or to delineate the tumor lesion for planning of surgery or radiation treatment *(50, 55–57)*. In infiltrating tumors such as glioblastomas, MRS may identify tumor load outside the Gd-enhancing area, which makes MRS especially useful in treatment planning *(56, 58)*. In all these cases the use of 3D multivoxel MRS approaches is essential. The tCho signal is most often used as a marker to assess the response to therapy of brain tumors by MRS *(39, 59)*. Of clinical interest in treatment follow-up of brain tumors is the discrimination of tumor recurrence from radiation necrosis by MRS, as there are few other ways to assess this properly *(60–67)*. The use of a multivoxel approach appears to work best for this purpose *(63)*.

As the analysis of MRS data of brain tumors may be rather complex to less experienced users in clinical routine, and also because the proper analysis of large datasets from multivoxel assessments is manually unpractical, there is need for decision support systems. Much attention has been given to automated and objective processing and classifying of voxels of MRS data by a variety of approaches *(25, 48, 55, 68, 69)*. In some studies MRI information has been included that generally improves the performance of the decision support systems *(70–74)*. Most of these studies have focused on the development of systems to separate brain tumor types and grades. To develop reliable and clinically useful classifiers of tumor type and grade it is necessary to have a sufficiently large dataset of these tumors available, which may require multicenter efforts, especially in the case of the rarer tumors. In such multicenter projects data should be acquired with some flexibility in acquisition modes and parameter settings, as the details of these will not be exactly the same for different MR systems. Proper system, spectral, clinical, and histopathological quality control should be part of these projects. An example is the multicenter EU project INTERPRET *(47, 48)*, which is currently expanded in a new project, eTUMOUR, which also includes other metabolomic and genomic approaches to assess brain tumors *(75)*.

The added diagnostic benefit of ^{1}H MRS to conventional MRI has been demonstrated in a number of studies, mostly assessing the added value of MRS to brain tumor typing and grading as compared to conventional MRI *(34, 48, 72, 76–80)*. The assessment of brain tumors in children by MRS has not been explicitly described here, but pediatric cases have to be considered as a separate group with specific clinical and diagnostic needs *(22, 81–84)*.

4. ASSESSMENT OF PROSTATE CANCER BY *IN VIVO* ^{1}H MAGNETIC RESONANCE SPECTROSCOPY

Functional imaging methods are much needed in the workup of patients suspected of having prostate cancer, to detect the presence of prostate cancer as well as for local staging and metastasis, localization of cancer tissue in the prostate, and treatment selection and assessment. The level (or change in the level) of the prostate-specific antigen (PSA) in serum is the most important biomarker currently used as an indication that a tumor of the prostate may be present, but it has a low specificity. In the detection of prostate cancer the analysis of ultrasound-guided biopsies from the prostate plays a major role, but due to sampling errors, negative biopsies often occur despite a positive PSA level. Thus better imaging of the presence of cancer tissue would be desirable to guide biopsies. The stage of prostate cancer (occurrence of extraprostatic cancer) is often decisive in therapy decisions, but the determination of stage is mostly based on the so-called Partin tables of clinical findings. These are valid only for an average patient population, and clearly the addition of a proper imaging examination might improve individual assessment. The proper localization of cancer tissue in the prostate is also becoming of interest due to the introduction of new focal therapies such as IMRT for local disease. Functional imaging to localize active tumors can be important for treatment assessment and for detection of recurrence. And finally, it would be extremely important if a functional imaging method could predict the progression of localized prostate cancer to more aggressive variants. Among the potential MR methods that may contribute to solving these diagnostic questions ^{1}H MRS is one of the promising candidates.

More than 10 years ago it was demonstrated that ^{1}H MR spectra of extracts of prostate tissue show a large number of metabolite signals, among which are signals for protons in citrate and choline compounds and that the (relative) signals for citrate may be decreased and that of choline compounds increased in prostate cancer tissue *(85, 86)*. After the introduction of endorectal coils it also became possible to obtain *in vivo* ^{1}H MR spectra of small volumes of the prostate with sufficient signal to noise *(87–89)*. Fortunately, the dominant peaks observed in these spectra are from protons in citrate, creatine, and choline compounds. Compared to healthy peripheral or BPH tissue the signals of citrate were reduced and those of choline compounds often increased in cancer tissue, and thus it was obvious that the tCho over citrate peaks could serve as a metabolic biomarker for prostate cancer. Weaker signals sometimes are also observed, for instance for protons in polyamines resonating between the creatine signal at about 3 ppm and the tCho peak at 3.2 ppm. In the interpretation of the data it is of note that citrate mainly occurs in the ducts of the prostate, and hence a lower citrate may indicate altered metabolism as well as a reduction of luminal space in cancer tissue. Because tumor tissue can occur anywhere in the prostate, it became clear that multivoxel methods would be essential in further clinical studies. As the prostate is relatively small and embedded in adipose tissue, this required the implementation of advanced radio-frequency (RF) pulses and sequences to suppress interfering strong lipid signals. In this way two- and three-dimensional MRSI sequences have been realized *(87, 90–92)*, of which 3D variants are now most favored, as these can cover the whole prostate. Three-dimensional acquisitions can be performed in about 10–15 min at a spatial resolution down to about 0.4 cm^3, with sufficient signal to noise, at 1.5 T. In the analysis of the data of patients, it should be taken into account that different regions of the healthy prostate such as the peripheral zone, central zone, and areas close to the urethra and the seminal vesicles have different amplitudes for citrate, creatine, and "choline" compound signals. In addition, MRS has to be performed at a time sufficiently after the time of biopsy to avoid possible interference of a hemorrhage with spectral quality, due to a magnetic field or morphological distortions.

Several studies have been devoted to an evaluation of the clinical potential of 3D ^{1}H MRSI to localize cancer tissue in the peripheral zone of the prostate *(93, 94)*. After radical prostatectomy step-section histopathology was performed and compared with the MRSI data in which the voxels were scored on a scale from malignant to benign using criteria based on the standard deviation of normal values. Because the signals of tCho and creatine are often not well resolved at 1.5 T, the common way of analyzing the data is by using the tCho plus creatine-over-citrate ratio, which ignores possible decreases in creatine in cancer tissue, but this can be taken into account in a refinement of the analysis. With sensitivities comparable to those obtained by standard T2-weighted MRI (about 70%), the specificity was significantly higher (up to about 85%), and by combining both methods sensitivity and specificity increased to about 90%. In a study that we recently completed on 34 patients using similar approaches, sensitivity and specificity in localizing prostate cancer both in the peripheral zone and central gland, by ^{1}H MRSI alone, were between 80 and 90% *(95)*. All these results are very promising, but the true clinical value can be judged from only results of multicenter trials. At present two trials are running that evaluate the properties of 3D ^{1}H MRSI to localize cancer tissue in the prostate: the International Multi-Centre Assessment of Prostate Spectroscopy (IMAPS) trial and a trial by the American College of Radiology Imaging Network (ACRIN 6659). Preliminary results of the IMAPS trial (seven clinical sites) show specificities and sensitivities comparable to single-site studies for tumors in the peripheral zone and central gland *(96, 97)*. Potential confounding conditions in the localization of cancer in the prostate are other prostate diseases like prostatitus *(98, 99)*, which may affect prostate metabolism, physiology, and morphology in the same way as cancer.

Although ^{1}H MRSI may be used to improve the reliability of diagnosing local staging, i.e., extracapsular extension *(100)*, it is not expected to be the prime MR approach for this purpose, as the very high resolution MRI obtainable at 3T may be more suitable to address this problem *(101)*.

MRSI can also contribute to the planning and assessment of various treatments of prostate cancer and in the detection of recurrence after treatment *(102–107)*. Hormone deprivation is a common procedure in prostate cancer treatment and during this procedure MRSI shows a remarkable, partly selective, decrease in metabolite levels (metabolic atrophy) over time, which may point to important cancer features *(108)*. Metabolic atrophy also occurs upon radiation treatment, but much more slowly. A major clinical issue is the determination of the aggressiveness of prostate cancer, and this is usually characterized by histology with the so-called Gleason score. It is of interest that the (tCho + cr)/citrate ratio is correlated with the Gleason score, although the overlap of the current data precludes that it can be used for individual decisions *(109, 110)*.

The clinical performance of MRSI of the prostate may be improved by still better shimming procedures (to decrease the number of low-quality spectra), better signal to noise, and better chemical shift dispersion. With the rapid implementation of higher field systems (3T) in the clinic, the prospects for improved clinical performance of MRSI of the prostate is very good, provided that proper adaptations of the technology are implemented *(111–114)*.

5. ASSESSMENT OF BREAST CANCER BY *IN VIVO* ^{1}H MAGNETIC RESONANCE SPECTROSCOPY

Currently the sensitivity for detecting invasive breast cancer by dynamic Gd contrast MRI is very high (up to 90% or higher), however, its specificity may be rather low (down to 40%), and this is a major reason why ^{1}H MRS is being explored as a complementary MR tool to discriminate malignant from benign lesions in the breast. In addition, ^{1}H MRS may have a unique role in therapy prediction and monitoring.

In vivo MRS of human breast cancer was first explored using the ^{31}P nucleus *(115)*, with typically high phosphomonoester and diester peaks present in spectra taken from cancer tissue. Spectra of extracts of this tissue showed that resonances from (glycero)phosphoethanolamine and (glycero)phosphocholine contributed to these peaks. In more recent years attention has switched to the ^{1}H nucleus, as it can be detected with a higher sensitivity, allowing smaller tumors to be analyzed within shorter measurement times, and as no special hardware is needed, it is rather easy to add to an MRI examination on a standard clinical system.

In the ^{1}H MR spectrum of the normal breast, without any signal suppression, the signals of lipids dominate, but in tumors a more pronounced water signal appears. Although some clinical studies have used these signals in the assessment of breast cancer *(116)*, most investigations focus on the peak at about 3.2 ppm, characteristic of tumor tissue. *Ex vivo* high-resolution NMR and so-called magic angle spectroscopy studies of tissue biopsies showed that this peak is mainly composed of resonances from methyl protons in choline compounds such as choline, phosphocholine, and glycerophosphocholine *(117, 118)* and is commonly referred to as the tCho. In a number of studies the clinical value of detecting a peak at 3.2 ppm was explored to identify various breast carcinomas and benign lesions at the common clinical field strength of 1.5 T *(119–122)*. The tCho peak was also seen in spectra of normal breasts of lactating women, which therefore has to be taken into account in the diagnosis of breast cancer. The sensitivities and specificities reported in some of these studies to discriminate malignant from benign lesions were in the order of 80–85%.

Although these initial *in vivo* ^{1}H MRS studies were promising, they were hampered by some shortcomings. Artifactual signals may arise at the 3.2 ppm position due to spurious sidebands of large lipid signals. Most importantly, the analysis in these studies was largely qualitative, as usually only the visual absence or presence of a peak at 3.2 ppm in the spectrum was used as a decisive biomarker. However, variable MRS sensitivity due to different RF coil positioning or loading and field strength may interfere with choline signal visibility. The false positives often occurring in the *in vivo* studies indicated that a more robust and quantitative approach to assess the 3.2 ppm peak was needed. It was demonstrated that artifactual lipid sidebands can be overcome by specific pulse sequences such as TE averaging *(123)*. Quantitative approaches have been introduced, either using an external reference signal *(124)* or the internal signal of water as a reference *(125)*. Currently a quantitative approach appears to be essential as a tCho peak can also be detected in spectra of asymptotic breast tissue, especially at higher field strengths (>1.5 T) and as malignant breast tissue is characterized by a generally higher, but variable, tissue content of tCho compounds. The addition of quantitative ^{1}H MRS to dynamic contrast-enhanced MRI has been shown to improve sensitivity, specificity, accuracy, and interobserver agreement between observer radiologists to discriminate malignant from benign breast lesions *(126)*. A more precise calibration of the resonance position of the tCho peak has also been proposed to separate benign tissue from malignant tissue in cases in which a choline signal is detected *(127)*.

In addition to the use of ^{1}H MRS to improve the discrimination between malignant and benign breast cancer, it may prove useful in the evaluation of treatments. This has not been extensively explored yet, but an interesting example is a study in which the change in the tCho signal was significantly different between patients with objective response and those with no response to a doxorubicin-based chemotherapy in locally advanced breast cancer *(128)*. In particular, in these studies a quantitative approach is essential.

In the current practice of ^{1}H MRS applied to breast cancer, mostly single-volume measurements are performed of one or several tumor locations in less than 10 min at a spatial resolution down to 1 cm^3. Positioning of the voxel at the proper tumor location is important, in particular in heterogeneous tumors such as invasive ductal carcinomas *(125)*. Therefore a Gd-enhanced MR image may be used for guidance as little effect of

Gd on the tCho signal is anticipated, at least at relatively short echo times. Recently multivoxel spectroscopic imaging methods have been introduced *(129)*. It remains to be evaluated how robust this can be performed in the presence of large lipid signals, and optimal field shimming strategies are likely to be crucial for this purpose *(130)*.

6. CONCLUSIONS

The potential of MR spectroscopy to contribute to MR examinations in the management of some human tumors has been convincingly demonstrated and a large number of clinical institutions are now routinely applying ^{1}H MRS in the assessment of brain, prostate, and breast cancer. But even with these demonstrations of the clinical use of MRS, the further translation into a widespread tool in routine clinical practice is not trivial. This depends on a large number of factors. Not only is a robust and automated measurement procedure necessary, but the rapid and easy digestible display of the results of an examination and proper training of the clinical users also are important. And above all it has to be clear that methods are generally applicable on major MR instruments in the production of reliable and significant clinical results compared to other approaches or modalities. Studies using evidence-based medicine (EBM) criteria to evaluate the diagnostic and therapy decision-making value of MRS applied to patients suspected of having a brain tumor *(131)* and a critical discussion of the results of these studies *(132, 133)* have made clear that carefully standardized multisite trials, complying to EBM criteria, are still needed to bring the assessment of brain tumors by MRS into general clinical practice *(134)*. The same holds true for the assessment of prostate and breast cancer by MRS. Thus, for the acceptance of MRS in routine clinical practice, it is important that prospective multisite trials, as described above, are performed. In these trials the selection of standardized (temporarily frozen) protocols may be critical, as MRS technology applicable to tumors is still continuously progressing. For instance, currently improvements in sensitivity are being investigated using new RF coil arrangements with parallel acquisition methods, and using higher field magnets, to exploit the potentially better signal to noise and chemical shift dispersion for more accurate assessment of metabolites. In addition, better automation in data acquisition and processing is being developed.

A particular advantage of MRS is that it provides quantitative data, which is not a common practice in the clinical assessment of tumors by most (conventional) MRI methods. A general trend now is to combine MRS data with that of other MR approaches with higher spatial resolution, such as conventional T1- and T2-weighted MRI, dynamic contrast MRI, and diffusion MRI, as this may improve the diagnostic performance beyond that of each single MR approach. Because of its noninvasive nature, it is expected that MRS, together with these other MR approaches, will be particularly useful in the evaluation and prediction of treatment response and disease progress.

Multivoxel MRS can be considered as molecular imaging "avant la lettre," although it does not involve the imaging of tailored probes for specific molecular or cellular targets, which is often the restricted definition used for molecular imaging. In contrast to the common "molecular imaging" approaches, MRS assesses the signals of endogenous compounds. Hence, no problems associated with the synthesis and injection of exogenous compounds aimed for targeted diagnostics are involved. The number of endogenous compounds that are visible by *in vivo* MRS is limited to about 40 (also including the use of nuclei other than ^{1}H), because of sensitivity reasons. However, new ways are being explored to enhance the sensitivity of MRS substantially with hyperpolarization of endogenous (or exogenous) compounds. This hyperpolarization is performed outside the body, and after the compounds are applied intravenously, their metabolic conversion can be monitored by fast high-resolution MRSI, for instance, to realize "real time metabolic imaging" for diagnostic purposes in oncology *(135)*.

ACKNOWLEDGMENTS

I thank Mark Rijpkema, Janneke Schuuring, and Marinette van der Graaf for acquiring and processing the data presented in Fig. 2. This chapter is also based on clinical research work and discussions with many other collaborators including Tom Scheenen, Dennis Klomp, Sjaak van Asten, Jannie Wijnen, Stijn Heymink, Jurgen Futterer, Jelle Barentsz, Carla Boetes, Hanneke van Laarhoven, Bozena Goraj, Yvonne Vermeulen, and Ivonne Loosbroek at the Radiology department of the Radboud University Nijmegen Medical Center (RUN-MC). This work has been and is supported by the RUN-MC, Dutch Cancer Society, Siemens, and EU projects IST-1999-10310 and FP6-2002-LIFESCIHEALTH 503094.

REFERENCES

1. Griffiths JR, *et al.* 31P-NMR studies of a human tumour in situ. *Lancet* 1983;1(8339):1435–1436.
2. Negendank W, *et al.* Phospholipid metabolites in 1H-decoupled 31P MRS in vivo in human cancer: Implications for experimental models and clinical studies. *Anticancer Res* 1996;16(3B):1539–1544.
3. Bruhn H, *et al.* Noninvasive differentiation of tumors with use of localized H-1 MR spectroscopy in vivo: Initial experience in patients with cerebral tumors. *Radiology* 1989;172(2):541–548.
4. Gillies RJ, Morse DL. In vivo magnetic resonance spectroscopy in cancer. *Annu Rev Biomed Eng* 2005;7:287–326.
5. Degani H, Eliyahu G, Maril N. Choline metabolism: Meaning and significance. Syllabus Educational Course International Society for Magnetic Resonance in Medicine, 2006. Experimental Methods in MR of Cancer.
6. Podo F. Tumour phospholipid metabolism. *NMR Biomed* 1999;12(7):413–439.
7. Glunde, K., Jacobs MA, Bhujwalla ZM. Choline metabolism in cancer: Implications for diagnosis and therapy. *Expert Rev Mol Diagn* 2006;6(6):821–829.
8. Gupta RK, *et al.* Relationships between choline magnetic resonance spectroscopy, apparent diffusion coefficient and quantitative histopathology in human glioma. *J Neurooncol* 2000;50(3):215–226.
9. Glunde K, Raman V, Bhujwalla Z. Hypoxia regulates phosphocholine and total choline concentrations in human prostate cancer cells. Proceedings of the International Society for Magnetic Resonance in Medicine 14th Scientific Meeting and Exhibition, Seattle, WA, 6–12 May 2006, p. 1261.
10. van Laarhoven HW, *et al.* Monitoring fluoropyrimidine metabolism in solid tumors with in vivo (19)F magnetic resonance spectroscopy. *Crit Rev Oncol Hematol* 2005;56(3):321–343.
11. Arias-Mendoza F, Smith MR, Brown TR. Predicting treatment response in non-Hodgkin's lymphoma from the pretreatment tumor content of phosphoethanolamine plus phosphocholine. *Acad Radiol* 2004;11(4):368–376.
12. Sijens PE, *et al.* 1H chemical shift imaging reveals loss of brain tumor choline signal after administration of Gd-contrast. *Magn Reson Med* 1997;37(2):222–225.
13. Murphy PS, Leach MO, Rowland IJ. Signal modulation in (1)H magnetic resonance spectroscopy using contrast agents: Proton relaxivities of choline, creatine, and N-acetylaspartate. *Magn Reson Med* 1999;42(6):1155–1158.
14. Lin AP, Ross BD. Short-echo time proton MR spectroscopy in the presence of gadolinium. *J Comput Assist Tomogr* 2001;25(5):705–712.
15. Leenders W, *et al.* Vascular endothelial growth factor-A determines detectability of experimental melanoma brain metastasis in GD-DTPA-enhanced MRI. *Int J Cancer* 2003;105(4):437–443.
16. van Dorsten FA, *et al.* Combined quantitative dynamic contrast-enhanced MR imaging and (1)H MR spectroscopic imaging of human prostate cancer. *J Magn Reson Imaging* 2004;20(2):279–287.

17. Futterer JJ, et al. Prostate cancer localization with dynamic contrast-enhanced MR imaging and proton MR spectroscopic imaging. *Radiology* 2006;241(2):449–458.
18. Leenders WP, et al. Antiangiogenic therapy of cerebral melanoma metastases results in sustained tumor progression via vessel co-option. *Clin Cancer Res* 2004;10(18 Pt 1):6222–6230.
19. Jain RK. Antiangiogenic therapy for cancer: Current and emerging concepts. *Oncology* 2005;19(4 Suppl 3):7–16.
20. Kugel H, et al. Human brain tumors: Spectral patterns detected with localized H-1 MR spectroscopy. *Radiology* 1992;183(3):701–709.
21. Negendank WG, et al. Proton magnetic resonance spectroscopy in patients with glial tumors: A multicenter study. *J Neurosurg* 1996;84(3):449–458.
22. Wilken B, et al. Quantitative proton magnetic resonance spectroscopy of focal brain lesions. *Pediatr Neurol* 2000;23(1):22–31.
23. Krouwer HG, et al. Single-voxel proton MR spectroscopy of nonneoplastic brain lesions suggestive of a neoplasm. *AJNR Am J Neuroradiol* 1998(9):1695–1703.
24. De Stefano N, et al. In vivo differentiation of astrocytic brain tumors and isolated demyelinating lesions of the type seen in multiple sclerosis using 1H magnetic resonance spectroscopic imaging. *Ann Neurol* 1998;44(2):273–278.
25. Poptani H, et al. Diagnostic assessment of brain tumours and non-neoplastic brain disorders in vivo using proton nuclear magnetic resonance spectroscopy and artificial neural networks. *J Cancer Res Clin Oncol* 1999;125(6):343–349.
26. Grand S, et al. Necrotic tumor versus brain abscess: Importance of amino acids detected at 1H MR spectroscopy–initial results. *Radiology* 1999;213(3):785–793.
27. Martinez-Perez I, et al. Diagnosis of brain abscess by magnetic resonance spectroscopy. Report of two cases. *J Neurosurg* 1997;86(4):708–713.
28. Manton DJ, et al. Determination of proton metabolite concentrations and relaxation parameters in normal human brain and intracranial tumours. *NMR Biomed* 1995;8(3):104–112.
29. Cho YD, et al. (1)H-MRS metabolic patterns for distinguishing between meningiomas and other brain tumors. *Magn Reson Imaging* 2003;21(6):663–672.
30. Castillo M, Smith JK, Kwock L. Correlation of myo-inositol levels and grading of cerebral astrocytomas. *AJNR Am J Neuroradiol* 2000;21(9):1645–1649.
31. Howe FA, et al. Metabolic profiles of human brain tumors using quantitative in vivo 1H magnetic resonance spectroscopy. *Magn Reson Med* 2003;49(2):223–232.
32. Galanaud D, et al. Use of proton magnetic resonance spectroscopy of the brain to differentiate gliomatosis cerebri from low-grade glioma. *J Neurosurg* 2003;98(2):269–276.
33. Bendszus M, et al. MR spectroscopy in gliomatosis cerebri. *AJNR Am J Neuroradiol* 2000;21(2):375–380.
34. Murphy M, et al. The contribution of proton magnetic resonance spectroscopy (1HMRS) to clinical brain tumour diagnosis. *Br J Neurosurg* 2002;16(4):329–334.
35. Barba I, et al. Magnetic resonance spectroscopy of brain hemangiopericytomas: High myoinositol concentrations and discrimination from meningiomas. *J Neurosurg* 2001;94(1):55–60.
36. Opstad KS, et al. Detection of elevated glutathione in meningiomas by quantitative in vivo 1H MRS. *Magn Reson Med* 2003;49(4):632–637.
37. Rijpkema M, et al. Characterization of oligodendrogliomas using short echo time 1H MR spectroscopic imaging. *NMR Biomed* 2003;16(1):12–18.
38. Herminghaus S, et al. Increased choline levels coincide with enhanced proliferative activity of human neuroepithelial brain tumors. *NMR Biomed* 2002;15(6):385–392.
39. Howe FA, Opstad KS. 1H MR spectroscopy of brain tumours and masses. *NMR Biomed* 2003;16(3):123–131.
40. Shimizu H, et al. Correlation between choline level measured by proton MR spectroscopy and Ki-67 labeling index in gliomas. *AJNR Am J Neuroradiol* 2000;21(4):659–665.
41. Stadlbauer A, et al. Preoperative grading of gliomas by using metabolite quantification with high-spatial-resolution proton MR spectroscopic imaging. *Radiology* 2006;238(3):958–969.
42. Auer DP, et al. Improved analysis of 1H-MR spectra in the presence of mobile lipids. *Magn Reson Med* 2001;46(3):615–618.
43. Kuesel AC, et al. 1H MRS of high grade astrocytomas: Mobile lipid accumulation in necrotic tissue. *NMR Biomed* 1994;7(3):149–155.

44. Barba I, Cabanas ME, Arus C. The relationship between nuclear magnetic resonance-visible lipids, lipid droplets, and cell proliferation in cultured C6 cells. *Cancer Res* 1999;59(8):1861–1868.
45. Opstad KS, et al. Differentiation of metastases from high-grade gliomas using short echo time 1H spectroscopy. *J Magn Reson Imaging* 2004;20(2):187–192.
46. Law M, et al. High-grade gliomas and solitary metastases: Differentiation by using perfusion and proton spectroscopic MR imaging. *Radiology* 2002;222(3):715–721.
47. INTERPRET. http://azizu.uab.es/INTERPRET/index.html.
48. Tate AR, et al. Development of a decision support system for diagnosis and grading of brain tumours using in vivo magnetic resonance single voxel spectra. *NMR Biomed* 2006;(4):411–434.
49. McKnight TR, et al. Histopathological validation of a three-dimensional magnetic resonance spectroscopy index as a predictor of tumor presence. *J Neurosurg* 2002;97(4):794–802.
50. Pirzkall A, et al. MR-spectroscopy guided target delineation for high-grade gliomas. *Int J Radiat Oncol Biol Phys* 2001;50(4):915–928.
51. Ganslandt O, et al. Proton magnetic resonance spectroscopic imaging integrated into image-guided surgery: Correlation to standard magnetic resonance imaging and tumor cell density. *Neurosurgery* 2005;56(2 Suppl):291–298; discussion 291–298.
52. Dowling C, et al. Preoperative proton MR spectroscopic imaging of brain tumors: Correlation with histopathologic analysis of resection specimens. *AJNR Am J Neuroradiol* 2001;22(4):604–612.
53. Hall WA, Truwit CL. 1.5 T: Spectroscopy-supported brain biopsy. *Neurosurg Clin North Am* 2005; 16(1):165–172, vii.
54. Stadlbauer A, et al. Integration of biochemical images of a tumor into frameless stereotaxy achieved using a magnetic resonance imaging/magnetic resonance spectroscopy hybrid data set. *J Neurosurg* 2004;101(2):287–294.
55. McKnightTR, et al. An automated technique for the quantitative assessment of 3D-MRSI data from patients with glioma. *J Magn Reson Imaging* 2001;13(2):167–177.
56. Nelson SJ, et al. In vivo molecular imaging for planning radiation therapy of gliomas: An application of 1H MRSI. *J Magn Reson Imaging* 2002;16(4):464–476.
57. Chan AA, et al. Proton magnetic resonance spectroscopy imaging in the evaluation of patients undergoing gamma knife surgery for grade IV glioma. *J Neurosurg* 2004;101(3):467–475.
58. Nelson SJ. Multivoxel magnetic resonance spectroscopy of brain tumors. *Mol Cancer Ther* 2003; 2(5):497–507.
59. Lichy MP, et al. [Application of (1)H MR spectroscopic imaging in radiation oncology: Choline as a marker for determining the relative probability of tumor progression after radiation of glial brain tumors.] *Röfo* 2006;178(6):627–633.
60. Tedeschi G, et al. Increased choline signal coinciding with malignant degeneration of cerebral gliomas: A serial proton magnetic resonance spectroscopy imaging study. *J Neurosurg* 1997; 87(4):516–524.
61. Wald LL, et al. Serial proton magnetic resonance spectroscopy imaging of glioblastoma multiforme after brachytherapy. *J Neurosurg* 1997;87(4):525–534.
62. Graves EE, et al. Serial proton MR spectroscopic imaging of recurrent malignant gliomas after gamma knife radiosurgery. *AJNR Am J Neuroradiol* 2001;22(4):613–624.
63. Chernov M, et al. Differentiation of the radiation-induced necrosis and tumor recurrence after gamma knife radiosurgery for brain metastases: Importance of multi-voxel proton MRS. *Minim Invasive Neurosurg* 2005;48(4):228–234.
64. Weybright P, et al. Differentiation between brain tumor recurrence and radiation injury using MR spectroscopy. *AJR Am J Roentgenol* 2005;185(6):1471–1476.
65. Rock JP, et al. Correlations between magnetic resonance spectroscopy and image-guided histopathology, with special attention to radiation necrosis. *Neurosurgery* 2002;51(4):912–919; discussion 919–920.
66. Rock JP, et al. Associations among magnetic resonance spectroscopy, apparent diffusion coefficients, and image-guided histopathology with special attention to radiation necrosis. *Neurosurgery* 2004;54(5):1111–1117; discussion 1117–1119.
67. Schlemmer HP, et al. Differentiation of radiation necrosis from tumor progression using proton magnetic resonance spectroscopy. *Neuroradiology* 2002;44(3):216–222.
68. Preul MC, et al. Using pattern analysis of in vivo proton MRSI data to improve the diagnosis and surgical management of patients with brain tumors. *NMR Biomed* 1998;11(4–5):192–200.

69. Herminghaus S, et al.: Determination of histopathological tumor grade in neuroepithelial brain tumors by using spectral pattern analysis of in vivo spectroscopic data. *J Neurosurg* 2003; 98(1):74–81.
70. De Edelenyi FS, et al. A new approach for analyzing proton magnetic resonance spectroscopic images of brain tumors: Nosologic images. *Nat Med* 2000;6(11):1287–1289.
71. Simonetti AW, et al. A chemometric approach for brain tumor classification using magnetic resonance imaging and spectroscopy. *Anal Chem* 2003;75(20):5352–5361.
72. Galanaud D, et al. Noninvasive diagnostic assessment of brain tumors using combined in vivo MR imaging and spectroscopy. *Magn Reson Med* 2006;55(6):1236–1245.
73. De Vos M, et al. Fast nosologic imaging of the brain. *J Magn Reson* 2006;Nov. 20 [Epub ahead of print].
74. Devos A, et al. The use of multivariate MR imaging intensities versus metabolic data from MR spectroscopic imaging for brain tumour classification. *J Magn Reson* 2005;173(2):218–228.
75. eTUMOUR. http://www.etumour.net/.
76. Moller-Hartmann W, et al. Clinical application of proton magnetic resonance spectroscopy in the diagnosis of intracranial mass lesions. *Neuroradiology* 2002;44(5):371–381.
77. Lin A, Bluml S, Mamelak AN. Efficacy of proton magnetic resonance spectroscopy in clinical decision making for patients with suspected malignant brain tumors. *J Neurooncol* 1999;45(1):69–81.
78. Butzen J, et al. Discrimination between neoplastic and nonneoplastic brain lesions by use of proton MR spectroscopy: The limits of accuracy with a logistic regression model. *AJNR Am J Neuroradiol* 2000;21(7):1213–1219.
79. Majos C, et al. Brain tumor classification by proton MR spectroscopy: Comparison of diagnostic accuracy at short and long TE. *AJNR Am J Neuroradiol* 2004;25(10):1696–1704.
80. Julia-Sape M, et al. Comparison between neuroimaging classifications and histopathological diagnoses using an international multicenter brain tumor magnetic resonance imaging database. *J Neurosurg* 2006;105(1):6–14.
81. Cecil KM, Jones BV. Magnetic resonance spectroscopy of the pediatric brain. *Top Magn Reson Imaging* 2001;12(6):435–452.
82. Taylor JS, Ogg RJ, Langston JW. Proton MR spectroscopy of pediatric brain tumors. *Neuroimaging Clin North Am* 1998;8(4):753–779.
83. Lazareff JA, et al. Pediatric low-grade gliomas: Prognosis with proton magnetic resonance spectroscopic imaging. *Neurosurgery* 1998;43(4):809–817; discussion 817–818.
84. Laprie A, et al. Longitudinal multivoxel MR spectroscopy study of pediatric diffuse brainstem gliomas treated with radiotherapy. *Int J Radiat Oncol Biol Phys* 2005;62(1):20–31.
85. Cornel EB, et al. Characterization of human prostate cancer, benign prostatic hyperplasia and normal prostate by in vitro 1H and 31P magnetic resonance spectroscopy. *J Urol* 1993;150(6):2019–2024.
86. Kurhanewicz J, et al. Citrate alterations in primary and metastatic human prostatic adenocarcinomas: 1H magnetic resonance spectroscopy and biochemical study. *Magn Reson Med* 1993;29(2):149–157.
87. Heerschap A, et al. Proton MR spectroscopy of the normal human prostate with an endorectal coil and a double spin-echo pulse sequence. *Magn Reson Med* 1997;37(2):204–213.
88. Kurhanewicz J, et al. Citrate as an in vivo marker to discriminate prostate cancer from benign prostatic hyperplasia and normal prostate peripheral zone: Detection via localized proton spectroscopy. *Urology* 1995;45(3):459–466.
89. Heerschap A, et al. In vivo proton MR spectroscopy reveals altered metabolite content in malignant prostate tissue. *Anticancer Res* 1997;17(3A):1455–1460.
90. Kurhanewicz J, et al. Three-dimensional H-1 MR spectroscopic imaging of the in situ human prostate with high (0.24–0.7-cm3) spatial resolution. *Radiology* 1996;198(3):795–805.
91. van der Graaf M, et al. Human prostate: Multisection proton MR spectroscopic imaging with a single spin-echo sequence–preliminary experience. *Radiology* 1999;213(3):919–925.
92. Scheenen TW, et al. Fast acquisition-weighted three-dimensional proton MR spectroscopic imaging of the human prostate. *Magn Reson Med* 2004;52(1):80–88.
93. Scheidler J, et al. Prostate cancer: Localization with three-dimensional proton MR spectroscopic imaging–clinicopathologic study. *Radiology* 1999;213(2):473–480.
94. Jung JA, et al. Prostate depiction at endorectal MR spectroscopic imaging: Investigation of a standardized evaluation system. *Radiology* 2004;233(3):701–708.

95. Futterer J, et al. Prostate cancer localization with dynamic contrast-enhanced MR imaging and proton MR spectroscopic imaging in localizing prostate cancer. *Rodiology* 2006;241(2):449–458.
96. Scheenen T, et al. Preliminary results of IMAPS: An international multi-centre assessment of prostate MR spectroscopy. Proceedings of the International Society for Magnetic Resonance in Medicine 13th Scientific Meeting and Exhibition, Miami, FL, 7–13 May 2005.
97. Scheenen T, et al. IMAPS: An international multi-centre assessment of prostate MR spectroscopy. Proceedings of the European Society Magnetic Resonance in Medicine and Biology, Basle, Switzerland, 15–18 September 2005.
98. Shukla-Dave A, et al. Chronic prostatitis: MR imaging and 1H MR spectroscopic imaging findings–initial observations. *Radiology* 2004;231(3):717–724.
99. van Dorsten F, et al. Differentiation of prostatitus from prostate carcinoma using 1H MR spectroscopic imaging and dynamic contrast-enhanced MRI. Proceedings of the International Society for Magnetic Resonance in Medicine 9th Scientific Meeting and Exhibition, Glasgow, Scotland, 21–27 April 2001.
100. Yu KK, et al. Prostate cancer: Prediction of extracapsular extension with endorectal MR imaging and three-dimensional proton MR spectroscopic imaging. *Radiology* 1999;213(2):481–488.
101. Futterer JJ, et al. Prostate cancer: Local staging at 3-T endorectal MR imaging–early experience. *Radiology* 2006;238(1):184–191.
102. Kurhanewicz J, et al. Prostate cancer: Metabolic response to cryosurgery as detected with 3D H-1 MR spectroscopic imaging. *Radiology* 1996;200(2):489–496.
103. Parivar F, et al. Detection of locally recurrent prostate cancer after cryosurgery: Evaluation by transrectal ultrasound, magnetic resonance imaging, and three-dimensional proton magnetic resonance spectroscopy. *Urology* 1996;48(4):594–599.
104. Coakley FV, et al. Endorectal MR imaging and MR spectroscopic imaging for locally recurrent prostate cancer after external beam radiation therapy: Preliminary experience. *Radiology* 2004;233(2):441–448.
105. Pickett B, et al. Use of MRI and spectroscopy in evaluation of external beam radiotherapy for prostate cancer. *Int J Radiat Oncol Biol Phys* 2004;60(4):1047–1055.
106. Pucar D, et al. Prostate cancer: Correlation of MR imaging and MR spectroscopy with pathologic findings after radiation therapy–initial experience. *Radiology* 2005;236(2):545–553.
107. Zaider M, et al. Treatment planning for prostate implants using magnetic-resonance spectroscopy imaging. *Int J Radiat Oncol Biol Phys* 2000;47(4):1085–1096.
108. Mueller-Lisse UG, et al. Time-dependent effects of hormone-deprivation therapy on prostate metabolism as detected by combined magnetic resonance imaging and 3D magnetic resonance spectroscopic imaging. *Magn Reson Med* 2001;46(1):49–57.
109. Zakian KL, et al. Correlation of proton MR spectroscopic imaging with Gleason score based on step-section pathologic analysis after radical prostatectomy. *Radiology* 2005;234(3):804–814.
110. Kurhanewicz J, et al. Combined magnetic resonance imaging and spectroscopic imaging approach to molecular imaging of prostate cancer. *J Magn Reson Imaging* 2002;16(4):451–463.
111. Chen AP, et al. High-resolution 3D MR spectroscopic imaging of the prostate at 3 T with the MLEV-PRESS sequence. *Magn Reson Imaging* 2006;24(7):825–832.
112. Scheenen T, et al. 3D proton-MR spectroscopic imaging of the human prostate at 3 tesla without an endorectal coil–feasibility. *Radiology* 2006, in press.
113. Futterer JJ, et al. Initial experience of 3 tesla endorectal coil magnetic resonance imaging and 1H-spectroscopic imaging of the prostate. *Invest Radiol* 2004;39(11):671–680.
114. Scheenen TW, et al. Optimal timing for in vivo 1H-MR spectroscopic imaging of the human prostate at 3T. *Magn Reson Med* 2005;53(6):1268–1274.
115. Leach MO, et al. Measurements of human breast cancer using magnetic resonance spectroscopy: A review of clinical measurements and a report of localized 31P measurements of response to treatment. *NMR Biomed* 1998;11(7):314–340.
116. Jagannathan NR, et al. Volume localized in vivo proton MR spectroscopy of breast carcinoma: Variation of water-fat ratio in patients receiving chemotherapy. *NMR Biomed* 1998;11(8):414–422.
117. Sitter B, et al. High-resolution magic angle spinning MRS of breast cancer tissue. *NMR Biomed* 2002;15(5):327–337.
118. Mountford CE, et al. Diagnosis and prognosis of breast cancer by magnetic resonance spectroscopy of fine-needle aspirates analysed using a statistical classification strategy. *Br J Surg* 2001;88(9):1234–1240.

119. Katz-Brull R, Lavin PT, Lenkinski RE. Clinical utility of proton magnetic resonance spectroscopy in characterizing breast lesions. *J Natl Cancer Inst* 2002;94(16):1197–1203.
120. Kvistad KA, *et al.* Characterization of neoplastic and normal human breast tissues with in vivo (1)H MR spectroscopy. *J Magn Reson Imaging* 1999;10(2):159–164.
121. Jagannathan NR, *et al.* Evaluation of total choline from in-vivo volume localized proton MR spectroscopy and its response to neoadjuvant chemotherapy in locally advanced breast cancer. *Br J Cancer* 2001;84(8):1016–1022.
122. Yeung DK, Yang WT, Tse GM. Breast cancer: In vivo proton MR spectroscopy in the characterization of histopathologic subtypes and preliminary observations in axillary node metastases. *Radiology* 2002;225(1):190–197.
123. Bolan PJ, *et al.* Eliminating spurious lipid sidebands in 1H MRS of breast lesions. *Magn Reson Med* 2002;48(2):215–222.
124. Bakken IJ, *et al.* External standard method for the in vivo quantification of choline-containing compounds in breast tumors by proton MR spectroscopy at 1.5 Tesla. *Magn Reson Med* 2001;46(1):189–192.
125. Bolan PJ, *et al.* In vivo quantification of choline compounds in the breast with 1H MR spectroscopy. *Magn Reson Med* 2003;50(6):1134–1143.
126. Meisamy S, *et al.* Adding in vivo quantitative 1H MR spectroscopy to improve diagnostic accuracy of breast MR imaging: Preliminary results of observer performance study at 4.0 T. *Radiology* 2005;236(2):465–475.
127. Stanwell P, *et al.* Specificity of choline metabolites for in vivo diagnosis of breast cancer using 1H MRS at 1.5 T. *Eur Radiol* 2005;15(5):1037–1043.
128. Meisamy S, *et al.* Neoadjuvant chemotherapy of locally advanced breast cancer: Predicting response with in vivo (1)H MR spectroscopy–a pilot study at 4 T. *Radiology* 2004;233(2):424–431.
129. Jacobs MA, *et al.* Combined dynamic contrast enhanced breast MR and proton spectroscopic imaging: A feasibility study. *J Magn Reson Imaging* 2005;21(1):23–28.
130. Maril N, *et al.* Strategies for shimming the breast. *Magn Reson Med* 2005;54(5):1139–1145.
131. Magnetic resonance spectroscopy for evaluation of suspected brain tumor. www.bcbs.com.tec/vol18/18_01.html. TEC Bull 2003;20(1):23–26.
132. Ross BD. Evidence-based medicine: What's wrong with spectroscopy papers. Proceedings of the International Society for Magnetic Resonance in Medicine 13th Scientific Meeting and Exhibition, Miami, FL, 7–13 May 2005, p. 126.
133. Lin A, *et al.* Efficacy of proton magnetic resonance spectroscopy in neurological diagnosis and neurotherapeutic decision making. NeuroRx 2005;2(2):197–214.
134. Hollingworth W, *et al.* A systematic literature review of magnetic resonance spectroscopy for the characterization of brain tumors. *AJNR Am J Neuroradiol* 2006;27(7):1404–1411.
135. Golman K, *et al.* Metabolic imaging by hyperpolarized 13C magnetic resonance imaging for in vivo tumor diagnosis. *Cancer Res* 2006;66(22):10855–10860.

14 Magnetic Resonance Probes for Tumor Imaging

Alexander S.R. Guimaraes, MD, PhD,
and Ralph Weissleder, MD, PhD

CONTENTS

    INTRODUCTION
    GADOLINIUM-CONTAINING AGENTS
    MAGNETIC NANOPARTICLES
    ANGIOGENESIS IMAGING
    MAGNETIC NANOPARTICLES AS LYMPHOTROPIC AGENTS
    IMAGING CELL TRACKING
    TARGETING TUMOR CELLS
    MAGNETIC NANOSENSORS

1. INTRODUCTION

Magnetic resonance imaging (MRI) is a noninvasive, high spatial resolution, multi-planar imaging modality that offers exquisite soft tissue contrast. Recent advances in MRI equipment (higher field strengths, optimized pulse sequences, and better coil design) have made this imaging modality a procedure of choice for evaluating many cancers. Coupled with the use of small molecule paramagnetic agents and magnetic nanoparticles, different tumor processes can now be probed. Imaging of angiogenesis, apoptosis, and specific targeting are all within the realm of experimental clinical imaging. This chapter summarizes different types of magnetic probes and their application in cancer.

Magnetic resonance imaging is based on the manipulation of the inherent nuclear magnetic moment of endogenous nuclei (most commonly ^{1}H in H_2O). Images can be obtained by exposing nuclei to a static magnetic field, and within that static field, perturbing a steady-state equilibrium with time- and space-varying magnetic fields. After perturbation, all nuclei relax by two unique and codepent relaxation mechanisms: T1 (spin–lattice relaxation), and T2 (spin–spin relaxation). By exploiting these relaxation mechanisms, chemists and physicists have been able to design contrast agents and pulse sequence algorithms to further specify the imaging patterns of many diseases

From: *Cancer Drug Discovery and Development
In Vivo Imaging of Cancer Therapy*
Edited by: A.F. Shields and P. Price © Humana Press Inc., Totowa, NJ

and add to the diagnostic acumen of MRI. Magnetic resonance imaging has therefore become an imaging modality of choice for disease states such as stroke, neurodegenerative states, trauma, and cancer.

Although MRI offers exquisite spatial resolution and high soft tissue contrast, it is of lower sensitivity for label detection when compared to other imaging modalities routinely used in molecular imaging (e.g., optical imaging and nuclear medicine). With ever increasing advances in MRI (higher field strengths, optimized pulse sequences, and better coil design) we are now poised to reduce this insensitivity and improve the combination of MRI with the development of more specific and sensitive magnetic probes. The purpose of this chapter is to focus on imaging probes that are specifically designed for MRI of molecular processes associated with cancer.

Magnetic resonance contrast agents can be divided into two classes, paramagnetic and superparamagnetic. The majority and most clinically utilized paramagnetic contrast agents utilize Gd(III), although Mn is also occasionally used because of its large magnetic moment and long electron spin relaxation time, which has the effect of shortening the T1 (spin–lattice) relaxation time *(1, 2)*. Dysprosium (Dy), another paramagnetic contrast agent, induces local magnetic field inhomogeneities, which can be measured by local shortening of the T2*. Chelates of Dy have been utilized to measure changes in cerebral blood flow and tissue injury in myocardial infarction *(3, 4)*, and although not routinely clinically utilized, as higher magnetic field systems become more routine, these agents may be revisited. Magnetic nanoparticles (MNP) contain superparamagnetic iron oxides and form the basis of susceptibility contrast either by shortening the T2 (spin–spin) relaxation time or the T1 (spin–lattice) relaxation time *(5–7)*.

A number of novel targeted MR imaging agents have employed either paramagnetic or superparamagnetic labels. Some examples utilizing MNP include asialoglycoprotein receptors for liver imaging *(8, 9)*, antimyosin-labeled MNP for detection of myocardial infarcts *(10)*, endothelial vascular adhesion molecule-1 *(11)*, and E-selectin *(12–16)*. Other exploited targets using paramagnetic contrast agents include the folate receptor with dendrimer-based paramagnetic contrast agents to image overexpression of folate receptor in ovarian tumor xenografts *(17)*, the fibrin receptor *(18)*, and direct labeling of monoclonal antibodies with gadolinium to image human tumors on nude mice *(19)*.

In addition to the group classification mentioned above, magnetic resonance agents can also be classified by their distribution and specificity into (1) compartmental agents (i.e., low-molecular-weight, extravascular, extracellular agents; or macromolecular weight-contrast agents, blood-pool, intravascular agents); (2) targeted agents (those agents that have been modified to bind to specific molecular targets); and (3) activatable agents (those agents that undergo a physicochemical process to "activate" their contrast mechanisms). The following discussion will summarize different types of imaging agents based on their composition and *in vivo* behavior. Finally we will review applications of the different agents for imaging cancer.

2. GADOLINIUM-CONTAINING AGENTS

Paramagnetic, low-molecular-weight contrast agents typically contain Gd(III) in a chelate such as diethylenetriaminepentaacetic acid (DTPA), gadoterate meglumine (DOTA–Dotarem®), or gadobenate dimeglumine (BOPTA–Multihance®) *(2)*. Gd chelates allow the evaluation of physiological parameters such as the status of the blood–brain barrier, perfusion with mathematical modeling, tumor enhancement, and renal function. Because of the relative nonspecificity of Gd chelates, the relatively poor relaxivity, as well as short intravascular half-life, there has been increased interest in gadolinium-based macromolecular contrast agents to attach more Gd(III) groups to each molecule *(2, 5)*.

Macromolecular contrast agents that utilize Gd(III) have been developed with varying protein based conjugates including (1) albumin, which has been demonstrated to have long-lived intravascular components, and as a result continues to be utilized both as a conjugate for other biomolecules as well as a primary imaging agent for angiogenesis *(5, 20–22)*; (2) avidin, which binds to streptavidin, the combination of which has been used as a prelabeling mechanism to bind to the biotin ligands *(5, 23–26)*; (3) poly-L-lysine *(19, 27)*; (4) polyamidoamine (PAMAM) dendrimers *(28–31)*; and (5) direct conjugation to monoclonal antibodies (Mab) *(32, 33)*. Another approach that has been attempted to increase delivery of a number of gadolinium groups to the target is cross-linking liposomes labeled with a large concentration of gadolinium, thus increasing the relaxivity of the target *(34)*. In all cases, the goal is to increase the contrast to noise after delivery of target to background.

With respect to "activatable" Gd agents, Louie and Meade *et al.* have recently demonstrated an example of a novel "smart" contrast probe that remains silent until activated by a specific transgene product *(35)*. By utilizing bacterial β-galactosidase (LacZ), because it is easily assayed and not expressed in most mammals, they developed a contrast agent that was associated with a substrate for LacZ, galactopyranose. They covalently linked galactopyranose to a chelated paramagnetic Gd^{3+} in a way that precluded access of water protons to the Gd^{3+} atom. This interaction with the LacZ substrate cleaved the galactopyranose, and thus allowed access of water protons to Gd^{3+}, which shortened T1 and thus produced contrast. With intravenous mRNA to allow β-galactosidase activity within organisms, injection of this novel smart probe produced visualization of those cells involved with LacZ activity.

3. MAGNETIC NANOPARTICLES

Magnetic nanoparticles (MNP) used in MRI usually consist of a 2- to 7-nm core of superparamagnetic iron (Fe) oxide (containing 2000–10,000 Fe atoms) and a polymer coating to which biomolecules can be attached *(36–38)*. Magnetic nanoparticles typically have R2 relaxivities ranging from 30 to 300 mM sec^{-1}, at least an order of magnitude higher than for Gd chelates.

Historically, polymer-coated iron oxide molecules have been used in the treatment of anemias *(39, 40)*. The first generation MNP, because of size heterogeneity and imperfect coating, was rapidly phagocytosed by macrophage, and served as imaging agents for the liver and spleen, demonstrating good sensitivity in distinguishing metastases from normal liver and splenic parenchyma *(41, 42)*. By refining the chemical structure and making the molecule smaller (25–30 nm) and homogeneous in size (termed monodisperse–one crystal per nanoparticle), second generation MNP were developed to have increased vascular half lives (>10 h in mice, and >24 h in humans) as well as lymphotrophic components *(7, 43–49)*.

Other derivatives of MNP involve iron oxide cores coated with lipid *(50)* and polyethylene glycol (PEG) *(51)*, which helps reduce binding of plasma proteins and phagocytosis and clearance by macrophages. Table 1 summarizes different MNP in clinical use. The most widely used agents contain dextran or dextran derivatives as a coating (Feridex®, Resovist®, Combidex®, and ferumoxytol) *(1, 6, 37, 38)*.

To make MNP more target specific, multiple strategies have been employed. Earlier work focused on creating Schiff bases between the amine of the biomolecule of attachment and aldehyde of the dextran coating of MNP *(8, 52)*. A second more recent approach cross-links and aminates the dextran of dextran-coated MNP to therefore provide an amino group for binding biomolecules. The molecule is termed amino-CLIO (cross-linked iron oxide). Each amino-CLIO bears approximately 40 amino groups for attachment of biomolecules, and is approximately 40–50 nm in size *(53)*. More recently, noncross-linked ultrastable MNPs have been developed. Examples of targeted MNP include the following: neuroblastoma antibody *(54)*, cardiac myosin antibody *(10)*, synaptotagmin *(55)*, E-selectin *(14–16)*, vascular cell adhesion molecule-1 (VCAM-1) *(11)*, asialoglycoprotein *(56)*, uMuc *(57)*, annexin V *(58)*, and the transferrin receptor *(59)*. Figure 1 represents an illustrative methodology toward this approach, with an example of MR imaging of transgene expression.

Activatable or smart MNPs are specifically engineered to undergo a physicochemical change after binding to their designated target, which then results in signal contrast amplification. Specific examples include conjugation of MNP to tat peptide *(60)*,

Table 1
Polymer-Coated Iron Oxides as Pharmaceuticals[a]

Drug	Composition	Major indication	Manufacturer/status
Ferumoxtrol® AMI-228	Superparamagnetic iron/ carboxymethyldextran	Anemia treatment MR angiograph, lymph node metastases	AMI/phase III (anemia)
Feridex IV® Ferumoxides®	Superparamagnetic iron/ dextran	Suspected liver metastases	AMI, Berlex/approved Europe, USA, Japan
Resovist® Ferucarbotra®	Superparamagnetic iron/ carboxydextran	Suspected liver metastases	Schering AG/approved EC and Japan
Combidex® Ferumoxtran	Superparamagnetic iron/ dextran	Suspected lymph node metastases	AMI, Cytogen/post phase III trials
Supravist® SHU555C	Superparamagnetic iron/ carboxydextran	Suspected liver metastases	Schering AG/in trials
Gastromark® Ferumoxsil®	Superparamagnetic iron/ silane	Bowel marker	AMI, Mallinckrodt/ approved USA and EC
Clariscan® Feruglose® NC 10050	Superparamagnetic iron/ PEG coating	MR angiography Blood pool imaging	Nycomed, Amersham/phase I/II trials

[a] MR, magnetic resonance; PEG, polyethylene glycol.

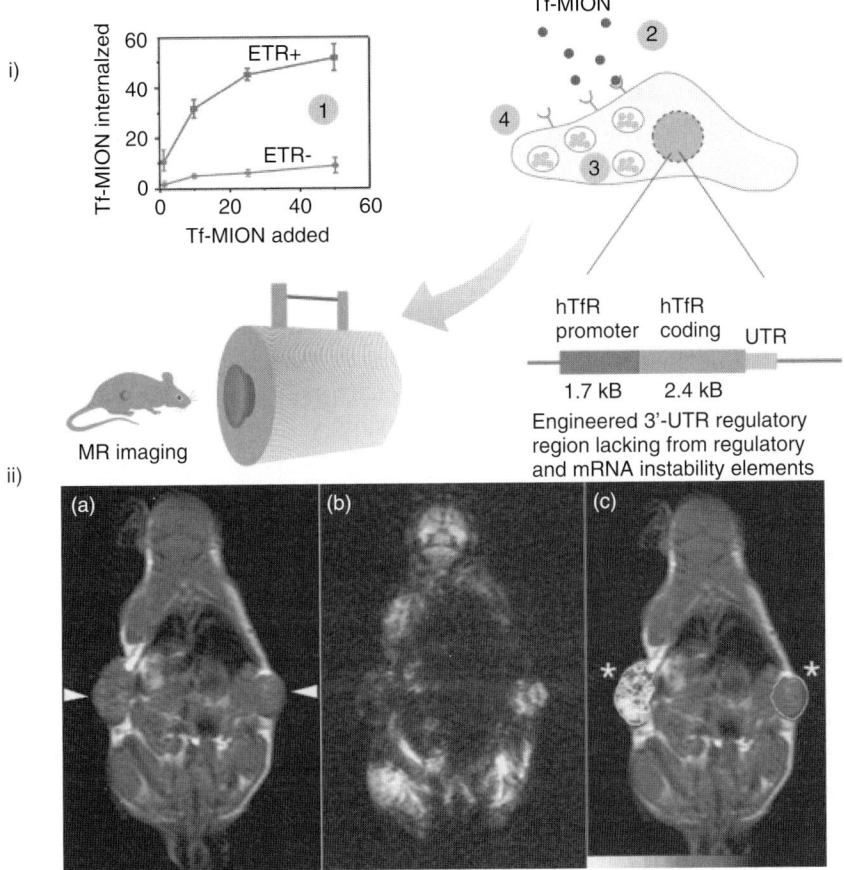

Fig. 1. (i) To demonstrate transgene expression in cells by MR imaging, several synergistic steps were used. Overexpression of ETR expression results in an approximately 500% more cell uptake of the Tf-MION probe per hour than in control cells (step 1). During each ETR-mediated internalization event, several thousand iron atoms (MION contains an average of 2,064 Fe molecules per 3-nm particle core, rather than just the two iron atoms in holo-Tf) accumulate in the cell (step 2). After cellular internalization and compaction in an endosome, the R2 and R2* "relaxivities" of superparamagnetic MION further increases approximately 400%, causing T2 to decrease and creating high local susceptibility gradients detectable by gradient-echo MR pulse sequences (step 3). Cellular internalization of iron does not down regulate the level of ETR expression (step 4). The ETR cDNA sequence consists of the hTfR promoter, the coding sequence, and the engineered 3 untranslated region (UTR) regulatory sequence. (ii) *In vivo MR* imaging of a single mouse with ETR$^+$ (left arrowheads) and ETR$^-$ (right arrowheads) flank tumors. (a) T1-weighted coronal spin echo image (imaging time, 3.5 min; voxel resolution, 300 × 300 × 3000 μm). ETR$^-$ and ETR$^+$ tumors have similar signal intensities. (b) T2-weighted gradient-echo image corresponding to the image in (a), showing substantial differences between ETR$^-$ and ETR$^+$ tumors (imaging time, 8 min.; voxel resolution, 300 × 300 × 3000 μm). As expected, ETR-mediated cellular accumulation of the superparamagnetic probe decreases signal intensity. These differences in MR signal intensity were most pronounced using T2 and T2* weighted imaging pulse sequences, consistent with the increased transverse relaxation (R2) after cellular internalization. (c) Composite image of T1-weighted spin-echo image obtained for anatomic detail with superimposed R2 changes after Tf-MION administration. *, difference in R2 changes between the ETR$^-$ and ETR$^+$ tumors. (Reproduced with permission from Weissleder *et al.* (59)).

oligomerization of MNP *(14)*, and magnetic relaxation switch mechanisms, which have been utilized to measure multiple different reversible molecular interactions at extremely low contrast agent concentration *(61–63)*.

4. ANGIOGENESIS IMAGING

Imaging angiogenesis with MRI has focused on three different arenas: (1) dynamic tracking of Gd chelates, (2) steady-state blood volume determinations using MNP, and (3) use of targeted imaging agents.

4.1 Dynamic Contrast-Enhanced Magnetic Resonance Imaging

Magnetic resonance imaging approaches of measuring angiogenesis have the advantage of providing noninvasive spatial assessment of angiogenic heterogeneity; however, most techniques are dynamic acquisitions resulting in serial data over single slices *(64–66)*. Malignant neovasculature has been shown to be hyperpermeable to low-molecular-weight molecules (e.g., macromolecules). Due to this hyperpermeability, dynamic contrast-enhanced magnetic resonance imaging (DCE MRI) offers a possible noninvasive, quantitative characterization of tumors, both morphologically and functionally *(64–66)*. This methodological approach uses a bolus administration of contrast agent, and Gd chelate is the most ubiquitous, FDA-approved contrast agent. Given the high concentration of Gd chelate within the first pass, inherent T2 relaxivity changes are proportional to blood volume and blood flow *(67)*. However, as a result of the highly permeable intratumoral vasculature, and low concentrations of contrast "leaking" into the extravascular, extracellular space, the T1 changes dominate initial and later phases of contrast administration *(64–66)*. Because the majority of contrast agents utilized in MRI leak out of the vascular space, but do not cross cellular membranes, extant kinetic models utilize a two-compartment system to analyze dynamic data sets, all of which are based on Kety modeling systems *(68)*. Agreed upon parameters that are measured include the following *(64)*: C_t = tracer concentration within the tissue, C_p = tracer concentration within the plasma, v_e = extracellular volume fraction, and K^{trans} = transendothelial permeability factor; these are related by the following first-order equation:

$$d\,C_t/dt = K^{trans}(C_p - C_t/v_e) = K^{trans}C_p - K_{ep}C_t$$

Utilizing this approach in humans suffering from breast cancer, Hulka *et al.* demonstrated a sensitivity of 86% and specificity of 93% for the diagnosis of malignancy *(64–66)*. Knopp *et al.* expanded on these results and were able to demonstrate, by correlative analysis with vascular endothelial growth factor (VEGF) and CD31 analysis, significantly faster enhancement characteristics between histological subtypes (invasive ductal carcinoma, invasive lobular carcinoma, and ductal carcinoma *in situ*) *(69)*. Subsequently, various groups have demonstrated, *in vivo* in animal models and clinical trials, statistically significant differences in permeability transfer constants following the administration of angiogenesis inhibitors *(70, 71)*. Recently Morgan *et al.* demonstrated a rapid reduction in enhancement within 26–33 hours after the first dose of the VEGF inhibitor phosphotyrosine kinase (PTK) 787/ZK 222584 in a liver metastasis from colorectal carcinoma *(71)*. This substantial reduction in enhancement is evident across all dose groups on day 2, with a mean reduction of permeability transfer constant of 43% (SE, 6.95%) *(71)*.

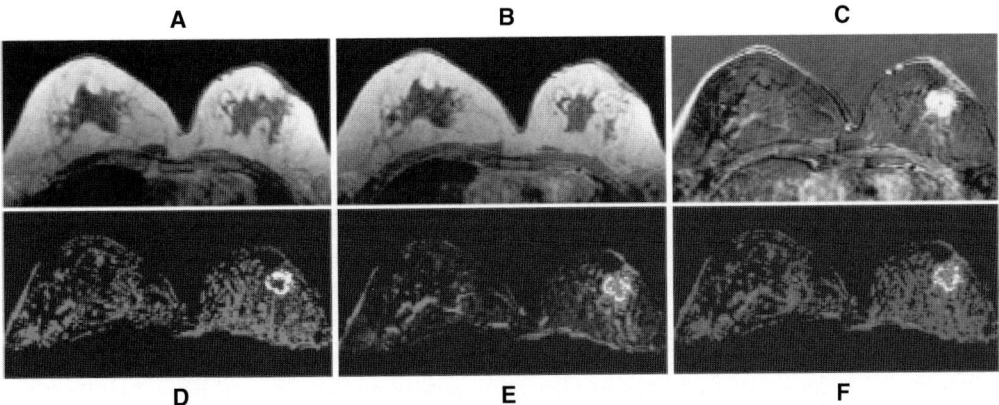

Fig. 2. The precontrast image (A), 5-min postcontrast image (B), and 5-min enhancement map (C) of a woman with breast cancer. Pharmacokinetic analysis was performed to analyze the enhancement kinetics obtained on a pixel-by-pixel basis from the entire bilateral breasts. The generated parameter maps, Vb (D), VeK1 (E), and K2 (F), are shown. The peripheral region had a higher vascularity (Vb) and a higher outflux transport rate (K2), but the entire cancer (except a very small central region) displayed a strong interstitial uptake (VeK1). [Reproduced with permission from Su et al. (73).]

Despite these sophisticated models and encouraging results, pharmacokinetic modeling has been utilized with varying success to calculate blood volume or fractional plasma volume, with reported values demonstrating a correlation coefficient of R^2 0.61, and most studies indicate high sensitivity (>90%), but wide variability in specificity, with published values as low as 30% (72). This variability is demonstrated well in the recent study by Su et al. (Fig. 2 and Table 2) who performed DCE MRI on 105 patients with breast cancer and correlated it to VEGF serum marker levels as well as microvascular density as assessed post-CD31 staining. Although patients with increased VEGF demonstrated higher CD31 microvessel densitites, no significant association between MRI parameters and these other surrogate markers was demonstrated (73).

Table 2
MRI Parameters Obtained Using Entire Tumor Analysis in High/Low VEGF Groups and High/Medium/Low CD31 Groups[a]

MRI parameter	High VEGF (N = 49)	Low VEGF (N = 22)	High CD31 (N = 12)	Med CD31 (N = 35)	Low CD31 (N = 24)
Vb	21 ± 20	17 ± 16	21 ± 20	21 ± 20	21 ± 20
K2	0.23 ± 0.09	0.23 ± 0.12	0.24 ± 0.09	0.21 ± 0.09	0.23 ± 0.11
VbK2/veK1	0.017 ± 0.02	0.019 ± 0.031	0.025 ± 0.022	0.011 ± 0.013	0.023 ± 0.032
1-min enhancement	326 ± 87	296 ± 94	345 ± 102	306 ± 92	321 ± 77
1-min enhancement	63 ± 25	55 ± 26	69 ± 31	57 ± 25	63 ± 22
1- to 3-min enhancement	94 ± 22	85 ± 23	99 ± 23	89 ± 24	92 ± 21

[a]MRI, magnetic resonance imaging; VEGF, vascular endothelial growth factor.

As a result of this high variance, investigators have employed more sophisticated mathematical modeling in an attempt to further dissect tumor physiology *(74, 75)*. Some of the variance in these results may also result from the size of the contrast agent as well as the inability to validate quantitatively derived parameters, such as K^{trans}, which are dependent on multiple variables (i.e., blood flow, blood volume, and permeability), and the inability to maintain an intravascular state. As a result, the diagnostic potential of DCE-MRI utilizing macromolecular contrast agents within breast malignancies has been studied *(76–80)*. The results indicate that macromolecular particulate MR imaging contrast agents, such as Gadomer-17, feruglose, Gd-PGC, and albumin-(Gd-DTPA)30, can be applied successfully to characterize tumor microvessels in animal models *(81)*. Derived estimates of microvascular permeability correlate strongly with the histopathological tumor grade, microvascular density, and microvascular permeability values derived by using albumin-(Gd-DTPA)30, (an experimental long-lived, intravascular agent) within animal models. However, albumin-(Gd-DTPA)30 has been shown to be immunogenic with retention within bone marrow and liver, limiting its clinical use *(22, 82)*.

4.2 Steady-State Assessment of Angiogenesis

An alternative approach to imaging angiogenesis utilizes the long-lived intravascular nature and inherent T2* contrast mechanisms of MNP, which offer a unique, steady-state approach to imaging blood volume over large areas of the body, offering evaluation of both primary malignancies and potentially metastases *(83–86)*. Bremer *et al.* first utilized intravital microscopy to determine whether a prototype MNP (MION) agent truly had intravascular distribution in a tumor microenvironment *(85)*. For these experiments a green fluorescence protein (GFP)-expressing 9L tumor model was utilized, in which tumor microvasculature is clearly outlined against fluorescent tumor cells, even at very high spatial resolutions, which demonstrated that (MION, a prototype MNP) selectively enhanced the vascularity without any significant leakage into tumor interstitium during the time of observation (30 min).

Figure 3 and Table 3 demonstrate four different tumor xenograft models varying in angiogenesis to assess the sensitivity of this steady-state approach to differentiate the degrees of angiogenesis. 9L rodent gliosarcoma, DU4475 human mammary adenocarcinoma, HT1080 human fibrosarcoma, and EOMA hemangioendothelioma were implanted into nude mice *(85)*. The 9L and the other chosen tumor models were char-

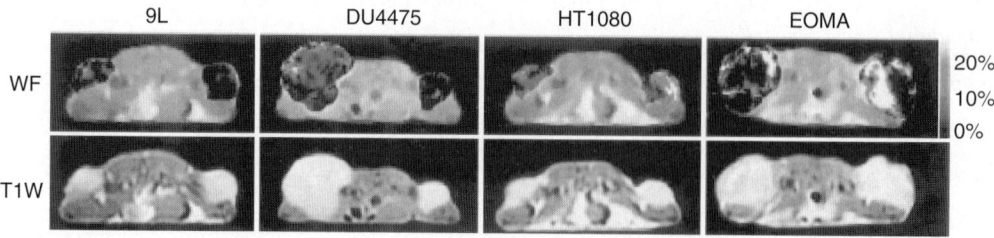

Fig. 3. MR images of the four experimental tumor models. Top row: Vascular volume fraction (VVF) tumoral vascularity maps are superimposed onto the tumors and derived from precontrast and postcontrast T2*-weighted MR imaging sequences. VVF values are from 0% to 30%. Note the heterogeneity of VVF among the tumor models. Bottom row: The different tumors are outlined on postcontrast T1-weighted spin–echo MR images (300/6). [Reproduced with permission from Bremer *et al. (85)*.]

Table 3
Summary of Experimental Measurements[a]

Tumor cell line	Cancer type	Radiotracer VVF (%)	MR imaging VVF (%)	MVD[b] (counts per field)	VEGF[b] (ng/mg protein)
9L	Glioma	$2.0 \pm 0.3^{c,d}$	$2.07 \pm 0.34^{c,d}$	$43.6 \pm 3.3^{c,d}$	$1.8 \pm 0.5^{c,d}$
DU4475	Breast cancer	3.0 ± 0.3^{d}	3.06 ± 0.43^{d}	$39.3 \pm 2.3^{c,d}$	2.3 ± 0.5^{d}
HT1080	Fibrosarcoma	5.2 ± 0.3^{e}	5.54 ± 0.82^{e}	$81.4 \pm 5.8^{d,e,f}$	5.5 ± 1.9
EOMA	Angiosarcoma	$6.1 \pm 1.2^{e,f}$	$6.64 \pm 0.94^{e,f}$	$150 \pm 1.3^{d,e,f}$	$7.7 \pm 1.3^{e,f}$

[a] All data are means ± standard errors of the mean. The vascular volume fraction (VVF) measurements obtained with MR imaging were almost identical to those obtained with nuclear imaging with a radiotracer, the reference standard for comparison with MR imaging measurements.
[b] MVD, microvessel density; VEGF, vascular endothelial growth factor.
[c] Value significantly different from corresponding value for HT1080 tumors ($p < 0.025$).
[d] Value significantly different from corresponding value for EOMA tumors ($p < 0.025$).
[e] Value significantly different from corresponding value for 9L tumors ($p < 0.025$).
[f] Value significantly different from corresponding value for DU4475 tumors ($p < 0.025$).

acterized by determining microvessel counts, VEGF production, and, in a separate set of experiments, global tumoral vascular volume fraction (VVF) by using a validated ^{99m}Tc marker of intravascular volume *(87, 88)*.

Steady-state tumoral blood volume maps were calculated from the precontrast and postcontrast MNP enhanced images as described in detail elsewhere *(83–85)*. A fundamental assumption is that the change in the transverse relaxation rate ($\Delta R2^*$) relative to the preinjection baseline is proportional to the perfused local blood volume per unit tumor volume (V) multiplied by a function (f) of the plasma concentration of the agent (P).

$$\Delta R2^* = k \cdot f(P) \cdot V$$

Assuming a steady state for iron oxide MNP distribution, the equation reduces to a simple linear relationship between $\Delta R2^*$ and the perfused blood volume fraction.

$$\Delta R2^*(t) = K \cdot V(t) \text{ or } V(t) = \Delta R2^*(t)/K$$

where the constant K includes the agent blood pool concentration and is therefore dose dependent. The enhancement of R2* can be expressed as

$$\Delta R2^* = 1/T2^*_{post} - 1/T2^*_{pre} \approx -1/TE \ \ln(S_{post}/S_{pre})$$

where S is the signal intensity and T2 the transverse relaxation time. Based on this formula $\Delta R2^*$ maps were calculated for all MR images using commercially available software. In addition, regions of interest (ROI) were collected from each tumor and adjacent muscle tissue to calculate tumoral vascular volume fractions (VVFs). Absolute tumoral VVFs were obtained by scaling measurements to muscle. Figure 3 demonstrates MR imaging of the four experimental tumor models. Row 1 shows coded tumoral vascularity maps superimposed onto the tumors, derived from precontrast and postcontrast T2*-weighted sequences (gray scale map ranges from 0 to 30% VVF). The accompanying table (Table 3) summarizes the results of radiotracer measurement of global VVF, as compared to MRI VVF%, histologically calculated microvascular density (MVD), and VEGF production. There was no statistically significant difference between radiotracer VVF and MRI VVF, with excellent correlation ($R > 0.9$) between

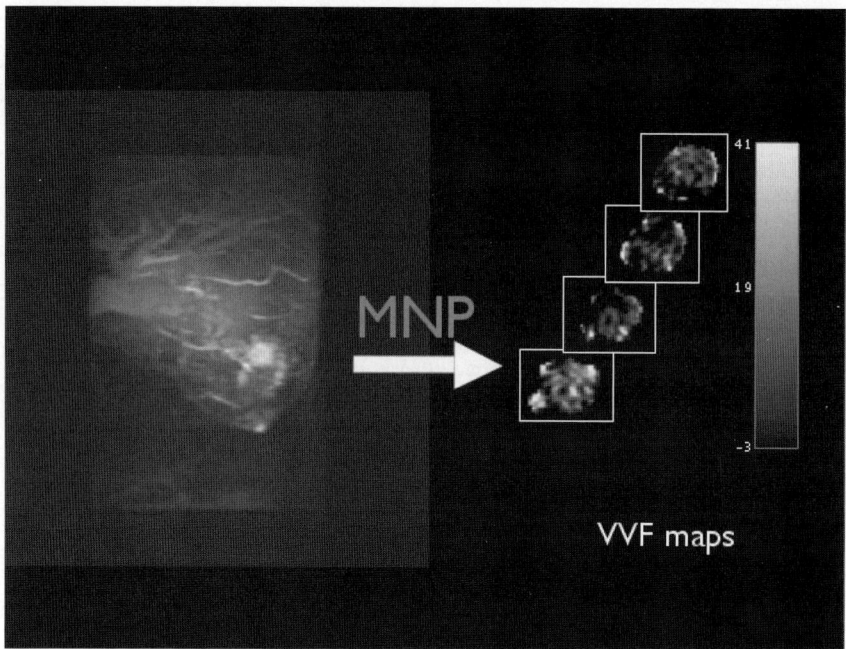

Fig. 4. Example of steady-state imaging of angiogenesis in a human suffering from breast cancer. The image on the left is a T1-weighted image with fat suppression post-Gd-DTPA enhancement. An enhancing mass is noted in the lateral aspect of the left breast. The images on the right demonstrate vascular volume fraction (VVF) maps from multiple slices of this same tumor obtained immediately following the administration of magnetic nanoparticles (MNP). The reference bar allows a correlation of grayscale to VVF.

VEGF and MRI VVF. These data confirm that steady-state measures of VVF with MRI allow a volumetric, *in vivo*, noninvasive assay of microvascular density in experimental tumor models. Experiments are ongoing to determine the sensitivity of this steady-state technique in investigating the role of antiangiogenic therapies *in vivo* in animal models and humans (Fig. 4).

4.3 Imaging Angiogenesis with Molecular Target-Selected Magnetic Resonance Imaging

Another potential means of imaging neovascular density could be performed through direct or indirect specific molecular targeting. One preferred target has been the integrin $\alpha_v\beta_3$. Although $\alpha_v\beta_3$ integrins are expressed on endothelial cells, they are also found on a wide range of tumor cells including the MDA-MB-435 breast and B16B15b melanoma cells *(89)* and human lung carcinoma *(90)* and melanoma *(91)*. This receptor has been shown to be upregulated in angiogenic endothelium *(92)*. Schmieder *et al.* demonstrated an antibody to the $\alpha_v\beta_3$ ligand and showed micromelanoma metastases in a melanoma mouse model at 1.5 T *(93)*. Figure 5 demonstrates early visualization of the angiogenic vasculature of C32 melanoma tumors implanted in athymic nude mice 2h after injection of $\alpha_v\beta_3$-labeled paramagnetic nanoparticles. The same ligand has been exploited in other MRI-targeted approaches either utilizing antibodies conjugated to liposome nanoparticles sequestering Gd, or other direct antibody conjugations to nanoparticles *(34, 94–96)*.

E-selectin offers another target that has been exploited by MRI using either paramagnetic *(12, 13)* or superparamagnetic MNP approaches *(15)*. Another exciting target that has just recently been utilized is VCAM-1. Kelly *et al.* recently utilized phage display-derived peptide sequences and multimodal MNP to develop a VCAM-1-targeted multimodal imaging agent that was internalized and therefore provided a novel amplification strategy, which demonstrated a 12-fold higher target-to-background ratio as compared to VCAM-1 monoclonal antibody approaches *(11)*. Their results may be useful for the design of other *in vivo* imaging markers involved with tumor angiogenesis *(11)*.

These approaches open up a novel means of addressing specific angiogenesis targets, and also demonstrate novel means of addressing the benefits of soft tissue contrast, and superior spatial resolution inherent to MRI, while solving some of the inherent low sensitivity associated with MRI.

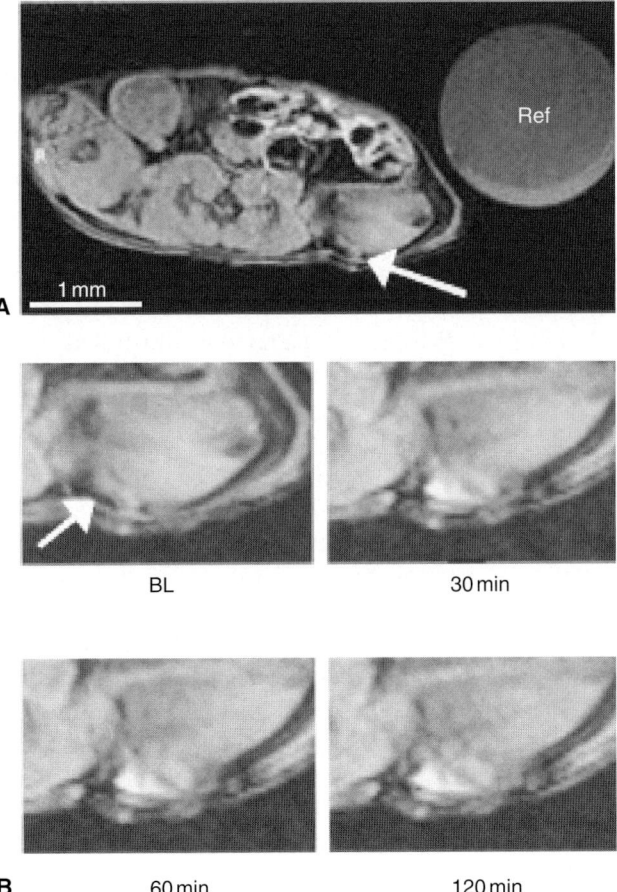

Fig. 5. (A) T1-weighted MR image (axial view) of an athymic nude mouse before injection of paramagnetic three-targeted nanoparticles. The arrow indicates a C32 tumor that is difficult to detect (Ref, Gd in a 10-cm^3 syringe). (B) Enlarged section of an MR image showing T1-weighted signal enhancement of angiogenic vasculature of early tumors over 2h as detected by three-targeted paramagnetic nanoparticles. (BL, baseline image.) [Reproduced with permission from Schmieder *et al.* *(93)*.]

5. MAGNETIC NANOPARTICLES AS LYMPHOTROPIC AGENTS

The accurate detection of nodal metastases remains a critically important step in cancer staging. The gold standard for determining lymph node involvement relies on invasive procedures such as biopsy, surgical dissection, or sentinel node biopsy. These are associated with cost and morbidity and are not infallible *(97, 98)*. Current imaging modalities that are utilized to diagnose metastatic involvement of lymph nodes include nuclear scintigraphic assessment of sentinel node involvement, which involves biopsy; positron emission tomography (PET), which may have size threshold limits; computed tomography, which relies on morphological and size criteria for determination of metastatic involvement; and MRI *(99)*. The key advantage of MRI approaches to imaging lymph node involvement in humans suffering from cancer is its ability to detect occult cancer in nonenlarged, nonregional lymph nodes that are typically below the detection threshold of PET.

The advent of lymphotropic magnetic nanoparticles (usually dextran T10 coated materials) offers a systemic approach toward identifying pathologically involved lymph nodes, which may supplant other more invasive approaches for recovering such information, such as lymphangiography, sentinel node biopsy, or mediastinoscopy. This is clinically relevant secondary to the possibility of finding nodes outside traditional surgical fields, in identifying, prior to biopsy, those patients who are node positive and thus direct them toward neoadjuvant chemotherapy or radiation, while providing a three-dimensional map for guiding surgical or radiation therapy.

The development *(7, 100)* and clinical introduction of lymph node-targeted MNP significantly improve diagnostic accuracies of MR imaging for nodal staging in prostate cancer *(46, 101)*. Within this technique, illustrated in Fig. 6, images are performed before and 24 h after the intravenous administration of contrast agents that are lymphotropic *(37, 44, 102–104)*, in particular Ferumoxtran-10 (Combidex®, Advanced Magnetics, Inc., Cambridge, MA). Secondary to their iron-oxide core, $T2^*$-weighted imaging is performed. As a result of being lymphotropic, these contrast agents enhance normal lymphatic tissue secondary to phagocytosis by macrophage *(37, 44, 102–104)*. There is reliable accumulation within normal lymph nodes, and the lack of contrast uptake, as determined by a lack of $T2^*$ decrease in signal, has been shown to be correlated with the presence of metastatic deposits *(7, 46, 53, 100, 103–105)*. This approach offers a global assessment of lymph node involvement from cancer. Preliminary studies in patients with prostate cancer show that lymphotrophic magnetic nanoparticles are highly accurate reporters for detecting tumor burden even in clinically occult disease *(46, 101)*. This methodological approach has increased the sensitivity of MRI detection of metastatic involvement of lymph nodes from values as low as 43% to >90%, with specificities approaching 100% *(46, 101)*. An example of metastatic deposit within the axilla of a patient with breast cancer, with histological correlation, is shown in Fig. 7.

In more recent work, semiautomated data analysis routines were instituted *(101)*. This is illustrated in Fig. 8. With this semiautomated approach, the combination of two variables was determined to increase the sensitivity and specificity of lymph node imaging with MNP to 94.3% and 93.5%, respectively, with positive and negative predictive values of 93.5% and 98%.

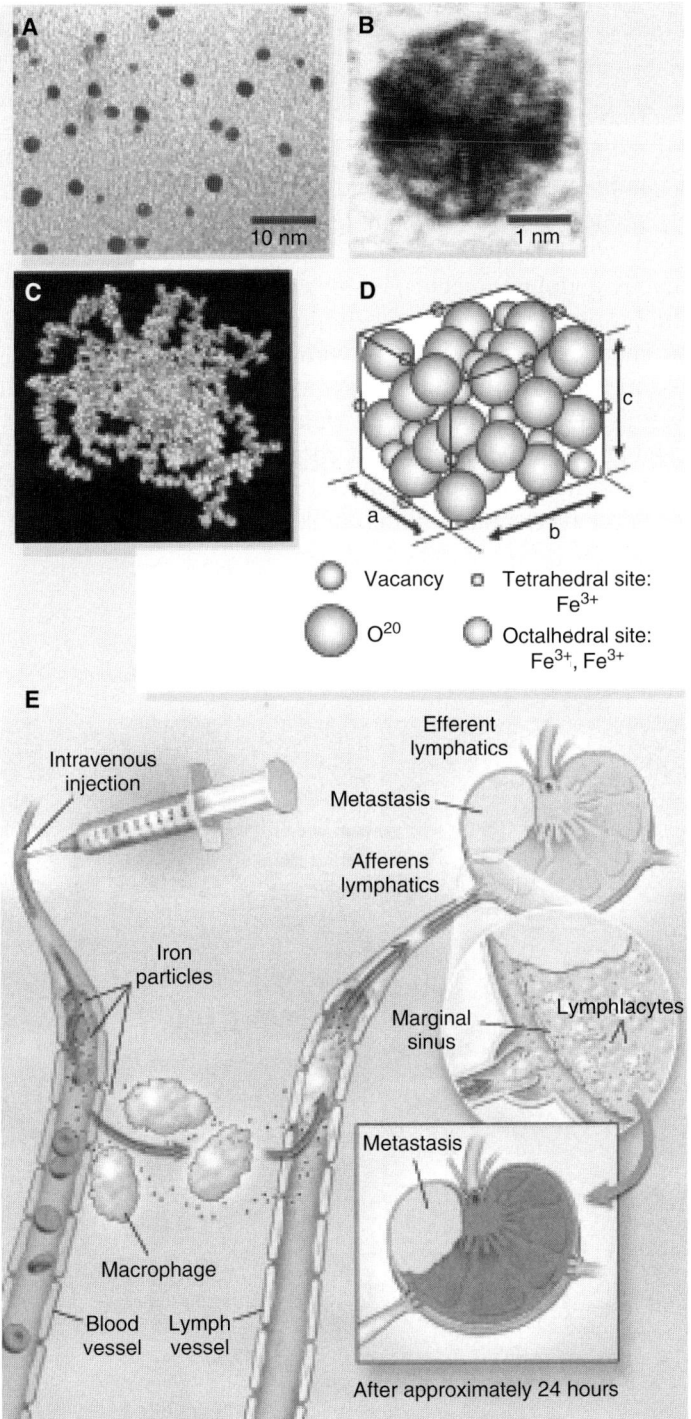

Fig. 6. Electron micrograph of hexagonal lymphotropic superparamagnetic nanoparticles (A and B), molecular model of surface-bound 10-kDa dextrans and packing of iron oxide crystals (C and D), and mechanism of action of lymphotropic superparamagnetic nanoparticles (E). The model lymphotropic superparamagnetic nanoparticles shown here measure 2–3 nm on average (A and B). The mean overall particle size of the 10-kDa dextrans is 28 nm (C and D). In (E), the systemically injected long-circulating particles gain access to the interstitium and are drained through lymphatic vessels. Disturbances in lymph flow or in nodal architecture caused by metastases lead to abnormal patterns of accumulation of lymphotropic superparamagnetic nanoparticles, which are detectable by MRI. [Based on Fig. 1 and reproduced with permission from Harisinghani et al. (46).]

Other lymphotropic MR agents based on gadolinium chelates have been developed. One example is a conjugate of Gd-DTPA to a polyglucose-associated macrocomplex (PGM), which combined the lymphotrophic properties of dextran with the T1 paramagnetic, relaxivity properties of Gd^{3+} *(103, 104)*. A more recent alternative approach to previous lipophilic compounds that form micelles, Gadofluorine 8, called Gadofluorine M, is a macrocyclic gadolinium chelate with a perfluorinated side chain, which results in the formation of micelles in aqueous solution *(102)*. In this study, Misselwitz demonstrated rapid changes in T1 relaxivity within lymph nodes plateauing at approximately 0.5 h within the lymph nodes of rabbits inoculated with VX2 carcinoma cells *(102)*. These results are experimental and were compared to Gadomer-17, an intravenous contrast agent being developed for T1 contrast blood pool imaging, which showed rapid T1 changes within lymph nodes, but did not plateau, and showed more heterogeneous contrast uptake within these lymph nodes *(102)*.

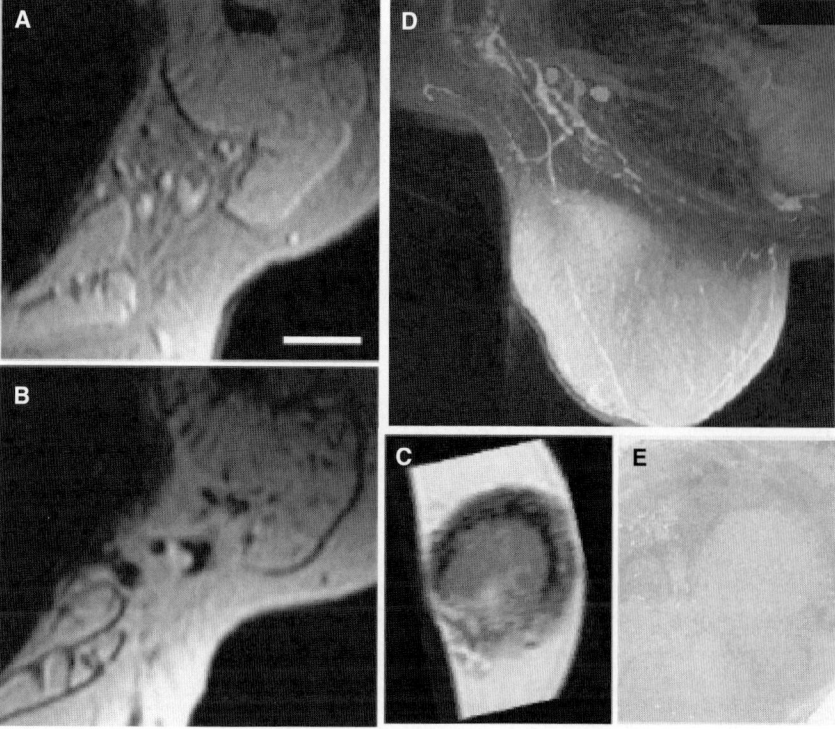

Fig. 7. Patient with breast cancer prior to sentinel lymph node biopsy. Conventional axillary MRI shows nonenlarged lymph nodes that do not meet the size criteria of malignancy (bar = 15 mm) (A). Following intravenous administration of nanoparticles, a single 3-mm intranodal metastasis was correctly identified (B). *Ex vivo* MR imaging of the sentinel node specimen (C) shows excellent correlation with histopathology (E). Semiautomated nodal analysis and reconstruction correctly juxtaposed solitary lymph node metastases adjacent to two normal lymph nodes (D). [Reproduced with permission Harisinghani and Weissleder *(101)*.]

Chapter 14 / MR Probes for Tumor Imaging

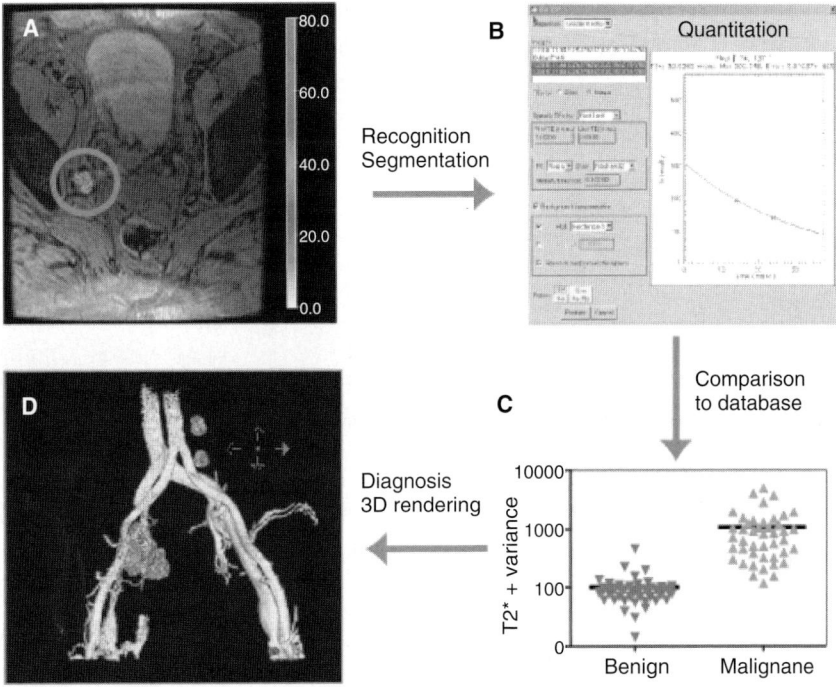

Fig. 8. Semiautomated image analysis involves recognition and automated segmentation of each lymph node (A), quantitation of magnetic tissue parameters (T2*, variance of pixel values) (B), comparison of the extracted tissue parameter with a data base (C), and a three-dimensional reconstruction of nodal anatomy onto vascular anatomy (D). [Reproduced with permission from Harisinghani and Weissleder (101).]

6. IMAGING CELL TRACKING

To track cells *in vivo* and visualize them by MRI, the cells must be tagged magnetically *(106, 107)*. Previous attempts at tagging cells with magnetic beads proved efficient for *in vitro* separation of cells, but because beads were recognized as foreign by macrophages and the reticuloendothelial system, they were rapidly eliminated from the blood when injected intravenously *in vivo (106, 107)*. Labeling lymphocytes with magnetic nanoparticles demonstrates a possible solution to this problem, but the low labeling efficiency exacerbates the inherently low sensitivity of MRI in cell trafficking studies as compared to fluorescence and nuclear medicine *(118–112)*. Unmodified magnetic nanoparticles have been utilized at high concentrations *in vitro* to label monocytes *(6, 113)*, T cells *(6, 114)*, glioma cells and macrophage *(6, 118, 114)*, and oligodendrocyte progenitors *(115)*.

Multiple methodological approaches have been utilized to induce internalization of MNP into nonphagocytic cells *(6)*. Linking amino CLIO to the human immunodeficiency virus (HIV) tat peptide, a membrane translocating signal, results in an MNP with high internalization into hematopoietic and neural progenitor cells (10–30 pg) per cell *(107)*. The same material has also been used to track cytotoxic T cells *(116)* in a B16-OVA melanoma model. High spatial three-dimensional imaging demonstrated the heterogeneity of T cell recruitment within this model (Fig. 9), and more significantly,

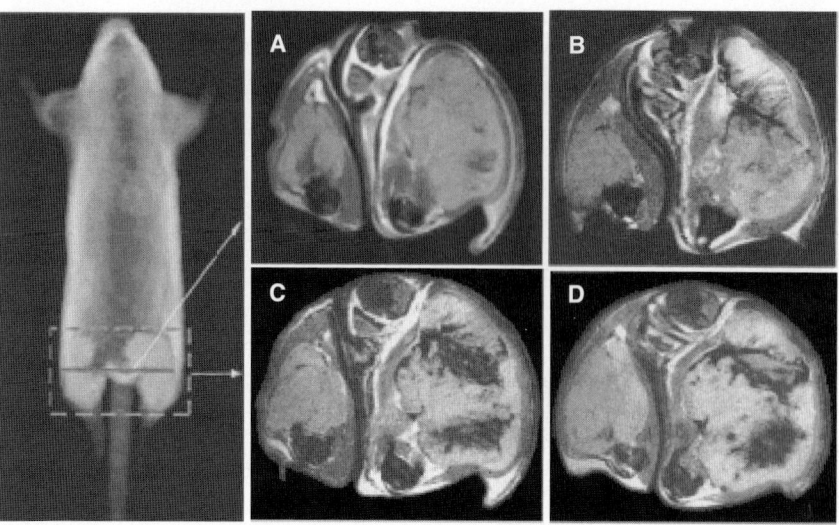

Fig. 9. Time course of CLIO-HD OT-I CD8 T cell homing to B16-OVA tumor. Serial MR imaging was performed after adoptive transfer into a mouse carrying both B16F0 (left) and B16-OVA (right) melanomas. (A–D) Axial slices through the mouse thighs at (A), before adoptive transfer; (B) 12 h; (C) 16 h; (D) 36 h after adoptive transfer of CLIO-HD-labeled OT-I CD8 T cells. Data are representative of eight individual animals. [Reproduced with permission from Kircher *et al.* *(116)*.]

the data indicate that serial administration of $CD8^+$ T cells appears to home to different intratumoral locations, which suggested that dose division may enhance the potency of T-cell based immunopotentiation therapies clinically.

Other approaches that have been utilized for cell labeling include the following: (1) dendritic cells utilizing MD-100, a magnetodendrimer, in a xenograft rat model of small cell lung cancer *(117, 118)*; (2) genetically engineered anti-Her2/neu directed NK cells to Her2/neu-positive mammary tumors implanted in mice *(119)*; and (3) labeled $Sca1^+$ bone marrow cells with superparamagnetic iron oxide MNP (ferumoxides–poly-L-lysine complexes) in glioma-bearing severe combined immunodeficient (SCID) mice *(120)*. In summary, these cell-based approaches offer an exciting potential to advance multiple areas of cell-based therapy including stem cell therapy, cell implantation therapy, and immunopotentiation therapies.

7. TARGETING TUMOR CELLS

The first approaches of molecular-targeted MRI directly linked to Mabs included paramagnetic and superparamagnetic contrast agent approaches. Early paramagnetic approaches to Mab using Gd-DTPA include 9L glioma *(5, 32)*, which showed increased contrast within tumors without conjugated control, and MM-138 melanoma xenografts, which showed retention of contrast at 24 h *(5, 24, 33)*. Conjugating Mab to poly-L-lysine Gd-DTPA *(5, 19)* demonstrated the capability of imaging mucin-like proteins within gastrointestinal carcinomas.

With the advent of ever-improving molecular biologial techniques receptor-targeted gadolinium contrast agents have demonstrated affinity for the folate receptor in folate-expressing ovarian tumor xenografts *(17)*. This contrast agent approach utilized a dendrimer (PAMAM) conjugated to Gd-DTPA. In a similar approach, breast cancer xenografts expressing HER-2/neu receptors were imaged with a two-step labeling protocol using biotinylated Herceptin Mab and avidin-Gd-DTPA conjugates *(5, 24–26)*.

Superparamagnetic iron oxide-based MNPs have also been successfully conjugated to Mab. One approach utilized the HER-2/neu receptor on the surface of malignant breast cancer cells using Herceptin Mab *(25, 26)*. By conjugating MNP to the C2 domain of the protein synaptotagmin, which binds to phosphatidylserine, a protein present on the plasma membrane of apoptotic cells, Zhao *et al* successfully imaged cellular apoptotic events in #L4 solid tumor models exposed to chemotherapy *(121)*.

8. MAGNETIC NANOSENSORS

Nanoparticles of metals and semiconductors have received significant attention in recent years because of their optical, electronic, and magnetic properties, the alteration of which, when coupled to ligands, allows detection of molecular interactions (e.g., DNA–DNA, protein–protein). Very recently, the application of this technology to MRI has demonstrated the production of stable nanoassemblies, which leads to a corresponding decrease in the T2 transverse relaxation of water molecules in the surrounding medium *(61–63, 122, 123)*.

This technology has been utilized to measure multiple different reversible molecular interactions at an extremely low contrast agent concentration (fM). Concentrations as low as 0.5 fM have been observed for DNA and proteins, while targets like viruses, with large, high multivalence, allow for detection of as few as five viral particles per 10 µl of herpes simplex virus-1 and adenovirus-5 *(61–63, 123)*. In a recent study, Perez *et al.* demonstrated a stable nanoassembly of complimentary oligonucleotides that was sensitive to the restriction endonuclease *Bam*H1. Alone, each nanoassembly had a representative T2, but when mixed, they formed a nanoassembly with a measurable difference in T2 relaxivity. This change in T2 relaxivity was specific, however, only in the presence of *Bam*H1, not in the presence of other restriction endonucleases (*Eco*R1, *Hin*dIII, and DPNI) *(62)*. It has also been shown that this is a reversible process, and thus these nanoassemblies can be disassembled and returned to their original dispersed state by methods including heat, enzyme cleavage, pH alteration, and disulfide bond reduction *(61–63, 123)*. This reversibility provides a powerful medium for distinguishing subtle changes in the environment for which they are applied, and have thus been termed magnetic relaxation switches (MRSW) *(61–63, 123)*. Efforts are currently underway to develop implantable sensors capable of measuring local concentrations of chemotherapeutic agents, oxygen, glucose, and tumor markers.

REFERENCES

1. Weinmann H, *et al*. Tissue-specific MR contrast agents. *Eur J Radiol* 2003;46(1):33–44.
2. Aime S, *et al*. Insights into the use of paramagnetic Gd(III) complexes in MR-molecular imaging investigations. *J Magn Reson Imaging* 2002;16(4):394–406.
3. Saeed M, *et al*. Demarcation of myocardial ischemia: Magnetic susceptibility effect of contrast medium in MR imaging. *Radiology* 1989;173(3):763–767.
4. Zhong J, *et al*. Measurements of transient contrast enhancement by localized water NMR spectroscopy. *J Magn Reson B* 1994;104(2):111–118.
5. Artemov D. Molecular magnetic resonance imaging with targeted contrast agents. *J Cell Biochem* 2003;90(3):518–524.

6. Bulte JW, Kraitchman DL. Iron oxide MR contrast agents for molecular and cellular imaging. *NMR Biomed* 2004;17(7):484–499.
7. Weissleder, R, *et al*. Ultrasmall superparamagnetic iron oxide: Characterization of a new class of contrast agents for MR imaging. *Radiology* 1990;175:489–493.
8. Weissleder R. Target-specific superparamagnetic MR contrast agents. *Magn Reson Med* 1991; 22(2):209–212; discussion 213–215.
9. Reimer P, *et al*. Asialoglycoprotein receptor function in benign liver disease: Evaluation with MR imaging. *Radiology* 1991;178(3):769–774.
10. Weissleder R, *et al*. Antimyosin-labeled monocrystalline iron oxide allows detection of myocardial infarct: MR antibody imaging. *Radiology* 1992;182(2):381–385.
11. Kelly KA, *et al*. Detection of vascular adhesion molecule-1 expression using a novel multimodal nanoparticle. *Circ Res* 2005;96(3):327–336.
12. Mulder WJ, *et al*. A liposomal system for contrast-enhanced magnetic resonance imaging of molecular targets. *Bioconjug Chem* 2004;15(4):799–806.
13. Barber PA, *et al*. MR molecular imaging of early endothelial activation in focal ischemia. *Ann Neurol* 2004;56(1):116–120.
14. Bogdanov A Jr, *et al*. Oligomerization of paramagnetic substrates result in signal amplification and can be used for MR imaging of molecular targets. *Mol Imaging* 2002;1(1):16–23.
15. Kang HW, *et al*. Magnetic resonance imaging of inducible E-selectin expression in human endothelial cell culture. *Bioconjug Chem* 2002;13(1):122–127.
16. Kang HW, Weissleder R, Bogdanov A Jr. Targeting of MPEG-protected polyamino acid carrier to human E-selectin in vitro. *Amino Acids* 2002;23(1–3):301–308.
17. Konda SD, *et al*. Specific targeting of folate-dendrimer MRI contrast agents to the high affinity folate receptor expressed in ovarian tumor xenografts. *Magma* 2001;12(2–3):104–113.
18. Flacke S, *et al*. Novel MRI contrast agent for molecular imaging of fibrin: Implications for detecting vulnerable plaques. *Circulation* 2001;104(11):1280–1285.
19. Gohr-Rosenthal S, *et al*. The demonstration of human tumors on nude mice using gadolinium-labelled monoclonal antibodies for magnetic resonance imaging. *Invest Radiol* 1993;28(9): 789–795.
20. Bhujwalla ZM, *et al*. Vascular differences detected by MRI for metastatic versus nonmetastatic breast and prostate cancer xenografts. *Neoplasia* 2001;3(2):143–153.
21. Bhujwalla ZM, *et al*. Reduction of vascular and permeable regions in solid tumors detected by macromolecular contrast magnetic resonance imaging after treatment with antiangiogenic agent TNP-470. *Clin Cancer Res* 2003;9(1):355–362.
22. Schmiedl U, *et al*. Albumin labeled with Gd-DTPA as an intravascular, blood pool-enhancing agent for MR imaging: Biodistribution and imaging studies. *Radiology* 1987;162(1 Pt 1):205–210.
23. Goldenberg DM, *et al*. Radioimmunotherapy: Is avidin-biotin pretargeting the preferred choice among pretargeting methods? *Eur J Nucl Med Mol Imaging* 2003;30(5):777–780.
24. Artemov D, Bhujwalla ZM, Bulte JW. Magnetic resonance imaging of cell surface receptors using targeted contrast agents. *Curr Pharm Biotechnol* 2004;5(6):485–494.
25. Artemov D, *et al*. MR molecular imaging of the Her-2/neu receptor in breast cancer cells using targeted iron oxide nanoparticles. *Magn Reson Med* 2003;49(3):403–408.
26. Artemov D, *et al*. Magnetic resonance molecular imaging of the HER-2/neu receptor. *Cancer Res* 2003;63(11):2723–2727.
27. Bogdanov AA Jr, *et al*. A new macromolecule as a contrast agent for MR angiography: Preparation, properties, and animal studies. *Radiology* 1993;187(3):701–706.
28. Kobayashi H, *et al*. Macromolecular MRI contrast agents with small dendrimers: Pharmacokinetic differences between sizes and cores. *Bioconjug Chem* 2003;14(2):388–394.
29. Bryant LH Jr, *et al*. Synthesis and relaxometry of high-generation (G = 5, 7, 9, and 10) PAMAM dendrimer-DOTA-gadolinium chelates. *J Magn Reson Imaging* 1999;9(2):348–352.
30. Kobayashi H, Brechbiel MW. Dendrimer-based nanosized MRI contrast agents. *Curr Pharm Biotechnol* 2004;5(6):539–549.
31. Kobayashi H, Brechbiel MW. Dendrimer-based macromolecular MRI contrast agents: Characteristics and application. *Mol Imaging* 2003;2(1):1–10.
32. Matsumura A, *et al*. MRI contrast enhancement by Gd-DTPA-monoclonal antibody in 9L glioma rats. *Acta Neurochir Suppl (Wien)* 1994;60:356–358.

33. Shahbazi-Gahrouei D, et al. In vivo studies of Gd-DTPA-monoclonal antibody and Gd-porphyrins: Potential magnetic resonance imaging contrast agents for melanoma. *J Magn Reson Imaging* 2001;14(2):169–174.
34. Sipkins DA, et al. Detection of tumor angiogenesis in vivo by alphaVbeta3-targeted magnetic resonance imaging. *Nat Med* 1998;4(5):623–626.
35. Louie AY, et al. In vivo visualization of gene expression using magnetic resonance imaging. *Nat Biotechnol* 2000;18(3):321–325.
36. Shen T, et al. Monocrystalline iron oxide nanocompounds (MION): Physicochemical properties. *Magn Reson Med* 1993;29(5):599–604.
37. Weissleder R, et al. Ultrasmall superparamagnetic iron oxide: An intravenous contrast agent for assessing lymph nodes with MR imaging. *Radiology* 1990;175(2):494–498.
38. Weissleder R, et al. Ultrasmall superparamagnetic iron oxide: Characterization of a new class of contrast agents for MR imaging. *Radiology* 1990;175(2):489–493.
39. Callender ST, Weatherall DJ. Iron chelation with oral desferrioxamine. *Lancet* 1980;2(8196):689.
40. Callender ST. Treatment of iron deficiency. *Clin Haematol* 1982;11(2):327–338.
41. Saini S, et al. Multicentre dose-ranging study on the efficacy of USPIO ferumoxtran-10 for liver MR imaging. *Clin Radiol* 2000;55(9):690–695.
42. Reimer P, et al. Hepatic lesion detection and characterization: Value of nonenhanced MR imaging, superparamagnetic iron oxide-enhanced MR imaging, and spiral CT-ROC analysis. *Radiology* 2000;217(1):152–158.
43. Weissleder H, Weissleder R. Interstitial lymphangiography: Initial clinical experience with a dimeric nonionic contrast agent. *Radiology* 1989;170(2):371–374.
44. Weissleder R, et al. Experimental lymph node metastases: Enhanced detection with MR lymphography. *Radiology* 1989;171(3):835–839.
45. Reimer P, Bader A, Weissleder R. Preclinical assessment of hepatocyte-targeted MR contrast agents in stable human liver cell cultures. *J Magn Reson Imaging* 1998;8(3):687–689.
46. Harisinghani M, et al. Noninvasive detection of clinically occult lymph-node metastases in prostate cancer. *N Engl J Med* 2003;348(25):2491–2499; erratum in: 2003;349(10):1010.
47. Harisinghani M, et al. MR imaging of lymph nodes in patients with primary abdominal and pelvic malignancies using ultrasmall superparamagnetic iron oxide (Combidex). *Acad Radiol* 1998;(Suppl 1):S167–169; discussion S183–184.
48. Harisinghani M, et al. MR imaging of pelvic lymph nodes in primary pelvic cancer with USPIO (Combidex). In 1997 Contrast Medical Research Conference. Kyoto, Japan: Academic Radiology.
49. Harisinghani M, et al. MR imaging of pelvic lymph nodes in primary pelvic carcinoma with ultrasmall superparamagnetic iron oxide (Combidex): Preliminary observatinons. *J Magn Reson Imaging* 1997;7:161–163.
50. Bulte JW, et al. Preparation of magnetically labeled cells for cell tracking by magnetic resonance imaging. *Methods Enzymol* 2004;386:275–299.
51. Kohler N, Fryxell GE, Zhang M. A bifunctional poly(ethylene glycol) silane immobilized on metallic oxide-based nanoparticles for conjugation with cell targeting agents. *J Am Chem Soc* 2004;126(23):7206–7211.
52. Molday RS, MacKenzie D. Immunospecific ferromagnetic iron-dextran reagents for the labeling and magnetic separation of cells. *J Immunol Methods* 1982;52(3):353–367.
53. Wunderbaldinger P, Josephson L, Weissleder R. Crosslinked iron oxides (CLIO): A new platform for the development of targeted MR contrast agents. *Acad Radiol* 2002;9(Suppl 2):S304–306.
54. Renshaw PF, et al. Immunospecific NMR contrast agents. *Magn Reson Imaging* 1986;4(4):351–357.
55. Jung HI, et al. Detection of apoptosis using the C2A domain of synaptotagmin I. *Bioconjug Chem* 2004;15(5):983–987.
56. Josephson L, Groman E, Weissleder R. Contrast agents for magnetic resonance imaging of the liver. *Targeted Diagn Ther* 1991;4:163–187.
57. Moore A, et al. In vivo targeting of underglycosylated MUC-1 tumor antigen using a multimodal imaging probe. *Cancer Res* 2004;64(5):1821–1827.
58. Schellenberger EA, et al. Annexin V-CLIO: A nanoparticle for detecting apoptosis by MRI. *Mol Imaging* 2002;1(2):102–107.

59. Weissleder R, et al. In vivo magnetic resonance imaging of transgene expression. *Nat Med* 2000;6(3):351–355.
60. Zhao M, et al. Differential conjugation of tat peptide to superparamagnetic nanoparticles and its effect on cellular uptake. *Bioconjug Chem* 2002;13(4):840–844.
61. Perez JM, et al. Magnetic relaxation switches capable of sensing molecular interactions. *Nat Biotechnol* 2002;20(8):816–820.
62. Perez JM, Josephson L, Weissleder R. Use of magnetic nanoparticles as nanosensors to probe for molecular interactions. *Chembiochem* 2004;5(3):261–264.
63. Perez JM, et al. DNA-based magnetic nanoparticle assembly acts as a magnetic relaxation nanoswitch allowing screening of DNA-cleaving agents. *J Am Chem Soc* 2002;124(12):2856–2857.
64. Tofts PS, et al. Estimating kinetic parameters from dynamic contrast-enhanced T(1)-weighted MRI of a diffusable tracer: Standardized quantities and symbols. *J Magn Reson Imaging* 1999;10(3):223–232.
65. Hulka C, et al. Dynamic echo-planar imaging of the breast: Experience in diagnosing breast carcinoma and correlation with tumor angiogenesis. *Radiology* 1997;205:837–842.
66. Hulka C, Smith B, Sgroi D. Benign and malignant breast lesions: Differentiation with echo-planar MR imaging. *Radiology* 1995;197:33–38.
67. Rosen B., et al. Perfusion imaging and NMR contrast agents. *Magn Reson Med* 1990;14(2):249–265.
68. Kety SS. Determinants of tissue oxygen tension. *Fed Proc* 1957;16(3):666–671.
69. Knopp MV, et al. Pathophysiologic basis of contrast enhancement in breast tumors. *J Magn Reson Imaging* 1999;10(3):260–266.
70. Pham CD, et al. Magnetic resonance imaging detects suppression of tumor vascular permeability after administration of antibody to vascular endothelial growth factor. *Cancer Invest* 1998;16(4):225–230.
71. Morgan B, et al. Dynamic contrast-enhanced magnetic resonance imaging as a biomarker for the pharmacological response of PTK787/ZK 222584, an inhibitor of the vascular endothelial growth factor receptor tyrosine kinases, in patients with advanced colorectal cancer and liver metastases: Results from two phase I studies. *J Clin Oncol* 2003;21(21):3955–3964.
72. Piccoli CW. Contrast-enhanced breast MRI: Factors affecting sensitivity and specificity. *Eur Radiol* 1997;7(Suppl 5):281–288.
73. Su M, et al. Correlation of dynamic contrast enhancement MRI parameters with microvessel density and VEGF for assessment of angiogenesis in a breast cancer. *J Magn Reson Imaging* 2003;18:467–477.
74. Dadiani M, et al. High-resolution magnetic resonance imaging of disparities in the transcapillary transfer rates in orthotopically inoculated invasive breast tumors. *Cancer Res* 2004;64(9):3155–3161.
75. Port RE, et al. Multicompartment analysis of gadolinium chelate kinetics: Blood-tissue exchange in mammary tumors as monitored by dynamic MR imaging. *J Magn Reson Imaging* 1999;10(3):233–241.
76. Turetschek K, et al. MR imaging characterization of microvessels in experimental breast tumors by using a particulate contrast agent with histopathologic correlation. *Radiology* 2001;218:562–569.
77. Turetschek K, et al. MRI monitoring of tumor response following angiogenesis inhibition in an experimental human breast cancer model. *Eur J Nucl Med Mol Imaging* 2002;30(3):448–455.
78. Turetschek K, et al. MRI monitoring of tumor response to a novel VEGF tyrosine kinase inhibitor in an experimental breast cancer model. *Acad Radiol* 2002;9(Suppl 2):S519–20.
79. Turetschek K, et al. Tumor microvascular characterization using ultrasmall superparamagnetic iron oxide particles (USPIO) in an experimental breast cancer model. *J Magn Reson Imaging* 2001;13:882–888.
80. Rydland J, et al. New intravascular contrast agent applied to dynamic contrast enhanced MR imaging of human breast cancer. *Acta Radiol* 2003;44:275–283.
81. Turetschek K, et al. Tumor microvascular changes in antiangiogenic treatment: Assessment by magnetic resonance contrast media of different molecular weights. *J Magn Reson Imaging* 2004;20(1):138–144.
82. Schmiedl U, et al. Comparison of initial biodistribution patterns of Gd-DTPA and albumin-(Gd-DTPA) using rapid spin echo MR imaging. *J Comput Assist Tomogr* 1987;11(2):306–313.

83. Boxerman J. et al. MR contrast due to intravascular magnetic susceptibility perturbations. *Magn Reson Med* 1995;34:555–566.
84. Dennie J, et al. NMR imaging of changes in vascular morphology due to tumor angiogenesis. *Magn Reson Med* 1998;40:793–799.
85. Bremer C, et al. Steady-state blood volume measurements in experimental tumors with different angiogenic burdens–a study in mice. *Radiology* 2003;226(1):214–220.
86. Tropres I, et al. Vessel size imaging. *Magn Reson Med* 2001;45:397–408.
87. Callahan RJ, et al. Preclinical evaluation and phase I clinical trial of a 99mTc-labeled synthetic polymer used in blood pool imaging. *AJR Am J Roentgenol* 1998;171(1):137–143.
88. Bogdanov AA, Lewin M, Weissleder R. Approaches and agents for imaging the vascular system. *Adv Drug Deliv Rev* 1999;37(1–3):279–293.
89. Pasqualini R, Koivunen E, Ruoslahti E. Alpha v integrins as receptors for tumor targeting by circulating ligands. *Nat Biotechnol* 1997;15(6):542–546.
90. Falcioni R, et al. Alpha 6 beta 4 and alpha 6 beta 1 integrins associate with ErbB-2 in human carcinoma cell lines. *Exp Cell Res* 1997;236(1):76–85.
91. Cheresh DA, et al. An Arg-Gly-Asp-directed receptor on the surface of human melanoma cells exists in an divalent cation-dependent functional complex with the disialoganglioside GD2. *J Cell Biol* 1987;105(3):1163–1173.
92. Brooks PC, Clark RA, Cheresh DA. Requirement of vascular integrin alpha v beta 3 for angiogenesis. *Science* 1994;264(5158):569–571.
93. Schmieder AH, et al. Molecular MR imaging of melanoma angiogenesis with alpha(nu)beta(3)-targeted paramagnetic nanoparticles. *Magn Reson Med* 2005;53(3):621–627.
94. Anderson SA, et al. Magnetic resonance contrast enhancement of neovasculature with alpha(v)beta(3)-targeted nanoparticles. *Magn Reson Med* 2000;44(3):433–439.
95. Winter PM, et al. Molecular imaging of angiogenesis in nascent Vx-2 rabbit tumors using a novel alpha(nu)beta3-targeted nanoparticle and 1.5 tesla magnetic resonance imaging. *Cancer Res* 2003;63(18):5838–5843.
96. Montet X, Funovics M, Montet-Abou K, Weissleder R, Josephson L. Multivalent effects of RGD peptides obtained by nanoparticle display. *J Med Chem* 2006;49:6087–6093.
97. Siegel BM, Mayzel KA, Love SM. Level I and II axillary dissection in the treatment of early-stage breast cancer. An analysis of 259 consecutive patients. *Arch Surg* 1990;125(9):1144–1147.
98. Senofsky GM, et al. Total axillary lymphadenectomy in the management of breast cancer. *Arch Surg* 1991;126(11):1336–41; discussion 1341–1342.
99. Stets C, et al. Axillary lymph node metastases: A statistical analysis of various parameters in MRI with USPIO. *J Magn Reson Imaging* 2002;16:60–68.
100. Weissleder R, et al. Ultrasmall superparamagnetic iron oxide: An intravenous contrast agent for assessing lymph nodes with MR imaging. *Radiology* 1990;175:494–498.
101. Harisinghani MG, Weissleder R. Sensitive, noninvasive detection of lymph node metastases. *PLoS Med* 2004;1(3):e66.
102. Misselwitz B, Platzek J, Weinmann HJ. Early MR lymphography with gadofluorine M in rabbits. *Radiology* 2004;231(3):682–688.
103. Harika L, et al. Macromolecular intravenous contrast agent for MR lymphography: Characterization and efficacy studies. *Radiology* 1996;198(2):365–370.
104. Harika L, et al. MR lymphography with a lymphotropic T1-type MR contrast agent: Gd-DTPA-PGM. *Magn Reson Med* 1995;33(1):88–92.
105. Wunderbaldinger P, et al. Detection of lymph node metastases by contrast-enhanced MRI in an experimental model. *Magn Reson Med* 2002;47(2):292–297.
106. Safarik I, Safarikova M. Use of magnetic techniques for the isolation of cells. *J Chromatogr B Biomed Sci Appl* 1999;722(1–2):33–53.
107. Lewin M, et al. Tat peptide-derivatized magnetic nanoparticles allow in vivo tracking and recovery of progenitor cells. *Nat Biotechnol* 2000;18(4):410–414.
108. Weissleder R, et al. Magnetically labeled cells can be detected by MR imaging. *J Magn Reson Imaging* 1997;7(1):258–263.
109. Schoepf U, et al. Intracellular magnetic labeling of lymphocytes for in vivo trafficking studies. *Biotechniques* 1998;24(4):642–646, 648–651.
110. Hawrylak N, et al. Nuclear magnetic resonance (NMR) imaging of iron oxide-labeled neural transplants. *Exp Neurol* 1993;121(2):181–192.

111. Bulte JW, et al. Neurotransplantation of magnetically labeled oligodendrocyte progenitors: Magnetic resonance tracking of cell migration and myelination. *Proc Natl Acad Sci USA* 1999; 96(26):15256–15261.
112. Lewin M, et al. In vivo assessment of vascular endothelial growth factor-induced angiogenesis. *Int J Cancer* 1999;83(6):798–802.
113. Zelivyanskaya ML, et al. Tracking superparamagnetic iron oxide labeled monocytes in brain by high-field magnetic resonance imaging. *J Neurosci Res* 2003;73(3):284–295.
114. Moore A, Weissleder R, Bogdanov A Jr. Uptake of dextran-coated monocrystalline iron oxides in tumor cells and macrophages. *J Magn Reson Imaging* 1997;7(6):1140–1145.
115. Franklin RJ, et al. Magnetic resonance imaging of transplanted oligodendrocyte precursors in the rat brain. *Neuroreport* 1999;10(18):3961–3965.
116. Kircher MF, et al. In vivo high resolution three-dimensional imaging of antigen-specific cytotoxic T-lymphocyte trafficking to tumors. *Cancer Res* 2003;63(20):6838–6846.
117. Bulte JW, et al. Magnetodendrimers allow endosomal magnetic labeling and in vivo tracking of stem cells. *Nat Biotechnol* 2001;19(12):1141–1147.
118. Bulte JW, Duncan ID, Frank JA. In vivo magnetic resonance tracking of magnetically labeled cells after transplantation. *J Cereb Blood Flow Metab* 2002;22(8):899–907.
119. Daldrup-Link HE, et al. In vivo tracking of genetically engineered, anti-HER2/neu directed natural killer cells to HER2/neu positive mammary tumors with magnetic resonance imaging. *Eur Radiol* 2005;15(1):4–13.
120. Anderson SA, et al. Noninvasive MR imaging of magnetically labeled stem cells to directly identify neovasculature in a glioma model. *Blood* 2005;105(1):420–425.
121. Zhao M, et al. Non-invasive detection of apoptosis using magnetic resonance imaging and a targeted contrast agent. *Nat Med* 2001;7(11):1241–1244.
122. Josephson L, et al. High-efficiency intracellular magnetic labeling with novel superparamagnetic-Tat peptide conjugates. *Bioconjug Chem* 1999;10(2):186–191.
123. Perez JM, et al. Viral-induced self-assembly of magnetic nanoparticles allows the detection of viral particles in biological media. *J Am Chem Soc* 2003;125(34):10192–10193.
124. Hogemann D, Basilion JP. "Seeing inside the body": MR imaging of gene expression. *Eur J Nucl Med Mol Imaging* 2002;29(3):400–408.
125. Tempany CM, McNeil BJ. Advances in biomedical imaging. *JAMA* 2001;285(5):562–567.

15 Fluorescent Imaging of Tumors

Kamiar Moin, PhD, Oliver J. McIntyre, PhD, Lynn M. Matrisian, PhD, and Bonnie F. Sloane, PhD

CONTENTS

INTRODUCTION
OPTICAL IMAGING AND ITS APPLICATIONS IN CANCER
  DIAGNOSIS AND THERAPY
SYSTEM DEVELOPMENT FOR *IN VIVO* OPTICAL IMAGING
CLINICAL IMPLICATIONS: ADVANTAGES AND LIMITATIONS
CONCLUSIONS AND FUTURE PROSPECTS

1. INTRODUCTION

One of the most difficult obstacles to early treatment of cancer is lack of sound methodologies for detection of the disease. By the time cancer is detected it has frequently progressed to the metastatic state. Because of this, the normal course of treatment, in addition to surgery, often consists of aggressive chemotherapy, radiation therapy, or both with potential for undesirable side effects *(1–6)*.

Traditionally, the difficulty in early detection of cancer has been a lack of specificity as well as sensitivity of current diagnostic imaging methods. Although various forms of noninvasive diagnostic imaging have been in clinical use for sometime, e.g., magnetic resonance imaging (MRI) and positron emission tomography (PET) (see Chapters 3–5 in this volume), they are not selective for cancer. In addition, the resolution of these modalities is at the millimeter level at best with poor contrast for imaging cancers. Optical imaging, on the other hand, is emerging as a promising high-resolution modality for cancer imaging in both diagnostic and therapeutic arenas. Recent advances in optical imaging, and in fluorescent imaging in particular, have made it possible to develop more sensitive imaging tools and protocols with increased selectivity for cancer diagnosis *(7–10)*. In this chapter we will discuss the benefits and advantages of optical imaging as well as some of the drawbacks as they apply to cancer diagnosis and therapy.

From: *Cancer Drug Discovery and Development
In Vivo Imaging of Cancer Therapy*
Edited by: A.F. Shields and P. Price © Humana Press Inc., Totowa, NJ

1.1 The Process of Tumor Progression

To develop strategies and mechanisms leading to improved imaging techniques, instrumentation, and protocols directed toward cancer diagnosis and therapy, it is critical to have a clear understanding of the process of tumor progression (development, invasion, and metastasis). As illustrated in Fig. 1, this is a multistage process that is highly controlled and regulated *(11–13)*. Briefly, after the onset of tumorigenesis, the newly transformed cell will divide for several generations to form the primary tumor. This results in adjacent epithelial/mesenchymal transitions that in turn lead to angiogenesis (to support tumor metabolism) and local invasion. Some of the cells from the primary tumor may then intravasate into the bloodstream, and/or the lymphatics, where they migrate to distant sites and then extravasate into the surrounding tissues and develop into metastatic foci.

All of these events are usually marked by specific changes, either in the tumor cell or the tumor cell microenvironment *(12)*, which may be measured and therefore targeted for diagnosis or therapeutic intervention. For example, there is a large body of work that has shown that the expression profile of proteolytic enzymes is altered in tumors *(14–16)*, suggesting a role for proteolysis in tumor progression. One hypothesis is that these enzymes are involved in the dissolution of the basement membrane aiding in the process of invasion [for review, see *(14)*]. Other proteins such as the markers for angiogenesis have also been implicated in this process *(13, 17–21)*. These events and alterations have been utilized by a number of investigators as targets for imaging of tumor progression in living systems *(22–25)*.

1.2 The Need for Noninvasive Imaging

The urgency for development of noninvasive methods for cancer diagnosis and evaluation of therapeutic efficacy (prognostic measures) is rather obvious. To date one of the few clinically accepted noninvasive measures that is somewhat predictive of the disease state is prostate specific antigen (PSA) titration for prostate cancer *(26–28)*. Predictive markers for other cancers are less satisfactory. Therefore, various imaging modalities may provide a viable alternative approach for early detection of the disease as well as therapeutic follow-up.

As mentioned above, options for noninvasive imaging modalities with the desired sensitivity and resolution are very limited. In addition to MRI and PET (see Chapters 3–5), X-ray imaging, particularly mammography, is a frequently utilized technique. Even though mammography is a well-accepted imaging practice for early detection of breast cancers, it is far from perfect. It lacks specificity, it is often painful (the breast needs to be flattened under extreme pressure to obtain clear images), and a biopsy and/or ultrasound follow-up are needed if an anomaly is found. Ultrasound is yet another frequently used imaging technique. However, it also suffers from lack of specificity and limited resolution.

Recent advances in optical imaging offer new opportunities and have generated tremendous interest for further development in the field. New model systems, probes (contrast agents), imaging devices, and methodologies for *in vivo* optical imaging are being developed at an accelerated rate. Although the application of optical imaging to cancer diagnostics and therapeutic strategies in the clinic will be somewhat limited, it may prove to be an invaluable tool for certain types of cancer (see below).

Chapter 15 / Fluorescent Imaging of Tumors

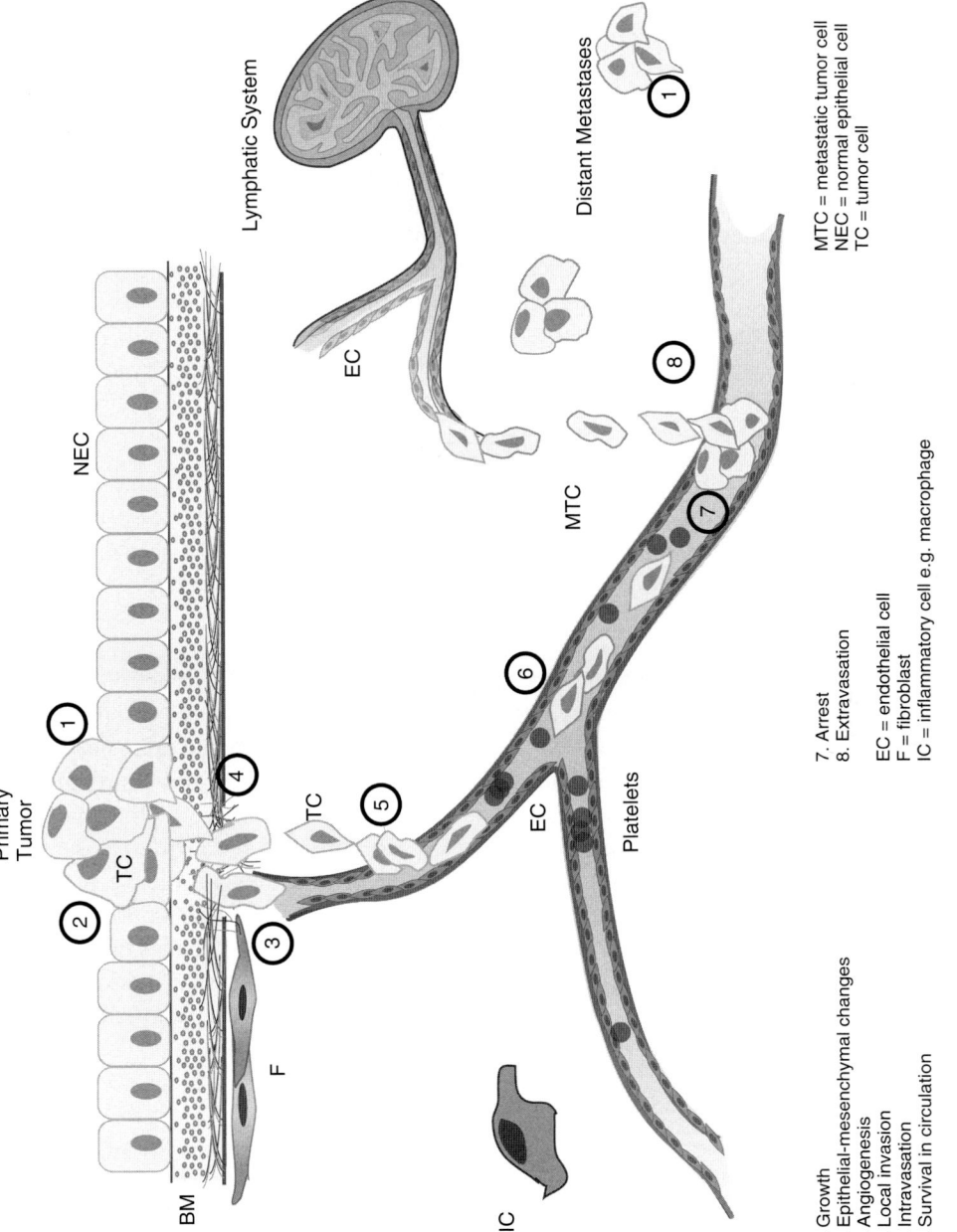

Fig. 1. Schematic representation of the process of tumor progression and metastasis.

1. Growth
2. Epithelial-mesenchymal changes
3. Angiogenesis
4. Local invasion
5. Intravasation
6. Survival in circulation
7. Arrest
8. Extravasation

EC = endothelial cell
F = fibroblast
IC = inflammatory cell e.g. macrophage

MTC = metastatic tumor cell
NEC = normal epithelial cell
TC = tumor cell

2. OPTICAL IMAGING AND ITS APPLICATIONS IN CANCER DIAGNOSIS AND THERAPY

Optical imaging techniques are methods in which electromagnetic radiation, i.e., light, is used to image an object. Any wavelength of light throughout the electromagnetic spectrum, from ultraviolet to near infrared, can be and has been utilized for this purpose. Until recently, optical imaging techniques have been limited to microscopic evaluations of fixed specimens for diagnostic and research purposes with almost no direct involvement in therapeutic evaluations. Recent breakthroughs in optical imaging have revolutionized the utility of these techniques for both research and clinical use *(7–10)*. This is of particular significance with respect to noninvasive imaging. In general, optical imaging is divided into three main categories: transmitted light, bioluminescence, and fluorescence. In this chapter only the latter two will be discussed.

Both bioluminescence and fluorescence involve the detection of emitted light from specimens. Sophisticated and highly sensitive imaging devices need to be designed and manufactured for the detection of the emitted light. Model systems will need to be developed and specific probes synthesized and tested in those model systems before they can be applied in the clinic.

2.1 Bioluminescence

Bioluminescence is the generation of light ($h\nu$) as the result of the enzymatic cleavage, in the presence of oxygen, of the substrate luciferin as shown in the following equation where P* is the electronically excited product *(29)*:

$$\text{Luciferin} \xrightarrow{\text{Luciferase} + O_2} P^* \rightarrow P + h\nu$$

As indicated in the above equation, the enzyme responsible for this reaction is luciferase. Luciferase is a designation given to a class of enzymes that is present in many organisms spanning a number of phylogenic kingdoms. These include, but are not limited to, protists, fungi, insects, bacteria, as well as some corals and chordates *(29)*. Luciferase from each phylogenic classification is a protein unique to that particular phylum. In fact, there is no homology between luciferases from different organisms *(30)*. Nonetheless, they are all functionally similar in that they all cleave a class of substrates known as luciferins, resulting in light emission that can be detected and quantified *(29, 30)*. Advances in molecular cloning in the past few decades have resulted in development of luciferase expression systems as a valid molecular marker for biological imaging *(31)*. The most common varieties of luciferase-luciferin currently utilized are the firefly, *Photinus* and *Luciona* sp., systems *(31)*.

2.1.1 DEVELOPMENT OF MODEL SYSTEMS

The models that have been developed to take advantage of the utility of luciferase are all expression systems in which luciferase expressed in cells functions as a reporter *(31, 32)*. There are generally two types of model systems in which luciferase is utilized. In one system, luciferase is expressed by itself, serving as a general reporter to detect a particular cell type (Fig. 2; *33–37)*. In the other, luciferase is expressed as a fusion pair with another protein *(38–41)*. In this case, light emission by the luciferase-luciferin reaction is utilized to study a specific gene of interest. Because luciferase is a xenogene,

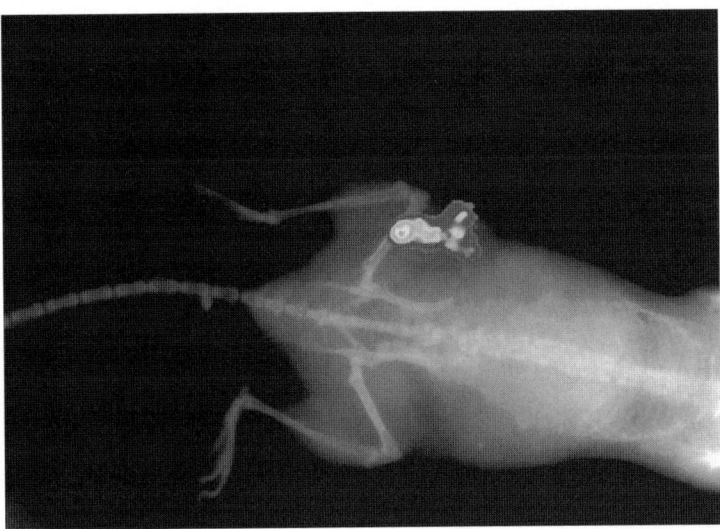

Fig. 2. *In vivo* multimodal bioluminescent and X-ray imaging of prostate cancer. LNCaP prostate cancer cells transfected with the firefly luciferase were injected into SCID mouse subcutaneously. Subsequent to tumor development the mice were injected with luciferin and imaged with an IS4000MM™ multimodal imager (Kodak, New Haven, CT). The bioluminescent tumor is clearly visible against the anatomic X-ray background. Tumor areas with high to low luciferase expression are indicated.

it cannot be used clinically. Luciferase can, however, be an invaluable tool in preclinical studies for the development and validation of therapeutic agents in cell culture as well as animal models *(36, 42, 43)*. For example, Shah and colleagues have developed a mouse model system to study tumor regression through specialized cellular targeting *(42)*. In this model neuronal precursor cells (NPCs) expressing both luciferase and S-TRAIL (secreted tumor necrosis factor related apoptosis-inducing ligand) are injected into mice bearing gliomas *(42)*. The NPCs expressing S-TRAIL are capable of tracking, finding, and killing glioma cells *(42)*. These investigators were able to track the migration of the NPCs and record the destruction of the tumor *in vivo* in real time by taking advantage of bioluminescent imaging *(42)*.

2.1.2 Development of Probes

In optical imaging, as in the other imaging modalities, probes are substances that provide some kind of contrast in an entity to be imaged. In bioluminescence as applied here, the contrast is provided by the action of a foreign gene product on a substrate, resulting in the generation of light that is then detected (see above). Therefore, generation of bioluminescent "probes" is essentially a two-stage process. First is the construction and expression of the luciferase gene in the target cell (either as a fusion product with another protein or by itself as a cellular identifier). The second is the introduction of luciferin as the target substrate for luciferase. In recent years numerous cell lines expressing luciferase, as well as luciferase fusion products, have been developed for *in vivo* bioluminescent imaging *(31)*.

2.1.3 Application to *In Vivo* Imaging

Luciferase can be utilized in small animals to study mechanisms of tumor progression *in vivo*, as shown in Fig. 2, and to measure therapeutic efficacy of drugs *in vivo* and therefore contribute to drug development *(31)*.

2.2 Fluorescent Imaging

Fluorescence is a two-stage phenomenon in which a fluorescent molecule (fluorophore) is first excited with high-energy (short wavelength) photons. Subsequently, as the excited state of the molecule decays to the ground state, it can fluoresce (emit light) at a longer wavelength (Fig. 3; *44*). The most significant advantage of fluorescence is its high sensitivity and high resolution, subcellular and even down to the level of single molecules *(45)*. In fluorescent imaging the target is labeled with a fluorophore and then observed with a device capable of detecting the fluorescence. Until recently fluorescent imaging was limited to fluorescent microscopy and gel electrophoresis. The latter is

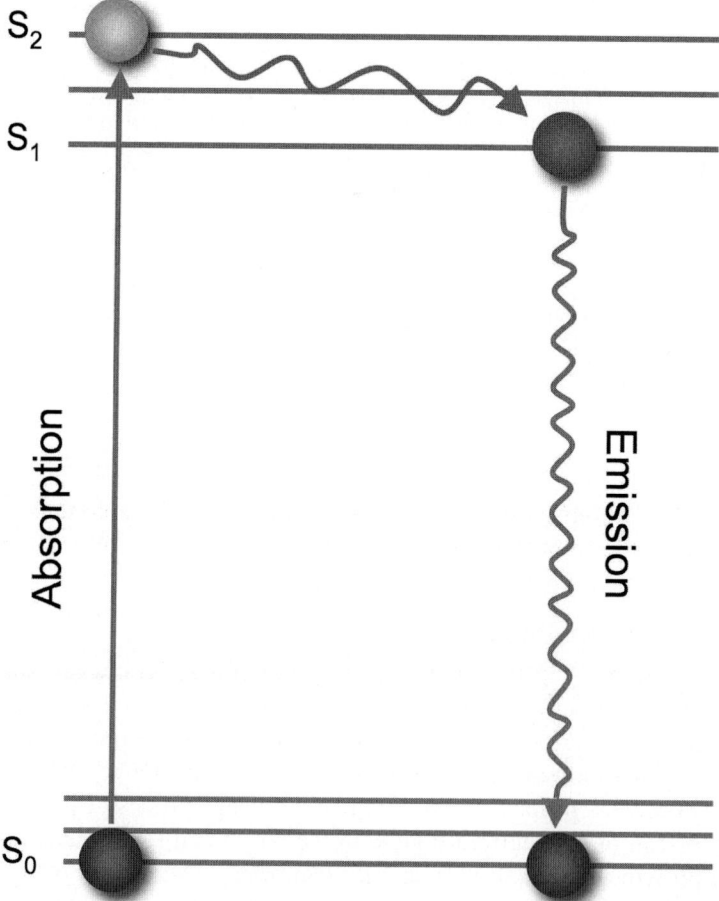

Fig. 3. Jablonski diagram illustrating the process of fluorescent excitation and emission. S_0, the ground state; S_1 and S_2, electronically excited states. S_2 represent the state of partial energy dissipation from S_1 before the onset of emission.

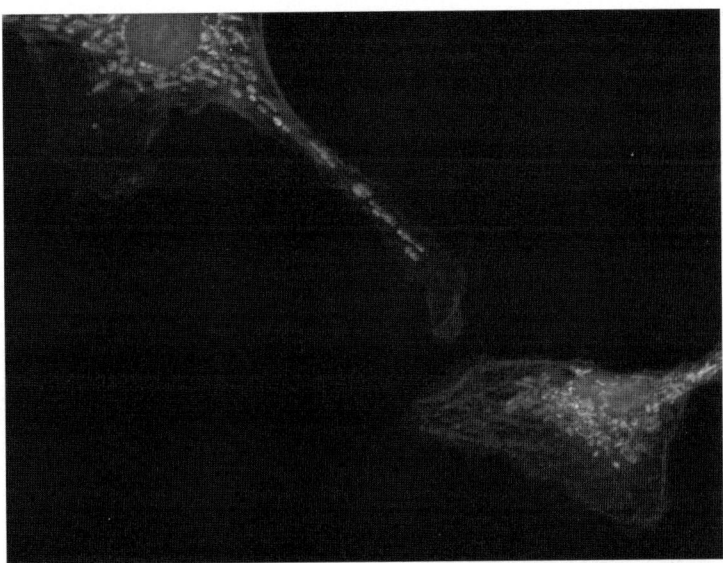

Fig. 4. Bovine pulmonary artery endothelial cells stained with DAPI and MitoTracker Red, illustrating the nuclei and the mitochondria. Magnification, 630×. (*See* color plate.)

beyond the scope of this chapter and therefore will not be discussed further. Since almost all of the methodologies for any fluorescent imaging are based on the techniques developed for fluorescent microscopy, a brief discussion is warranted.

In early fluorescent microscopy the target was labeled with a free dye that showed affinity for specific cellular organelles. For example, one of the earliest fluorescent dyes to be used is Acridine Orange (excitation at 502 nm, with emission at >600 nm). It was utilized as a marker for lysosomes because of its accumulation in vesicles with acidic pH as well as in mitochondrion *(46)*. Other dyes such as 4′-6-diamidino-2-phenylindole (DAPI, excitation at 350 nm, with emission at 450 nm) and chloromethyl-X-rosamine (MitoTracker Red, excitation at 568 nm and emission at 665 nm) are used routinely to stain nuclei and mitochondria, respectively (Fig. 4). DAPI has an affinity for DNA and MitoTracker Red will bind to the inner membranes of mitochondria *(47, 48)*.

The next step in the evolution of fluorescent imaging was the targeting of specific protein molecules to observe cellular events. Antibodies have been the most common targeting agents and are routinely utilized to image other proteins. In this technique, an antibody against a protein is conjugated to a fluorophore and the conjugate is then utilized to target and image the protein of interest (Fig. 5). The main drawback with antibody staining has been the fact that the staining is normally done on fixed specimens, or frozen sections that are subsequently fixed and mounted. Therefore, observations are static rather than dynamic.

The discovery of the green fluorescent protein (GFP) from the jellyfish *Aequoria victoria (49)* and its subsequent cloning *(50)* have revolutionized fluorescent imaging, opening new avenues into imaging of living systems *(51)*. Like luciferase, GFP is expressed in living cells either as a tracker to identify the transfected cells or as a fusion product with other proteins to serve as a marker for those proteins. Unlike luciferase, GFP's fluorescent properties require excitation with blue light to be detected *(49)*.

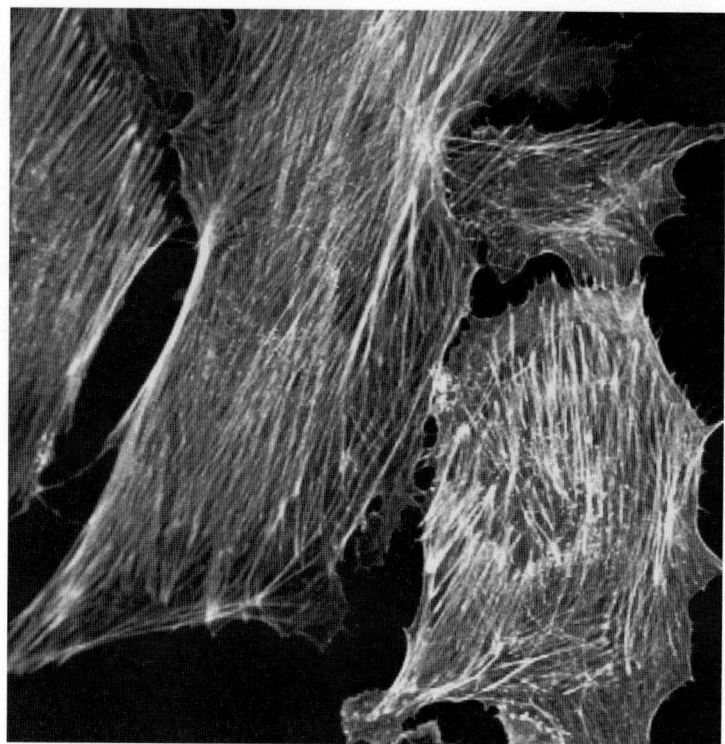

Fig. 5. An example of immunocytochemical/immunohistochemical staining of bovine pulmonary artery endothelial cells with monoclonal antibody against bovine tubulin as the primary antibody. Goat anti-mouse IgG conjugated to BODIPY was used as the secondary antibody. The nuclei were stained with DAPI. Magnification, 630×. (*See* color plate.)

Various GFP mutants and other fluorescent proteins such as DsRed from *Discosoma* coral and its mutants *(52, 53)* are now available.

Another key development in the optical field has been the availability of synthetic substrates for proteolytic enzymes that can be used in living systems as markers for functional imaging. These are normally quenched. Upon activation by the enzyme, the fluorescence is released and detected. Early attempts to define the protease activity in tumors and other tissues, such as those pioneered by R.E. Smith, used histochemical techniques *(54)*. His protease probes were designed primarily to assess the activities of lysosomal proteases. In this technique cryostat sections of the tumors were subjected to histochemical analyses employing the substrates in solution or later in a cellulose membrane overlay *(55)*. Another such group is the DQ-substrates (Invitrogen, Carlsbad, CA). These are large nonspecific protein-based substrates (e.g. DQ-gelatin™, DQ-BSA™) that have incorporated into them large numbers of fluorescein isothiocyanate (FITC) molecules that are situated very close to each other on the protein backbone. This molecular proximity causes the substrate to be self-quenched due to a Förester Resonance Energy Transfer (FRET) effect. Cleavage of the protein backbone by a protease will result in fluorescent emission *(54)*. The same principle has also been applied to another set of proteolytic substrates designed to be more selective for a particular protease (see Development of Probes below; *56*).

2.2.1 DEVELOPMENT OF MODEL SYSTEMS

Models developed for fluorescence imaging of tumors and tumor cells involve the introduction of a fluorophore. In general there are two main categories: a transcription system where the cells are actively expressing the fluorophores, namely the fluorogenic proteins (e.g., GFP and DsRED), and a passive system in which an external fluorescence tag is brought into the vicinity of the tumor. In the first instance, as in the case for luciferase, the fluorogenic protein is expressed (see Section 3.1.1) in tumor cells. The differences here are that the fluorophore needs to be excited and that there is no substrate requirement. Several laboratories have been involved in the development of model systems based on GFP expression. For example, Hoffman and colleagues have developed a number of mouse model systems, including a transgenic mouse expressing GFP in all cells, to image tumor angiogenesis and progression *(58–64)*. Whereas the Hoffman laboratory's models usually involve observations of whole animals (see Section 3.2.2) and/or excised tissues, Lin and colleagues have developed a skin chamber model to image tumor angiogenesis in mice *(25, 65)*. In this system the window chamber in placed on the dorsal skin fold of a mouse. One side of the epidermis is removed allowing the exposure of the underlying vasculature. Tumor cells expressing GFP are transplanted onto this surface. The chamber is then sealed with a glass coverslip allowing direct fluorescent imaging of subsequent events *(65)*. Using this model they were able to record tumor development and angiogenesis induced by a single tumor cell *(65)*.

In the second instance, the fluorophore is presented as a "probe" that needs to be transported toward the target and either attaches to it as an identifier (static) or serves as a functional substrate to be activated and subsequently fluoresce (dynamic). Either case has been utilized in both *in vivo* and *in vitro* models *(21, 56, 66–69)*. In our laboratory we have developed a quantitative 3D model system to study tumor proteolysis and tumor stromal interactions *in vitro* under living conditions *(56, 66)*. In this model a substratum of reconstituted basement member is mixed with a quenched fluorescent substrate, e.g., DQ-collagen IV™, and applied to a glass coverslip. Cells (with or without diluted Matrigel) are seeded on the matrices and incubated in culture media to follow proteolysis of the quenched fluorescent substrate. The cells and their associated matrices are periodically observed with a confocal microscope to image the release of fluorescence due to proteolytic activity *(56, 66, 70)*.

2.2.2 DEVELOPMENT OF PROBES

Probe development for fluorescent imaging is critical to successful imaging. In the case of luciferase (see above), a foreign gene is introduced into cells. Fluorescent proteins may also be either expressed in cells alone as markers to identify a particular cell type, or as fusion proteins to study specific molecular events *(51, 52)*. As in the case with luciferase, since these have very little direct significance in the clinical arena (see below), they will not be discussed further. Instead, our focus will be the development of fluorescent probes as molecular beacons with the potential to monitor diagnosis and therapeutic regimens for clinical applications.

In general, there are two types of fluorescent probes, static and functional. In static probes a ligand for the protein of interest is tagged with a fluorophore that will attach to the desired target. Traditionally these have been antibody based, utilizing immunocytochemical/immunohistochemical methods (see Fig. 5). Furthermore, these are always in an "ON" configuration, i.e., fluorescence is emitted upon excitation regardless of whether the probe is bound to the target. Because of this, the main issue with these types of probes is that excess unbound probe has to be cleared. Otherwise the signal would be contaminated with high non-specific background. They also suffer from the finite presence of their targets, i.e., if the target molecule is present only in a small amount, signal strength may be so weak that detection may not be possible. Therefore, although these probes may be adequate for imaging of fixed specimens, they are not ideal for *in vivo* imaging because of a low signal-to-noise ratio.

Functional probes, on the other hand, require activation as a result of some biological events, e.g., enzymatic reaction, to be detected *(22–24, 57, 69)*. They are ideal for *in vivo* imaging as they are designed to be silent before they reach their target, hence there is less of an issue with background noise. These have gained popularity in recent years in part due to the pioneering work by R. Weissleder and colleagues. This group designed and developed quenched fluorescent probes that have been successfully used for *in vivo* imaging of tumors in mice *(8, 9, 57, 69)*. The probes are based on activity of proteases that cleave the quenched molecule resulting in fluorescence emission, similar to the DQ-substrates mentioned above *(56, 66)*. These types of probes can serve a dual function. As diagnostic markers they can serve to detect the presence of tumors. As therapeutic indicators they can be utilized to monitor the efficacy of a given drug.

There are two major considerations in the development of functional fluorescent probes: the chemical structure of the probe itself, which is critical for the probe's selectivity and specificity, and the choice of a suitable fluorophore. Both cases are heavily dependent on the eventual utility of the probe. In cancer imaging, proteases have become the enzymes of choice as targets for quenched fluorescent probe development due to several important parameters. One factor, as mentioned above, is that proteolytic enzymes have been shown to have altered profiles in cancer and cancer cells, including elevated expression and secretion into the extracellular milieu *(15, 16)*. This allows a prospective probe (or beacon) to target and concentrate in the tumor and/or tumor vicinity where there is elevated concentrations of proteases. Another parameter is that these probes, by virtue of being a substrate for an active enzyme, possess a built-in signal amplification property. As the new probes accumulate at the site of enzyme activity, they are cleaved, resulting in elevated fluorescent emission *(8, 9, 22–24)*.

There are a number of methods for the generation of fluorescent probes. There are two that are more commonly utilized for *in vivo* imaging *(69, 71–75)*. One is based on the original linear structure pioneered by C. Tung *(69)*. The other is the use of branched dendrimers as the probe backbone *(72–75)*. In the first approach, a peptide linker sequence corresponding to a protease cleavage site is attached to a polylysine backbone to which polyethylene glycol (PEG) molecules are also attached (Fig. 6). The PEGs provide bulk to increase tissue retention and minimize rapid clearance from the system *(69)*. Fluorophores are attached to the peptide linkers at the N-terminus. The linkers are situated such that the attached fluorophores lie in close proximity to each other, resulting in self-quenching due to a FRET effect (Fig. 5; *69*). When the peptide is cleaved by an appropriate protease, the fluorophore is released and fluorescence emitted (Fig. 7; *69*).

The second approach, as stated above, is the use of dendrimers *(72–75)*. These are polymeric compounds based on a PAMAM (PolyAmido Amino) structure presenting numerous branched sidearms ranging in size from ~500 Da to ~900 kDa (Fig. 8). The

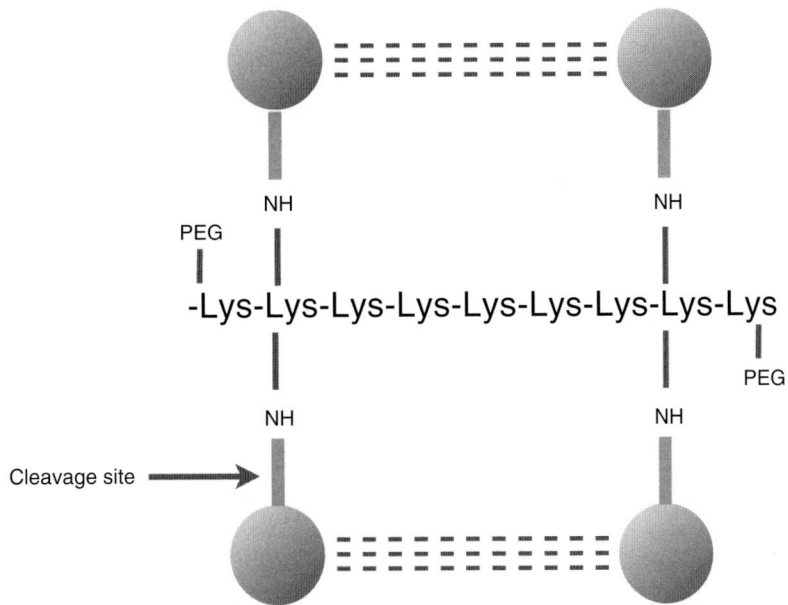

Fig. 6. Schematic representation of protease sensitive Near Infrared Fluorescent (NIRF) probes for *in vivo* imaging. The grey circles represent the near infrared fluorescent dye. The gray bars depict the site of proteolytic cleavage. Triple dashed lines represent fluorescent quenching due to close proximity of the dye molecules. (Adapted from C. Tung, 57).

advantage here is each sidearm can be attached to a separate functional group. For example, R. Kannan and colleagues have tested the efficacy of dendrimers as a drug delivery tool for targeting lung carcinoma cells by attaching ibuprofen and FITC (as a tracer) molecules on different branches of the dendrimer *(75)*. By imaging FITC emission, they showed that dendrimers were able to efficiently enter the cells and deliver their drug cargo *(75)*. To take this step further, it may be possible to generate a beacon in which a drug and a quenched fluorophore are attached to different arms of the same dendrimer via identical linkers. In this way when the linkers are cleaved due to an enzymatic reaction not only is the drug released, but the site of release can be monitored. Drawing on this premise, O. McIntyre and colleagues have recently reported the development of a matrix metalloproteinase-7 (MMP-7, also known as matrilysin)-sensitive fluorogenic probe for *in vivo* imaging *(73)*. The probe is based on the Generation-4 Starburst™ PAMAM decorated with fluorescein and tetramethyl rhodamine (TMR). In this probe TMR is attached directly to the dendrimer, serving as an internal reference (Fig. 8). Spacing is in such a way that no quenching is permitted, resulting in the TMR always being in the ON position. This provides for the tracking of the probe regardless of proteolytic activation. Fluorescein, on the other hand, is attached to the backbone via a peptide linker specific for cleavage by MMP-7 (Fig. 8). As in the case with the linear probe, the fluorophores attached to the linkers are positioned to promote self-quenching. Upon cleavage by the enzyme, in this case MMP-7, green fluorescence is emitted *(73)*.

In contrast to probes based on substrates, M. Bogyo and colleagues have popularized yet another method in fluorescent probe development directed against proteolytic

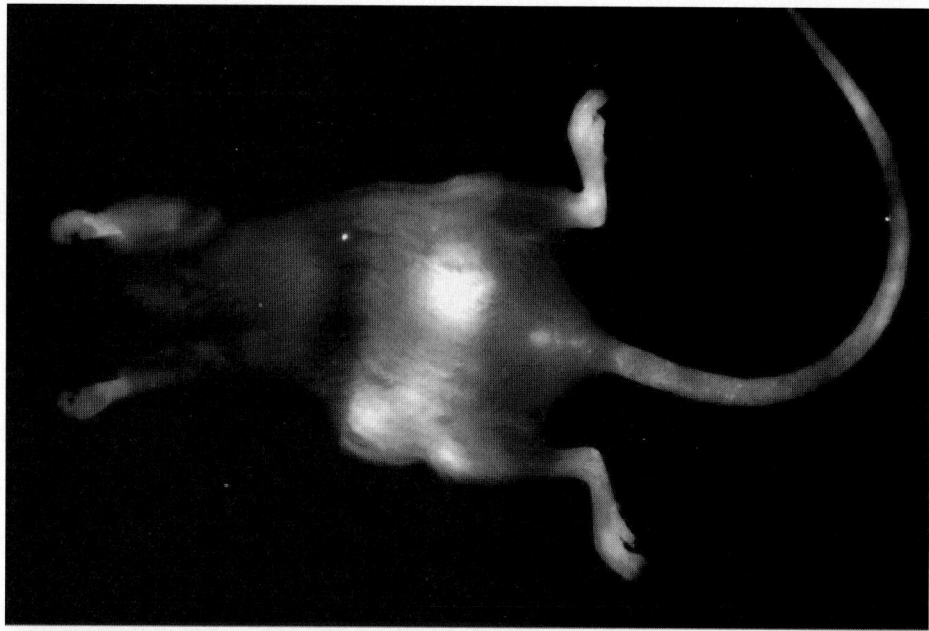
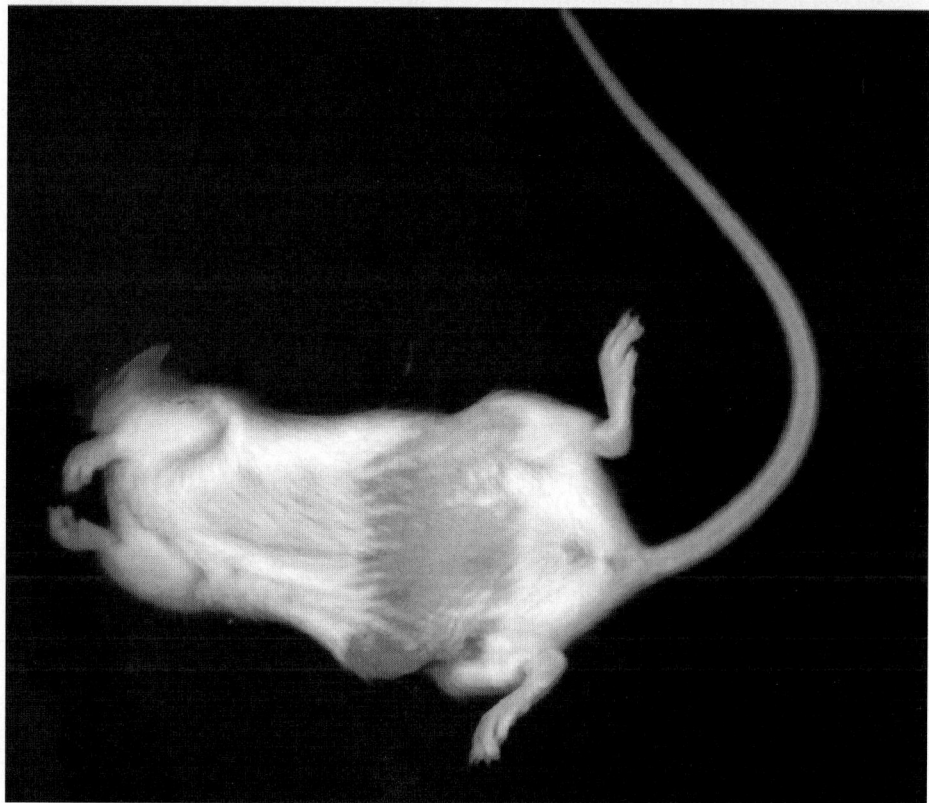

Fig. 7. *In vivo* NIRF imaging of breast cancer in mice. MDA-231 human breast tumor cells were injected into mammary fat pads of SCID mice. Subsequent to tumor development, the mice were injected (via tail vein) with 2 nmoles of a protease cleavable NIRF probe (see Fig. 6 legend). After 16 hours, mice were imaged with an IS4000MM™ multimodal imager (Kodak, New Haven, CT). Left panel represents the white light image. Right panel represents the NIRF image. Multiple tumors are clearly visible in the NIRF image.

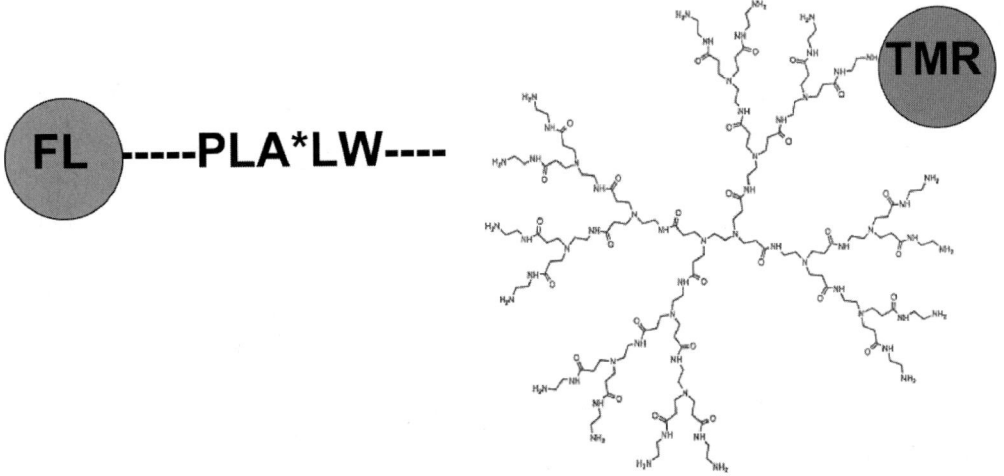

Fig. 8. Schematic representation of MMP-7 sensitive dendrimer based probe. Fl, fluorescine; TMR, tetramethyl rhodamine. The asterisk denotes the site of cleavage by MMP-7. (Adapted from McIntyre et al., 73).

enzymes. They have developed small molecular weight probes with a fluorescent tag to image proteases based on an inhibitor *(76–78)*. These probes are designed to target the active site of the enzyme, hence the name activity-based probes (ABPs). In fact, they are specific to the mature active enzyme and will not bind to the target if the active site is blocked *(76–78)*. For example, based on the molecular structure of the epoxide-derived E-64, a potent inhibitor of cysteine proteases, the Bogyo group has developed probes that will specifically target these enzymes *(76–78)*. Therefore, in a tumor where these enzymes are expressed at high levels the ABPs can prove to be of significant utility. The Bogyo group has also developed quenched ABPs by including a quencher on the probes that can be removed by proteolytic cleavage *(79)*. A concern is that due to their small size the ABPs may clear the system too quickly before being sufficiently accumulated in the tumor. On the other hand, since the probes bind to their targets covalently, this is less of an issue. In addition, B. Cravatt and colleagues have successfully utilized ABPs *in vivo (80)* showing in principle that the system does work.

Recently R. Tsien and colleagues have introduced an exciting new strategy to the development of fluorescent probes for *in vivo* imaging of tumors *(81)*. In this approach a cationic cell penetrating peptide (CPP) carrying a fluorogenic cargo (e.g., Cy 5) is fused to a polyanionic peptide via a protease-cleavable linker sequence. Normally, this complex cannot enter the cell due to hindrance caused by the anionic piece. When the linker is cleaved by an appropriate protease, the CPP is released (hence activatable CPP) and can then enter the cell carrying its payload *(81)*. Utilizing an HT-1080 fibrosarcoma model system Tsien and co-workers were able to image these tumors *in vivo (81)*. This approach has an added advantage in that the same concept can be utilized to deliver drugs to the tumor *(81)*. In fact, it is possible to envision a scenario in which drug and reporter can both be delivered to the tumor site, therefore allowing for monitoring of drug delivery.

2.2.3 Application to *in vivo* Imaging

The main advantage of fluorescence over other modalities for *in vivo* imaging is the high resolution that is afforded (down to subcellular levels). Until recently the utility of fluorescent imaging *in vivo* had not been realized. Traditionally, the main hindrances for fluorescent imaging *in vivo* have been 3-fold. One was our inability to selectively label targets in living systems. The second is the poor penetration of living tissue by light in the visible spectrum. This is due mostly to the absorption of light and its scattering as the result of high-energy (short wavelength) light interactions with tissue components and water in living systems *(82)*. The third problem is that certain tissue components (e.g, hemoglobin, NADP/NADPH) have autofluorescent properties in the lower end of the spectrum, causing severe background issues *(80)*. Recent technological advances in the field have helped to reduce some of these issues and have resulted in an increased application of fluorescence for *in vivo* imaging *(9, 82, 83)*.

As stated previously, the increased interest in *in vivo* imaging has been due in part to the discovery of GFP and its homologs *(51)* as well as new synthetic fluorophores, particularly the ones with absorbance in the far red and near infrared regions of the spectrum *(9, 52, 53)*. Although there is no clinical application for GFP, like luciferase it has been utilized extensively in recent years for small animal *in vivo* imaging *(58–65)*. Our ability to express GFP in tumor cells has made it possible to design experiments in which tumors can be monitored *in vivo*. Hoffman and colleagues have successfully developed several unique mouse models to image tumors and tumor angiogenesis utilizing GFP fusion products of specific marker proteins *(58–65)*. They have shown that metastatic nodules can be detected in whole animals *in vivo* by either tail vein injection of GFP expressing tumor cells or orthotopic transplantation of tumor cells into appropriate animals. Furthermore, the Hoffman laboratory has developed a transgenic mouse that ubiquitously express GFP in all organs *(63)*. The advantage of such a model is that it may be possible to study tumor host interactions directly and over extended periods of time *in vivo* by injecting tumor cells expressing a different color fluorescent protein (RFP, for example) into the GFP mouse *(63)*. Others have also utilized GFP expression systems to study cancer-related events in mice *(65)*.

Another milestone in fluorescent imaging has been the increased efforts in probe development utilizing the newly available far red and near infrared fluorescent (NIRF) dyes *(57)*. The main advantage of these dyes is their ability to be imaged deeper in living tissues. This is due to their longer excitation wavelengths, thus low energy incident light requirements, in the range of 680–800 nm. At this end of the spectrum there is much less interaction of light rays with water and other tissue components, which results in less light scattering, reduced background, and therefore cleaner and sharper images *(71, 82)*. As indicated above, the Weissleder group at Harvard pioneered the development of *in vivo* fluorescent imaging in small animals with NIRF probes *(71)*. They have successfully utilized a number of their functional probes to image a variety of tumors in mice *(69)*. For example, they were able to image fibrosarcomas, gliosarcomas, and colon and breast tumors in living mice with some of their protease-sensitive probes *(69)*, albeit the selectivity and specificity of these probes in some settings remain to be validated *(70)*.

3. SYSTEM DEVELOPMENT FOR *IN VIVO* OPTICAL IMAGING

To adapt optical imaging principles to the *in vivo* arena relevant to the present discussion, new imaging systems had to be developed. In general, there are two major categories involved: whole body imaging, where the entire living organism is imaged, and localized or focal imaging, where specific regions within an organism are imaged.

3.1 Whole Body Imaging

As the name implies, in whole body imaging our efforts are directed toward collecting optical signals (emitted light) from the entire body. To date almost all such efforts have been concentrated on the development of systems for small animal imaging. This is for the most part because of the fact that optical imaging in large animals and patients will be limited due to depth of penetration of light (see clinical implications below).

There are currently two basic commercially available designs used for whole body optical imaging instruments (Fig. 9). The imaging principle for both systems is the same in that the animal is placed in a light-tight box and imaged via a CCD camera *(32, 71)*. The difference is whether the animal is imaged from below *(71)* or from above *(32)*. In one design, the subject (while under anesthesia) is placed on a glass platform inside the instrument and the image is reflected onto a CCD camera via a mirror placed at a 45° angle under the platform (Fig. 9A). In the other, the subject is placed on a platform inside the instrument and imaged directly by a CCD camera from above (Fig. 9B). In either case the resolution is rather low and limited to the millimeter range *(32, 71)*.

Recently, a new device capable of tomographic multichannel fluorescent detection for *in vivo* imaging of mice has been developed. The design includes a holding chamber for the subject and a modular scanner capable of acquiring transillumination, reflectance, and absorption data utilizing two diode laser lines as excitation sources. The main advantage here is the ability to obtain noninvasive optical slices that can be used for three-dimensional reconstruction and volumetric analysis. Using this device, investigators were able to collect data for quantitative three-dimensional imaging *(83)*.

3.2 Localized (Focal) Imaging

Here the imaging is restricted to a small area within a subject. This is of particular interest for imaging of large animals and patients. It has to be noted that our discussion here deals primarily with fluorescence and not bioluminescence, since there is no clinical application for bioluminescence (see Section 3.1.3). As mentioned above, whole body optical imaging of large subjects is not possible at this time. This is due to the fact that under the best of circumstances the ability of light to penetrate tissue (even when considering near infrared wavelengths) is limited to a narrow range (a few hundred micrometers at the most). Also, in larger subjects thicker skin is a formidable barrier to light penetration. Therefore, unless the object to be imaged (a tumor, for example) is located superficially, it is difficult to image. Although in the past decade fluorescent bronchoscopy has been in clinical practice for lung cancer diagnostics, the outcome has not been ideal *(84)*. Both autofluorescence and drug-induced fluorescence have been utilized *(84)*. With the former, clinicians have been relying on differential

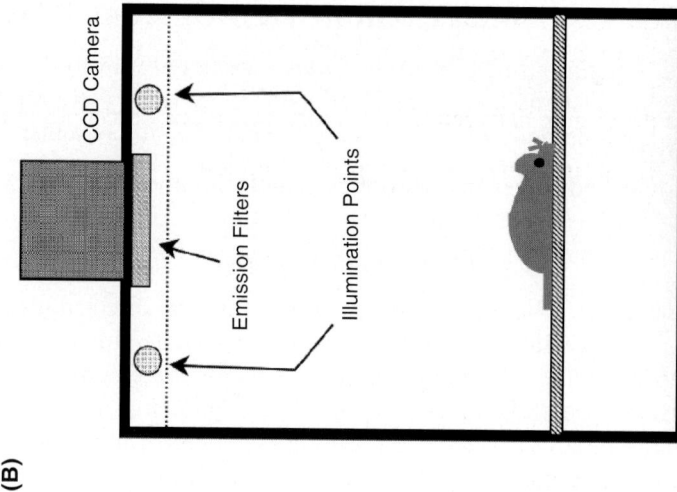
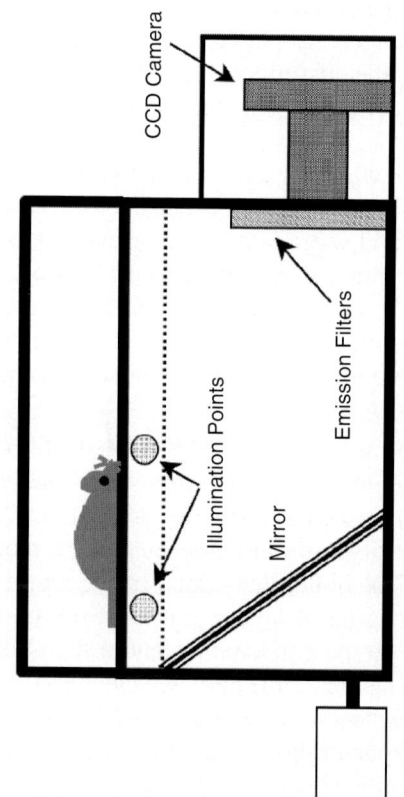

Fig. 9. Schematic representation of two commercially available *in vivo* small animal imaging devices capable of imaging mice from (A) below or (B) above.

autofluorescence of tumor versus normal tissues when exposed to blue light. With the latter, they rely on the preferential deposition of a blue light-excitable fluorescent drug in the tumor *(85)*. In either case, the major problem has been the lack of specificity due to the fact that the difference between tumor fluorescence and surrounding tissue fluorescence is marginal.

Recent technological advances in fiber optics, nanotechnology, and laser optics have made it possible to adapt previously available internal imaging devices such as laparoscopes, bronchoscopes, and endoscopes to fluorescent imaging. Several groups have been developing endoscope-based confocal microscopy for *in vivo* fluorescent imaging *(86–90)*. These are essentially miniaturized confocal microscopes utilizing micro lenses, microscanners, and fiberoptics that are fitted onto an endoscope. The advantage here is that it is possible to image down to subcellular resolution and take advantage of confocal optics. In the past, one of the problems with fluorescent imaging, particularly in thicker specimens, has always been the presence of a background haze due to interference by out-of-focus light. This issue was significantly reduced with the advent of confocal optics in which a pinhole is placed in the optical path at the detector *(91)*. In this way the interference due to out-of-focus light is reduced, and sharper images representing only the plane of focus are obtained *(91)*. Alternatively, it is possible to utilize two-photon (also known as multiphoton) imaging principles to overcome the problems caused by out-of-focus light *(92–94)*. In this technique a fluorophore is excited by simultaneous absorption of two or more photons of high wavelengths (thus of low energy) generated by a pulsed laser, e.g., a titanium-sapphire laser *(92–94)*. Since two/multiphoton excitation phenomenon occurs only at the plane of focus, the resulting image is inherently confocal, therefore eliminating the need for a pinhole. An added advantage here is that because near infrared illumination is used, deeper tissue penetration with much reduced scattering effects and photo damage is realized *(82, 84)*. More importantly, both confocal and two-photon fluorescence image only the focal plane, therefore multiple images can be obtained throughout the sample volume. These images can then be reconstructed in three dimensions and analyzed *(91–94)*.

4. CLINICAL IMPLICATIONS: ADVANTAGES AND LIMITATIONS

Optical imaging methods for clinical application have been receiving increasing attention based on recent research developments in this area. In addition to optical surface imaging such as in ophthalmology with and without the use of fluorescent dyes *(95)* or in endoscopy, newer imaging modalities based on the propagation of light through tissues are emerging, particularly in the areas of brain, muscle, and breast imaging *(96)*. New developments in NIR optical tomography research *(9, 96)* are yielding promising optical approaches for imaging in clinical practice particularly as a complementary modality for breast cancer detection *(97, 98)*. The development of new kinds of targeted optical reagents including those providing for both imaging and therapy *(99)* will likely provide new optical paradigms for the clinician.

The most significant advantage of bioluminescent and fluorescent imaging is the ability for selective targeting. This together with the increased sensitivity and resolving power that is usually associated with optical imaging makes bioluminescence and fluorescence attractive imaging modalities for clinical cancer diagnostics. The major limitation of optical imaging in the clinical arena has been the limited ability of light to penetrate thick tissues. This is especially true in the area of whole body imaging. As mentioned above, unlike MRI and PET imaging, direct clinical application of whole body optical imaging is essentially nonexistent at this juncture. Indirectly through major advancements in small animal imaging it is having a significant impact. Small animal models for *in vivo* imaging have been developed that can serve as cost-effective surrogates for studying the efficacy of anticancer therapeutics (see above). For example, human tumor cells expressing GFP or luciferase may be injected into mice and their development into tumors can be monitored with whole body *in vivo* imaging *(32, 61)*. Because this is noninvasive imaging, the same subject can be imaged multiple times throughout the course of the experiment to measure a given drug's effectiveness against the tumor.

Localized *in vivo* fluorescent imaging on the other hand is showing great potential for use in the clinical setting *(87)*. Through utilization of specialized instruments it is possible to harness the increased sensitivity and subcellular resolution of optical imaging as a diagnostic tool to detect minute changes associated with certain types of cancer that are accessible to these devices (e.g., digestive tract, respiratory tract, and urinary and reproductive tracts). Furthermore, this utility can be extended throughout the therapeutic regimen to follow up on a patient's response to treatment and therefore measure the efficacy of a given drug as an anticancer agent.

5. CONCLUSIONS AND FUTURE PROSPECTS

New discoveries and technical advances in the past two decades have revitalized optical imaging and its biological applications. This has resulted in a number of new developments in recent years:

1. Development of a new model system for *in vivo* optical imaging.
2. Synthesis of new fluorescent dye, especially in the near infrared region of the spectrum.
3. Development of new functional probes using the above dyes.
4. Development of new optical imaging devices for small animal imaging.
5. Development of endoscope-based optical devices for clinical use.
6. Development of combination ultrasound/optical imaging devices for mammography.

The most significant direct impact of optical imaging in the clinic, however, is in the area of focal/localized fluorescent imaging. There has been a burst of activity on endoscope-based fluorescent devices for clinical applications that has resulted in the development of several such devices *(86–89)*. Moreover, it is in this area that most likely we will see further advances and innovations in the near future. As stated before, this is due to the nature of optical imaging and its inherent limitations for deep tissue and whole body imaging.

ACKNOWLEDGMENTS

This work was supported in part by U.S. Public Health Service Grants CA 36481 and CA 56586 and the following awards from the Department of Defense: a Breast Cancer Center of Excellence (DAMD17–02–1-0693) and PC991261. The Microscopy and Imaging Resources Laboratory is supported in part by National Institutes of Health Center Grants P30ES06639 and P30CA22453 and a National Institutes of Health

Roadmap Grant U54RR020843. We thank Drs. Michael Cher and Daniel Bonfil for providing the animals with luciferase expressing tumors. We also thank Ms. Mary Olive for technical assistance.

REFERENCES

1. Belani C, Langer C. First-line chemotherapy for NSCLC: An overview of relevant trials. *Lung Cancer* 2002;38:S13–S19.
2. Adjei A, Rowinsky E. Novel anticancer agents in clinical development. *Cancer Biol Ther* 2003;2: S5–S15.
3. Eriguchi M, Levi F, Hisa T, Yanagie H, Nonaka Y, Takeda Y. Chronotherapy for cancer. *Biomed Pharmacother* 2003;57:92s–95s.
4. Van Laarhove H, Punt C. Systemic treatment of advanced colorectal carcinoma. *Eur J Gastroentrol Hepatol* 2004;16:283–289.
5. Yokoba M, Yanase N, Masusa N. New anticancer agents—from cytotoxic systemic chemotherapy to target-based agents. *Gan To Kagaku Ryoho* 2005;32:783–788.
6. Gelimelius B, Nordenskjold B, Kjellen E, Zackrisson B, Swedish Cancer Investigation Group. Interactions between chemotherapy, endocrine therapy and radiation. *Acta Oncol* 2002;41:635–638.
7. Emptage N. Fluorescent imaging in living systems. *Curr Opinion Pharmacol* 2001;1:521–525.
8. Weissleder R. Scaling down imaging: Molecular mapping of cancer in mice. *Nature Rev* 2002; 2:1–8.
9. Ntziachriston V, Ripoll J, Wand L, Weissleder R. Looking and listening to light: The evolution of whole-body photonic imaging. *Nature Biotech* 2005; 23: 313–320.
10. Jaffer F, Weissleder R. Molecular imaging in the clinical arena. *JAMA* 2005;293:855–862.
11. Crnic I, Christofori G. Novel technologies and recent advances in metastasis research. *Int J Dev Biol* 2004;48:573–581.
12. Micke P, Östman A. Tumor-stroma interaction: Cancer associated fibroblasts as novel targets in anti-cancer therapy. *Lung Cancer* 2004;45:S163–S175.
13. Folkman J. Role of angiogenesis in tumor growth and metastasis. *Semin Oncol* 2002;29:15–18.
14. Skrzydlewska E, Sulkowska M, Koda M, Sulkowski S. Proteolytic-antiproteolytic balance and its regulation in carcinogenesis. *World Gastroenterol* 2005;11:1251–1266.
15. Brunner N, Matrisian L, Dano K, eds. Proteases and Protease Inhibitors in Cancer, Vol 107. Copenhagen: APMIS, 1999.
16. Suzuki M, Hiwasa T, eds. Proteases Involved in Cancer. Monduzzi Editore, 1994.
17. Fox S, Harris A. Markers of tumor angiogenesis: Clinical applications in prognosis and anti-angiogenic therapy. *Invest New Drugs* 1997;15:15–28.
18. Zetter B. Angiogenesis and tumor metastasis. *Annu Rev Med* 1998;49:407–424.
19. Cavallaro U, Christofori G. Molecular mechanisms of tumor angiogenesis and progression. *J Neuro-Oncol* 2000;50:63–70.
20. Ellis L, Liu W, Ahmad S, Fan F, Jung Y, Shaheen R, Reinmuth N. Overview of angiogenesis: Biologic implications for antiangiogeneic therapy. I. 2001;28:94–104.
21. Allessi P, Ebbinghaus C, Neri D. Molecular targeting of angiogenesis. *Biochim Biophys Acta* 2004;1654:39–49.
22. Bremer C, Tung C, Weissleder R. In vivo molecular target assessment of matrix metalloproteinase inhibition. *Nature Med* 2001;7:743–748.
23. Bremer C, Bredow S, Mahmood O, Weissleder R, Tung C. Optical imaging of matrix metalloproteinase-2 activity in tumors: Feasibility study in a mouse model. *Radiology* 2001;221:523–529.
24. Bremer C, Tung C, Bogdanov A, Weissleder R. Imaging of differential protease expression in breast cancers for detection of aggressive tumor phenotypes. *Radiology* 2002;222:814–818.
25. Lin P. Optical imaging and tumor angiogenesis. *J Cell Biochem* 2003;90:484–491.
26. Catalona W, Smith D, Ratliff T, Dodds K, Coplen D, Yuan J, Andriole G. Measurement of prostate-specific antigen in serum as a screening test for prostate cancer. *N Engl J Med* 1991;324: 1156–1161.
27. Paul B, Dhir R, Landsittel D, Hitchens M, Getzenberg R. Detection of prostate cancer with a blood-based assay for early prostate cancer antigen. *Cancer Res* 2005;65:4097–4100.

28. Leach F, Koh M, Chan Y, Bark S, Ray R, Morton R, Remaley A. Prostate specific antigen as a clinical biomarker for prostate cancer: What's the take home message? *Landes Biosci* 2005;4:371–375.
29. Wilson T, Hastings J. Bioluminescence. *Annu Rev Cell Dev Biol* 1988;14:197–230.
30. Day J, Tisi L, Bailey M. Evolution of beetle bioluminescence: The origin of beetle luciferin. *Luminescence* 2004;19:8–20.
31. Greer III L, Szalay A. Imaging of light emission from the expression of luciferases in living cells and organisms: A review. *Luminescence* 2002;17:43–74.
32. Contag P. Whole-animal cellular and molecular imaging to accelerate drug development. *Drug Discovery Today* 2002;7:555–562.
33. Edinger T, Sweeney T, Tucker A, Olomu A, Negrin R, Contag C. Non-invasive assessment of tumor cell proliferation in animal models. *Neoplasia* 1999;1:303–310.
34. Contag C, Jenkins D, Contag P, Negrin R. Use of reporter genes for optical measurements of neoplastic disease *in vivo*. Neoplasia 2000;2:41–52.
35. Rehmtulla A, Stegman L, Cardozo S, Gupta G, Hall D, Contag C, Ross B. Rapid and quantitative assessment of cancer treatment response using *in vivo* bioluminescence imaging. *Neoplasia* 2000; 2:491–495.
36. Rosol T, Tannenhil-Gregg S, LeRoy B, Mandl S, Contag C. Animal models for bone metastasis. *Cancer* 2003;97:748–757.
37. Hyoudou K, Nishikawa, M, Umeyama Y, Kobayasi Y, Yamashita F, Hashida M. Inhibition of metastatic tumor growth in mouse lung by repeated administration of glycol-conjugated catalase: Quantitative analysis by Firefly luciferase-expressing melanoma cells. *Clin Cancer Res* 2004;10:7685–7691.
38. Adams J, Johnson M, Sato M, Burger F, Gambhir S, Carey M, Irueal-Arispe L, Wu L. Visualization of advanced human prostate cancer lesions in living mice by a targeted gene transfer vector and optical imaging. *Nature Med* 2002;8:891–896.
39. Wu J, Inobushi M, Sundaresan G, Schelbert H, Gambhir S. Optical imaging of reporter gene expression in living rats. *Circulation* 2002;105:1631–1634.
40. Massoud T, Paulmurugan R, Gambhir S. Molecular imaging of homodimeric protein-protein interactions in living subjects. *FASEB J* 2004;10:1105–1107.
41. Gross S, Piwnica-Worms D. Spying on cancer: Molecular imaging in vivo with genetically encoded reporters. *Cancer Cell* 2005;7:5–15.
42. Shah K, Bureau E, Kim D, Yang K, Tang Y, Weissleder R, Breakfield X. Glioma therapy and real-time imaging of neural precursor cell migration and tumor regression. *Ann Neurol* 2005;57: 34–41.
43. Scatena C, Hepner M, Oei Y, Dusich J, Yu S, Purchio T, Contag P, Jenkins D. Imaging of bioluminescent LNCaP-Luc-M6 tumors: A new animal model for the study of metastatic human prostate cancer. *Prostate* 2004;59:292–303.
44. Jamison D, Croney J, Moens P. Fluorescence: Basic concepts, practical aspects, and some anecdotes. *Methods Enzymol* 2003;360:1–43.
45. Pierce, D, Vale R. Single-molecule fluorescent detection of green fluorescent protein and application to single protein dynamics. *Methods Cell Biol* 1999;58:49–73.
46. Traganos F, Darzynkiewicz Z. Lysosomal proton pump activity: Supravital cell staining with acridine orange differentiates leukocyte subpopulations. *Methods Cell Biol* 1994;41:185–194.
47. Larsen T, Goodsell D, Cascio D, Grzeskowiak K, Dickerson R. The structure of DAPI bound to DNA. *J Biomol Struct Dyn* 1989;7:477–491.
48. Pendergrass W, Wolf N, Poot M. Efficacy of MitoTracker Green and CMRXRosamine to measure changes in mitochondrial membrane potential in living cells and tissues. *Cytometry Part A* 2004; 61A:162–169.
49. Morin J, Hastings J. Energy transfer in a bioluminescent system. *J Cell Physiol* 1971;77:313–318.
50. Prasher D, Echenrode V, Ward W, Prendergast F, Comier M. Primary structure of the Aequorea victoria green fluorescent protein. *Gene* 1992;111:229–233.
51. Lippincott-Schwartz J, Patterson G. Development and use of fluorescent protein markers in living cells. *Science* 2003;300:87–90.
52. Fradkov A, Verkhusha V, Staroverov D, Bulina M, Yanushevich Y, Lukyonov S, Lukyonov K. Far-red fluorescent tag for protein labelling. *Biochem J* 2002;368:17–21.
53. Shaner N, Campbell R, Steinback P, Giepmans B, Palmer A, Tsien R. Improved monomeric red, orange and yellow fluorescent proteins derived from Discosoma sp. red fluorescent protein. *Nat Biotech* 2004;22:1567–1572.

54. Smith RE, van Frank RM. The use of amino acid derivatives of 4-methoxy-beta-naphthylamine for the assay and subcellular localization of tissue proteinases. *Front Biol* 1975;43:193–249.
55. Garrett JR, Kidd A, Kyriacou K, Smith RE. Use of different derivatives of D-Val-Leu-Arg for studying kallikrein activities in cat submandibular glands and saliva. *Histochem J* 1985;17:805–818.
56. Sameni M, Moin K, Sloane BF. Imaging proteolysis by living human breast cancer cells. *Neoplasia* 2000;2:496–504.
57. Tung C. Fluorescent peptide probes for in vivo diagnostic imaging. *Biopolymers* 2004;76:391–403.
58. Yang M, Barnov E, Jiang P, Sun F, Li X, Li L, Hasegawa S, Bouvet M, Al-Towaijri M, Chishima T, Shimada S, Moossa A, Penman S, Hoffman R. Whole-body imaging of green fluorescent protein-expressing tumors and metastasis. *Proc Natl Acad Sci USA* 2000;97:1206–1211.
59. Yang M, Baranov E, Moossa A, Penman S, Hoffman R. Visualizing gene expression by whole-body fluorescent imaging. *Proc Natl Acad Sci USA* 2000;97:12278–12282.
60. Hoffman R. Green fluorescent protein imaging of tumour growth, metastasis and angiogenesis in mouse models. *Lancet Oncol* 2002;3:546–556.
61. Bouvt M, Wang J, Nardin S, Nassirpour R, Yang F, Barnov E, Jiang P, Moossa A, Hoffman R. Real-time optical imaging of primary tumor growth and multiple metastatic events in a pancreatic cancer orthotopic model. *Cancer Res* 2002;62:1534–1540.
62. Yamamoto N, Jiang P, Yang M, Xu M, Yamauchi L, Tsuchia H, Tomita K, Whal G, Moossa A, Hoffman R. Cellular dynamics visualized in live cells *in vitro* and *in vivo* by differential dual-color nuclear-cytoplasmic fluorescent-protein expression. *Cancer Res* 2004;64:4251–4256.
63. Yang M, Raynoso J, Jiang P, Li L, Moossa A, Hoffman R. Transgenic nude mouse with ubiquitous green fluorescent protein expression as a host for human tumors. *Cancer Res* 2004;64:8651–8656.
64. Yang M, Jiang P, Yamamoto N, Geller J, Moossa A, Hoffman R. Real-time whole-body imaging of an orthotopic metastatic prostate cancer model expressing red fluorescent protein. *The Prostate* 2005;62:374–379.
65. Li C, Shan S, Huang Q, Braun R, Lanzen J, Hu K, Lin P, Dewhirst M. Initial stages of tumor cell-induced angiogenesis: Evaluation via skin window chambers in rodent models. *J Natl Cancer Inst* 2000;92:143–147.
66. Sameni M, Dosescu J, Moin K, Sloane BF. Functional imaging of proteolysis: Stromal and inflammatory cells increase tumor proteolysis. *Mol Imaging* 2003;2:1–17.
67. Sonnichsen B, Renzis S, Nielsen E, Reitdorf J, Zerial M. Distinct membrane domains on endosomes in recycling pathway visualized by multicolor imaging of Rab4, Rab5, and Rab11. *J Cell Biol* 2000;149:901–913.
68. Bogdanov A, Lin C, Simonova M, Matuszewski L, Weissleder R. Cellular activation of self-quenched fluorescent reporter probe in tumor microenvironment. Neoplasia 2002;4:228–236.
69. Funovics M, Weissleder R, Tung C. Protease sensors for bioimaging. *Anal Bioanal Chem* 2003; 377:956–963.
70. Sloane BF, Sameni M, Podgorski I, Cavalo-Medved D, Moin K. Functional imaging of tumor proteolysis. *Annu Rev Pharmacol Toxicol* 2006;46:301–315.
71. Mahmood U, Tung C, Bogdanov A, Weissleder R. Near-infrared optical imaging of protease activity for tumor detection. *Radiology* 1999;213:866–870.
72. Weiner E, Shadron L, Brechbiel M, Gansow O. Targeting dendrimer-chelates to tumors and tumor cells expressing the high-affinity folate receptor. *Invest Radiol* 1997;32:748–754.
73. McIntyre J, Fingleton B, Wells S, Piston D, Lynch C, Gautm S, Matrisian L. Development of a novel fluorogenic proteolytic beacon for in vivo detection and imaging of tumour-associated matrix metalloproteinase-7 activity. *Biochem J* 2004;377:617–628.
74. Khandare J, Kolhe P, Pillai O, Kannan S, Lieh-Lai M, Kannan R. Synthesis, cellular transport, and activity of polyamidoamine dendrimer-methylprednisolone conjugates. *Bioconjugate Chem* 2005; 16:330–337.
75. Kolhe P, Khandare J, Pillai O, Kannan S, Lieh-Lai M, Kannan R. Preparation, cellular transport, and activity of polyamidoamine-based dendritic nanodevices with a high drug payload. *Biomaterials* 2006;27(4):660–669.
76. Berger A, Vitorino P, Bogyo M. Activity-based protein profiling: Application to biomarker discovery, in vivo imaging and drug discovery. *Am J Pharmacogenom* 2004;4:371–381.
77. Kato D, Boatright K, Berger A, Nazif T, Blum G, Ryan C, Chehade K, Salvesen G, Bogyo M. Activity-based probes that target diverse cysteine protease families. Nature Chem Biol *Nature Chem Biol* 2005;1:33–38.

78. Veerhelst S, Bogyo M. Solid-phase synthesis of double-headed epoxysuccinyl activity-based probes for selective targeting of papian family cysteine proteases. *ChemBioChem* 2005;6:824–827.
79. Blum G, Mullins S, Keren K, Jedesko C, Rice M, Sloane B, Bogyo M. Dynamic imaging of protease activity with fluorescently quenched activity-based probes. *Nature Chem Biol* 2005;1:203–209.
80. Speers A, Cravatt B. Activity-based protein profiling in vivo using a copper(i)-catalyzed azide-alkyne [2+3] cycloaddition. *J Am Chem Soc* 2003;125:4686–4687.
81. Jiang T, Olson E, Nguyen Q, Roy M, Jennings P, Tsien R. Tumor imaging by means of proteolytic activation of cell-penetrating peptides. *Proc Natl Acad Sci USA* 2004;101:17867–17872.
82. Rubart M. Two-photon microscopy of cells and tissue. *Circ Res* 2004;95:1154–1166.
83. Montet X, Ntziachristos V, Gimm J, Weissleder R. Tomographic fluoresecence mapping of tumor targets. *Cancer Res* 2005;65:6330–6336.
84. Konig K. Multiphoton microscopy in life sciences. *J Microsc* 2000;200:83–104.
85. Stanzel F. Fluorescent bronchoscopy: Contribution for lung cancer screening? *Lung Cancer* 2004;45: S29–S37.
86. Helmchen F, Fee M, Tank D, Denk W. A miniature head mounted two-photon microscope: High-resolution brain imaging in freely moving animals. *Neuron* 2001;31:903–912.
87. Sokolov K, Aaron J, Hsu B, Nida D, Gillenwater A, Follen M, MacAullay C, Adler-Storthz K, Korgel B, Descour M, Pasqualini R, Arap W, Lam W, Richards-Kortum R. Optical systems for *in vivo* molecular imaging of cancer. *Technol Cancer Res Treat* 2003;2:491–504.
88. Funovics M, Alencar H, Su H, Khazaie K, Weissleder R, Mahmood U. Miniaturized multichannel near infrared endoscope for mouse imaging. *Mol Imaging* 2003;2:350–357.
89. Wang T, Contag C, Mandella M, Chan N, Kino G. Confocal fluorescence microscope with dual-axis architecture and biaxial postobjective scanning. *J Biomed Opt* 2004;9:735–742.
90. Laemmel E, Genet M, Le Goualher G, Perchant A, Le Gargasson J, Vicaut E. Fibered confocal fluorescence microscopy (Cell-viZio) facilities extended imaging in the field of microcirculation. *J Vasc Res* 2004;41:400–411.
91. Folds-Papp Z, Demel U, Tilz G. Laser scanning confocal fluorescence microscopy: An overview. *Int Immunopathopharmacol* 2003;3:1715–1729.
92. Piston D. When two is better than one: Elements of intravital microscopy. *PLoS Biol* 2005;3:e207.
93. So P, Dong C, Masters B, Berland K. Two-photon excitation fluorescence microscopy. *Annu Rev Biomed Eng* 2000;2:399–429.
94. White N, Errington R. Fluorescence techniques for drug delivery research: Theory and practice. *Adv Drug Del Rev* 2005;57:17–42.
95. Dzurinko VL, Gurwood AS, Price JR. Intravenous and indocyanine green angiography. *Optometry* 2004;75:743–755.
96. Nioka S, Chance B. NIR spectroscopic detection of breast cancer. *Technol Cancer Res Treat* 2005;4:497–512.
97. Zhu Q, Cronin EB, Currier AA, Vine HS, Huang M, Chen N, Xu C. Benign versus malignant breast masses: Optical differentiation with US-guided optical imaging reconstruction. *Radiology* 2005; 237:57–66.
98. Chance B, Nioka S, Zhang J, Conant EF, Hwang E, Briest S, Orel SG, Schnall MD, Czerniecki BJ. Breast cancer detection based on incremental biochemical and physiological properties of breast cancers: A six-year, two-site study. *Acad Radiol* 2005;12:925–933.
99. Chen Y, Gryshuk A, Achilefu S, Ohulchansky T, Potter W, Zhong T, Morgan J, Chance B, Prasad PN, Henderson BW, Oseroff A, Pandey RK. A novel approach to a bifunctional photosensitizer for tumor imaging and phototherapy. *Bioconjug Chem* 2005;16:1264–1274.

16 Imaging of Apoptosis

*Francis G. Blankenberg, MD, and
H. William Strauss, MD*

CONTENTS

INTRODUCTION
WATER-SUPPRESSED LIPID PROTON MAGNETIC RESONANCE
  SPECTROSCOPY, DIFFUSION-WEIGHTED IMAGING, AND
  MAGNETIC RESONANCE CONTRAST AGENTS
DETECTION OF APOPTOSIS WITH ULTRASOUND
  AND COMPUTED TOMOGRAPHY
RADIONUCLIDE IMAGING OF APOPTOSIS
SUMMARY

1. INTRODUCTION

Many diseases are associated with an abnormal increase or decrease in apoptosis (programmed cell death). A variety of newer drugs have been designed to enhance apoptosis (such as cancer therapy) or decrease programmed cell death (such as agents interrupting the immune inflammatory pathway in arthritis). Until recently apoptosis could be assessed only *in vitro* or by histological assay of biopsied material. To determine the effectiveness of therapy, it would be very helpful to have an *in vivo* imaging technique. Characteristic changes of apoptosis can be identified by ultrasound, magnetic resonance, and radionuclide approaches. The status of these approaches is outlined in this chapter with possible clinical uses listed in Table 1.

2. WATER-SUPPRESSED LIPID PROTON MAGNETIC RESONANCE SPECTROSCOPY, DIFFUSION-WEIGHTED IMAGING, AND MAGNETIC RESONANCE CONTRAST AGENTS

Water-suppressed lipid proton magnetic resonance spectroscopy (^{1}H-MRS) can detect the selective mobilization of intracellular lipids of cells undergoing apoptosis both *in vitro* (1–4) and *in vivo* (5–7). Water-suppressed proton spectroscopic pulse sequences can image these increases in membrane and cytoplasmic neutral mobile lipid domains. The precise origin of these mobile lipid domains is not clear and may be due

From: *Cancer Drug Discovery and Development
In Vivo Imaging of Cancer Therapy*
Edited by: A.F. Shields and P. Price © Humana Press Inc., Totowa, NJ

Table 1
Potential Clinical Uses for Apoptosis Imaging

Clinical use	References
Stroke/myocardial infarction (ischemic-related damage and postischemic inflammation)	*26, 37, 55, 56, 65, 66, 77, 78*
Inflammation of the central nervous system (i.e., multiple sclerosis, Alzheimer's, ADE)	*7, 36*
Rheumatoid diseases and soft tissue infection	*79, 80, 81*
Inflammatory bowel disease	*82, 83*
Organ and bone marrow transplant rejection	*46, 47, 84, 85*
Myelodysplastic diseases	*86*
Ophthalmological diseases affecting the retina	*87, 88, 89, 90*
Pulmonary inflammatory processes	*91*
Dermatological disease processes	*92, 93, 94, 95*
Imaging of vulnerable atherosclerotic plaques	*57, 58*
Monitoring cancer treatment	*1–5, 9, 10, 12–14, 18, 19, 48, 49, 53, 54, 59–63*
Targeted delivery of radioisotopes and drugs	*96*

to the intracellular partitioning of and/or the enzymatic formation of polyunsaturated fatty acids, cholesterol esters, and neutral triglycerides. Both the cytoplasm (cytoplasmic lipid droplets) and the plasma membrane (mobile lipid rafts and caveolae) contribute to the formation of MR visible intracellular mobile lipids in cells undergoing apoptosis *(8)*. Neutral triglyceride resonances seen at 1.3 ($-CH_2-$, methylene) and 0.9 ($-CH_3$, methyl) ppm are the largest contributors to the nuclear magnetic resonance (NMR) visible lipid proton signal. Polyunsaturated fatty acids, in particular the 18:1 and 18:2, that resonate at 5.3 and 2.8 ppm, respectively, however, also generate a significant NMR visible signal *(9)*. The lysosomal processing of damaged mitochondria by catabolic lipid enzymes including sphingomyelinase and phospholipases A1 and A2, which rapidly generate fatty acids, glycerol, and phosphodiesters, may be the source of the mobile lipid signal that arises within the cytoplasm during apoptosis *(10)*. Lysosomally processed mitochondrial lipids subsequently form cytoplasmic droplets, also known as myelinoid bodies (Oil-Red O positive), and contain markedly osmiophilic membranes (at electron microscopy) that are believed to be end-stage autophagic vacuoles (apoptotic bodies). Outside the brain, however, water-suppressed lipid proton MRS remains a challenge due to physiological motion and the nonspecific "bleeding in" of the very strong lipid signal from normal adipose tissue.

Another approach to image apoptosis with MR is the use of diffusion-weighted pulse sequences known collectively as diffusion-weighted imaging (DWI) *(11)*. This is a relatively new MR technique that takes advantage of the differences between the extracellular, intracellular, and transcellular motion (diffusion) of water molecules in the local cellular environments within a region of interest or voxel. Proton spins that move quickly out of a voxel (i.e., diffuse in a nonrandom fashion) will cause a loss of MR signal as compared to stationary spins that have a relatively higher MR signal. The majority of the DWI signal relates to extracellular space and perfusion. Therefore any contraction of the extracellular environment, such as seen with cellular swelling (restricted diffusion), will cause a signal loss that can be displayed as a bright signal on DWI images (by convention) or as a dark signal on a map of diffusion, i.e., the so-called "average diffusion coefficient (ADC)" mapping. Diffusion-weighted imaging can therefore be used to distinguish between viable and necrotic tumor, as the latter will have more free water and thus a higher signal compared to viable tissue. It has been used to determine the efficacy of treatment of marrow or soft tissue tumor because a treated (presumably necrotic) tumor will have higher signal on DWI compared to a viable treatment-resistant tumor *(12, 13)*.

The relationship to DWI changes after therapy and apoptosis specifically (as opposed to necrosis) is unclear. An early characteristic of apoptosis, seen both *in vitro (14)* and *in vivo (15)* within treated tumor cells, is the contraction of cytoplasmic volume with an associated decrease in ADC and T2 values. There is a balance over time after tissue injury (or treatment) between necrosis (which shows increases in ADC) and apoptosis (which shows a decrease in ADC) as damaged apoptotic cells that are not cleared by adjacent cells or phagocytes eventually swell and mimic necrotic cells as they lose both energy and membrane integrity *(16)*. The use of DWI as a marker of apoptosis could therefore be confusing and give conflicting results, depending on the time and precise mechanisms of cell death *(17)*.

More recent DWI work by Valonen *et al. (18)* and Carano *et al. (19)*, however, seems to validate the use of *in vivo* multispectral MR analyses to distinguish viable from necrotic tumors in animal models of treated glioma and human colorectal carcinoma, respectively. Carano *et al.* also found an increase in proton density (M_0) of subcutaneous adipose tissue with respect to viable tumor that can allow for the separation of the signal of the tumor, which can have ADC and T2 values similar to fat, both prior to and after treatment.

An intriguing new set of MR pulse sequences has been developed that focuses on the imaging of ^{23}Na nuclei (quadrapolar nuclei that resonant at 106 MHz at 9.4T) and might prove useful for the imaging of apoptosis *(20)*. While ^{23}Na nuclei generate 9.25% of the NMR signal of ^{1}H (protons), they present in 100% abundance in living tissues. ^{23}Na binds strongly to membranes that contain both phosphatidylcholine (PC) and phosphatidylserine (PS) but not to membranes of PC alone. This high selectivity may permit an alternative MR method to detect apoptotic and/or necrotic cells, as both conditions generate significant (greater than 2- to 5-fold) increases in bound versus free ^{23}Na nuclei as deduced by ^{23}Na NMR relaxation curve analyses.

Finally, it maybe possible to use intravenously administered MR contrast agents labeled with iron particles or gadolinium chelates to localize apoptotic tissue *in vivo*. One possible method utilizes an iron nanoparticulate that has a positive charge that is selective, at least *in vitro*, for apoptotic cells *(21)*. Another iron particulate tracer developed for MR is based on synaptotagim I, a human protein that selectively binds to PS on the surface of apoptotic cells *in vitro* and *in vivo (22, 23)*. Both these and other MR tracers, however, suffer from the inherently low sensitivity of iron- or gadolinium-based agents *(24)*. MR tracers typically require concentrations in the micromolar to millimolar range for imaging that can dramatically increase the potential cost and chances for adverse reactions compared to single-photon emission computed tomography (SPECT) or positron emission tomography (PET) tracers, which give satisfactory signals at the nanomolar to picomolar range *(23)*.

3. DETECTION OF APOPTOSIS WITH ULTRASOUND AND COMPUTED TOMOGRAPHY

High-frequency ultrasound (40 MHz or greater) has been used to detect the unique specular reflections of apoptotic cells *in vitro* and *in vivo (25)*. Backscatter from apoptotic nuclei is up to 6-fold greater compared to nonapoptotic cellular nuclei. The specific nuclear features resolved at 40 MHz include fragmentation of DNA and chromatin condensation, which occur relatively late in the apoptotic cascade. Unfortunately there is significant energy loss with the soft tissues at these higher frequencies that currently limits high-frequency ultrasound to the study of the skin and other superficial structures. High-frequency ultrasound can be useful to study the brain of infants. The open fontanelles provide excellent sonographic windows for the high-frequency ultrasonographic study of apoptosis known to be associated with hypoxic ischemic injury *(26)*.

Contrast-enhanced ultrasound may also be applied to the study of apoptosis in a fashion similar to MR agents. The development of novel microbubble-based contrast agents for ultrasound, however, has focused on blood pool and macrophage/reticuloendothelial system (RES) for liver/spleen/lymph node and atherosclerotic plaque imaging *(27–29)*. Most of these blood pool agents are composed of lipid, albumin, or perfluorocarbon shells encapsulating microbubbles <5 µm in diameter, permitting easy access to all portions of the microcirculation. Because of their size and physical characteristics, these agents are confined to the imaging of the vascular space. There is, however, the potential to direct biotinylated coated microbubbles with a number of avidin-labeled molecules, including antiintegrin $\alpha_v\beta_3$, anti-P-selectin, and antiintercellular adhesion molecule-1 (ICAM-1) antibodies *(30, 31)*. Although it should be possible to label microbubbles with apoptotic-specific agents such as annexin V, it is unlikely that a sufficient concentration would localize at the areas of interest to permit reliable *in vivo* imaging.

There has been little progress in the development of CT contrast agents beyond lipophilic and nanoparticulate iodinated agents for blood pool, liver, spleen, lymph node, and bone marrow imaging *(32–34)*. Of the various imaging modalities, CT requires at least millimolar concentrations of radiopaque material for imaging. This requirement makes it doubtful that CT agents could specifically identify changes in PS expression on small groups of cells. As a result, the use of CT to detect apoptosis appears to be limited.

4. RADIONUCLIDE IMAGING OF APOPTOSIS

Since Blankenberg described the use of radiolabeled annexin V for *in vivo* imaging of apoptosis *(35)*, there have been multiple studies utilizing this agent as a noninvasive marker of cellular injury in a number of human diseases *(36)*. Annexin V [one of more than 13 annexins identified thus far *(37)*] is a 36-kDa human protein with a nanomolar affinity for apoptotic cells, based on the expression of PS on the outer leaflet of the plasma membrane *(38)*. A more complete discussion of the structure and function of annexin V and its binding to PS-expressing membrane lipid bilayers can be found in several recent review articles *(39–42)*.

Human imaging studies used recombinant human annexin V labeled with ^{99m}Tc to detect thrombi in the atria. This work was a direct extension of the experimental studies in pigs with atrial thrombi *(43)*. Annexin V was labeled with 4,5-bisthioacetamidopentanoyl (BTAP, also referred to as N_2S_2) as linker *(44)*. This method transchelates the ^{99m}Tc from glucoheptonate to the active ester 2,3,5,6-tetrafluoro-4,5-bis-*S*-(1-ethoxyethyl)mercaptoacetamidopentanoate *(45)*. Subsequently, the ^{99m}Tc active ester is conjugated to the lysine functional groups on annexin V. The preparation of the ^{99m}Tc-rh-annexin V tracer with the N_2S_2 linker required five time-consuming steps: (1) preparation of the ^{99m}Tc-glucoheptonate; (2) formulation of the phenthioate ligand; (3) conjugation of the [^{99m}Tc]technetium ligand ester to lysine functional groups on rh-annexin V; (4) purification of the conjugate on a Sephadex G-25 gel filtration column; and (5) a final dilution for patient administration.

Even with the technical complexity of preparing the radiopharmaceutical, ^{99m}Tc-rh-annexin V labeled with the N_2S_2 linker was employed in two clinical trials. The first trial by Narula *et al. (46)* examined the efficacy of radiolabeled annexin V for the screening of heart transplant recipients for acute rejection. The rationale for utilizing annexin imaging in these patients is the induction of immunologically mediated apoptotic cell death in the cardiac myocytes of the transplanted heart. Vriens *et al.* had demonstrated the feasibility of this imaging approach in a laboratory study *(47)*. Narula *et al.* studied 18 cardiac allograft recipients: 13 patients had negative and five had positive myocardial uptake of annexin V as seen by ECG-gated SPECT imaging. Endomyocardial biopsies obtained within 2 days of the scan demonstrated histological evidence of at least moderate transplant rejection and caspase-3 staining, an enzyme activated early in the apoptotic cascade, suggesting apoptosis in their biopsy specimens.

Belhocine *et al. (48)* describe their findings in 15 cancer patients with late stage small cell and non-small-cell lung cancers (SCLC and NSCLC), Hodgkin's and non-Hodgkin's lymphomas (HL and NHL), and metastatic breast cancers (BC). Annexin V SPECT was performed immediately prior to starting chemotherapy (day −2 and day −1) and immediately after the first course of treatment (day +1 and day +2). A negative annexin V study posttherapy, that is no change in tumor uptake of tracer from pretreatment baseline, correlated well with no tumor response in six of eight patients. Two women (two BC) of the eight total patients with negative posttreatment annexin V studies actually had a clinically significant response to Taxol-based chemotherapy. On the other hand, all seven patients with increased tumor uptake over baseline (positive annexin V study) had an objective tumor response. Five of these patients showed increased annexin V uptake at 40–48 h postchemotherapy (one NHL, one HL, one SCLC, and two NSCLC), and two patients had increases in annexin V uptake observed at 20–24 h posttreatment (one NSCLC and one SCLC). Taken together, these results suggest a variability in optimal timing with regard to the cancer type and emphasize the need to determine the best time in which to administer radiolabeled annexin V to determine therapeutic response in the design of all future oncology trials *(49)*.

To eliminate the difficulty in preparing the material, alternative labeling approaches were sought. Recent human studies with ^{99m}Tc-annexin V utilized hydrazino nicotinamide (HYNIC) as a coupling molecule *(50)*. This approach uses HYNIC [succinimidyl (6-hydrazinopyridine-3-carboxylic acid)], also known as succinimidyl (6-hydrazinonicotinic acid), which is covalently attached to rh-annexin V; this can later be labeled with ^{99m}Tc, performed simply by reacting the conjugate with [^{99m}Tc]pertechnetate in the presence of stannous tricine for 5–10 min at room temperature. The whole procedure has been reduced to a standardized two-vial kit that can be ready for patient use within 30 min of receiving 20–30 mCi of sterile [^{99m}Tc]pertechnetate from a local radiopharmacy or generator.

The HYNIC method of labeling overcomes one of the major disadvantages of the N_2S_2 method: the large degree of hepatic uptake and excretion of BTAP-annexin V into the bowel, which effectively precludes imaging in the abdomen. Both animal and human studies with HYNIC-annexin V have shown a more favorable biodistribution with little to no gut excretion as compared with BTAP-annexin V. Unfortunately, although ^{99m}Tc HYNIC-annexin V is not concentrated in the liver or excreted in the bowel, it concentrates in the cortex of the kidney, limiting visualization of any structures in this region *(51)*.

Multiple new clinical trials are ongoing with HYNIC-annexin V including the imaging of the efficacy of chemotherapy in oncology patients *(52–54)*, acute myocardial infarction *(55, 56)*, rheumatoid arthritis (R. Hustinx and C. Beckers, Liege, Belgium, personal communication), atherosclerosis (vulnerable plaque) *(57, 58)*, and acute stroke (F. Blankenberg, Stanford, personal communication).

A follow-up phase II–III study in patients with late stage (IIIB and IV) small-cell and non-small-cell lung cancer with HYNIC-annexin V has been undertaken by Belhochine *et al. (59)*. Preliminary results of the first 22 evaluable patients showed that late imaging (24 h posttracer injection or 48 h postchemotherapy) is likely unnecessary to obtain an optimal signal as was done in the previous trial using N_2S_2-labeled annexin V. At 24 h after the start of treatment, in the subset of patients with a partial response to platinum-based chemotherapy ($n = 5$), only one patient had increased tumor uptake of ^{99m}Tc-Hynic-annexin V over pretreatment baseline, while the four remaining patients showed an unexpected decrease in tracer uptake. The imaging pattern observed in these four patients having a tumor response but without an increase in annexin V uptake stresses the importance of determining the optimal timing for the imaging of apoptosis in the clinical setting.

Interestingly, ^{99m}Tc annexin V uptake in tumor immediately prior to chemotherapy was strongly correlated with tumor response, that is 100% of responding patients had some degree of tracer uptake above soft tissue background before treatment, thereby suggesting the presence of ongoing apoptosis in the tumor, and presumably the ability of these tumors to respond apoptotically to chemotherapy. As there is a significantly increased expression of PS in vascular endothelial cells seen *in vitro* during neoangiogenesis, annexin V could also be an imaging marker of tumor vessels *(60)*. Tumor vessels may indeed be the first cell population affected by chemotherapy prior to actual tumor cell death, which may in part explain at least one of the peaks of annexin V seen after the start of treatment *(61)*.

The 24 h time point in Belhocine's human study may in fact represent one of the three nadirs of the biphasic time course of annexin V uptake analogous to that seen in the diseased spleens of Doxorubicin treated lymphoma-bearing BALB/c mice observed by Mandl *et al. (62)*. In another study with cyclophosphamide-treated rats with flank allogeneic hepatomas (KDH-8) it was found that the peak of annexin V uptake occurred 20 h after administration of the drug *(63)*. The timing of imaging after treatment appears to be critical for the proper use of annexin V as a marker of therapeutic efficacy.

Timing is also an important factor in imaging apoptosis following an acute myocardial infarct in both animal models and humans *(64, 65)*. Thimister's clinical study of patients with acute infarction *(55)* demonstrated the highest annexin V localization within the first day after infarction, with partial resolution by day 3–4 and complete resolution by day 8 in regions of ischemic injury (as defined by a persistent perfusion deficit with ^{99m}Tc-Sestamibi SPECT). These results suggest that apoptotic cells that concentrated tracer were removed from the ischemic zone or that these cells recovered in terms of both function and viability with loss of PS positivity. The reduction of perfusion abnormalities with restoration of regional wall motion 1 week following infarction suggests the latter explanation. If it is true, then annexin V imaging may be vastly more sensitive to cellular stress than previously thought and may be a true marker of tissues at risk that have the potential for salvage with prompt therapeutic intervention *(66)*.

Alternative methods to radiolabel annexin V include the use of self-chelating annexin V mutants that have 50–75% less uptake in the kidneys in mice and rats as compared with HYNIC-annexin V *(67–69)*. These approaches to labeling annexin would allow higher doses of activity to be safely administered, as well as permit the imaging of renal apoptosis. The best studied annexin V mutant with an endogenous site for ^{99m}Tc chelation is known as V117. The protein contains six amino acids added at the N-terminus, followed by amino acids 1–320 of wild-type annexin V. The amino acid Cys-316 is also mutated to serine in this molecule. Technetium-99m chelation is thought to occur via formation of an N_3S structure involving the N-terminal cysteine and the immediately adjacent amino acids. The purified protein is then reduced and can be stored for later labeling with ^{99m}Tc using glucoheptonate as the exchange reagent.

A newer form of self-chelating annexin V that is easier to produce as compared with V117 is the V128 mutant, a fusion protein with an endogenous Tc chelation site (Ala-Gly-Gly-Cys-Gly-His) added to the N-terminus of annexin V *(70, 71)*. Both V117 and V128 have major advantages over the HYNIC chelator with regard to renal retention of ^{99m}Tc, with attendant decreased abdominal background and renal radiation dose (Figs. 1 and 2).

In another approach designed specifically for PET imaging, annexin V has been successfully labeled with fluorine-18 (^{18}F) using *N*-succinimidyl 4-fluorobenzoate *(72–74)*. ^{18}F-annexin V offers an advantageous biodistribution with much lower uptake in the liver, spleen, and kidney compared to HYNIC-annexin V. The use of PET imaging with annexin V will allow absolute quantitation of uptake in the tumor before and after the initial dose of therapy. This will be particularly important when serial images are required for evaluation of the effectiveness of therapy in sepsis, clinical flares of autoimmune disease, myocardial or cerebral ischemic/reperfusion injury, or acute organ transplant rejection.

Another intriguing possibility for improving target uptake of annexin V is being offered by labeling with a longer lived radionuclide that could permit a longer imaging window. Two approaches to this problem have been tested in mice. The first approach uses radioiodine ^{124}I-labeled annexin V for PET imaging *(75)*. The ^{124}I isotope has a half-life of 4.1 days but a higher positron energy (2.1 meV, max) compared to ^{18}F (633 keV, max), which limits both the resolution of images recorded with the agent and the dose that can be administered. ^{111}In in parallel with the use of a PEGylated form of the protein is another potentially useful form of long-lived annexin V *(76)*. Labeling of annexin V with ^{111}In consists of a one-step procedure to introduce both polyethylene glycol (PEG) and the metal chelator diethylenetriaminepentaacetic acid (DTPA) to annexin V through a heterofunctional PEG precursor. The PEG precursor contains DTPA at one end and an amine-reactive isothiocyanate (SCN–) functional group at the other end. Protein conjugation is achieved by mixing the proteins and the PEG precursor SCN-PEG-DTPA in an aqueous solution. Unlike the unPEGylated annexin V, the PEGylated annexin V penetrates further in depth, thereby reaching superficial as well as central zones of apoptotic tissues.

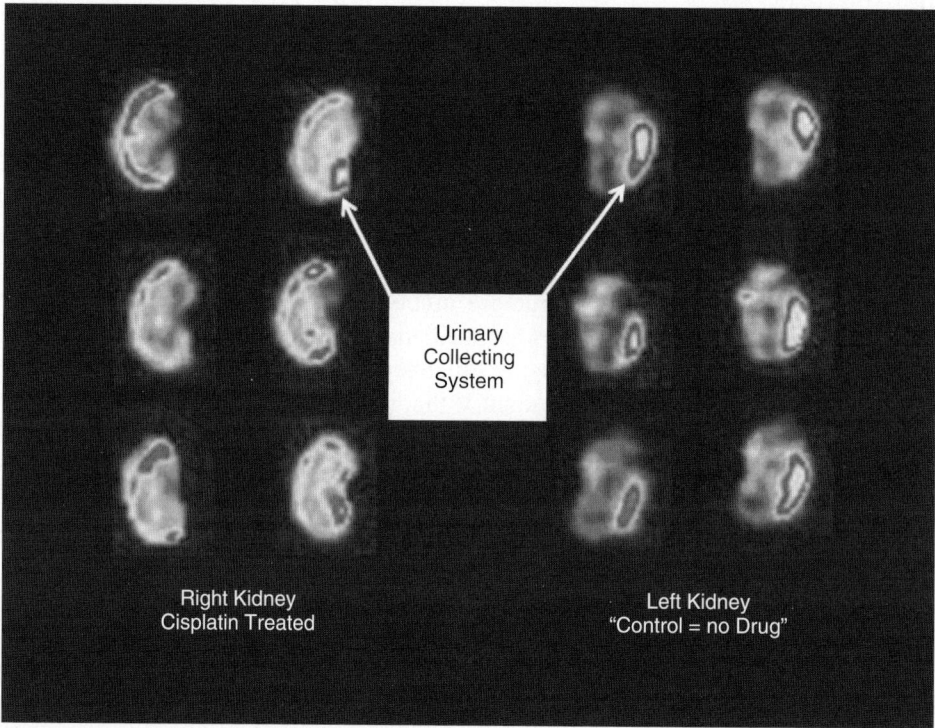

Fig. 1. ^{99m}Tc-annexin V128 imaging of cisplatin-induced nephropathy. Serial coronal 1.2-mm SPECT slices are shown of the right and left kidneys of an adult male BALB/c mouse 24 h after intravenous injection of cisplatin (5 mg/kg, renal cortical apoptosis inducing, nonnecrotic dose). During injection of the drug the vascular pedicle of the left kidney was transiently occluded (15 min ischemic time) with a microaneurysm clip thereby preventing the drug from reaching the left (control) kidney without any renal damage. As the circulatory half-life of cisplatin is only several minutes in mice, the majority of this renal tubular excreted drug passed through the nonoccluded right kidney generating a differential effect with respect to the left control kidney. SPECT images were obtained 20 min after tail vein injection of 1–2 mCi of ^{99m}Tc-annexin V128 (10–20 μg/kg of protein) with a single-headed A-SPECT-dedicated animal system (Gamma Medica, Inc., Los Angeles, CA) equipped with a 1-mm pinhole collimator (64 × 64 matrix, 20 sec/step, 64 steps, 360° rotation, 0.5 mm resolution). Note the marked heterogeneous uptake of tracer in the cortex of the right drug-treated kidney as compared to the left "control" kidney. Also note that unbound tracer is excreted into the renal collecting system (arrows mark the renal pelvis bilaterally). (*See* color plate.)

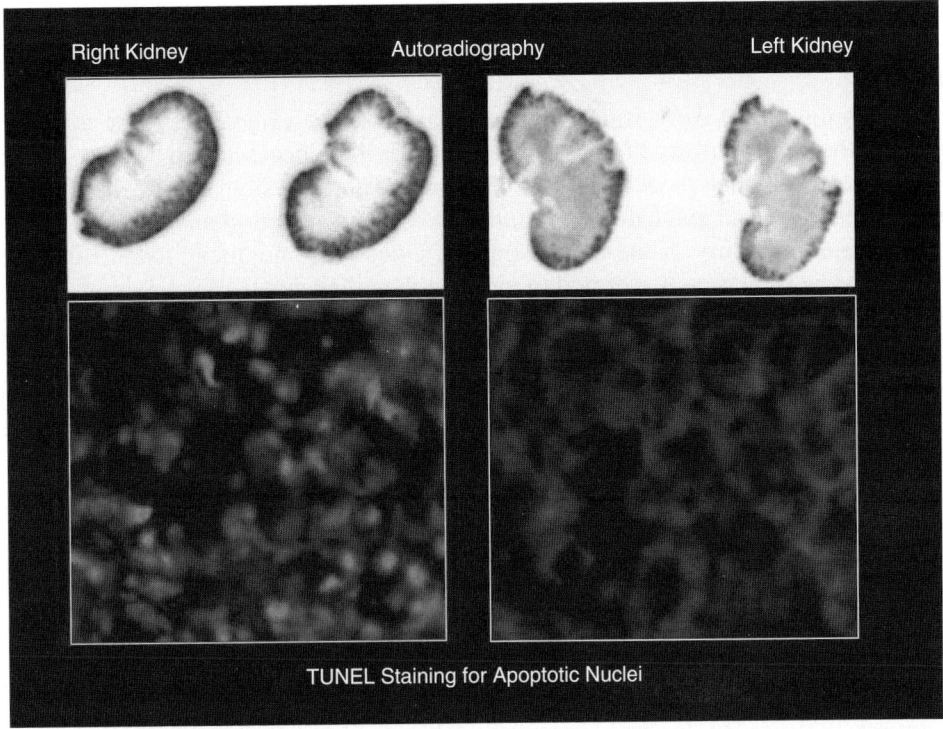

Fig. 2. Autoradiographic and histological analyses of drug and control kidneys. Digital images of 60-μm coronal frozen slices through the hila of the right (drug) and left (control) kidneys from the animal shown in Fig. 1 are shown. Images were obtained after exposure overnight on image phosphor. Note the marked heterogeneous increased tracer uptake of the renal cortex of the right drug-treated kidney as compared with the left. Fluorescent TUNEL staining for apoptotic nuclei from the right and left kidneys is shown below the autoradiographs (40×). Note the numerous TUNEL-positive cells in the treated versus untreated renal cortex (red). (*See* color plate.)

5. SUMMARY

In vivo imaging of apoptosis identifies the status of disease in evolution. Inflammatory cells, including granulocytes, lymphocytes and macrophages, undergo apoptosis when they have completed their assigned tasks. Although apoptosis can be identified by a number of imaging techniques, only MR and radionuclide approaches appear to provide reliable data. Unfortunately, in spite of its excellent spatial resolution, MR detection of apoptosis is difficult to apply in routine practice. Radiolabeled annexin imaging, on the other hand, appears to be a safe and effective way to localize apoptosis *in vivo*.

To date, over 300 patients have been imaged with radiolabeled annexin, without a major adverse event attributable to the imaging agent. These data suggest the agent is safe. Preliminary human studies suggest that for patients with subacute to chronic inflammation, imaging with radiolabeled annexin V permits identification of active, severe inflammation. The technique can distinguish active from fibrotic disease in patients with rheumatoid arthritis, and preliminary evidence suggests it will play a significant role in distinguishing atheroma likely to progress from those lesions that are stable. In patients with neoplasia, an intriguing finding is the apparent importance of some annexin uptake in tumors prior to therapy, as an indication of the likelihood of response.

There is significant work still be done to maximize the value of imaging apoptosis. To define the clinical utility of annexin imaging it will be necessary to develop specific quantitative techniques to define the relationship of total lesion size to the extent of annexin uptake and to standardize the interval between injection and imaging to optimize the reproducibility of the measurements. Once these points are addressed, large clinical studies should be performed to validate the clinical role of annexin imaging in patient management.

ACKNOWLEDGMENT

Supported in part by NIH Grant EB000898.

REFERENCES

1. Blankenberg FG, Katsikis PD, Storrs RW, Beaulieu C, Spielman D, Chen JY, Naumovski L, Tait JF. Quantitative analysis of apoptotic cell death using proton nuclear magnetic resonance spectroscopy. *Blood* 1997;89:3778–3786.
2. Al-Saffar NM, Titley JC, Robertson D, Clarke PA, Jackson LE, Leach MO, Ronen SM. Apoptosis is associated with triacylglycerol accumulation in Jurkat T-cells. *Br J Cancer* 2002;86:963–970.
3. Huang Z, Tong Y, Wang J, Huang Y. NMR studies of the relationship between the changes of membrane lipids and the cisplatin-resistance of A549/DDP cells. *Cancer Cell Int* 2003;3:5.
4. Bezabeh T, Mowat MR, Jarolim L, Greenberg AH, Smith IC. Detection of drug-induced apoptosis and necrosis in human cervical carcinoma cells using (1)H NMR spectroscopy. *Cell Death Differ* 2001;8:219–224.
5. Hakumaki JM, Poptani H, Sandmair AM, Yla-Herttuala S, Kauppinen RA. 1H MRS detects polyunsaturated fatty acid accumulation during gene therapy of glioma: Implications for the in vivo detection of apoptosis. *Nat Med* 1999;5:1323–1327.
6. Hakumaki JM, Brindle KM. Visualizing apoptosis using nuclear magnetic resonance. *Trends Pharmacol Sci* 2003;24:146–149.
7. Brauer M. In vivo monitoring of apoptosis. *Prog Neuropsychopharmacol Biol Psychiatry* 2003;27:323–331.
8. Ferretti A, Knijn A, Raggi C, Sargiacomo M. High-resolution proton NMR measures mobile lipids associated with triton-resistant membrane domains in haematopoietic K562 cells lacking or expressing caveolin-1. *Eur Biophys J* 2003;32:83–95.
9. Griffin JL, Lehtimaki KK, Valonen PK, Grohn OH, Kettunen MI, Yla-Herttuala S, Pitkanen A, Nicholson JK, Kauppinen RA. Assignment of 1H nuclear magnetic resonance visible polyunsaturated fatty acids in BT4C gliomas undergoing ganciclovir-thymidine kinase gene therapy-induced programmed cell death. *Cancer Res* 2003;63:3195–3201.
10. Delikatny EJ, Cooper WA, Brammah S, Sathasivam N, Rideout DC. Nuclear magnetic resonance-visible lipids induced by cationic lipophilic chemotherapeutic agents are accompanied by increased lipid droplet formation and damaged mitochondria. *Cancer Res* 2002;62:1394–1400.
11. Bammer R. Basic principles of diffusion-weighted imaging. *Eur J Radiol* 2003;45:169–184.
12. Byun WM, Shin SO, Chang Y, Lee SJ, Finsterbusch J, Frahm J. Diffusion-weighted MR imaging of metastatic disease of the spine: Assessment of response to therapy. *Am J Neuroradiol* 2002;23:906–912.
13. Geschwind JF, Artemov D, Abraham S, Omdal D, Huncharek MS, McGee C, Arepally A, Lambert D, Venbrux AC, Lund GB. Chemoembolization of liver tumor in a rabbit model: Assessment of tumor cell death with diffusion-weighted MR imaging and histologic analysis. *J Vasc Interv Radiol* 2000;11:1245–1255.
14. Hortelano S, Garcia-Martin ML, Cerdan S, Castrillo A, Alvarez AM, Bosca L. Intracellular water motion decreases in apoptotic macrophages after caspase activation. *Cell Death Differ* 2001;8:1022–1028.

15. Schmitz JE, Kettunen MI, Hu DE, Brindle KM. 1H MRS-visible lipids accumulate during apoptosis of lymphoma cells in vitro and in vivo. *Magn Reson Med* 2005;54:43–50.
16. Abe O, Nakane M, Aoki S, Hayashi N, Masumoto T, Kunimatsu A, Mori H, Tamura A, Ohtomo K. MR imaging of postischemic neuronal death in the substantia nigra and thalamus following middle cerebral artery occlusion in rats. *NMR Biomed* 2003;16:152–159.
17. Brauer M. In vivo monitoring of apoptosis. *Progr Neuro-Psychopharmacol Biol Psychiatry* 2003; 27:323–331.
18. Valonen PK, Lehtimaki KK, Vaisanen TH, Kettunen MI, Grohn OH, Yla-Herttuala S, Kauppinen RA. Water diffusion in a rat glioma during ganciclovir-thymidine kinase gene therapy-induced programmed cell death in vivo: Correlation with cell density. *J Magn Reson Imaging* 2004;19:389–396.
19. Carano RA, Ross AL, Ross J, Williams SP, Koeppen H, Schwall RH, Van Bruggen N. Quantification of tumor tissue populations by multispectral analysis. *Magn Reson Med* 2004;51:542–551.
20. Lupu M, Ojcius D, Perfettini JL, Patry J, Dimicoli JL, Mispelter J. Evidences on sodium ions compartmentalization in biological systems due to pathological states. A noninvasive NMR study. *Biochimie* 2003;85:849–861.
21. Schellenberger EA, Reynolds F, Weissleder R, Josephson L. Surface-functionalized nanoparticle library yields probes for apoptotic cells. *Chembiochem* 2004;5:275–279.
22. Brindle KM. Molecular imaging using magnetic resonance: New tools for the development of tumour therapy. *Br J Radiol* 2003;76(Spec No 2):S111–S117.
23. Blankenberg FG, Eckelman WC, Strauss HW, et al. Role of radionuclide imaging in trials of antiangiogenic therapy. *Acad Radiol* 2000;7:851–867.
24. Zhao M, Beauregard DA, Loizou L, Davletov B, Brindle KM. Non-invasive detection of apoptosis using magnetic resonance imaging and a targeted contrast agent. *Nature Med* 2001;7:1241–1244.
25. Czarnota GJ, Kolios MC, Abraham J, Portnoy M, Ottensmeyer FP, Hunt JW, Sherar MD. Ultrasound imaging of apoptosis: High-resolution non-invasive monitoring of programmed cell death in vitro, in situ and in vivo. *Br J Cancer* 1999;81:520–527.
26. Chamnanvanakij S, Margraf LR, Burns D, Perlman JM. Apoptosis and white matter injury in preterm infants. *Pediatr Dev Pathol* 2002;5:184–189.
27. Yucel C, Ozdemir H, Gurel S, Ozer S, Arac M. Detection and differential diagnosis of hepatic masses using pulse inversion harmonic imaging during the liver-specific late phase of contrast enhancement with Levovist. *J Clin Ultrasound* 2002;30:203–212.
28. Harvey CJ, Pilcher JM, Eckersley RJ, Blomley MJK, Cosgrove DO. Advances in ultrasound. *Clin Radiol* 2002;57:157–177.
29. Hohmann J, Albrecht T, Hoffmann CW, Wolf KJ. Ultrasonographic detection of focal liver lesions: Increased sensitivity and specificity with microbubble contrast agents. *Eur J Radiol* 2003;46:147–159.
30. Lanza GM, Wallace KD, Scott MJ, Cacheris WP, Abendschein DR, Christy DH, Sharkey AM, Miller JG, Gaffney PJ, Wickline SA. A novel site-targeted ultrasonic contrast agent with broad biomedical application. *Circulation* 1996;94:3334–3340.
31. Lindner JR. Detection of inflamed plaques with contrast ultrasound. *Am J Cardiol* 2002;21; 90(10C):32L–35L.
32. Choi BI, Han JK, Kim YI, Kim HC, Park JH, Kim CW, Han MC. Combined hepatocellular and cholangiocarcinoma of the liver: Sonography, CT, angiography, and iodized-oil CT with pathologic correlation. *Abdom Imaging* 1994;19:43–46.
33. Gazelle GS, Wolf GL, McIntire GL, Bacon ER, Na G, Halpern EF, Toner JL. Hepatic imaging with iodinated nanoparticles: A comparison with iohexol in rabbits. *Acad Radiol* 1995;2:700–704.
34. Li C, Yu D, Kan Z, Yang DJ, Tansey W, Kuang LR, Wallace S. Biodistribution of cyclic carbonate of ioxilan: A radiopaque particulate macrophage imaging agent. *Acad Radiol* 1996;3:500–506.
35. Blankenberg FG, Katsikis PD, Tait JF, Davis RE, Naumovski L, Ohtsuki K, Kopiwoda S, Abrams MJ, Darkes M, Robbins RC, Maecker HT, Strauss HW. In vivo detection and imaging of phosphatidylserine expression during programmed cell death. *Proc Natl Acad Sci USA* 1998; 95:6349–6354.
36. Blankenberg F, Mari C, Strauss HW. Imaging cell death in vivo. *Q J Nucl Med* 2003;47:337–348.
37. Camors E, Monceau V, Charlemagne D. R Annexins and Ca(2+) handling in the heart. *Cardiovasc Res* 2005;65:793–802.
38. Allen RT, Hunter WJ 3rd, Agrawal DK. Morphological and biochemical characterization and analysis of apoptosis. *J Pharmacol Toxicol Methods* 1997;37:215–228.

39. Bohm I, Schild H. Apoptosis: The complex scenario for a silent cell death. *Mol Imaging Biol* 2003; 5:2–14.
40. Rand JH. The annexinopathies: A new category of diseases. *Biochim Biophys Acta* 2000;1498(2–3): 169–173.
41. Russo-Marie F. Annexin V and phospholipid metabolism. *Clin Chem Lab Med* 1999;37:287–291.
42. van Engeland M, Nieland LJ, Ramaekers FC, Schutte B, Reutelingsperger CP. Annexin V-affinity assay: A review on an apoptosis detection system based on phosphatidylserine exposure. *Cytometry* 1998;31:1–9.
43. Stratton JR, Dewhurst TA, Kasina S, Reno JM, Cerqueira MD, Baskin DG, Tait JF. Selective uptake of radiolabeled annexin V on acute porcine left atrial thrombi. *Circulation* 1995;92:3113–3121.
44. Kemerink GJ, Boersma HH, Thimister PWL, Hofstra L, Liem IH, Pakbiers M-TW, Janssen D, Reutelingsperger CPM, Heidendal GAK. Biodistribution and dosimetry of 99mTc-BTAP-annexin-V in humans. *Eur J Nucl Med* 2001;28:1373–1378.
45. Kasina S, Rao TN, Srinivasan A, et al. Development and biologic evaluation of a kit for preformed chelate technetium-99m radiolabeling of an antibody fab fragment using a diamide dimercaptide chelating agent. *J Nucl Med* 1991;32:1445–1451.
46. Narula J, Acio ER, Narula N, Samuels LE, Fyfe B, Wood D, Fitzpatrick JM, Raghunath PN, Tomaszewski JE, Kelly C, Steinmetz N, Green A, Tait JF, Leppo J, Blankenberg FG, Jain D, Strauss HW. Annexin-V imaging for noninvasive detection of cardiac allograft rejection. *Nat Med* 2001;7:1347–1352.
47. Vriens PW, Blankenberg FG, Stoot JH, Ohtsuki K, Berry GJ, Tait JF, Strauss HW, Robbins RC. The use of technetium Tc 99m annexin V for in vivo imaging of apoptosis during cardiac allograft rejection. *J Thorac Cardiovasc Surg* 1998;116:844–852.
48. Belhocine T, Steinmetz N, Hustinx R, Bartsch P, Jerusalem G, Seidel L, Rigo P, Green A. Increased uptake of the apoptosis-imaging agent (99m)Tc recombinant human annexin V in human tumors after one course of chemotherapy as a predictor of tumor response and patient prognosis. *Clin Cancer Res* 2002;8:2766–2774.
49. Blankenberg F. To scan or not to scan, it is a question of timing: Technetium-99m-annexin V radionuclide imaging assessment of treatment efficacy after one course of chemotherapy. *Clin Cancer Res* 2002;8:2757–2758.
50. Kemerink GJ, Liu X, Kieffer D, Ceyssens S, Mortelmans L, Verbruggen AM, Steinmetz ND, Vanderheyden J-L, Green A, Verbeke K. Safety, biodistribution, and dosimetry of 99mTc-HYNIC-annexin V, a novel human recombinant annexin V for human application. *J Nucl Med* 2003;44:947–952.
51. Boersma HH, Liem IH, Kemerink GJ, Thimister PW, Hofstra L, Stolk LM, van Heerde WL, Pakbiers MT, Janssen D, Beysens AJ, Reutelingsperger CP, Heidendal GA. Comparison between human pharmacokinetics and imaging properties of two conjugation methods for 99mTc-annexin A5. *Br J Radiol* 2003;76:553–560.
52. Blankenberg FG. Molecular imaging: The latest generation of contrast agents and tissue characterization techniques. *J Cell Biochem* 2003;90:443–453.
53. Haas RL, de Jong D, Valdes Olmos RA, Hoefnagel CA, van den Heuvel I, Zerp SF, Bartelink H, Verheij M. In vivo imaging of radiation-induced apoptosis in follicular lymphoma patients. *Int J Radiat Oncol Biol Phys* 2004;59:782–787.
54. Kartachova M, Haas RL, Olmos RA, Hoebers FJ, van Zandwijk N, Verheij M. In vivo imaging of apoptosis by 99mTc-annexin V scintigraphy: Visual analysis in relation to treatment response. *Radiother Oncol* 2004;72:333–339.
55. Thimister PW, Hofstra L, Liem IH, Boersma HH, Kemerink G, Reutelingsperger CP, Heidendal GA. In vivo detection of cell death in the area at risk in acute myocardial infarction. *J Nucl Med* 2003; 44:391–396.
56. Narula J, Strauss HW. Invited commentary: P.S.* I love you: Implications of phosphatidyl serine (PS) reversal in acute ischemic syndromes. *J Nucl Med* 2003;44:397–399.
57. Kolodgie FD, Petrov A, Virmani R, Narula N, Verjans JW, Weber DK, Hartung D, Steinmetz N, Vanderheyden JL, Vannan MA, Gold HK, Reutelingsperger CP, Hofstra L, Narula J. Targeting of apoptotic macrophages and experimental atheroma with radiolabeled annexin V: A technique with potential for noninvasive imaging of vulnerable plaque. *Circulation* 2003;108:3134–3139.
58. Kiestelaer BLJH, Reutelingsperger CPM, Heidendal GAK, Daemen MJAP, Mess WH, Hofstra L. Noninvasive detection of plaque instability with use of radiolabeled annexin A5 in patients with carotid-artery atherosclerosis. *New Engl J Med* 2004;350:1472–1473.

59. Belhocine T, Steinmetz N, Li C, Green A, Blankenberg FG. The imaging of apoptosis with the radiolabeled annexin V: Optimal timing for clinical feasibility. *Technol Cancer Res Treat* 2004;3: 23–32.
60. Ran S, Downes A, Thorpe PE. Increased exposure of anionic phospholipids on the surface of tumor blood vessels. *Cancer Res* 2002;62:6132–6140.
61. van de Wiele C, Lahorte C, Vermeersch H, Loose D, Mervillie K, Steinmetz ND, Vanderheyden JL, Cuvelier CA, Slegers G, Dierck RA. Quantitative tumor apoptosis imaging using technetium-99m-HYNIC annexin V single photon emission computed tomography. *J Clin Oncol* 2003;21:3483–3487.
62. Mandl SJ, Mari C, Edinger M, Negrin RS, Tait JF, Contag CH, Blankenberg FG. Multi-modality imaging identifies key times for annexin V imaging as an early predictor of therapeutic outcome. *Mol Imaging* 2004;3:1–8.
63. Takei T, Kuge Y, Zhao S, Sato M, Strauss HW, Blankenberg FG, Tait JF, Tamaki N. Time course of apoptotic tumor response after a single dose of chemotherapy: Comparison with 99mTc-annexin V uptake and histologic findings in an experimental model. *J Nucl Med* 2004;45:2083–2087.
64. Flotats A, Carrio I. Non-invasive in vivo imaging of myocardial apoptosis and necrosis. *Eur J Nucl Med Mol Imaging* 2003;30:615–630.
65. Taki J, Higuchi T, Kawashima A, Tait JF, Kinuya S, Muramori A, Matsunari I, Nakajima K, Tonami N, Strauss HW. Detection of cardiomyocyte death in a rat model of ischemia and reperfusion using 99mTc-labeled annexin V. *J Nucl Med* 2004;45:1536–1541.
66. Strauss HW, Narula J, Blankenberg FG. Radioimaging to identify myocardial cell death and probably injury. *Lancet* 2000;356:209–212.
67. Tait JF, Brown DS, Gibson DF, Blankenberg FG, Strauss HW. Development and characterization of annexin V mutants with endogenous chelation sites for (99m)Tc. *Bioconjug Chem* 2000;11: 918–925.
68. Belhocine TZ, Tait JF, Vanderheyden JL, Li C, Blankenberg FG. Nuclear medicine in the era of genomics and proteomics: Lessons from annexin V. *J Proteome Res* 2004;3:345–349.
69. Lahorte CM, Vanderheyden JL, Steinmetz N, Van de Wiele C, Dierckx RA, Slegers G. Apoptosis-detecting radioligands: Current state of the art and future perspectives. *Eur J Nucl Med Mol Imaging* 2004;31:887–919.
70. Jin M, Smith C, Hsieh HY, Gibson DF, Tait JF. Essential role of B-helix calcium binding sites in annexin V-membrane binding. *J Biol Chem* 2004;279:40351–40357.
71. Tait JF, Smith C, Blankenberg FG. Structural requirements for in vivo detection of cell death with ^{99m}Tc-annexin V. *J Nucl Med* 2005;46:807–815.
72. Grierson JR, Yagle KJ, Eary JF, Tait JF, Gibson DF, Lewellen B, Link JM, Krohn KA. Production of [F-18]fluoroannexin for imaging apoptosis with PET. *Bioconjug Chem* 2004;15:373–379.
73. Murakami Y, Takamatsu H, Taki J, Tatsumi M, Noda A, Ichise R, Tait JF, Nishimura S. 18F-labelled annexin V: A PET tracer for apoptosis imaging. *Eur J Nucl Med Mol Imaging* 2004; 31:469–474.
74. Yagle KJ, Eary JF, Tait JF, Grierson JR, Link JM, Lewellen B, Gibson DF, Krohn KA. Evaluation of 18F-annexin V as a PET imaging agent in an animal model of apoptosis. *J Nucl Med* 2005;46: 658–666.
75. Collingridge DR, Glaser M, Osman S, Barthel H, Hutchinson OC, Luthra SK, Brady F, Bouchier-Hayes L, Martin SJ, Workman P, Price P, Aboagye EO. In vitro selectivity, in vivo biodistribution and tumour uptake of annexin V radiolabelled with a positron emitting radioisotope. *Br J Cancer* 2003;89:1327–1333.
76. Ke S, Wen X, Wu QP, Wallace S, Charnsangavej C, Stachowiak AM, Stephens CL, Abbruzzese JL, Podoloff DA, Li C. Imaging taxane-induced tumor apoptosis using PEGylated, 111In-labeled annexin V. *J Nucl Med* 2004;45:108–115.
77. D'Arceuil H, Rhine W, de Crespigny A, Yenari M, Tait JF, Strauss WH, Engelhorn T, Kastrup A, Moseley M, Blankenberg FG. 99mTc annexin V imaging of neonatal hypoxic brain injury. *Stroke* 2000;31:2692–2700.
78. Mari C, Karabiyikoglu M, Goris ML, Tait JF, Yenari MA, Blankenberg FG. Detection of focal hypoxic-ischemic injury and neuronal stress in a rodent model of unilateral MCA occlusion/reperfusion using radiolabeled annexin V. *Eur J Nucl Med Mol Imaging* 2004;31:733–739.
79. Post AM, Katsikis PD, Tait JF, Geaghan SM, Strauss HW, Blankenberg FG. Imaging cell death with radiolabeled annexin V in an experimental model of rheumatoid arthritis. *J Nucl Med* 2002;43: 1359–1365.

80. Tokita N, Hasegawa S, Maruyama K, Izumi T, Blankenberg FG, Tait JF, Strauss HW, Nishimura T. 99mTc-Hynic-annexin V imaging to evaluate inflammation and apoptosis in rats with autoimmune myocarditis. *Eur J Nucl Med Mol Imaging* 2003;30:232–238.
81. Blankenberg FG, Tait JF, Blankenberg TA, Post AM, Strauss HW. Imaging macrophages and the apoptosis of granulocytes in a rodent model of subacute and chronic abscesses with radiolabeled monocyte chemotactic peptide-1 and annexin V. *Eur J Nucl Med* 2001;28:1384–1393.
82. Bennink RJ, Peeters M, Rutgeerts P, Mortelmans L. Evaluation of early treatment response and predicting the need for colectomy in active ulcerative colitis with 99mTc-HMPAO white blood cell scintigraphy. *J Nucl Med* 2004;45:1698–1704.
83. Ringheanu M, Daum F, Markowitz J, Levine J, Katz S, Lin X, Silver J. Effects of infliximab on apoptosis and reverse signaling of monocytes from healthy individuals and patients with Crohn's disease. *Inflamm Bowel Dis* 2004;10:801–810.
84. Ogura Y, Martinez OM, Villanueva JC, Tait JF, Strauss HW, Higgins JP, Tanaka K, Esquivel CO, Blankenberg FG, Krams SM. Apoptosis and allograft rejection in the absence of CD8+ T cells. *Transplantation* 2001;71:1827–1834.
85. Ogura Y, Krams SM, Martinez OM, Kopiwoda S, Higgins JP, Esquivel CO, Strauss HW, Tait JF, Blankenberg FG. Radiolabeled annexin V imaging: Diagnosis of allograft rejection in an experimental rodent model of liver transplantation. *Radiology* 2000;214:795–800.
86. Blankenberg FG, Naumovski L, Tait JF, Post AM, Strauss HW. Imaging cyclophosphamide-induced intramedullary apoptosis in rats using 99mTc-radiolabeled annexin V. *J Nucl Med* 2001;42:309–316.
87. Yang P, Smith JR, Damodar KS, Planck SR, Rosenbaum JT. Visualization of cell death in vivo during murine endotoxin-induced uveitis. *Invest Ophthalmol Vis Sci* 2003;44:1993–1997.
88. Podesta F, Romeo G, Liu WH, Krajewski S, Reed JC, Gerhardinger C, Lorenzi M. Bax is increased in the retina of diabetic subjects and is associated with pericyte apoptosis in vivo and in vitro. *Am J Pathol* 2000;156:1025–1032.
89. Jiang S, Moriarty-Craige SE, Orr M, Cai J, Sternberg P Jr, Jones DP. Oxidant-induced apoptosis in human retinal pigment epithelial cells: Dependence on extracellular redox state. *Invest Ophthalmol Vis Sci* 2005;46:1054–1061.
90. Howes KA, Liu Y, Dunaief JL, Milam A, Frederick JM, Marks A, Baehr W. Receptor for advanced glycation end products and age-related macular degeneration. *Invest Ophthalmol Vis Sci* 2004;45:3713–3720.
91. Blankenberg FG, Robbins RC, Stoot JH, Vriens PW, Berry GJ, Tait JF, Strauss HW. Radionuclide imaging of acute lung transplant rejection with annexin V. *Chest* 2000;117:834–840.
92. Xu B, Bulfone-Paus S, Aoyama K, Yu S, Huang P, Morimoto K, Matsushita T, Takeuchi T. Role of Fas/Fas ligand-mediated apoptosis in murine contact hypersensitivity. *Int Immunopharmacol* 2003;3:927–938.
93. Messadi DV, Le A, Berg S, Jewett A, Wen Z, Kelly P, Bertolami CN. Expression of apoptosis-associated genes by human dermal scar fibroblasts. *Wound Repair Regen* 1999;7:511–517.
94. Mendonca MS, Howard KL, Farrington DL, Desmond LA, Temples TM, Mayhugh BM, Pink JJ, Boothman DA. Delayed apoptotic responses associated with radiation-induced neoplastic transformation of human hybrid cells. *Cancer Res* 1999;59:3972–3979.
95. Ozawa M, Ferenczi K, Kikuchi T, Cardinale I, Austin LM, Coven TR, Burack LH, Krueger JG. 312-nanometer ultraviolet B light (narrow-band UVB) induces apoptosis of T cells within psoriatic lesions. *J Exp Med* 1999;189:711–718.
96. Blankenberg FG. Recent advances in the imaging of programmed cell death. *Curr Pharm Des* 2004;10:1457–1467.

Index

A

Abdominal tumors
  labeled thymidine imaging of, 128
  tumor perfusion measurement in, 53
N-Acetylaspartate metabolite, 245, 246, 247
Acridine Orange, 287
Adenocarcinoma, angiogenesis assessment in, 266–268
Adjuvant therapy, for resected cancer, 6
Adriamycin, 97
Albumin, as gadolinium-based contrast agent conjugate, 261
Amino-CLIO, 262, 273–274
Anatomical imaging, of tumors, 2, 33–34
  with computed tomography, 35, 37–44, 45, 122
    baseline examination in, 38–40
    contrast agents for, 40–44
    with dual slice CT, 38
    limitations to, 121–122
    with multislice CT, 38–44, 45
    with single slice CT, 38
  confirmation of, 37
  with magnetic resonance imaging, 35, 44–45
  Response Evaluation Criteria in Solid Tumors (RECIST) criteria for, 36–37, 38, 39
  with ultrasound, 35, 36
  World Health Organization criteria for, 35–37
Angiogenesis, in tumors, 282
  definition of, 47–48, 88
  effect on computed tomography-based tumor enhancement, 88
  endothelial precursor cells in, 228–229
  histological measurement of, 88
  hypoxia-related, 48
  magnetic resonance imaging of, 263–269
    dynamic contrast-enhanced, 264–266
    molecular target-selected, 268–269
    steady-state, 266–268
  in metastasized cells, 17
  protein markers of, 282
  treatment strategies for, 88
Animal models
  imaging in, 26
  immunodeficient, 15–16
Annexin V
  radiolabeled, for apoptosis imaging, 306–310, 311–312
  as targeted magnetic nanoparticle, 262

Antiangiogenesis treatment, 88
  targeted, 55
Antimetabolite drugs. *See also specific antimetabolite drugs*
  effect on FLT retention, 135–136
Apoptosis, *in vivo* imaging of, 23–24, 303–316
  with computed tomography, 306
  with magnetic resonance imaging
    diffusion-weighted, 304–305
    with magnetic nanoparticles, 275
  with radionuclide imaging, 306–312
  with ultrasound, 306
  with water-suppressed lipid proton magnetic resonance spectroscopy, 303–304
Apparent diffusion coefficient (ADC), 24, 25
Aromatase inhibitors, 151
Asialoglycoprotein, 262
Asialoglycoprotein receptors, 260
Astrocytoma, 247
Autochthonous models, of tumors, 15, 17
Avian leukosis virus (ALV) receptor, 18–19
Avidin, 261
Azidothymidine (AZT), 132
Azomycin-based imaging agents, 60–63

B

N-Benzoyl straurosporine, 129
Bidirectional promoters, in gene imaging, 222, 223
Biological target volumes (BTV), 8
Bioluminescence, 284
Bioluminescence reporter genes, 219–220, 221
Bioluminescent optical imaging, 20, 284–286, 298
  of apoptosis, 23–24
  of hematopoietic stem cells, 230
  in vivo applications of, 286
  in pharmacodynamic analysis, 23
  probes for, 286
1,3-Bis-(2-chloroethyl-1-nitrosourea) (BCNU), radiolabeled, 9
Blood flow, in tumors. *See* Tumor perfusion
Bovine pulmonary artery endothelial cells, fluorescent dye staining of, 287, 288
Brain tumors
  apparent diffusion coefficient (ADC) in, 24
  gene imaging of, 209–210, 211
  labeled thymidine imaging of, 129
  magnetic resonance imaging of

Brain tumors (cont.)
  diffusion-weighted, 247
  perfusion-weighted, 247
  magnetic resonance spectroscopy imaging of, 242, 243, 244, 245–248
    N-acetylaspartate metabolites in, 245, 246, 247
    choline compound metabolites in, 245, 246, 247, 249, 250, 251–252
    for differentiation of nontumors, 246–247
  marrow stromal cell targeting in, 229
  positron emission tomography imaging of, 53, 54, 96
  radiotherapy for, as necrosis cause, 6
  treatment response assessment in, 96
  tumor perfusion assessment in, 53, 54
Breast cancer
  autochthonous tumor models of, 15
  detection of, 3, 135, 282
  estrogen-receptor imaging of, 145–152
    for hormonal therapy monitoring, 5, 148–152
    with positron emission tomography, 148–152
    with single-photon gamma scintigraphy, 146
    tumor perfusion assessment, 53–54
  FDG uptake in, 147, 149, 150, 151–152
  FES uptake in, 147–148
  hormonal therapy for, estrogen-receptor imaging in, 5, 148–153
  magnetic resonance imaging of, 3, 270, 272
    for angiogenesis assessment, 264–265, 266–268
    dynamic contrast-enhanced, 264–265
    with lymphotropic magnetic nanoparticles, 270, 272
    molecular-targeted, 275
    steady-state, 264–265, 266–268
  magnetic resonance spectroscopy imaging of, 243, 250–252
  mammography of, 3, 282
  metastatic, 109
    apoptosis imaging in, 309
    magnetic resonance imaging of, 270, 272
    tamoxifen treatment of, 109
  near infrared fluorescent imaging of, 292
  neoadjuvant therapy for, 4, 114–115
  positron emission tomography imaging of, 3, 135
    for hormonal therapy assessment, 5, 148–153
    for neoadjuvant therapy assessment, 114–115
    for tumor perfusion assessment, 53, 54, 99
  treatment response assessment in
    with positron emission tomography, 133, 134, 143–153
    standardized uptake value (SUV) in, 133
    tumor perfusion assessment-based, 99
  tumor perfusion assessment in, 53–54, 99

  ultrasound imaging of, 3
5-Bromodeoxyuridine (BUdR), 124–125, 130

C
Caliper measurements, of tumors, 19
Cancer. See also specific types of cancer
  predictive markers for, 282
Cancer treatment. See also Treatment response, imaging of
  role of imaging in, 1–12
Capecitabane, oral administration of, 170
Carboplatin, 173
Cardiac myosin, as targeted magnetic nanoparticle, 262
Caspase-3, 23–24
CD31, as breast cancer marker, 264–265
Cell implantation therapy, 274
Cell labeling and tracking
  in adoptive immune cell therapies, 224–228
  with magnetic resonance imaging, 225, 273–274
  with positron emission tomography, 227–228
Cervical cancer
  treatment response assessment in, 24, 111, 113
  tumor hypoxia assessment in, 59
  tumor perfusion assessment in, 53, 54
Chemotherapeutic agents. See also specific chemotherapeutic agents
  development of, use of imaging in, 8–9
Chemotherapy. See also specific chemotherapeutic agents
  aggressive, 33
  cytotoxicity of, 33, 34
  drug administration routes in, 170
  FDG uptake during, 107, 108
  new drug developments in, 33–34
  tumor response to, 95–97
1,3-bis-(2-Chloroethyl-1-nitrosourea) (BCNU), radiolabeled, 9
Chromatography, high-performance liquid, 170
Cisplatin, as nephropathy cause, 312
Colon/colorectal cancer
  autochthonous tumor models of, 15
  metastatic, 9, 43, 53
  screening for, 3
  staging of, 4
  treatment response assessment in, 24, 95, 134
  tumor perfusion assessment in, 53, 95
Colonoscopy, virtual, 3
Combretstatin, 5–6, 55
Compartmental analysis, of tumor perfusion measurement, 91–93
Computed tomography (CT)
  for anatomical measurement of tumors, 37–44, 45
    baseline examination in, 38–40
    contrast agents for, 40–44
    with dual slice CT, 38

with multislice CT, 38–44, 45
with single slice CT, 38
for apoptosis imaging, 308
contrast agents in, 40–44
of preclinical tumor models, 20, 21
radiation dose in, 41
for treatment response assessment, 5, 35, 37–44, 45
for tumor diagnosis, 20
for tumor perfusion assessment, 85–102
contrast enhancement determinants in, 86–88
Computed tomography (CT) colonography, 3
Contrast agents. *See under specific types of imaging*
Copper-pyruvaldehyde bis *N*-4-methylthiosemicarbazone, 49, 52, 55
Cyclophosphamide, oral administration of, 170

D
Deconvolution analysis, of tumor perfusion, 93
Dendrimers, 290, 293
Deoxy-2′-fluoro-1-b-D-arabinofuranosyl-5-bromouracil (FBAU), 131
Deoxy-2′-fluoro-D-arabinofuranosyl thymidine (FMAU), 136, 137
Deuterium-based magnetic resonance imaging, 73–74
Dextran, as magnetic nanoparticle coating, 261–262, 270, 271
4′-6-Diamidino-2-phenylindole (DAPI), 287, 288
Dihydrofolate reductase, 214
N-[2-(Dimethylamino)ethyl]acridine-4-carboxamide, kinetic studies of, 181–186
DNA (deoxyribonucleic acid), synthesis and proliferation, measurement of
with flow cytometry, 123–124, 125
with Ki-67 antigen, 126, 131, 133, 134
labeling index (LI) in, 124, 125
mitotic index (MI) in, 123
with radiolabeled thymidine, 122, 124, 126–128
with unlabeled 5-bromodeoxyuridine (BUdR), 124–126
DNA (deoxyribonucleic acid) damage
bioluminescence imaging of, 23
in hypoxic cells, 58
Dopamine D2 receptor gene, 218–219
Doxorubicin, 310
DQ-substrates, 288
Drug metabolism. *See also* Pharmacodynamics; Pharmacokinetics
positron emission tomography of, 178–179

E
Endothelial precursor cells, 228–230
Endothelial vascular adhesion molecule-1, 260
Epoxide-derived E-64, 294
E-selectin, 262, 269

Esophageal cancer
neoadjuvant therapy for, 4, 115
staging of, with positron emission tomography, 4
treatment response assessment in, with positron emission tomography, 24, 105, 111, 112–113, 134
Estrogen-receptor imaging, 5
eTUMOUR project, 248
Ewing's sarcoma, 114

F
FBAU *See* deoxy-2′-fluoro-1-b-D-arabinofuranosyl-5-bromouracil
FDG. *See* Fluorodeoxyglucose
FIAU (fluoro-iodo-1-b-D-arabinofuranosyluracil), 209–211
Fibrosarcoma, angiogenesis assessment in, 266–268
Fick principle, 91
Fireflies, as luciferase-luciferin source, 284, 285
Firefly luceriferase reporter gene systems, 219–220
FLT (3′-fluoro-3′-deoxythymidine), as treatment response tracer, 135–136
Fluorescence, 286
Fluorescence reporter gene imaging, 221
Fluorescent optical imaging, 20, 286–299
activity-based probes in, 293–294
advantages of, 286
antibody staining in, 287–288
DQ-substrates in, 288, 289, 290
fluorescent dyes in, 287
fluorophores in, 290, 291, 292
green fluorescent protein in, 288, 289, 294–295
in vivo applications of, 20, 294–295, 298
model systems in, 289
in pharmacodynamic analysis, 23
probes in, 289–294
activity-based, 293–294
cationic cell penetrating peptide-based, 294
dendrimer-based, 290, 293
development of, 289–294
functional, 289, 290
linear structure-based, 290, 291–292
static, 289–290
process of, 286
protein targeting agents in, 287–289
whole-body, 220, 221
Fluorine-18, 175
Fluorodeoxyglucose (FDG). *See also* Positron emission tomography (PET), fluorodeoxyglucose (FDG) in
uptake and retention of, 181
Fluorodeoxythymidine (FLT), 131, 132–136, 135–136
Fluoroerythronitroimidazole (FETNIM), 57, 63

Fluoroestradiol (FES), in estrogen-receptor imaging, 147–148, 149–150, 151
Fluoroethyl spiperone, 218, 219
Fluoroiodo-1-b-D-arabinofuranosyluracil (FIAU), 209–211
Fluoromisonidazole (FMISO), 8, 61–63, 99
5-Fluorouracil (5-FU), 130, 175
  effect on FLT retention, 135–136
  in positron emission tomography pharmacokinetic studies, 186–195
    biomodulatory studies, 187–188
    proof of principle studies, 188–191
    tissue pharmacokinetic modeling studies, 191–195
  radiolabeled, 9
  as tumor proliferation tracer, 130–131
FMAU [1'-(2'-deoxy-2'-fluoro-beta-D-arabinofuranosyl) thymine], 136, 137
FMISO (fluoromisonidazole), 8
Foreign bodies, metallic, 44
Forester resonance energy transfer (FRET), 288, 289
5-FU. *See* 5-Fluorouracil
Fulvestrant, 151
Fusion gene constructs, in gene imaging, 221–223

G

Gadolinium-containing contrast agents, 44
  in ^{1}H magnetic resonance spectroscopy, 244, 245, 247, 250, 251–252
  in magnetic resonance imaging, 260–261, 264–266, 272, 273
  receptor-targeted, 274–275
b-Galactosidase, 261
Gastric cancer, 108, 115
Gastrointestinal stromal tumors, 5, 116
Gene expression profiling, 48
Gene imaging
  in adoptive immune cell therapies, 224–228
    ex vivo radiolabeling and nuclear imaging, 224–225
    with magnetic resonance imaging, 225
    with supermagnetic agent labeling, 225
    of T cell activation, 228
  biomarker/surrogate marker imaging, 208
  direct imaging probes in, 230–231
  direct molecular imaging strategies in, 207
  indirect molecular imaging strategies in, 207
  optical imaging genes in, 219–221
    bioluminescence reporter genes, 219–220, 221
    fluorescence reporter genes, 221
  receptor imaging genes in, 218–219
  reporter genes in, 207–224, 230–231
  therapeutic/reporter genes in, 209
    enzyme-encoding genes, 209–214
    herpes simplex virus 1 thymidine kinase, 207, 209–214
    sodium iodide symporter (NIS), 214–216
    somatostatin receptor, 216–218
    transporter-encoding genes, 214–216
  vector delivery systems in, 221–224
    bicistronic vectors, 222, 224, 227
    bidirectional promoters, 222, 223
    fusion gene constructs, 221–223
    internal ribosome entry site (IRES)-linked, 222, 224
  vectors in, 230–231
Gene therapy, for cancer, 205–206. *See also* Gene imaging
  T cell-mediated, 225–228
GFP. *See* Green fluorescent protein
Glioblastoma, 247
Glioblastoma multiforme, 53
Glioma
  angiogenesis assessment in, 266–268
  in animal models, 19
  bioluminescent optical imaging of, 285
  endothelial precursor cells in, 229
  grading of, computer tomography-based, 88
  tumor hypoxia assessment in, 59
  tumor proliferation assessment in, 126
Gliomatosis cerebri, 247
Glucose metabolism, in tumors. *See also* Fluorodeoxyglucose (FDG)
  relationship to hypoxia, 98–99
Green fluorescent protein (GFP), in fluorescent optical imaging, 288, 289, 294–295
Green fluorescent protein (GFP)-based reporter gene systems, 221
Green fluorescent protein (GFP)-expressing 9L tumor model, 266–267

H

Head and neck cancer
  chemotherapy for, FDG uptake during, 108
  hypoxia assessment in, 59
  neoadjuvant therapy for, 4
  radiotherapy for, 7
  treatment response assessment in
    with FDG positron emission tomography, 111
    with perfusion computed tomography, 96
  tumor perfusion assessment in, 53, 54
Heart transplants, apoptosis imaging in, 309
Hemangioendothelioma, 266–268
Hemangioma, 40–41
Hemangiopericytoma, 247
Hematopoietic stem cells, 229–230
Hepatocellular carcinoma, 53, 54
Herpes simplex virus 1-thymidine kinase, 207, 209–214, 222–223, 224
Herpes simplex virus 1-thymidine kinase/green fluorescent protein fusion gene, 222–223, 226

Hodgkin's disease, treatment response assessment in, 110–111, 112
Hollow fiber assay, 16
Human immunodeficiency virus (HIV) infection, 132
Human immunodeficiency virus (HIV) tat peptide, 273
Hypoxia, in tumors, 57–63
　as cancer treatment resistance cause, 95
　effect on clinical outcome, 58–59, 95
　effect on tumor biology, 58
　evaluation of, 59–63
　　ex vivo assay of, 59
　　ideal assay of, 60
　　with positron emission tomography, 60–63
　　in vivo assay of, 59
　relationship to glucose metabolism, 98–99
　relationship to tumor perfusion, 56–57, 98–99
Hypoxia-inducible factors (HIFs), 48, 58, 98, 212–213

I

Imaging, of cancer. *See also specific types of imaging*
　in chemotherapeutic agent development, 8–9
　techniques in, 1–3
Imatinib, 5–6
Immunodeficiency. *See also* Human immunodeficiency virus (HIV) infection
　in animal models, 15–16
Immunopotentiation therapy, cell-based approach in, 274
Infants, cerebral apoptosis imaging in, 306
Inflammatory reactions, to radiotherapy, 8, 109, 110
Integrins, 48
INTERPRET project, 247, 248
Intravenous administration, of chemotherapeutic agents, 170
Iodide, radioactive, as thyroid cancer treatment, 214
Iodine allergy, 40
5-Iododeoxyuridine (IUdR), 130
Iron oxide
　as endothelial precursor cell label, 229
　as magnetic nanoparticle, 261–262, 275

K

Ki-67 antigen, 126, 131, 133, 134
Kidney cancer. *See* Renal cancer

L

Labeling index (LI), 124, 125
LacZ, 261
Leukemia, transplantable syngeneic models of, 14–15

Li-Fraumeni familial cancer predisposition syndrome, 18
Linear system analysis, of tumor perfusion, 93
Lipiodol, 97
Liver cancer, 53, 97
Liver metastases, 17, 53, 54
Luciferase, 23, 213–214, 284–286, 288
　comparison with green fluorescent protein, 221
　estrogen receptor regulatory domain-linked, 23–24
　as hematopoietic stem cell marker, 230
Luciferase genes, in bioluminescence reporter systems, 219–220
Luciferin, 20, 284
Lung cancer
　antiangiogenic treatment of, 55
　apoptosis imaging in, 307, 308
　hypoxia assessment in, 57, 59
　marrow stromal cell targeting in, 229
　neoadjuvant therapy for, 4
　palliative chemotherapy for, 108–109
　radiotherapy for, 7
　treatment response assessment in
　　with perfusion computed tomography, 96, 97, 99
　　with positron emission tomography, 24, 99, 111, 113, 134
　tumor proliferation assessment in, 126
　vascular endothelial growth factor expression in, 88
Lung cancer cells, dendrimer-based drug delivery to, 293
Lung metastases, models of, 17
Lymphocytes, labeling and tracking of, 224–226
Lymphoma
　curative chemotherapy for, 108–109
　treatment response assessment in, 105, 110–112, 134
Lymphotropic agents, in magnetic resonance imaging, 270–273

M

Magnetic resonance imaging (MRI), 1
　of angiogenesis, 264–269
　　dynamic contrast-enhanced, 264–266
　　molecular target-selected, 268–269
　　steady-state, 266–268
　avoidance of ferrous materials during, 44
　cell labeling and tracking applications of, 225, 273–274
　contrast agents in, 259–280
　　activatable, 260, 261
　　for angiogenesis imaging, 264–269
　　compartmental, 260
　　dysprosium-containing, 260
　　gadolinium-containing, 260–261, 264–266, 272, 273

Magnetic resonance imaging (MRI) (*cont.*)
   lymphotropic, 270–273
   macromolecular particulate, 266
   manganese-based, 260
   molecular-targeted, 274–275
   paramagnetic, 260–261
   superparamagnetic, 260, 271
   targeted, 260
  diffusion-weighted, 242
   for apoptosis imaging, 306–307
   apparent diffusion coefficient (ADC) in, 24, 25
   of brain tumors, 247
   for tumor response assessment, 24–25
  lymphotropic agents in, 270–273
  magnetic nanoparticles in, 260, 261–262
   activatable, 262–263
   for cell labeling and tracking, 273–274
   lymph node-targeted, 270–273
   for molecular targeting, 270–275
  magnetic nanosensors in, 275
  molecular targeting in, 268–269
  patients' claustrophobia during, 44
  perfusion-weighted, 242
   of brain tumors, 247
  of preclinical tumor models, 20
  T1, 259
   shortening of, 260
  T2, 259
  technical basis for, 259–260
  for treatment response assessment, 5, 35, 44–45
  for tumor diagnosis, 20
  of tumor perfusion and vascularity, 73–84
   contrast agent-based, 74–81
   deuterium-based, 73–74
   dynamic contrast-enhanced, 74–81
   gadolinium chelate contrast agent-based, 74–76
Magnetic resonance spectroscopy
  deuterium, 73–74
  dynamic contrast-enhanced
   change measurement in, 78
   relation to physiology, 76–78
   transcytolemmal water exchange in, 80–81
   of tumor perfusion and vascularity, 76–81
  ^{1}H
   for apoptosis imaging, 305–306
   3D, for prostate cancer assessment, 249
   data acquisition protocols in, 244–245
   in vivo, in clinical oncology, 241–258
   multi-voxel approach in, 244, 247–248
   phosphocholine compounds in, 242–243
   single-voxel approach in, 244
  in pharmacokinetics, 9
  of preclinical tumor models, 20
Mammography, 3, 282
Manganese-containing contrast agents, 44

Marrow stromal cells, tumor targeting of, 229
Matrix metalloprotinease-6, 293
MDR1 transporter, 220
Melanoma, 268
Meningioma, 97, 247
Metabolic flare reactions, 109, 149, 150–151
Metabolism
  of drugs, 170, 171
  relationship to perfusion, 56–57
Metastases
  models of, 17–18
  nodal, magnetic nanoparticle-based detection of, 270–273
  positron emission tomography detection of, 155
  process of, 282
  "seed and soil" hypothesis of, 17
  visceral, contrast-enhanced computed tomography of, 40, 41–44
Methotrexate, 135, 173
Mice
  immunodeficient, 15–16
  in vivo imaging in
   with tomographic multichannel fluorescent devices, 297
   whole-body optical imaging, 295, 296, 298
  transgenic
   with germline mutations, 18
   green fluorescent protein expression in, 295
   with somatic cell mutations, 18–19
Misonidazole, 60–61
Mitotic index (MI), 123
Molecular imaging
  in anticancer drug development, 9, 10
  in radiotherapy, 8
Molecular targeting
  assessment of drug effects on, 22–23
  in magnetic resonance imaging, 268–269
Monoclonal antibodies
  as gadolinium-based contrast agent conjugates, 261
  in molecular-targeted magnetic resonance imaging, 274–275
Mucin-like proteins, 274
Myeloma, 215

N

Nanoparticles, magnetic, 260, 261–263
  activatable, 262–263
  for cell labeling and tracking, 273–274
  as cell labels, 273–274
  lymph node-targeted, 270–273
  for molecular targeting, 270–275
Nanosensors, magnetic, 275
Near Infrared Fluorescent (NIRF) probes, 295
  protease-positive, 291
Necrosis, radiation-related, differentiated from tumor recurrence, 6, 246, 247–248

Neoadjuvant therapy, 4
Nephropathy, cisplatin-related, 312
Neuroblastoma antibody, as targeted magnetic nanoparticle, 262
Nolatrexed, 129–130
Nuclear factor of activated T cells (NFAT), 228

O

Oligodendroglioma, 244, 245, 247
  differentiated from astrocytoma, 247
  tumor perfusion assessment in, 53, 54
  tumor perfusion/metabolism relationship in, 56
Optical imaging, 1, 281, 284–286. *See also* Bioluminescent optical imaging; Fluorescent optical imaging
  advantages of, 298
  bioluminescence, 20
  definition of, 284
  in vivo
    localized (focal) imaging, 297–298
    system development for, 295–298
    whole-body imaging, 295–297, 298
  limitations of, 297
  new developments in, 298–299
Orthoptic models, of tumors, 16–17
Osteosarcoma, 104, 114

P

Pancreatic cancer, neoadjuvant therapy for, 4
Patency rights, to drugs, 34
Patlak/Gjedde analysis, 93, 107, 161–162, 162, 163, 164, 165–166
PEG (polyethylene glycol), 261–262
PET. *See* Positron emission tomography (PET)
Pharmaceutical industry, 10
Pharmacodynamics, 8–9
  definition of, 170
  of drug target modulation, 22–23
Pharmacogenetics, 171
Pharmacokinetic-pharmacodynamic optimization, 173
Pharmacokinetics, 8–9
  autoradiography in, 22
  definition of, 22, 170
  dose-response curves in, 173
  linear and nonlinear, 175–176
  plasma, 171–172
    area under the concentration-time curve (AUC), 172, 173, 174, 175–176, 177, 178
    drug clearance, 172
    drug volume of distribution, 172
    modeling in, 172–173
    plasma concentration and half-life, 171–172
    relationship with drug toxicity, 173, 174
    tumor response/toxicity relationship, 173, 174

positron emission tomography in, 22, 169, 175–199
  application levels of, 176–177
  area under the plasma concentration-time curve in, 177, 178
  of drug half-life and clearance, 178
  of drug uptake, 178
  of drug volume of distribution, 178
  partition coefficients in, 178
  of radioactive decay, 177–178
  with temozolomide, 195–198
  of tissue pharmacokinetic parameters, 177–178
processes in, 170–171
single-photon emission computed tomography (SPECT) in, 22
tissue, 174, 177–178
Phase I clinical trials, 9
Phase II clinical trials, 9, 34
Phase III clinical trials, 9, 34
  anticancer drug failure rate in, 10
Physiologic imaging, 2
  for tumor treatment response assessment, 5–6
Polyamidoamine dendrimers, 261
Polyethylene glycol (PEG), 261–262, 290, 291
Poly-L-lysine, 261
Polyvinylidene fluoride hollow fiber assay, 16
Positron emission tomography/computed tomography scanners, 155
Positron emission tomography (PET), 1
  in cancer staging, 4
  in drug development, 175
  with fluorodeoxyglucose (FDG), 2, 24, 155–167
    blood flow measurement with, 165
    European Organisation for Research and Treatment of Cancer (EORTC) criteria for, 104, 107, 163–164
    for functional processes measurement, 155–156
    glucose metabolism measurement with, 155–156, 157–158, 160, 161, 162, 164–165
    glucose transporter expression in, 160, 161, 162
    hexokinase activity in, 160, 161, 162
    indications for, 109
    for molecular interactions evaluation, 155, 156
    nonlinear regression analysis of, 159–161, 163
    Patlak/Gjedde analysis of, 107, 161–162, 163, 164, 165–166
    qualitative approach in, 157
    quantification for response monitoring in, 162–163
    quantitative approach in, 155–167

Positron emission tomography (PET) (cont.)
   in radiotherapy, 6–8, 109, 110
     significance of metabolic response in, 107–109
     simplified kinetic method (SKM) of, 162, 163, 164, 165
     standardization of, 163–164
     standardized uptake value (SUV) in, 107–108, 157–159, 163–164
     T/N ratio of, 157, 163
     for treatment response assessment, 103–120
   with fluorodeoxythymidine (FLT), 21, 165, 166
   with fluoromisonidazole (FMISO), 8, 53, 61–63
   in gene imaging, 210–214, 226–228
   for hypoxia imaging, 8, 60–64
   with labeled thymidine, 129–130
   micro, 21, 26
   in pharmacodynamic analysis, 23, 169
   in pharmacokinetic analysis, 22, 169, 175–199
     of anticancer agents, 181–199
     application levels of, 176–177
     area under the plasma concentration-time curve in, 177, 178
     of drug distribution, 9
     of drug half-life and clearance, 178
     of drug uptake, 178
     of drug volume of distribution, 178
     with 5-fluorouracil, 186–195
     graphic analysis in, 179–180
     modeling applications of, 179–181
     with N-[2-(dimethylamino)ethyl]acridine-4-carboxamide, 181–186
     partition coefficients in, 178
     of radioactive decay, 177–178
     spectral analysis in, 180–181
     with temozolomide, 195–198
     of tissue pharmacokinetic parameters, 177–178
   qualitative approach in, 156
   quantitative approach in, 155–167
   for treatment response assessment
     anatomical measurements in, 45
     in breast cancer hormonal therapy, 143–153
     FDG-based, 103–120
     of tumor perfusion measurement, 54–55
   for tumor diagnosis, 20
   for tumor perfusion assessment, 47–57
     advantages and disadvantages of, 49
     in cancer patients, 53–57
     chemical microspheres in, 49, 50
     in combination with computed tomography, 98–99
     with Cu-pyruvaldehyde bis N-4-methylthiosemicarbazone tracers, 49, 52, 55
     with FDG tracers, 532
     with FIMSO tracers, 53
     of metabolism and hypoxia, 56–57
     with ^{13}N-labeled ammonia tracers, 52
     with ^{15}O[H_2O] tracers, 49, 50–52, 54–57
     quantitative approaches in, 49–50
   for tumor proliferation assessment, 121–142
Prephase I clinical trials, 9
Prostate cancer
   antiangiogenic treatment of, 55
   bioluminescent optical imaging of, 285
   Gleason score in, 250
   intensity-modulated radiotherapy for, 248
   magnetic resonance imaging of, 4, 270, 271
   magnetic resonance spectroscopy of, 243, 248–250
   positron emission tomography of, 135, 136
     for tumor perfusion assessment, 53, 54
   prostate-specific antigen in, 55, 99, 248, 282
   staging of, 4
   x-ray imaging of, 285
Prostate-specific antigen (PSA), 99, 248, 282
Prostate-specific antigen (PSA) promoter, 213–214
Prostheses, metallic, 44
Protease probes, in fluorescent imaging, 288
Protein kinase C inhibitors, 129
Protein kinase inhibitors, 115–116
Proteolysis, in tumor progression, 282
Proteolytic enzymes
   expression in tumors, 282
   fluorescent probes for, 293–294
   synthetic substrates for, 288–289
Pyrimidine analogs, fluorinated, as tumor proliferation tracers, 130–131
Pyrimidines
   brominated, 124–125, 130
   iodinated, 130

Q

Quality of life, of cancer patients, 33–34

R

Radiation dose, in computed tomography, 41
Radiolabeling, of anticancer drugs, 9
Radionuclide imaging, of apoptosis, 308–313
Radiotherapy
   imaging in, 6–8
   as inflammation cause, 8, 109, 110
   intensity-modulated (IMRT), 246, 248
   positron emission tomography monitoring of, 6–8
   targeted, with sodium iodide symporter (NIS) gene, 216
   tumor response assessment in, 95, 97
Rats, immunodeficient, 15
Receptor imaging genes, 218–219
Rectal cancer. See also Colon/colorectal cancer
   neoadjuvant therapy for, 4

Renal cancer
  tumor perfusion measurement in, 53, 54
  vascular endothelial growth factor expression in, 88
Renilla luceriferase reporter gene systems, 219–220
Respiratory motion, during perfusion computed tomography, 90–91
Response Evaluation Criteria in Solid Tumors (RECIST), 36–37, 38, 39
Rhabdosarcoma, 242
RMP-7, 96

S
Sarcoma, 134
  Ewing's, 114
  soft tissue, 111, 113–114
Schwannoma, 247
Screening, role of imaging in, 3
Signal transduction pathways, as anticancer drug targets, 17
Single-photon emission computed tomography (SPECT), 1
  micro, 26
  in pharmacodynamic analysis, 23
  in pharmacokinetic analysis, 22
  for tumor diagnosis, 20
Smith, Robert E., 288
Sodium iodide reporter-internal ribosome entry site-enhanced green fluorescent protein, 216, 217
Sodium iodide symporter (NIS) gene, 214–216
Solid tumors, transplantable syngeneic models of, 14–15
Somatostatin receptor genes, 216–218
Spectrometry, liquid mass, 170
Staging, of cancer, 4
Standardized perfusion value (SPV), 92
Standardized uptake value (SUV)
  in breast cancer treatment, 133
  errors in measurement of, 106–107
  in FDG positron emission tomography, 107–108, 157–159, 163–164
Stem cells, imaging of, 228–230
Stem cell therapy/transplantation, 112, 274
Stromal tumors, gastrointestinal, 5, 116
Stroma-tumor interactions, 16
Subcutaneous models, of metastases, 17
Subcutaneous xenografts, 16
Subrenal capsule xenograft assay, 15
Synaptotagmin, 262

T
Tamoxifen, 150
  estrogenic effect of, 151
  as metabolic flare phenomenon cause, 109
  oral administration of, 170

Targeted therapies, 174
T cell receptor-dependent cell activation, 228
T cells, labeling and tracking of, 225–228
Temozolomide, 195–198
Tetracycline, 223
Tetrazolium dye MTT, 122
Thalidomide, 55
Thorax, computed tomography scan through, 39, 41
Thymidine
  catabolism of, 127
  radiolabeled, 9, 122, 124, 126–128
  retention and excretion of, 131
  structure of, 125
Thymidylate synthase inhibitors, 9, 129–130
Thyroperoxidase gene, 215
Time-to-progression (TTP) monitoring, 45
Tirapazamine, 59
Transferin receptor, 262
Transgenic tumor models, 17, 18–19
Treatment response, imaging of, 4–6, 34–35
  with anatomical imaging, 2, 33–34
    with computed tomography, 35, 37–44, 45
    with magnetic resonance imaging, 35, 44–45
    Response Evaluation Criteria in Solid Tumors (RECIST) criteria for, 36–37, 38, 39
    with ultrasound, 35, 36
    World Health Organization criteria for, 35–37
  definition of, 34
  with FDG positron emission tomography, 103–120
    clinical studies in, 110–116
    European Organisation for Research and Treatment of Cancer (EORTC) criteria for, 104, 107
    factors influencing, 106–107
    indications for, 109
    metabolic flare phenomenon in, 109
    Patlak/Gjedde analysis of, 107
    during radiotherapy, 109, 110
    significance of metabolic response in, 107–109
    standardized uptake value (SUV) in, 106, 107–108
    of tumor response after treatment, 110–114
    of tumor response during treatment, 114–115
    visual interpretation *versus*, 105
  with FLT positron emission tomography, 135–136
  histopathological, 104–105
  labeled thymidine imaging of, 129–130
  limitations of, 104–105
  Response Evaluation Criteria for Solid Tumors (RECIST) criteria for, 5, 104
  for tumor perfusion assessment, 54–55
  World Health Organization criteria for, 5, 104

Tumor burden, assessment of, 19, 21–22
Tumorigenesis, 282
Tumor markers, 4
Tumor models, preclinical *in vivo*, 13–32
   endpoints and measurements for, 19–25
      assessment of change in tumor burden, 21–22
      drug effects at the molecular targets, 22–23
      drug-induced physiological change, 23–24
      pharmacokinetics of, 22
      tumor response prediction, 24–25
   types of, 13–32
      human tumor xenografts, 15–16
      in situ models, 16–17
      models of metastases, 17–18
      orthotopic models, 16–17
      spontaneous and autochthonous models, 15
      transgenic, 13, 18–19
      transplantable, 13–19
      transplantable syngeneic models, 14–15
Tumor perfusion
   computed tomography of, 48–49, 85–102
      in combination with positron emission tomography, 98–100
      contrast enhancement determinants in, 86–88
      data processing in, 91–93
      image acquisition in, 88–91
      technical limitations and advantages of, 94–95
      technical validation and reproducibility in, 93–94
      treatment response measurement with, 96–97
      treatment response prediction with, 95–96
      x-ray exposure factors in, 90
   definition of, 73
   Doppler ultrasound of, 48–49
   dynamic contrast-enhanced magnetic resonance spectroscopy of
      change measurement in, 78
      input function in, 78–80
      relation to physiology, 76–78
   labeled thymidine imaging of, 127–128
   magnetic resonance imaging of, 48–49
   positron emission tomography imaging of, 47–57
      in cancer patients, 53–57
      with FDG, 532
      with FMISO, 53
      of metabolism and hypoxia, 56–57
      with ^{13}N-labeled ammonia, 52
      precision of, 53
      relationship to hypoxia, 98–99
      single-positron emission tomography of, 48–49
   in tumor models, 23
Tumor perfusion imaging, 2
Tumor proliferation
   doubling time of, 122
   positron emission tomography assessment of, 121–142
      with FLT, 132–136
      with fluorinated pyrimidine analogs, 130–131
      with FMAU, 136
      with iodinated and brominated pyrimidines, 124–125, 130
   process of, 282, 283
Tumor volume delineation (TVD), 6

U

Ultrasound, 1
   for apoptosis imaging, 308
   for breast cancer detection, 3
   limitations to, 282
   microbubble-based contrast agents in, 308
   for tumor response to cancer treatment monitoring, 35, 36
uMuc, 262

V

Vascular cell adhesion molecule-1, 262
Vascular endothelial growth factor, 58, 212–213
   as breast cancer marker, 264–265
   expression in lung tumors, 88
   expression in renal tumors, 88
Vascularity, of tumors, magnetic resonance imaging measurement of, 73–84
Vascular volume fraction, 266–268
Von Hippel-Lindau syndrome, 48

W

Water, radiolabeled (^{15}O[H$_2$O]), 9, 49, 50–52, 54–57
Will Rogers' effect, 4

X

Xenografts, of human tumors, 15–16
   in immunodeficient animal models, 15–16
   implanted beneath subrenal capsule, 15
Xenotransplantation, definition of, 15
X-ray imaging, 1, 282
   of chest, for lung cancer detection, 3